Pain management: Evidence, outcomes, and quality of life
A sourcebook

Pain Research and Clinical Management

Other volumes in this series:

PAIN RESEARCH AND
CLINICAL MANAGEMENT

Pain management: Evidence, outcomes, and quality of life

A sourcebook

Edited by

Harriët M. Wittink, PhD PT
Professor and Chair,
Lifestyle and Health Research
Faculty of Health Care
University of Applied Sciences
Utrecht, The Netherlands

Daniel B. Carr, MD DABPM FFPMANZCA(Hon)
Saltonstall Professor of Pain Research
Department of Anesthesia
Tufts-New England Medical Center
Boston and
Chief Executive Officer and Chief Medical Officer
Javelin Pharmaceuticals Inc
Cambridge
Massachusetts, USA

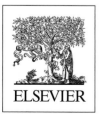

Edinburgh   London   New York   Oxford   Philadelphia   St Louis   Sydney   Toronto   2008

ELSEVIER

© 2008, Elsevier BV. All rights reserved.

The right of Harriët M. Wittink and Daniel B. Carr to be identified as editors of this work has been asserted by them in accordance with the Copyright, Designs and Patents Act 1988

First published 2008

ISBN-13: 978-0-444-51414-1

British Library Cataloguing in Publication Data
A catalogue record for this book is available from the British Library

Library of Congress Cataloging in Publication Data
A catalog record for this book is available from the Library of Congress

Notice
Knowledge and best practice in this field are constantly changing. As new research and experience broaden our knowledge, changes in practice, treatment and drug therapy may become necessary or appropriate. Readers are advised to check the most current information provided (i) on procedures featured or (ii) by the manufacturer of each product to be administered, to verify the recommended dose or formula, the method and duration of administration, and contraindications. It is the responsibility of the practitioner, relying on their own experience and knowledge of the patient, to make diagnoses, to determine dosages and the best treatment for each individual patient, and to take all appropriate safety precautions. To the fullest extent of the law, neither the Publisher nor the Editors assume any liability for any injury and/or damage to persons or property arising out or related to any use of the material contained in this book.

The Publisher

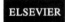

For Elsevier:

Commissioning Editor: Mary Law, Timothy Horne
Development Editor: Hannah Kenner
Project Manager: Jess Thompson
Designer: Stewart Larking

Printed in China

The publisher's policy is to use **paper manufactured from sustainable forests**

II

Preface

Pain research and practice in the developed nations have undergone a sea change in the past decade as the entire healthcare enterprise responds to pressures to become more patient-centered yet also to trim unnecessary costs. As a result, the "outcomes movement" increasingly permeates pain research and clinical care. Practicing healthcare in a cost-effective fashion also involves the mustering of unbiased evidence for (or against) treatments: "evidence-based healthcare."

Some time ago, we chatted about these trends with colleagues at the Elsevier booth at an International Pain Congress. To our surprise, we were encouraged to consider publication of an innovative monograph to explore these trends and serve as a practical resource for pain clinicians and researchers. Professor Patrick Wall, then lead editor of the Elsevier series on *Pain Research and Clinical Management*, suggested that we assemble an outstanding group of contributors to guide practitioners and researchers in advancing from the old ways of conducting pain research and practice, to a new evidence-based, outcomes-oriented model. Professor Wall's subsequent illness and death deprived the pain research community of a giant, and our project of a uniquely visionary supervisory editor. Yet, after an interim delay while Elsevier carefully selected a successor to Professor Wall, we again were able to move forward with the project, now under the distinguished editorial leadership of Professor Gerald Gebhart.

We are lucky to have enlisted as collaborators many global leaders in the application of evidence-based healthcare and outcomes research – two dynamic, evolving disciplines that interdigitate at many levels with the fields of pain research and care. Like us, they were all familiar with the ceaseless encroachment of clinical or research responsibilities upon their days and nights. Yet each one – selected because of their accomplishments in the specific research and clinical areas in which they were asked to contribute – accepted our invitation to contribute, seduced by the possibility that the end product might have enduring practical influence and benefit not only for their colleagues, but also for patients with pain.

In the years that this project required to complete, around the world a number of exciting developments for those involved in pain relief, evidence-based practice and outcomes assessment have taken place. The US Joint Commission for the Accreditation of Healthcare Organizations added effective pain assessment and treatment to its list of standards.

Governmental agencies and professional organizations in many countries prepared and disseminated evidence-based pain treatment guidelines, and gauged the quality of care according to clinicians' adherence to these guidelines, and their patients' achievement of optimal outcomes. New outcomes instruments were developed that were better suited to monitoring health-related quality of life in patients with pain, and their response to therapies. The Cochrane Collaboration, through collaborative review groups such as those concerned with pain, palliative and supportive care, prepared increasing numbers of systematic reviews of methods for pain relief. The World Health Organization (WHO) inaugurated a comprehensive international effort to categorize and classify function. Most recently, WHO in collaboration with IASP and the European Federation of IASP Chapters convened a Global Day Against Pain. At this event, these organizations mutually recognized the huge impact of pain upon the global burden of disease, and described the ways in which pain relief is increasingly acknowledged as a basic human right. Distinguished thought leaders – participants in each of these sentinel events and many other important initiatives – are contributors to the present volume. On the other hand, we thought it would be premature to include a stand-alone chapter on the internet. To date, although it has served as a powerful vehicle to disseminate evidence and instruments and (for some populations) to collect data, it has not in our view generated new primary content such as assessment tools. Internet-based healthcare is a rapidly evolving field in which websites may become outdated, inactive, or convey information affected by subtle or not-so-subtle bias. When and if this promising area differentiates so as to provide novel content in outcomes and quality of life research, we may devote a separate chapter to it (if given the opportunity!). In the present edition, however, relevant websites and web-based resources are provided on an ad hoc basis within each chapter.

Is the quest to practice healthcare on the basis of sound, unbiased knowledge of what works and what does not simply a reaction to recent external pressures? We think not: across the millennia, there are many testaments that practice according to the best available evidence, followed by unbiased appraisal of how well treatments work, are not behaviors into which the best clinicians must be pushed. Rather, the innate human drives towards distillation of truth from chaos or complexity have often (though not always) pulled clinicians into seeking more effective treatments, derived on a quasi-scientific basis.

Socrates, quoted in Plato's *Dialogs* and in turn by Osler in an essay that surveyed medical practice in ancient Greece, had contempt for the formulaic practice of the lower of its two-tiered medical system: "And did you ever observe that there are two classes of patients in states, slaves and freemen; and the slave doctors run about and cure the slaves, or wait for them in the dispensaries – practitioners of this sort never talk to their patients individually, or let them talk about their individual complaints? The slave-doctor prescribes what mere experience suggests, as if he had exact knowledge; and when he has given his orders, like a tyrant, he rushes off with equal assurance to some other servant who is ill…But the other doctor, who is a freeman, attends and practices upon freemen. And he carries his inquiries far back, and goes into the nature of the disorder; he enters into discourse with the patient and his friends, and is at once getting information from the sick man, and also instructing him as far as he is able, and he will not prescribe for him until he has first convinced him…Now which is the better way of proceeding? Is he the better who accomplishes his ends in a double way, or he who works in one way, and that the ruder and inferior?"

Socrates also insisted upon practical appraisal of the outcomes of care, such as in his description of evaluating a candidate for a municipal physician: "Would you not ask me, and should I not ask you, well, what about Socrates himself, has he good health? And was anyone ever treated by him known to get better?" Osler also described how each municipal physician in ancient Greece was appointed for a term of one year at a time, at the end of which his performance was reviewed publicly by the citizens he had cared for (or their survivors, when the clinical outcomes were poor).

The Bible, in the Book of Daniel, recounts an early, investigator-initiated, parallel design, controlled clinical trial with an initial 10-day efficacy phase, followed by a long-term effectiveness assessment. Qualitative measures were used in the first phase, while a quantitative measure was applied in the second phase. "And the king appointed them a daily provision of the king's food, and of the wine which he drank…But Daniel purposed in his heart that he would not defile himself with the portion of the king's food, nor with the wine which he drank: therefore he requested of the prince of the eunuchs that he might not defile himself…And the prince of the eunuchs said to Daniel, I fear my lord the king, who hath appointed your provision and your drink: for why should he see your faces more meager than the children who are of your sort? Then will ye make me endanger my head to the king. Then said Daniel to Melzar, whom the prince of the eunuchs had set over Daniel, prove [i.e., test] thy servants, I beseech thee, ten days; and let them give us pulse [i.e., coarse food] to eat, and water to drink. Then let our countenances be looked upon before thee, and the countenances of the children that eat of the portion of the king's provision: and as thou seest, deal with thy servants. So he consented to them in this matter, and proved them ten days. And at the end of ten days their countenances appeared fairer and fatter in flesh than all the children who ate the portion of the king's provision. Thus Melzar took away the portion of their food, and the wine that they should drink, and gave them pulse...And in all matters of wisdom and understanding, that the king inquired of them, he found them ten times superior to all the magicians and astrologers that were in all his realm."

Maimonides took a cautious approach to accepting data from individuals with a conflict of interest: "If anyone declares to you that he has actual proof, from his own experience, of something that he requires for the confirmation of his theory – even though he be considered a man of great authority, truthfulness, earnest words and morality – yet, just because he is anxious for you to believe his theory, you should hesitate."

In the last century Shaw, who had undergone many operations to excise recurrent tibial osteomyelitis in the pre-antibiotic area, observed in *The Doctor's Dilemma* that: "Doctors are not trained in the use of evidence, nor in biometrics, nor in the psychology of human credulity, nor in the incidence of economic pressure. [Yet] there is no harder scientific fact than the fact that belief can be produced in practically unlimited quantity and intensity, without observation or reasoning, and even in defiance of both, by the simple desire to believe founded on a strong interest in believing."

What do we hope to accomplish as stewards of the good will and substantial efforts of the distinguished contributors to this volume? We believe that this handbook can introduce healthcare professionals at all levels to the concepts that underlie the current approaches to assessing the evidence for or against medical interventions to relieve pain. It includes sections on qualitative methods as well as the all-powerful placebo. It also presents the basis for current efforts to assess the outcomes of care in daily practice, pain research, and in the approval of new analgesic drugs and other therapies – not just for certain types of pain in homogeneous subpopulations, but in a variety of pain conditions and in diverse sufferers. It presents methods for evidence synthesis and outcomes assessment in the context of what drives the healthcare enterprise – the improvement of quality of life. And, in the Glossary, it tabulates key outcomes instruments that have been applied in pain research and clinical management. To us, the three concepts of evidence, outcomes and quality of life have always been intertwined in patient-centered decision-making. They are crucial components of the cognitive software that channels our innate human drives into behavior that is – usually – purposeful, just, and humane.

Harriët M. Wittink
Daniel B. Carr

Dedication

To my family; my Quality of Life is much enhanced by their presence, warmth and laughter; and to Dan Carr MD and Bill Rogers PhD; two truly extraordinary men that I owe immeasurable thanks for being my mentors and friends.

HMW

To my dear family (past, present and future); the select handful of colleagues to who I owe a lifelong debt for expanding my vistas in pain studies (Professors Michael Cousins, Joseph Lau, Bill Rogers and the late Louis Lasagna); and my remarkable co-editor Harriët Wittink PT PhD without whose energy, insights, cheerfulness and determination this volume would have remained a dream.

DBC

Acknowledgments

Thanks to Elly Tjoa, Evelyn Hall and Heirich Wurm MD. Also, many thanks to all the clinicians and researchers who do outcomes research. Without them, this book would not have been possible. We hope we did their work justice.

Contents

Contributors

Benjamin C. Amick III, PhD
Scientific Director,
The Institute for Work and Health, Toronto, Ontario,
Canada; Southwest Center for Occupational and
Environmental Health. Professor, The University of Texas
School of Public Health, Health Science Center at Houston,
Texas, USA

Ann Berger, MSN MD
Bethesda, Maryland, USA

Sir Michael Bond, MD PhD FRSE
Past President of IASP, Emeritus Professor of Psychological
Medicine, Glasgow, UK

Harald Breivik, MD DMSc FRCA (elected)
Professor of Medicine/Anesthesiology, University of Oslo,
Rikshospitalet Medical Center,
Department of Anesthesiology, Oslo, Norway

Daniel B. Carr, MD DABPM FFPMANZCA(Hon)
Saltonstall Professor of Pain Research, Department of
Anesthesia, Tufts-New England Medical Center, Boston,
Massachusetts, USA; Chief Executive Officer, Javelin
Pharmaceuticals Inc, Cambridge, Massachusetts, USA

Alarcos Cieza, PhD, MPH
Senior Researcher of Health and Rehabilitation Sciences
ICF Research Branch of the WHO CC FIC (DIMDI), IMBK,
Ludwig-Maximilians-University, Munich, Germany

Charles S. Cleeland, PhD
McCullough Professor of Cancer Medicine, Chairman of
Department of Symptom Research, Division of Internal
Medicine, The University of Texas M.D. Anderson Cancer
Center, Houston, Texas, USA

Raymond A. Dionne, DDS PhD
Scientific Director, National Institute of Nursing Research,
National Institutes of Health, Bethesda, Maryland, USA

Robert H. Dworkin, PhD
Professor of Anesthesiology, Neurology, Oncology, and
Psychiatry, University of Rochester School of Medicine and
Dentistry, Rochester, New York, USA

Elon Eisenberg, MD
Professor, Pain Relief Unit, Rambam Medical Center, Haifa
Pain Research Group, Technion – Israel Institute of
Technology, Haifa, Israel

Christopher J. Evans, PhD MPH
Senior Project Director, Mapi Values, Massachusetts, USA

Keri L. Fakata, PharmD
Postdoctoral Fellow in Pain and Palliative Care
Pharmacotherapy, Clinical Instructor in Pharmacotherapy,
College of Pharmacy, University of Utah, Salt Lake City,
Utah, USA

Liana Fraenkel, MD MPH
Associate Professor of Medicine, Yale University School of
Medicine, New Haven, Connecticut, Chief of
Rheumatology, VA, Connecticut Healthcare System, West
Haven Campus, West Haven, Connecticut, USA

Rollin M. Gallagher, MD MPH
Departments of Psychiatry and Anesthesiology, University
of Pennsylvania School of Medicine; Pain Medicine Service,
Philadelphia Veterans Affairs Medical Center;
Department of Epidemiology and Biostatistics, School of
Public Health, Drexel University, Philadelphia, Pennsylvania,
USA

Nathalie Gauthier, BA
Département de psychologie, Université de Montréal,
Montréal, Québec, Canada

Maurice J.M.M. Giezeman, PhD MD
Department of Anesthesiology, University Medical Center
Utrecht, Utrecht, The Netherlands

David Gimeno, PhD
Senior Research Fellow, Department of Epidemiology &
Public Health, University College London, London, UK;
Formerly at Southwest Center for Occupational and
Environmental Health. The University of Texas School of
Public Health, Health Science Center at Houston, Texas, USA

Nathalie Horowicz-Mehler, MS
PhD Candidate, Cancer Epidemiology Department, Columbia
University, New York, USA

Mark P. Jensen, PhD
Professor of Rehabilitation Medicine, Department of
Rehabilitation Medicine, University of Washington, Seattle,
WA, USA

Vijay N. Joish, PhD
Adjunct Faculty, University of Utah, Salt Lake City, UT, USA

Tina Koch, PhD RN
Professor of Nursing, Older Person Care, School of Nursing
and Midwifery, University of Newcastle, Australia

Debbie Kralik, PhD RN
Associate Professor and Director, Research Unit of the Royal
District Nursing Service, Glenside, South Australia

Ron C. Kupers, PhD
PET Unit & Dept. Surgical Pathophysiology, Rigshospitalet,
Copenhagen, Denmark

Alvin E. Lake III, PhD
Michigan Head-Pain and Neurological Institute, Ann Arbor,
Michigan, USA

Joseph Lau, MD
Professor of Medicine, Center for Clinical Evidence
Synthesis, Institute for Clinical Research and Health Policy
Studies, Tufts-New England Medical Center, Massachusetts,
USA

Arthur G. Lipman, PharmD
Professor of Pharmacotherapy, College of Pharmacy;
Adjunct Professor of Anesthesiology, School of Medicine;
Director of Clinical Pharmacology, Pain Management Center,
University Hospitals and Clinics, University of Utah, Salt
Lake City, Utah, USA

Douglas C. McCrory, MD MHS FACP
Center for Clinical Health Policy Research, Department of
Medicine, Duke University Medical Center and the Center
for Health Services Research in Primary Care,
Durham Veterans Affairs Medical Center, North Carolina,
USA

Jana M. Mossey, PhD MPH MSN
Professor of Epidemiology, Department of Epidemiology and
Biostatistics, School of Public Health, Drexel University,
Philadelphia, Pennsylvania, USA

Roberto S.G.M. Perez, PhD
Assistant Professor, Pain & Pain therapy research,
Department of Anesthesiology and the Trauma Related
Neuronal Dysfunction research consortium (TREND),
VU University Medical Center, Amsterdam, The Netherlands

Kay Price, PhD RN
Senior Lecturer, School of Nursing and Midwifery, University
of South Australia, Adelaide, South Australia

Hans Rasmussen, MPsych MSc
Psychiatric Centre Glostrup, Copenhagen University
Hospital, Glostrup, Denmark

Joel R. Saper, MD FACP FAAN
Michigan Head Pain and Neurological Institute, Ann Arbor,
Michigan, USA

Scott A. Strassels, PharmD BCPS
Assistant Professor, Division of Pharmacy Practice,
University of Texas at Austin, College of Pharmacy, Division
of Pharmacy Practice, Austin, Texas, USA

Gerold Stucki, MD MS
Professor of Physical Medicine and Rehabilitation,
Department of Physical Medicine and Rehabilitation,
Ludwig-Maximilians-University, Munich, Germany and Swiss
Paraplegic Research, Switzerland

Michael J.L. Sullivan, PhD
Department of Psychology, McGill University, Montreal,
Quebec, Canada

Athina Tatsioni, MD
Post-doctoral research fellow, Center for Clinical Evidence
Synthesis, Institute for Clinical Research and Health Policy
Studies, Tufts-New England Medical Center, Massachusetts,
USA

Isabelle Tremblay, BA
Département de psychologie, Université de Montréal,
Montréal, Québec, Canada

Dennis C. Turk, PhD
John and Emma Bonica Professor of Anesthesiology & Pain Research, Department of Anesthesiology, University of Washington, Seattle, USA

Henrica C.W. de Vet, PhD
Professor of Clinimetrics, Institute for Research in Extramural Medicine, VU University Medical Center, Amsterdam, The Netherlands

Suellen M. Walker, MBBS MM(PM) PhD FANZCA FFPMANZCA
Clinical Senior Lecturer and Consultant in Paediatric Anaesthesia and Pain Medicine, Portex Anaesthesia Unit, UCL Institute of Child Health and Great Ormond Street Hospital for Children, London, UK

Gwenyth R. Wallen, PhD RN
Chief, Clinical Nurse Scientist, National Institutes of Health, Bethesda, Maryland, USA

Xin Shelley Wang, MD MPH
Associate Professor of Medicine, Department of Symptom Research, Division of Internal Medicine, The University of Texas M. D. Anderson Cancer Center, Texas, USA

Erwin van Wegen, PhD
Senior Scientist, Department of Physical Therapy, VU University Medical Center, Amsterdam, The Netherlands

James Witter, MD PhD
Food and Drug Administration, Center for Drug Evaluation and Research, Bethesda, Maryland, USA

Dick R. Wittink,[§] PhD
George Rogers Clark Professor of Management and Marketing, School of Management, Yale University and co-director, Yale Center for Health Care Management and Policy, Connecticut, USA

Harriët M. Wittink, PhD PT
Professor and Chair, Health and Lifestyle Research, Faculty of Health Care, University of Applied Sciences, Utrecht, The Netherlands

[§]Deceased

Disclaimers and Acknowledgments

Daniel B. Carr gratefully acknowledges support from the Saltonstall Fund for Pain Research, as ably represented and guided by Dudley Willis; and the Evenor Armington Fund. The views expressed are those of the author.

Chapter 3: Sincere thanks is extended to the research participants and research team. This project has been funded by a Discovery grant from the Australian Research Council (ARC).

Chapter 5: Support for the preparation of this manuscript was provided in part by the Initiative on Methods, Measurement, and Pain Assessment in Clinical Trials (IMMPACT) and by funding from the American Pain Society's Clinical Practice Guideline Program.

Chapter 6: The authors would like to thank Paul Cumming for English revision. Parts of this work were made possible thanks to a grant from the Danish Medical Research Council, the Lundbeck foundation and the Svend Anderson Foundation.

Chapter 9: The views expressed are those of the authors. No official support or endorsement by the US Food and Drug Administration or the National Institutes of Health is provided or should be inferred.

Chapter 11: The authors are thankful to the editors of the Journal of Rehabilitation Medicine for granting permission to use extracts and tables of previously published materials in this article.

Chapter 18: The IMMPACT meetings have been supported by unrestricted educational grants to the University of Rochester Office of Professional Education by Abbott Laboratories, Allergan, Alpharma, AstraZeneca, Celgene, Elan Pharmaceuticals, Endo Pharmaceuticals, GlaxoSmithKline, Johnson & Johnson, Lilly, Merck, NeurogesX, Novartis Pharmaceuticals, Ortho-McNeil Pharmaceuticals, Pfizer, Purdue Pharma, and Schwartz Pharma. The views expressed in this chapter are those of the authors. No official endorsement by the US Department of Veterans

Affairs (VA), US Food and Drug Administration (FDA), US National Institutes of Health (NIH), or the pharmaceutical companies that provided unrestricted grants to the University of Rochester Office of Professional Education should be inferred.

Chapter 19: Research from our center summarized in this chapter was supported by grants from the Canadian Institutes of Health Research awarded to Michael J. Sullivan.

Chapter 20: David Gimeno was supported by the Fogarty International Center Training Grant 3 D43 TW00644.

Chapter 23: The chapter was written outside the official National Institutes of Health duties of Dr Wallen and Dr Berger. The opinions expressed are those of the authors and do not necessarily reflect those of the National Institutes of Health, the Public Health Service, or the Department of Health and Human Services.

Chapter 24: Reprinted with permission from PAIN; Clinical Updates® Volume XII, No. 4 September 2004. INTERNATIONAL ASSOCIATION FOR THE STUDY OF PAIN®. For permission to reprint or translate this article, contact: International Association for the Study of Pain, 909 NE 43rd St., Suite 306, Seattle, WA 98105-6020 USA Tel: 206-547-6409; Fax: 206-547-1703; email: iaspdesk@iasp-pain.org; Internet: www.iasp-pain.org and HYPERLINK "http://www.painbooks.org" www.painbooks.org Copyright© 2004, International Association for the Study of Pain®. All rights reserved. ISSN 1083-0707.

CHAPTER 1

Health outcomes and treatment effectiveness in pain medicine

Harriët M. Wittink • Scott A. Strassels • Daniel B. Carr

INTRODUCTION

Patients and their families have always been concerned with the expertise and qualifications of the healthcare providers caring for them, as well as the likely outcomes of proposed treatments. This concern is well articulated in Plato's dialogs (Osler 1932; Carr 1994), and numerous other historical letters, books, plays and poems over the past centuries. For many centuries the arbitrariness of medical care certainly warranted concern. Beralde, a character in Molière's comic drama *Le Malade Imaginaire* (1673), observed that "medicine is only for those who are fit enough to survive the treatment as well as the illness." Benjamin Franklin (1706–1790) also had his doubts: "God heals, and the doctor takes the fee," and Voltaire (1694–1778) famously wrote "Doctors are men who prescribe medicines, of which they know little, to cure diseases of which they know less, in human beings of whom they know nothing."

The individual healthcare provider traditionally has been the focus and the main decision maker of the healthcare delivery system in the Western world. The passive, obedient patient, however, has shifted to the educated consumer of healthcare, in part through access to information through the internet. The emerging concept of quality of care, and other factors such as the decrease and actual reversal of the proportion of care rendered for acute illnesses versus chronic diseases, technological advancements in healthcare, rising healthcare costs, and adoption of an evidence-based approach to healthcare (Carr et al. 1999; Sackett et al. 1999; Mulrow and Lohr 2001), have been accompanied by a recognition of the importance of patients' views about their care and health and a shift towards emphasis upon patient-centered health outcomes (Gerteis et al. 1993). Patient-centered outcome measures are indicators of patients' evaluations of changes in patient health status, including health-related quality of life (HRQoL) and indicators of or patients' evaluations of the quality of healthcare.

All of these trends have created the need to change from a provider-centered healthcare delivery culture to a patient-centered culture (Stryer et al. 2004). What this means is that outcomes measures are chosen that are important to the *patient*. One might even argue that the increased interest in palliative care and pain control in recent years is the direct result of a power shift according to which patients and their families – the consumers of healthcare – have much greater autonomy and power than under the previous disease-centered model of care (Carr 2001). Clinicians taking the patient's view into account is associated with greater patient satisfaction with care (Hall et al. 1988), better compliance with treatment programs (Becker 1985) and increased likelihood to maintain a continuous relationship during healthcare (Kaplan et al. 1989).

Challenged not only to eradicate disease but to improve health, today's healthcare professionals must examine the structure, process and outcomes of care to ensure that optimal care is provided (Gouveia et al. 1991). Understanding the efficacy and effectiveness of healthcare interventions and the assessment of and improvement in the quality of healthcare have posed vexing difficulties for decades (Patrick and Chiang 2000). Health outcomes information to gauge treatment effectiveness continues to be important for all stakeholders in healthcare. Policy makers, purchasers, clinicians and patients all want to know from their different perspectives whether treatments that are being considered or are being delivered have value. The main purpose of the evaluation of treatment effectiveness is to identify the degree to which interventions intended to improve health or quality of life actually succeed in producing the desired "end result" outcomes, that in practice are a balance between benefits and harm (Patrick and Chiang 2000).

Health outcomes information focuses on the consequences, rather than on the process, of care. If the process is sound, then the outcomes should be good. On an individual patient level, health outcomes information can help monitor the individual's response to care, empower consumers and involve them in service evaluation and planning. From a health services point of view, health outcomes information provides ways to monitor actual results of care, evaluate new services and eliminate services that are poor or unnecessary. Health status outcomes help in priority setting, resource allocation and communication between purchasers and providers. Finally, outcomes research, by informing the content of policy positions, payment rules and practice guidelines, presumably solves the problems of both quality and cost that beset healthcare and does so by scientific rather than political means (Tanenbaum 1993, p. 1268).

In this chapter we describe the historical context of the outcomes movement, the difference between efficacy and effectiveness studies, outcomes measures and present a number of frequently used generic health status instruments.

WHAT IS OUTCOME RESEARCH?

Donabedian (1966) coined the term "outcome" as part of his *structure, process* and *outcome* paradigm for quality assessment in healthcare. Structure refers to the physical aspects of how care is provided, process refers to what is done and to whom, and the outcomes are simply the results. Donabedian had a broad definition of outcome: "Although some outcomes are generally unmistakable and easy to measure (death, for example), other outcomes, not so clearly defined, can be difficult to measure. These include patient attitudes and satisfactions, social restoration and physical disability, and rehabilitation." He believed that "outcomes, by and large, remain the ultimate validators of the effectiveness and quality of medical care."

The terms "outcomes research" and "effectiveness research" have been used to refer to a wide range of studies, and there is no single definition for either that has gained widespread acceptance. As these fields evolved, it appears that "outcomes research" emerged from a new emphasis on measuring a greater variety of impacts on patients and patient care (function, quality of life, satisfaction, readmissions, costs, etc.). The term "effectiveness research" is used to emphasize the contrast (see below) with efficacy studies, that employ randomized controlled trials to estimate the effect of active treatment versus another treatment or placebo. This term underscores the goal of learning how medical interventions affect real patients in "typical" practice settings (Office of Technology Assessment 1994).

Mendelson et al. (1998) defined health outcomes and treatment effectiveness research (OER) as "the evaluation of the impact of healthcare (including discrete interventions such as particular drugs, medical devices, and procedures as well as broader programmatic or system interventions) on the health outcomes of patients and populations. OER may include evaluation of economic impacts linked to health outcomes, such as cost-effectiveness and cost utility. OER emphasizes health problem- (or disease-) oriented evaluations of care delivered in general, real-world settings; multidisciplinary teams; and a wide range of outcomes, including mortality, morbidity, functional status, mental wellbeing, and other aspects of health-related quality of life." Others define outcome research as "the study of the end results of medical care." It involves "the rigorous determination of what works in medical care and what does not" (Tanenbaum 1993, p. 1268). It is "a rapidly evolving field that incorporates epidemiology, health services research, health economics, and psychometrics" (Epstein and Sherwood 1996), or broader: "Outcomes research is fundamentally concerned with improving the practice of medicine as applied to patients treated outside clinical trials" (Lee et al. 2000). The Agency for Healthcare Research and Quality (AHRQ 2003), the successor to the Agency for Health Care Policy and Research (AHCPR; see below), has a highly practical definition which states that outcomes research was developed to address basic questions confronting clinicians and patients:

- What works and what does not?
- For which patients?
- When in the course of an illness?
- At what cost?

Clearly, definitions for outcome research range from the narrow to the very broad. Mendelson's definition of outcome research is remarkably similar to that used for health services research (Bowling 2000) and it is no surprise the two terms are used interchangeably. In the dictionary of epidemiology (Last 1995) outcomes are defined as "all possible results that may stem from exposure to a causal factor, or from a preventative or therapeutic intervention." "Outcomes" are thus distinct from "services," meaning the structure or process of a program or intervention (such as processes of care). In other words, services refer to what kind, or how much, care is provided and in which setting. It is often necessary to measure structure and process in order to interpret the outcome of care (Bowling 2000). In this chapter we define "outcome research" as the measurement of the result of healthcare interventions.

HISTORICAL CONTEXT OF OUTCOME RESEARCH

For decades healthcare expanded in the USA and other free market economies with few limits. More recently, the earlier revolutions of healthcare expansion have been followed by a backlash of cost-containment efforts that appear to grow more grim with each passing year. In the early 1970s in the USA, at a time of increased focus upon reducing the cost of medical care, researchers discovered that for surgical procedures "geography is destiny." John Wennberg and Alan Gittelsohn (1973) published a seminal article in *Science* that reported a wide geographical variation in resource utilization, expenditures and rates of hospitalization and procedures. Studies documented that medical practices as commonplace as hysterectomy and hernia repair were performed much more frequently in some areas than in others, even when there were no differences in the underlying rates of disease or severity (McPherson et al. 1982). Furthermore, the quality of medical evidence was poor: often there was little or no information about the end results for patients who received a particular procedure, and few comparative studies to show which interventions were most effective (Eddy and Billings 1988). These findings challenged researchers, clinicians and health systems leaders to develop new tools to assess the impact of healthcare services (AHRQ 2000).

William Roper, M.D., a former Health Care Financing Administration administrator, coined the phrase "what works in the practice of medicine" to characterize the questions that researchers in medical effectiveness might address (Roper et al. 1988). At about the same time the Omnibus Budget Reconciliation Act of 1989

(P.L. 101–239) established the Agency for Health Care Policy and Research (AHCPR) within the Department of Health and Human Services and appropriated funds for outcomes research and particularly for the establishment of the Patient Outcomes Research Teams (PORTs). In response to payers' and policymakers' concerns that widely demonstrated practice variations represented important sources of "cost without benefit," fourteen PORTs were established with each a focus on specific conditions that were common, costly, and for which there was known to be well-documented evidence on substantial variation in practice. The PORTs were designed to be multidisciplinary enterprises involving not only specialist and generalist clinicians but also epidemiologists, survey researchers, statisticians, quality-of-life experts, health economists and experts in other related disciplines (Freund et al. 1999). These teams were to include literature synthesis activities, analysis of administrative databases, prospective cohort studies and efforts to disseminate research findings to the larger practice community. For many PORTs, the rallying cry was "finding out what works in medicine" (Deyo 1995).

The PORTs were required to follow a very specific sequence and approach over a five-year period. The effectiveness initiative itself represented an important hypothesis: guidance for optimal medical practice could be gleaned from analysis of data routinely gathered in the process of delivering and paying for patient care. Although these studies often involve rigorous design and statistical methods, by intent they were usually not randomized trials that required massive primary data collection but instead relied upon information on healthcare that already had been collected and stored in data files (Committee on Regional Health Data Networks 1994). Database analysis, systematic literature review, decision analysis and guideline development were the methodologic staples of early OER. PORT researchers used data from Medicare, Medicaid, insurance claims and other large administrative databases to characterize patterns of care, develop general and disease-specific outcome measures and disseminate important outcome information to patients and physicians so as to reduce inappropriate practice variation and improve outcomes. The Low Back research team, for instance, documented wide geographic variations in rates of back surgery at the international, national and state levels and identified important variations in surgical outcomes according to the type of surgical procedure. This team also developed outcome measures that could be incorporated into future research. Yet, in 1995, Deyo (1995) argued for a greater role of randomized clinical trials as part of the outcomes research portfolio as he felt the team was unable to establish "what works" in medicine. In 1993, AHCPR published its second Request for Proposals for PORT studies, so-called PORT-IIs. These projects differed somewhat from the original PORTs in that they encouraged generation of primary data about the effectiveness of interventions, through either randomized trials or prospective, longitudinal study designs. Since the end of the initial PORT grants in 1995 and 1996, the private sector, including healthcare organizations, has adopted findings from the PORTs in many of its day-to-day workings (Mendelson et al. 1998). Over the past decade there has been a proliferation of generic and disease-specific outcomes tools. Many clinical trials now include these outcomes measures as endpoints. Centers for (clinical) outcomes research have been and continue to be established widely in the Western world, at governmental levels and within universities and hospitals. The "Global Consultation on Increasing Investments in Health Outcomes for the Poor" took place in October 2003 at the World Health Organization headquarters in Geneva. One of the three themes that were addressed was how to better the effectiveness of health delivery systems and monitor outcomes, underlining the global challenge to improve health and healthcare delivery.

Outcomes studies have led to a number of advances, among them the development of outcomes instruments for clinical research, refinement and clarification of clinical hypotheses, involvement of professional health organizations in outcomes research and dissemination of findings, new expectations for clinical care and an explosion of interest in outcomes and effectiveness research by the private sector (Stryer et al. 2004). However, reality has not fully met expectations to the extent that the uptake of outcomes research findings into daily practice has often been incomplete or delayed (AHCPR 1999).

Despite observations that adhering to evidence-based practice improves long term outcomes, reduces costs and improves consumer satisfaction (McGuirk et al. 2001), routine care of patients often fails to follow evidence-based guidelines. The main purpose of evidence-based medicine (EBM) is to improve patient care and to achieve optimal outcomes. Misconceptions, myths, established attitudes and practices stand in the way of effective adoption of EBM (Carr 2001). Improved clinical effectiveness can only be achieved by the presence of routine mechanisms by which individual and organizational change can occur. For this reason considerable effort has been devoted in the past decade to questions about clinical behavior and changing clinical practice (Wittink and Carr 2003). In this context, disease management programs appear promising. A recent meta-analysis (Weingarten et al. 2002) on published evidence regarding the characteristics and effectiveness of disease management programs concluded that provider education, feedback and reminders each significantly increased improvements in provider adherence to guidelines. Evidence should guide not only EBM, but also inform decision making about the administrative and organizational aspects of healthcare as they relate to the quality and outcomes of care, i.e., evidence-based *healthcare* (Stryer et al. 2004).

EFFICACY VERSUS EFFECTIVENESS STUDIES

The distinction between disease-based clinical investigation and patient-centered outcomes research is analogous to that between measures of *efficacy* versus measures of *effectiveness*. In an ideal setting, such as a randomized controlled clinical trial, the *efficacy* of a treatment may be derived as the dose–response relationship for a specific intervention upon a given physiologic effect assessed under well-controlled conditions. In controlled trials the end points of interest are usually biologic measures, such as changes in blood glucose levels, or blood pressure. Although the randomized controlled trial (RCT) is the best method for evaluating efficacy, it frequently requires an enormous expenditure of economic and structural resources. Current evidence indicates that approximately 80% of commonly used medical treatments have not been shown to be efficacious, primarily because the necessary randomized controlled trials have not been conducted because of methodologic problems, the time required for their execution, the expense, or ethical reasons (Coyle 2000). In addition, individuals differ in their responses to many interventions. Just as it may be invalid to generalize from small-scale observations to large groups, one can never say with certainty that an aggregate conclusion drawn from a large group applies well to each subgroup (Lau et al. 1998) or individual within the group (Carr 1996; Jadad 1998; McQuay and Moore 1998).

At least as important to practitioners and patients is the *effectiveness* of a treatment, meaning the outcomes of this treatment when applied in a realistic clinical setting, measured over the course of disease and including patient-centered outcomes (Pransky and Himmelstein 1996). Outcome research is more likely to be generalizable to typical medical practice than are controlled clinical trials and asks the question: does it work in the "real world"? As a general rule effectiveness studies emphasize external validity, whereas efficacy studies are more concerned with internal validity.

An important goal of outcome research is the evaluation of the effects of the selected practice patterns on the outcomes of interest. In outcomes research, practice patterns range from the use of medication, diagnostic tests and therapeutic procedures to the length of hospital stay, transfer to other facilities and/or scheduled visits to physicians. Consequently, any inference made about this association must be evaluated as a function of the potential selection, information (measurement error) and confounding biases (Pilote and Tager 2002). Other important reasons to perform research outside of the rigorous controlled clinical trial setting are:

- to examine treatment effects of subgroups not often found or excluded from trials;

- to define variations in the utilization and outcome among geographic region, ages, races or genders;
- to study a condition or outcome in which a large number of patients are needed;
- to study subjects who cannot be ethically subjected to a randomized design;
- to restrict costs when economic and structural resources are limited; and
- to generate hypotheses or provide estimates in the design of RCTs (Canto et al. 1999).

The emergence of an effectiveness perspective reflects an underlying paradigm shift towards greater concern with societal impacts of treatment and toward a corresponding reexamination of what is considered relevant scientific evidence on the value of treatments (Wells 1999).

The distinction between effectiveness and efficacy is critical to disease management; treatments with proven efficacy do not always offer great effectiveness when applied under conditions of typical clinical practice. In most efficacy studies, highly specialized practitioners treat selected patients according to tight protocols in a setting in which both patients and practitioners have economic incentives to comply. In contrast, effectiveness studies apply treatments as they would be in usual settings (Epstein and Sherwood 1996). Thus, while efficacy studies tell us something about the maximum effects of specific treatments under experimental conditions, effectiveness studies evaluate the real world validity of these conclusions. Effectiveness research can be seen as complementary to efficacy research because it explores the "ecological validity" of the latter findings (Lambert 2001).

Effectiveness trials are more heterogeneous in design than controlled clinical trials. Some effectiveness studies are controlled experiments, but ones that often modify or sacrifice design features that protect internal validity, such as blinding or treatment standardization (Wells 1999). Other designs include retrospective analyses, observational studies, quasi-experimental designs or hybrid forms of effectiveness and efficiency research. Outcomes research has been facilitated by the application of computers and electronic medical records in the healthcare arena. Some modern observational databases (such as dedicated clinical registries) share many methodologic strengths with randomized studies, including standard definitions for data, complete and prospective data collection, use of computerized data management and comprehensive patient follow-up (Hlatky et al. 1984). A substantial debate about whether the results of nonrandomized studies are consistent with the results of randomized controlled trials on the same topic is ongoing (Concato et al. 2000; Ioannidis et al. 2001; Victora et al. 2004). To merge the strengths of both approaches, hybrid studies are emerging that use features of both efficacy and efficiency studies, such as prospective, randomized efficacy studies (Zatzick et al. 2004) or "real world" randomized trials (Simon et al. 1999). As in other clinical trials, these designs include the development of a protocol with a priori hypotheses, recruitment of participants who provide informed consent, randomization to eliminate selection bias and routine collection of data at pre-specified time periods. Prospective effectiveness trials differ, however, from typical clinical trials in that the former enroll heterogeneous participants, use providers more similar to those who treat the disease, impose few protocol-driven interventions, and incorporate outcome measures relevant to the disease and delivery system. Such trials attempt to reduce biased resulting from selection factors while still addressing outcomes and effectiveness (Epstein and Sherwood 1996).

HEALTH OUTCOMES INSTRUMENTS AND MEASURES

Until the first part of the 20th century, health was defined as the absence of disease and was measured in terms of morbidity and mortality. This simple definition of health was rejected in 1948 with the expansion of the concept of health by the World Health Organization (WHO), defining it as "A state of complete *physical*, *mental* and *social* well being and not merely the absence of disease or infirmity" (World Health Organization 1948). This definition reflects the multidimensionality of the concept of health and considers not only biologic markers, but also the ability to perform physically, psychologically and socially in the everyday environment. Central to the evaluation of healthcare services today is the measurement of health. Health outcomes focus on two broad categories of measures: traditional biologic or clinical measures, and patient-centered measures that can be general ("generic") or disease specific. Recently, the field of health outcomes research has broadened the utilization of HRQoL instruments to document economic, clinical and humanistic outcomes (ECHO) (see Table 1.1).

Traditional biologic measures may be primary, such as morbidity and mortality, or surrogate, such as a decrease in blood pressure in patients given an antihypertensive drug. Measures used for patient-centered outcomes generally estimate persons' HRQoL and their ability to function and to do the things they want to do. These measures may be generic and evaluate overall health status, or they may be disease-specific and focus upon the effect of a given condition on a person's life.

HRQoL assessment is the measurement or evaluation of the health of an individual or a patient. HRQoL may include biologic markers, but it emphasizes indicators of physical functioning, mental health, social functioning and other health-related concepts, such as pain, fatigue and perceived well-being (Greenfield and

Table 1.1 Types of outcome measures

Outcomes	Types	Measures
Biologic/clinical measures	Clinical events Physiologic or metabolic measures Mortality	Stroke, myocardial infarction Blood pressure, glucose levels Death
Economic	Direct medical costs Indirect medical costs	Cost of healthcare Cost-effectiveness Cost benefit Cost minimization Cost utility Cost of work loss, sick time
Patient centered/humanistic	Generic measures Disease-specific measures Topic-specific measures	Symptoms HRQoL Patient satisfaction Mental health, functional status

Modified from Epstein and Sherwood (1996).

Nelson 1992). Concepts included in some commonly applied HRQoL instruments are presented in Table 1.2.

The use of HRQoL as a clinical outcome measure extends consideration of the impact of the condition and its treatment to encompass the person's emotional, physical and social functioning and lifestyle. It addresses the question of whether a treatment leads to a life worth living, and it provides a more subjective, patient-led baseline against which the effects of an intervention can be evaluated (Bowling 2000). *Quality of life* includes HRQoL, but is a broader term that includes nonmedical aspects of life that reflect the aggregate impact of food, shelter, safety, living standards, and social and physical environmental factors (Greenfield and Nelson 1992). Systematic measurement and documentation of HRQoL is also a useful, clinically relevant

Table 1.2 Domains used in health-related quality of life measurements

Domains	QWB	SIP	NHP	QLI	COOP	EQ-5D	DUKE	MOS SF-36	WHO QOL
Physical functioning	X	X	X	X	X	X	X	X	X
Social functioning	X	X	X	X	X	X	X	X	X
Role functioning	X	X	X	X	X	X	X	X	X
Psychological distress		X	X	X	X	X	X	X	X
Health perceptions (general)		X	X	X	X	X	X	X	X
Pain (bodily)		X	X		X	X	X	X	X
Energy/fatigue	X		X				X	X	X
Psychological well-being							X	X	X
Sleep		X	X				X		X
Cognitive functioning		X					X		
Quality of life				X					X
Reported health transition						X			

COOP = Dartmouth Function Charts; DUKE = Duke Health Profile; EQ-5D = European Quality of Life Index; MOS SF-36 = MOS 36 item Short-Form Health Survey; NHP = Nottingham Health Profile; QLI = Quality of Life Index; QWB = Quality of Well-Being Scale; SIP = Sickness Impact Profile; WHO QOL = World Health Organization Quality of Life Assessment.
Modified from Ware J. The status of health assessment 1994. Ann Rev Public Health 1995; 16:327–354.

approach to incorporate patient preferences into front line medical decision making. Monitoring HRQoL validates the importance of patients' subjective experiences to their care providers, and may thereby also improve overall patient satisfaction with care (Marvel et al. 1999).

The pressing need for tools to monitor and adjust treatment and to approach clinical decision making from a viewpoint that is evidence-based and patient-centered (Marvel et al. 1999), the need to know which treatments reduce pain, improve functional status, social functioning and mental health, and in particular which treatments are worth paying for, has fueled the development of numerous instruments. These instruments are intended to quickly and conveniently capture the health status of patients (Rucker et al. 1996). No single instrument is ideal for all intended uses and questionnaires are available in a variety of forms that can be readily incorporated into clinical care and research. Outcomes assessment is a dynamic area, particularly as it stands at the interface between routine practice and standards for pain assessment and treatment applied (in the USA) by the Joint Commission for the Assessment of Healthcare Organizations. The comprehensiveness and validity of outcome measures for the treatment of all types of pain, however, lags behind those of equally high-impact conditions that affect the public's health; a lag is even more pronounced for cancer pain than for noncancer pain (Goudas et al. 2001). Much more research has addressed functional assessment, and how pain management influences function, in patients with acute or chronic noncancer pain than in those whose pain results from malignancy (McQuay and Moore 1998).

Outcomes instruments are well-suited to monitor health over time with repeated measurements and should be linked to the process of the healthcare intervention while any mediating factors are identified. A prerequisite, of course, is that the outcome measurement tool is reliable, valid, precise, specific, responsive to change and sensitive (Bowling 2000) (see also Chapter 2). Selection of a specific outcomes tool will depend on the specific population and outcome of interest and the ability of the measurement tool to detect changes within the domain of interest. The selection of an instrument consists of three phases. The first phase is to determine which outcomes are important to the study or clinical context. While pain studies used to center on pain intensity reduction as the paramount criterion for success, their focus is shifting to increases in functional activities and participation. The second phase has to do with the condition(s) that this instrument will be used for; the third has to do with the psychometric properties of the instrument.

Choosing a domain-specific, condition-specific or generic instrument depends on the aim of the study. If one specific domain is of interest, such as pain

intensity or depression, a domain-specific instrument can be used (e.g., the McGill Pain Questionnaire or the Beck Depression Inventory). In general, a condition (or disease) specific instrument will have a narrow focus, but will provide considerable detail in the area of interest. If the interest is in general HRQoL, comparison across different conditions, or with healthy people, a generic instrument can be used. Using a condition-specific survey or module together with a generic scale may provide more insight into aspects of health that are not well measured by either type of instrument (Rogers et al. 2000a,b). The dissemination of ever-simpler and more powerful means to capture data electronically in everyday healthcare opens new opportunities for understanding which treatments are effective, and for whom, and may provide irrefutable evidence that we who treat pain do add patient-centered value to the healthcare enterprise (Wittink et al. 2004).

Over the past decade much attention has been paid to what makes a "good" instrument in terms of psychometrics. The debate on how to measure change is ongoing, with many different statistical interpretations being put forward. HRQoL and other outcomes measures are increasingly used to supplement objective clinical or biologic measures of disease to assess the quality of services, the effectiveness of interventions and in cost–utility analyses (Carr and Higginson 2001). Scientific papers and monographs have been dedicated to the discussion of various forms of reliabilities and validities and how to best measure these. The interpretability of the score, the clinical relevance of the attribute being measured, and the feasibility of scoring were raised as barriers to the use of patient-based measures in clinical practice in 1992 (Deyo and Carter 1992). Yet today, outcome measures have become mainstream in the sense that they are being used by clinicians, not only to monitor progress, but to direct therapy based on the initial and subsequent score(s) on a measurement tool. The routine application in daily clinical practice of outcomes instruments to guide treatment for the individual patient has to date been under researched, although there is a rising trend to use questionnaires as a prognostic tool. For instance, Nederhand et al. (2004) showed that a combination of Neck Disability Index and Tampa Scale of Kinesiophobia scores could predict chronic disability with a probability of 83.3% in a sample of acute motor vehicle accident victims. Equally, Fritz and George (2002) found that a score of 34 or greater of the Fear Avoidance Questionnaire (FAQ) predicted a likelihood of 59% of not returning to work in patients with acute work-related back pain (see also Chapter 17). Implications for treatment in acute back pain might be to implement a cognitive behavioral approach if the patient scores greater than 34 on the FAQ. Outcome measures may thus assist in individualizing treatment. When using an outcome instrument to direct therapy and/or estimate prognosis of treatment for the individual patient, some of the questions to ask are: 1. Is this instrument sensitive to change in an individual patient? 2. Do the questions on the instrument and the resulting score adequately reflect the concerns of my patient? 3. How does it guide my treatment?

In recent years, a debate has started on whether HRQoL and other outcome measures are sufficiently patient centered and to what extent they actually represent the concerns of individual patients. If a measure does not cover domains that are important to the individual patient then it may not be a valid measure for that patient. It is then unlikely to be responsive to change after treatment because it did not measure the patient's specific problem or problems. One approach is to simply ask patients if they are better (Wright 2000). The validity of this approach is uncertain because patients have difficulty recalling their health before treatment and patients' expectations may affect their perceptions of treatment benefit. A number of studies have compared measurement at two points in time to the patients' retrospective assessment of change made at one point in time. In general there is poor agreement and low correlation between these two commonly used methods for assessing change (Baker 1998; Fischer et al. 1999; Elliott et al. 2002). Kaplan et al. (2000) feel that the use of a retrospective patient-reported measure of health perceptions, as advocated by some researchers, represents a tautology, especially in the evaluation and effectiveness of care. Fischer et al. (1999), however, conclude that because retrospective assessments appear to provide information that is different from serial change data, are more sensitive to change and are more highly correlated with patients' satisfaction with change, they may be considered an independent outcome measure and should be used in conjunction with serial measures. The question remains why real-time and retrospective measures differ. One possibility is that a single retrospective answer to the question "are you better?" may yield the patients' "Gestalt" on what getting better means, which may or may not include improvements in pain intensity, function and/or mental health. The question, however, assumes that all patients have the same meaning for being "better." Beaton et al. (2001) explored the meaning of the concept of recovery (getting better) in a group of people with upper limb musculoskeletal disorders by means of a qualitative study. Unsurprisingly, they found that two patients could mean very different things when saying that they are better. Some patients may not actually have a change in disease state as measured by symptoms, impairments or function, yet consider themselves "better." It is clear more research is needed in this area.

Another option allows patients essentially to develop their own questionnaires. Patient-originated outcomes measures have been developed so as to be derived from patients' individual concerns (see Table 1.3).

Guyatt et al. (1987) suggest tailoring the outcome measure to the individual patient by asking each patient which activities are both important and difficult to perform. The advantages of this patient-specific approach are that only changes in activity limitations

Table 1.3 Selected patient-specific measurement tools

Name of instrument	Author
Patient-specific complaints	Beurskens et al. (1999)
Patient Specific Index (PASI)	Wright et al. (1994)
Patient Specific Symptom Distress Index (PSSDI)	Testa & Simonson (1988)
McMaster Toronto Arthritis Patient Preference Disability Questionnaire (MACTAR)	Tugwell et al. (1987)
Canadian Occupational Performance Measure	Law et al. (1990)
Discretized Analogue Scale	Singh & Bilsbury (1989)
Schedule for the Evaluation of Individual Quality of Life (SEIQOL)	O'Boyle et al. (1992)
Goal attainment methods	Kiresuk & Sherman (1968)
Patient Generated Index	Ruta et al. (1994)
Disease Repercussion Profile	Carr & Thompson (1994)
Measure Yourself Medical Outcome Profile (MYMOP). For instrument see: http://www.hsrc.ac.uk/mymop/main.htm	O'Boyle et al. (1992); Paterson (1996)

that have the potential to improve are assessed, and that improvement is assessed with respect to activities experienced as most important by the patient (Feinstein et al. 1986; Tugwell et al. 1987). A practical problem, nevertheless, is that patients often have difficulty defining their main functional problem. Beurskens et al. (1999) developed a patient-specific questionnaire and found that only 32% of the patients selected the same three principal functional complaints during the first and second intake. They further found this method was labor intensive as patients needed help selecting the appropriate activities. Several other methodologic issues remain unresolved, such as who identifies the goals of treatment, how concerns are identified, how to accommodate unrealistic expectations of treatment and how to interpret mean scores in clinical trials on measures which focus on the concerns of individual patients (Wright 2000).

DESCRIPTIONS OF SELECTED GENERIC HEALTH-RELATED QUALITY OF LIFE INSTRUMENTS

According to Kirshner and Guyatt (1985) and Guyatt et al. (1987) health status measures have three broad applications: (1) discrimination between individuals or groups, (2) prediction of outcomes and (3) evaluation of change over time. Generic HRQoL instruments are mostly epidemiologic tools and as such are able to measure change in large samples of patients. By design they are not intended, nor are they always sufficiently sensitive, to measure changes in a single subject. Furthermore, these instruments do not provide information on items frequently assessed in pain management such as solicitous responses, coping ability, life control, catastrophizing, fear avoidance or the extent of disablement from pain. As mentioned earlier, it is recommended to complement a generic HRQoL instrument with a disease-specific instrument. Ideally the instrument should provide relevant information to all clinicians within an inter- or multidisciplinary team, have a low respondent burden and be sensitive enough to detect changes at both group and individual levels. Guidelines for "how to use articles about health-related quality of life measurements" are provided by Guyatt (1997).

A 1998 systematic review on the frequency and quality of reporting on quality of life in randomized controlled trials found that while during 1980–1997 reporting on HRQoL increased from 0.63 to 4.2% for trials from all disciplines, fewer than 5% of all randomized trials reported on HRQoL and even for cancer trials this proportion was below 10% (Sanders et al. 1998). Garratt et al. (2002) assessed the growing use of HRQoL measures in a systematic review. They found 3921 reports that described the development and evaluation of patient assessed measures. Disease or population specific measures comprised 46%, generic measures 22%, dimension-specific measures 18%, utility measures 10% and individualized measures 1% of the total sample. During 1990–1999 the number of new reports of development and evaluation rose from 144 to 650 per year and reports of disease-specific measures rose exponentially. The most frequently used generic HRQoL measure was the SF-36 (10.4%), followed by the Sickness Impact Profile (2.8%), the Nottingham Health Profile (2.4%), the EORTC QLQ-C30 (2.1%) and the EUROQOL/EQ-5D (2%).

We will survey these instruments in the following sections, except for the EORTC QLQ-C30, which is also discussed in Chapters 22 and 23. The eight characteristics of an instrument addressed in this review are: (1) conceptual and measurement model; (2) reliability; (3) validity; (4) responsiveness; (5) interpretability; (6) respondent and administrative burden; (7) alternative forms; and (8) cultural and language adaptations as recommended by the Scientific Advisory Committee of the Medical Outcomes Trust (Lohr and SAC 2002).

THE 36-ITEM SHORT FORM MEDICAL OUTCOMES STUDY QUESTIONNAIRE (SF-36)

The SF-36 is a generic measure of general health status, designed for use in populations. Developed from data acquired by the Rand Corporation in the Medical Outcomes Study (MOS) (Tarlov et al. 1989), the SF-36 contains eight scales of general health and functioning that are thought to be important to all people: physical functioning, role-physical (limitations in physical roles due to health problems), bodily pain, general health, vitality, social functioning, role-emotional (limitations in emotional roles due to health problems) and mental health (Ware and Sherbourne 1992). All items are scored on scales from 0 to 100 such that a higher score indicates better health. Individual values are expressed as percentages of the total possible score. Scaling is variable for different questions including: excellent, very good, good, fair, poor; limited a lot, limited a little, not limited at all; yes/no; not at all, slightly, moderately, quite a bit, extremely; none, very mild, mild, moderate, severe, very severe; all of the time, most of the time, a good bit of the time, some of the time, a little of the time, none of the time; and others.

The SF-36 can be administered quickly, during a face-to-face interview, over the telephone, or by the patient. Its internal reliability in both general populations and chronic disease sufferers ranges from 0.78 to 0.93 (McHorney et al. 1994). Internal reliabilities in a sample of 424 patients with chronic pain in a pain management program in Boston ranged from alpha = 0.79 for bodily pain to 0.91 for physical functioning (Wittink et al. 2004). With an alpha > 0.90 the physical functioning domain is reliable for comparison within individuals (Nunnally 1978). Test–retest reliability was more than 0.80 across all domains.

Numerous studies have shown associations between the SF-36 and other general health status instruments (e.g., Essink-Bot et al. 1997; Bronfort and Bouter 1999; Skevington et al. 2001) (see also Chapter 17). In fact, the SF-36 has become the "gold standard" against which new HRQoL outcomes instruments are compared.

Normative SF-36 scores for a variety of populations and medical conditions have been published in a number of countries. There are two main versions: the Rand 36 item Health Survey version by the Rand Corporation, and the SF-36 (Ware and Sherbourne 1992). Although the questions used in these two instruments are the same, the item responses and scoring methods differ somewhat. The Rand 36 item Health Survey is in the public domain, as are the scoring methods. Ware and his colleagues have further developed several forms of the SF-36. The SF-36 version 2 is a revised and improved version of the original questionnaire that is now recommended for use. Other versions include the one-week recall version (also called the "acute" version), the SF-8 (Turner-Bowker et al. 2003) and the SF-12 (Gandek et al. 1998; Ware et al. 1996, 2003): 8- and 12-item subsets of the SF-36, respectively. The SF-12 offers an opportunity to collect health status information when time and resources are limited (Ware et al. 1996). The SF-36 has been translated into more than 40 languages. Wagner et al. (1998) performed cross-cultural comparisons of the content of SF-36 translations across 10 countries and determined that "the translations are culturally appropriate and comparable in their content."

The SF-36 has been validated for use in many pain patient populations, such as osteoarthritis and rheumatoid arthritis (Kosinski et al. 1999; Ruta et al. 1998), headache and migraine (Essink-Bot et al. 1997; Solomon 1997), neck pain (Riddle and Stratford 1998) and in patients participating in functional restoration programs (Leidy et al. 1998). The SF-36 is increasingly being used in epidemiologic studies on chronic pain (Elliott et al. 2003; Eriksen et al. 2003; Bergman et al. 2004; Dysvik et al. 2004; Kerr et al. 2004), and to a lesser, but still growing, extent to measure outcomes in pain management programs (Becker et al. 1997, 1998, 2000; Brown et al. 1999; Rogers et al. 2000a,b; Ho and LaFleur 2004; Wittink et al. 2004). Elliott et al. (2003) found that the Mental Health Composite scale (MCS) t-score and most subscale scores of the SF-36 were significantly correlated with type of depression (major depressive disorder, minor depression) in a sample of 242 patients with chronic pain. A dose–effect relationship was found between depression severity and SF-36 scorers, with patients having major depressive disorder having the lowest scores. The SF-36 was not helpful in detecting minor depression, but very effective in detecting major depression and no depression.

Shortcomings of the SF-36 for use on its own (i.e., without the supplementation of a disease-specific tool) in the chronic pain population include the lack of sufficient upper body functional items, the lack of differentiation between work disability and disability in other activities, and the lack of sensitivity of the Bodily Pain scale to change in an individual patient (Rogers et al. 2000a).

Information on the Rand 36-Item Survey can be found at: http://www.rand.org/health/surveys/sf36item/ (tool, permission and scoring of the instrument). The SF-36 version 2 can be obtained from the Medical Outcomes Trust, 20 Park Plaza, Suite 1014, Boston, MA 02116; phone: 1–617–426–4046; fax: 617–426–4131; email: info@outcomes-trust.org; URL:www.outcomes-trust.org.

NOTTINGHAM HEALTH PROFILE (NHP)

The Nottingham Health Profile (NHP) (Hunt and McEwen 1980) is a generic measure of general health designed for use in primary care settings. It was developed to reflect lay rather than professional perceptions of health. It has been widely used in Europe, particularly before the advent of the SF-36 (McDowell and Newell 1996). The NHP resulted from a revision of the Nottingham Health Index (NHI), which was similar in design and content to the NHP. The NHP provides an estimate of physical, social and health problems (Hunt et al. 1980). The NHP was influenced by the Sickness Impact Profile; however, the NHP asks about feelings and emotions, and the SIP examines changes in behavior. The NHP is a 38-item questionnaire with responses compiled into 6 domains: physical mobility (8 items), pain (8 items), social isolation (5 items), emotional reactions (9 items), energy (3 items) and sleep (5 items). Each item is weighted; weights were derived from patients and nonpatients. Dimension scores range from 0 to 100, with higher scores indicative of greater health problems. Scores are presented as a profile rather than as a unidimensional, overall number. A second section includes 7 optional questions about work, social and sex life, interests and hobbies, and holidays. The scaling of the items is dichotomous (yes/no answers). The NHP takes about 10 to 15 minutes for patients to complete.

Test–retest correlations coefficients for repeated administrations of the NHP over a 4-week period were reported as 0.75–0.88 for Part 1 and 0.44–0.86 for Part 2 (Carr 2003). In patients with musculoskeletal disease ICC = 0.95 (Beaton et al. 1997). Cronbach alphas were reported from 0.77 to 0.85 for the first section and 0.44 to 0.86 for the second section in a sample of patients with osteoarthritis (Hunt et al. 1981). Meyer-Rosberg et al. (2001) compared the psychometric properties of the SF-36 and the NHP in a group of 126 patients with chronic peripheral neuropathic pain (PNP). The SF-36 had higher internal consistency (reliability) coefficients (alpha = 0.79, range 0.70–0.90) than the NHP (alpha = 0.68, range 0.49–0.79). Correlations between comparable dimensions of the two instruments were significant (range from −0.79 for the physical and mental dimensions to −0.29 for the social dimension) indicating a moderate degree of convergent validity. Overall, the SF-36 performed somewhat better on psychometric testing than did the NHP. The NHP might have better content validity than the SF-36 because it contains dimensions such as sleep and more pain items that might be of particular importance in the PNP population.

The NHP shows moderate correlations with other measures of health status such as the SF-36, AIMS and Dartmouth COOP charts (e.g., Essink-Bot et al. 1997; Prieto et al. 1997; Coons et al. 2000; Post et al. 2001) and demonstrates discriminant validity (Kind and Gudex 1994; Prieto et al. 1997; Uutela et al. 2003). However, although the NHP was able to discriminate between healthy and non-healthy subjects in the community (Kind and Gudex 1994), it was unable to differentiate between subjects in the range of low and medium levels of complaints. The NHP energy category appeared to have a high detection threshold for fatigue in patients with postpoliomyelitis syndrome (Horemans et al. 2004).

Data on the responsiveness to change of the NHP are mixed (Fitzpatrick et al. 1992; Taylor et al. 1998; Wells et al. 1999; Falcoz et al. 2002). It does not seem to respond to small changes in health (probably because of the dichotomous response scaling) (Carr 2003). There is some indication, acknowledged by Hunt, that the NHP has a floor effect, whereby it does not identify low levels of disability (McDowell and Newell 1996, p. 442). In patients with chronic obstructive pulmonary disease the score distribution was very skewed, with more than 50% of the patients achieving the best score (Jans et al. 1999), suggesting the NHP suffers from ceiling effects as well.

This tool should be used with caution in the healthy population or in health surveys because of the floor effects and its inability to discriminate between low levels of disability. Its system of weighting and scoring has been criticized, particularly in people whose disabilities limit their roles. The norms are considered of limited value as standards because there are no smooth trends in health status across expected groups (Carr 2003).

The NHP has been translated into most European languages, as well as Turkish, Japanese, Arabic and Urdu.

Reference scores for the NHP are available for healthy people (by age, sex and social class) and for various categories of patients (Hunt et al. 1985).

To obtain the NHP contact Dr. Stephen McKenna, Galen Research Enterprise House, Manchester Science Park, Lloyd Street North, Manchester M15 6SE, UK; email: 100663.1650@compuserve.com.

SICKNESS IMPACT PROFILE (SIP)

The Sickness Impact Profile (SIP) is a generic measure used to evaluate the impact of disease on both physical and emotional functioning. The SIP was designed for use in population surveys, evaluative studies of the outcomes of care and in clinical practice to monitor patients. The SIP is used to estimate behavioral changes due to illness (Bergner 1976a,b). In this context, sickness encompasses the effects of being ill upon a person's everyday activities, as well as on his or her feelings and attitudes (McDowell and Newell 1996). Thus, the SIP examines how sickness affects a person's behavior and the ability to carry out daily activities. The SIP contains 136 yes/no statements in 12 categories, and patients complete the survey by checking the items that describe them on a particular day. It takes about 20–30 minutes to complete the SIP, and 5 to 10 minutes to score it. Each of the 12 categories is scored on a 0–100 scale. Each item is individually weighted to indicate the severity of the impact. The overall score ranges from 0 to 100 and is calculated by summing the weighted values of the selected items, dividing them by the scale values for all items and multiplying the results by 100. The lower the score, the better the respondent's health status.

Test–retest reliability was shown to be high ($r = 0.92$), as was internal consistency (Cronbach alpha 0.94) in the original study (Bergner et al. 1981). Test–retest reliability has consistently been high (0.88–0.92) for the overall scores. Reliability was higher for the interviewer-administered version than for the self-administered version (McDowell and Newell 1996). Cronbach's alpha from several studies range from 0.91 to 0.95 for overall score, 0.84 to 0.93 for the 2 subscales and 0.60 to 0.90 for the 12 categories (McDowell and Newell 1996).

The SIP has established good face and content validity in the development phase by deriving items from a literature review and interviews with patients, professionals and a healthy population. Good concurrent validity with other health status instruments was shown in a number of studies (de Bruin et al. 1992; Essink-Bot et al. 1996; Martin et al. 1997; Lipsett et al. 2000). Essink-Bot et al. (1996) found that the SIP emphasizes physical functioning, whereas the NHP emphasizes mental functioning.

The SIP has been validated in many populations, including the elderly (Morishita et al. 1995), those with rheumatoid arthritis (Sullivan et al. 1990), back pain (Follick et al. 1985; Deyo 1986), chronic pain (Jensen et al. 1992) and after trauma (Jurkovich et al. 1995). Studies have demonstrated discriminant validity (Parkerson et al. 1981; Read et al. 1987; Farrell et al. 1996; Hutter and Wurtemberger 1997; Damiano et al. 1999; Tate et al. 1999). In one trial, the SIP was used with the Medical Examination and Diagnostic Information Coding System (MEDICS) to try to identify subgroups of persons with chronic pain and to evaluate responses to rehabilitation programs (Sanders and Brena 1993). Multidimensional cluster analyses using SIP and MEDICS data identified 4 replicable subgroups: cluster A, highly dysfunctional with moderate levels of physical pathology; cluster B, moderately dysfunctional with moderate levels of physical pathology; cluster C, highly functional with low levels of physical pathology; and cluster D, highly dysfunctional with low levels of physical pathology. Cluster A and D patients showed significantly higher levels of depression, more medication usage, less activity and were less likely to be working at pretreatment. These 2 clusters also showed the largest improvement in subjective pain intensity, medication usage, activity level and return to work post-treatment. Patients in cluster B exhibited the least amount of improvement across outcome measures and, unlike the other 3 clusters, failed to show any significant improvement in work status at post-treatment.

Data on the responsiveness of the SIP are mixed. An effect size of 0.52 was reported for musculoskeletal patients, somewhat lower than that of the SF-36 or the NHP (Beaton et al. 1997). Deyo and Inui (1984) compared changes in SIP scores over time with clinicians' ratings of change in the status of arthritic patients. The SIP showed only a 50% sensitivity to clinically estimated improvement and a 43% sensitivity in detecting clinical deterioration. De Bruin et al. (1997a) compared the SIP-136 and the SIP-68 in terms of effect sizes, and found they do not differ significantly in their responsiveness. They reported that changes detected by both SIPs appear to be valid representations of changes in health-related functional status.

The SIP has been translated in a number of European languages. A Chicano version exists.

Abbreviations of the SIP have been proposed. A 68-item generic tool (SIP-68) was designed (de Bruin et al. 1994, 1997). A 64-item tool (SIP-RA) was designed for patients with rheumatoid arthritis (Sullivan et al. 1993). A 66-item tool (SIP-NH) was developed for use in nursing homes (Gerety et al. 1994). Roland and Morris (1983a,b) selected 24 items from the SIP to construct the Roland-Morris Disability Questionnaire, a disease-specific back pain questionnaire (see also Chapter 17).

The SIP is reliable and valid and is used in many studies as the "gold standard" against which other instruments are validated. More work needs to be done on establishing responsiveness of the SIP. The instrument is time consuming to complete and score. Alternative methods of scoring have been proposed (Pollard and Johnston 2001; Lindeboom et al. 2004).

THE EUROQOL INSTRUMENT: THE EQ-5D

The EQ-5D is a generic health status measurement developed by the EuroQoL group and is a utility measure that has been specifically designed to complement other health status instruments or disease-specific measures. The EuroQoL group is an international, multicenter, multidisciplinary organization founded in 1987. The EQ-5D can give three different scores: a profile, a weighted health index and the general health status score. The EQ-5D consists of 5 dimensions: mobility, self care, usual activities, pain/discomfort and depression/anxiety. Each dimension is subdivided into three levels: 1, no problems; 2, some problems; 3, extreme problems. Participants are asked to indicate their level of health by checking one of three boxes for each domain. To produce the profile score, the levels for each item are simply represented as a five-digit number, each digit representing the level of difficulty on one of the dimensions. To calculate the weighted index across the 5 dimensions, population weights are assigned for each level of difficulty selected and are subtracted from 1. Scores range from 0 to 1 (where a score of 1 represents a perfect state). A standardized extended version of EQ-5D was designed for the collection of health state values using a visual analogue scale (VAS) rating: a vertical 20 cm VAS with the end points labeled best imaginable health state at the top and worst imaginable health state at the bottom, assigned numeric values of 100 and 0 respectively (EQ-VAS). Participants draw a line to the point on the thermometer-like scale corresponding to their health state, 0–100 (100 = best health state). Scores for the VAS reflect the position where a participant's line crosses the thermometer-like scale, yielding the general health status score. The EQ-VAS should not be used in routine clinical or economic studies or population health surveys. By combining the different levels of each of the dimensions a total of 243 health states can be defined. Self-reported, observer, proxy and telephone versions are available. The instrument takes several minutes to complete.

The descriptive data of the EQ-5D can be converted into values suitable for cost-effectiveness analysis by linking patient's health state descriptions to empirical valuations of health states from the general population.

Test–retest reliability was reported as 0.86 for group level coefficients calculated for each state and averaged over health states and 0.90 for a coefficient derived from individual states simultaneously (van Agt et al. 1994). ICC = 0.93 was reported in patients with epilepsy (Stavem et al. 2001). Other studies have found the reliability of the EQ-5D acceptable (Dorman et al. 1998; Stavem 1999; Salkeld et al. 2000; Ankri et al. 2003; Luo et al. 2003a,b; Perkins et al. 2004).

Evidence for construct validity is demonstrated by the expected patterns of responses across recent users of healthcare, age group, gender and socioeconomic groups. Concurrent validity of the EQ-5D is supported by moderate correlations with, for example, the COOP-WONCA charts (Stave and Jodalen 2002), the SF-36 (Brazier et al. 1996; Konig et al. 2002), the SF-12 (Johnson and Coons 1998; Johnson and Pickard 2000; Brazier et al. 2004; Franks et al. 2004), the SF-6 (Brazier et al. 2004) and the Health Utilities Index mark 3 (Luo et al. 2003a). The EQ-5D demonstrated moderate to high correlations with measures of impairment and high correlations with disability measures in patients with rheumatoid arthritis. Stepwise regression models showed that EQ-5D utility values and visual analogue scores were explained best as a function of pain, disability, disease activity and mood (R^2 approximately 70%), although other variables (side effects, years of education) were required to explain the visual analogue scores. The EQ-5D health index and visual analogue scale are more responsive than any of the other measures, except pain and doctor-assessed disease activity (Hurst et al. 1994, 1997). Essink-Bot et al. (1997) compared the EQ-5D with the SF-36, the NHP and the COOP/WONCA charts (van Weel, 1993) in a sample of migraine patients and a matched control group. The SF-36 exhibited the best ability to discriminate between groups.

Data on the responsiveness of the EQ-5D are mixed. Some have reported good responsiveness (Tidermark et al. 2003), while others have not (Harper et al. 1997; Haywood et al. 2002; Wu et al. 2002; Brazier et al. 2004). Patient-based measures are, as expected, more responsive than the EQ-5D (Dawson et al. 2001).

The EQ-5D has been reported to have stronger ceiling effects than the SF-36 (Johnson and Pickard 2000; Wu et al. 2002; Oga et al. 2003; Brazier et al. 2004) in various populations.

Because of the coarseness of the categories, this measure is likely not suitable for clinical use in the individual patients if the intent is to measure change. Because of its brevity it should be supplemented, as its authors recommend, by other measures of interest. It is well suited to measuring the health in populations with major morbidity.

The EQ-5D has been translated into multiple languages and many cultural adaptations of the EQ-5D are available.

For use contact Dr. Frank de Charro, EuroQol Business Manager, PO Box 4443, 3006 AK Rotterdam, The Netherlands; email: fdecharro@compuserve.com. There is no charge for its use in clinical research. See also their website: http://www.euroqol.org/accessed May 15, 2007.

THE FUTURE

In the past several decades great progress has been made in the measurement of patient-based outcomes. Although such advances in measurement have served many useful purposes, a crucial drawback is that the various assessment tools cannot speak to one another (McHorney 2003).

The proliferation of generic and disease specific measures that differ in breadth and depth of measurement preclude comparisons across measures, because of their differences in number of items, type of rating scale and item difficulty. This near-chaos was evident in the evidence report prepared by Tufts-New England Medical Center Evidence-based Practice Center (EPC), sponsored by the AHRQ. The T-NEMC group performed a systematic review on the management of cancer pain (Goudas et al. 2001) and, later, updated the results on the management of cancer pain and added new reviews on depression and fatigue (Carr et al. 2002). Within the 218 retrieved randomized controlled analgesic trials, *125 distinct tools to assess pain* were employed. The assessment challenge is to identify an optimal set of functional items that is relevant for the diverse group of patients who receive pain management services yet is feasible for use in the current healthcare environment (see also Chapter 18). A variety of issues are encountered when trying to meet this challenge. Data from outcomes assessments may be compromised or not even collected if the response burden on clinicians or patients is too high (Haley et al. 2004). If not developed properly, static clinical forms or interviews with a fixed number of items may not capture the impact of pain of every patient's health status.

By far, most quality-of-life measures have been created under the umbrella of classic test theory, a set of assumptions and procedures that has been used to develop tests for much of the 20th century (Bowling 2001). Classic test theory has two major shortcomings. The first is test dependency: different items assessing the same construct cannot be linked to a common metric. The second is group dependency: different samples yield different item and scale parameter estimates, thereby limiting the usefulness of a given set of item parameters for different samples. One way to overcome such test dependency is test equating, which relates scores from different measures to a common metric (McHorney and Cohen 2000). Item response theory (IRT) methods, of which Rasch modeling is one example, can be used to calibrate items from existing instruments onto a common scale, thus developing a structure and order of domain-specific items (Hays et al. 2000; Ware et al. 2000). Once the structure and ordering of items is determined, items can then be selected to create short forms based on a number of criteria, including comprehensiveness of content, item fit to the construct, item precision, correlation to the total item score and practical considerations of length.

Computer-adaptive testing (CAT), an extension of IRT, is a technologically advanced method of assessment in which the computer selects and presents test items to patients according to the estimated level of the patients' ability. The basic notion of an adaptive test is to mimic automatically what experienced healthcare providers would normally do in their assessment of patients. For instance, in trying to understand the level of physical ability of a patient, the provider might ask "can you walk one mile?" If the patient says no, there is no point in asking if the patient can walk two miles. It makes much more sense to then focus on lower levels of ability. This approach stems from the realization that we learn little about an individual's ability if we persist in asking questions relating to too high a level of functioning or too low a level of functioning. We learn the most about a patient's ability when we accurately direct our questions at the current level of the patient's ability or "zoom in." Thus, in a CAT, the first item is usually of a medium-difficulty level for the patients. A patient who responds positively to a given ability (e.g., walk one mile) will then receive a more difficult item. A patient who responds negatively will be given a less challenging ability question. And so it goes, with the computer algorithm adjusting the selection of the items interactively to hone in on the physical ability of the patient. CAT makes it possible to ask only the most informative questions at each person's individual level of health. Other practical advantages are the virtual elimination of ceiling and floor effects that plague many widely used measures (Ware 2003). The depth and breadth of the item pool from which individual items are drawn strongly affects the validity and utility of the resulting CAT scores (Dunkel 1999). An item pool is a collection of items that represent a range of performance or difficulty levels of a particular functional domain (Velozo et al. 1999). Item pools are developed by equating outcome items from different sources so that they can be meaningfully compared on a common underlying metric.

McHorney (2003) warns that despite the promise of IRT and CAT much needs to be done before developers and users can confidently take the next step towards CAT. Clear conceptual frameworks and guidelines for the inclusion and exclusion of items into the data bank need to be developed. IRT methods need to be compared and commercialization of CATs questioned.

Howard et al. (1996) have suggested a research paradigm that is complementary to efficacy and effectiveness research, but also unique in its focus on the outcomes of individual patients. This patient-focused paradigm seeks to identify empirical methods to improve outcomes for the individual patient in ongoing clinical practice (Lambert 2001). It is an extension of quality assurance efforts which involves repeated patient measurement and feedback to the clinician. The methodology and research results draw heavily on the power of newer statistical techniques, which allow monitoring of individual patients. Specific techniques include the use of probit analysis, survival analysis and hierarchical linear modeling which allow

researchers to plot the course of improvement (or lack thereof) for each patient in relation to the comparison groups. An additional methodology underlying patient-focused research is the development of statistical methods to discern clinically significant change in a single patient (Lambert 2001). Much of this research has taken place in psychotherapy. Lueger et al. (2001) describe the development of a tracking system to accurately monitor the progress of an individual patient and objectively assess key benefits of psychotherapy. They decided the outcome instrument should meet several criteria: (1) the measurement scheme should be based on models of patient response to treatment, (2) the outcomes assessed should be important to the patient, (3) the outcomes assessed should be important to the purchaser of services, (4) the data should clinically inform the therapist, (5) the length of the instrument should allow repeated administration during treatment and (6) the measures should be normed to be representative of outpatients in psychotherapy. Their model of quality assurance has focused on the detection of eventual treatment failures within the first 10–15 sessions. Clinicians receive feedback on their patient's scores with supportive tips. This "smart" feedback system thus has the potential to facilitate clinician learning.

As patients with (chronic) pain can be widely divergent in many respects, including their goals, it makes sense to monitor them on an individual basis. The utility of any measure depends on the purpose to which it will be put. One purpose of an outcomes instrument is to document the performance of a particular clinic or clinicians. For that purpose, it is good to have measures with a large response to treatment. Another purpose, to measure the progress of an individual patient, requires a measure that is more accurate at the individual level. A dimension useful for tracking change in an individual patient will ordinarily have a high value of Cronbach's alpha (greater than 0.90, ideally 0.95 or as close to 1.0 as possible) (Nunnally 1978) and a low ratio of the standard error of change to the standard deviation of the concept (Rogers et al. 2000b). Other than the TOPS (see also Chapter 17), no pain-specific outcomes instrument has reported sensitivity to change in an individual patient (Ho and LaFleur 2004; Rogers et al. 2000a,b).

CONCLUSION

Outcomes studies have led to a number of advances, among them the development and refinement of instruments for clinical research and practice, numerous insights into current practice and practice variations, clarification and evolution of clinical hypotheses, involvement of health professional organizations in capturing outcomes data and dissemination of their findings, new expectations for clinical care and an explosion of interest in clinical outcomes and effectiveness by the private sector (Stryer et al. 2004). The impact of these findings on routine (nonresearch) clinical practice, however, has been incomplete or delayed (Agency for Health Care Policy and Research 1999). Better ways must be found to disseminate and implement research findings into healthcare, aiming for evidence-based healthcare (Stryer et al. 2004).

Accumulating data support the greatly reduced health status of patients with chronic pain, but few trials have reported effects on health-related quality of life in patients treated with multidisciplinary biopsychosocial rehabilitation for chronic low back pain (Guzman 2002). As pain clinicians we must examine whether our outcomes measurements tools are sufficiently patient focused, both in terms of whether they ask the right questions and in terms of their ability to measure change in the individual patient. Qualitative research (see Chapter 3) can assist us in asking the right questions, while psychometrics can help us develop sensitive instruments. As a group, clinicians either need to agree on which measurement tools we want to use, based on scientific rather than emotional or financial arguments, so we can start comparing our research outcomes, or start contributing to an item data bank in order to develop a (chronic) pain-specific CAT. We must further examine what tools and methods are available to support patient decision-making to enhance our quality of care, as we have an ethical and moral obligation to our patients to provide patients with the best care possible within the current financial constraints.

REFERENCES

Agency for Health Care Policy and Research. The outcome of outcomes research at AHCPR. AHCPR Publication No. 99-R044. AHCPR, Rockville, MD, 1999.

Ankri J, Beaufils B, Novella JL, et al. Use of the EQ-5D among patients suffering from dementia. J Clin Epidemiol 2003; 56:1055–1063.

Baker R. Measuring change in health in general practice: a comparison of a simple transition question with the Nottingham Health Profile. Int J Qual Health Care 1998; 10:207–212.

Beaton DE, Hogg-Johnson S, Bombardier C. Evaluating changes in health status: reliability and responsiveness of five generic health status measures in workers with musculoskeletal disorders. J Clin Epidemiol 1997; 50:79–93.

Beaton DE, Tarasuk V, Katz JN, et al. "Are you better?" A qualitative study of the meaning of recovery. Arthritis Rheum 2001; 45:270–279.

Becker MH. Patient adherence to prescribed therapies. Med Care 1985; 23:539–555.

Becker N, Bondegaard TA, Olsen AK, et al. Pain epidemiology and health related quality of life in chronic non-malignant pain patients referred to a Danish multidisciplinary pain center. Pain 1997; 73:393–400.

Becker N, Hojsted J, Sjogren P, et al. Sociodemographic predictors of treatment outcome in chronic non-malignant pain patients. Do patients receiving or applying for disability pension benefit from multidisciplinary pain treatment? Pain 1998; 77:279–287.

Becker N, Sjogren P, Bech P, et al. Treatment outcome of chronic non-malignant pain patients managed in a Danish multidisciplinary pain centre compared to general practice: a randomised controlled trial. Pain 2000; 84:203–211.

Bergman S, Jacobsson LT, Herrstrom P, et al. Health status as measured by SF-36 reflects changes and predicts outcome in chronic musculoskeletal pain: a 3-year follow up study in the general population. Pain 2004; 108:115–123.

Bergner M, Bobbitt RA, Carter WB, et al. The Sickness Impact Profile: development and final revision of a health status measure. Med Care 1981; 19:787–805.

Beurskens AJ, de Vet HC, Koke AJ, et al. A patient-specific approach for measuring functional status in low back pain. J Manipulative Physiol Ther 1999; 22:144–148.

Bowling A. Research Methods in Health. Investigating Health and Health Services. Open University Press, Buckingham, 2000.

Bowling A. Measuring Disease: A Review of Disease-Specific Quality of Life Measurement Scales. Open University Press, Buckingham, 2001.

Brazier J, Roberts J, Tsuchiya A, et al. A comparison of the EQ-5D and SF-6D across seven patient groups. Health Econ 2004; 13:873–884.

Brazier JE, Walters SJ, Nicholl JP, et al. Using the SF-36 and Euroqol on an elderly population. Qual Life Res 1996; 5:195–204.

Bronfort G, Bouter LM. Responsiveness of general health status in chronic low back pain: a comparison of the COOP charts and the SF-36. Pain 1999; 83:201–209.

Brown J, Klapow J, Doleys D, et al. Disease-specific and generic health outcomes: a model for the evaluation of long-term intrathecal opioid therapy in noncancer low back pain patients. Clin J Pain 1999; 15:122–131.

Canto JG, Kiefe CI, Williams OD, et al. Comparison of outcomes research with clinical trials using preexisting data. Am J Cardiol 1999; 84:923–927, A6.

Carr A. Adult measures of quality of life. Arthritis Rheum 2003; 49:S113–S133.

Carr AJ, Higginson IJ. Are quality of life measures patient centred? Br Med J 2001; 322:1357–1360.

Carr AJ, Thompson PW. Towards a measure of patient-perceived handicap in rheumatoid arthritis. Br J Rheumatol 1994; 33:378–382.

Carr D, Goudas L, Lawrence D, et al. Management of Cancer Symptoms: Pain, Depression, and Fatigue. Agency for Healthcare Research and Quality, Rockville, MD, 2002: Evidence Report/Technology Assessment No. 61, AHRQ publication No, 02–E032.

Carr DB. The evolving practice of regional anesthesia. Curr Opin Anesthesiol 1994; 7:427–429.

Carr DB. Pain therapy: evidence, explanation – or "the power of myth"? Curr Opin Anesthesiol 1996; 9:420.

Carr DB. The development of national guidelines for pain control: synopsis and commentary. Eur J Pain 2001; 5(suppl A):91–98.

Carr DB, Wiffen P, Fairman F, et al. The Cochrane collaboration and its Pain, Palliative and Supportive Care review group. In: Max M (ed.). Pain 1999 – an updated review. Refresher course syllabus. IASP Press, Seattle, WA, 1999: 399–410.

Committee on Regional Health Data Networks, DoHCS. Health Data in the Information Age. Use, Disclosure, and Privacy. Institute of Medicine, National Academy Press, Washington, DC, 1994.

Concato J, Shah N, Horwitz RI. Randomized, controlled trials, observational studies, and the hierarchy of research designs. N Engl J Med 2000; 342:1887–1892.

Coons SJ, Rao S, Keininger DL, et al. A comparative review of generic quality-of-life instruments. Pharmacoeconomics 2000; 17:13–35.

Damiano AM, Patrick DL, Guzman GI, et al. Measurement of health-related quality of life in patients with amyotrophic lateral sclerosis in clinical trials of new therapies. Med Care 1999; 37:15–26.

Dawson J, Fitzpatrick R, Frost S, et al. Evidence for the validity of a patient-based instrument for assessment of outcome after revision hip replacement. J Bone Joint Surg Br 2001; 83:1125–1129.

de Bruin AF, de Witte LP, Stevens F, et al. Sickness Impact Profile: the state of the art of a generic functional status measure. Soc Sci Med 1992; 35:1003–1014.

de Bruin AF, Buys M, de Witte LP, et al. The sickness impact profile: SIP68, a short generic version. First evaluation of the reliability and reproducibility. J Clin Epidemiol 1994; 47:863–871.

de Bruin AF, Diederiks JP, de Witte LP, et al. Assessing the responsiveness of a functional status measure: the Sickness Impact Profile versus the SIP-68. J Clin Epidemiol 1997; 50:529–540.

Deyo RA. Comparative validity of the sickness impact profile and shorter scales for functional assessment in low-back pain. Spine 1986; 11:951–954.

Deyo RA. Promises and limitations of the Patient Outcome Research Teams: the low-back pain example. Proc Assoc Am Physicians 1995; 107:324–328.

Deyo RA, Carter WB. Strategies for improving and expanding the application of health status measures in clinical settings. A researcher-developer viewpoint. Med Care 1992; 30:MS176–MS186.

Deyo RA, Inui TS. Toward clinical applications of health status measures: sensitivity of scales to clinically important changes. Health Serv Res 1984; 19:277–289.

Donabedian A. Evaluating the quality of medical care. Milbank Mem Fund Q 1966; 44(suppl):206.

Dorman P, Slattery J, Farrell B, et al. Qualitative comparison of the reliability of health status assessments with the EuroQol and SF-36 questionnaires after stroke. United Kingdom Collaborators in the International Stroke Trial. Stroke 1998; 29:63–68.

Dunkel PA. Considerations in Developing and Using Computer-Adaptive Tests to Assess Second Language Proficiency, 1999; http://www.cal.org/resources/digest/cat.html.

Dysvik E, Lindstrom TC, Eikeland OJ, et al. Health-related quality of life and pain beliefs among people suffering from chronic pain. Pain Manag Nurs 2004; 5:66–74.

Eddy DM, Billings J. The quality of medical evidence: implications for quality of care. Health Aff (Millwood) 1988; 7:19–32.

Elliott AM, Smith BH, Hannaford PC, et al. Assessing change in chronic pain severity: the chronic pain grade compared with retrospective perceptions. Br J Gen Pract 2002; 52:269–274.

Elliott TE, Renier CM, Palcher JA. Chronic pain, depression, and quality of life: correlations and predictive value of the SF-36. Pain Med 2003; 4:331–339.

Epstein RS, Sherwood LM. From outcomes research to disease management: a guide for the perplexed. Ann Intern Med 1996; 124:832–837.

Eriksen J, Jensen MK, Sjogren P, et al. Epidemiology of chronic non-malignant pain in Denmark. Pain 2003; 106:221–228.

Essink-Bot ML, Krabbe PF, Bonsel GJ. NHP or SIP: a comparative study in renal insufficiency associated anemia. Qual Life Res 1996; 5:91–100.

Essink-Bot ML, Krabbe PF, Bonsel GJ, et al. An empirical comparison of four generic health status measures. The Nottingham Health Profile, the Medical Outcomes Study 36-item Short-Form Health Survey, the COOP/WONCA charts, and the EuroQol instrument. Med Care 1997; 35:522–537.

Falcoz PE, Chocron S, Mercier M, et al. Comparison of the Nottingham Health Profile and the 36-item health survey questionnaires in cardiac surgery. Ann Thorac Surg 2002; 73:1222–1228.

Farrell MJ, Gibson SJ, Helme RD. Measuring the activity of older people with chronic pain. Clin J Pain 1996; 12:6–12.

Feinstein AR, Josephy BR, Wells CK. Scientific and clinical problems in indexes of functional disability. Ann Intern Med 1986; 105:413–420.

Fischer D, Stewart AL, Bloch DA, et al. Capturing the patient's view of change as a clinical outcome measure. JAMA 1999; 282:1157–1162.

Fitzpatrick R, Ziebland S, Jenkinson C, et al. Importance of sensitivity to change as a criterion for selecting health status measures. Qual Health Care 1992; 1:89–93.

Follick MJ, Smith TW, Ahern DK. The sickness impact profile: a global measure of disability in chronic low back pain. Pain 1985; 21:67–76.

Franks P, Lubetkin EI, Gold MR, et al. Mapping the SF-12 to the EuroQol EQ-5D Index in a national US sample. Med Decision Making 2004; 24:247–254.

Freund D, Lave J, Clancy C, et al. Patient Outcomes Research Teams: contribution to outcomes and effectiveness research. Annu Rev Public Health 1999; 20:337–359.

Fritz JM, George SZ. Identifying psychosocial variables in patients with acute work-related low back pain: the importance of fear-avoidance beliefs. Phys Ther 2002; 82:973–983.

Gandek B, Ware JE, Aaronson NK, et al. Cross-validation of item selection and scoring for the SF-12 Health Survey in nine countries: results from the IQOLA Project. International Quality of Life Assessment. J Clin Epidemiol 1998; 51:1171–1178.

Garratt A, Schmidt L, Mackintosh A, et al. Quality of life measurement: bibliographic study of patient assessed health outcome measures. Br Med J 2002; 324:1417.

Gerety MB, Cornell JE, Mulrow CD, et al. The Sickness Impact Profile for nursing homes (SIP-NH). J Gerontol 1994; 49:M2–M8.

Gerteis M, Edgman-Levitan S, Daley J, et al. Through the Patient's Eyes: Understanding and Promoting Patient-Centered Care. Jossey-Bass, San Francisco, 1993.

Goudas LC, Carr DB, Balk E, et al. Management of Cancer Pain, Evidence Report/Technology Assessment 35. Agency for Healthcare Research and Quality, Public Health Service, US Department of Health and Human Services, Rockville, MD, 2001.

Gouveia WA, Bungay KM, Massaro FJ, et al. Paradigm for the management of patient outcomes. Am J Hosp Pharm 1991; 48:1912–1916.

Greenfield S, Nelson EC. Recent developments and future issues in the use of health status assessment measures in clinical settings. Med Care 1992; 48:MS23–MS41.

Guyatt G, Walter S, Norman G. Measuring change over time: assessing the usefulness of evaluative instruments. J Chronic Dis 1987; 40:171–178.

Guyatt GH, Naylor CD, Juniper E, et al. Users' guides to the medical literature: XII. How to use articles about health-related quality of life. Evidence-Based Medicine Working Group. JAMA 1987; 277:1232–1237.

Guzman JE. Multidisciplinary bio-psycho-social rehabilitation for chronic low back pain (Cochrane review). Cochrane Database Syst Rev 2002: (1) CD000963.

Haley SM, Andres PL, Coster WJ, et al. Short-form activity measure for post-acute care. Arch Phys Med Rehabil 2004; 85:649–660.

Hall JA, Roter DL, Katz NR. Meta-analysis of correlates of provider behavior in medical encounters. Med Care 1988; 26:657–675.

Harper R, Brazier JE, Waterhouse JC, et al. Comparison of outcome measures for patients with chronic obstructive pulmonary disease (COPD) in an outpatient setting. Thorax 1997; 52:879–887.

Hays RD, Morales LS, Reise SP. Item response theory and health outcomes measurement in the 21st century. Med Care 2000; 38:II28–II42.

Haywood KL, Garratt AM, Dziedzic K, et al. Generic measures of health-related quality of life in ankylosing spondylitis: reliability, validity and responsiveness. Rheumatology (Oxford) 2002; 41:1380–1387.

Hlatky MA, Lee KL, Harrell FE Jr. Tying clinical research to patient care by use of an observational database. Stat Med 1984; 3:375–387.

Ho MJ, LaFleur J. The treatment outcomes of pain survey (TOPS): a clinical monitoring and outcomes instrument for chronic pain practice and research. J Pain Palliat Care Pharmacother 2004; 18:49–59.

Horemans HL, Nollet F, Beelen A, et al. A comparison of 4 questionnaires to measure fatigue in postpoliomyelitis syndrome. Arch Phys Med Rehabil 2004; 85:392–398.

Howard KI, Moras K, Brill PL, et al. Evaluation of psychotherapy. Efficacy, effectiveness, and patient progress. Am Psychol 1996; 51:1059–1064.

Hunt SM, McEwen J, McKenna SP. Measuring health status: a new tool for clinicians and epidemiologists. J R Coll Gen Pract 1985; 35:185–188.

Hurst NP, Jobanputra P, Hunter M, et al. Validity of Euroqol: a generic health status instrument in patients with rheumatoid arthritis. Economic and Health Outcomes Research Group. Br J Rheumatol 1994; 33:655–662.

Hurst NP, Kind P, Ruta D, et al. Measuring health-related quality of life in rheumatoid arthritis: validity, responsiveness and reliability of EuroQol (EQ-5D). Br J Rheumatol 1997; 36:551–559.

Hutter BO, Wurtemberger G. [Quality of life in patients with chronic obstructive lung diseases: psychometric criteria of the German version of the Sickness Impact Profile and initial results of its application]. Pneumologie 1997; 51:108–114.

Ioannidis JP, Haidich AB, Pappa M, et al. Comparison of evidence of treatment effects in randomized and nonrandomized studies. JAMA 2001; 286:821–830.

Jadad AR. Meta-analysis in pain relief: a valuable but easily misused tool. Curr Opin Anesthesiol 1998; 9:426–429.

Jans MP, Schellevis FG, van Eijk JT. The Nottingham Health Profile: score distribution, internal consistency and validity in asthma and COPD patients. Qual Life Res 1999; 8:501–507.

Jensen MP, Strom SE, Turner JA, et al. Validity of the Sickness Impact Profile Roland scale as a measure of dysfunction in chronic pain patients. Pain 1992; 50:157–162.

Johnson JA, Coons SJ. Comparison of the EQ-5D and SF-12 in an adult US sample. Qual Life Res 1998; 7:155–166.

Johnson JA, Pickard AS. Comparison of the EQ-5D and SF-12 health surveys in a general population survey in Alberta, Canada. Med Care 2000; 38:115–121.

Jurkovich G, Mock C, MacKenzie E, et al. The Sickness Impact Profile as a tool to evaluate functional outcome in trauma patients. J Trauma 1995; 39:625–631.

Kaplan SH, Greenfield S, Ware JE. Assessing the effects of physician-patient interactions on the outcomes of chronic disease. Med Care 1989; 7(suppl):S110–S127.

Kaplan SH, Kravitz RL, Greenfield S. A critique of current uses of health status for the assessment of treatment effectiveness and quality of care. Med Care 2000; 38:II184–II191.

Kerr S, Fairbrother G, Crawford M, et al. Patient characteristics and quality of life among a sample of Australian chronic pain clinic attendees. Intern Med J 2004; 34:403–409.

Kind P, Gudex CM. Measuring health status in the community: a comparison of methods. J Epidemiol Community Health 1994; 48:86–91.

Kiresuk T, Sherman R. A general method for evaluating comprehensive community mental health programs. Com Mental Health J 1968; 4:443–453.

Kirshner B, Guyatt G. A methodological framework for assessing health indices. J Chronic Dis 1985; 38:27–36.

Konig HH, Ulshofer A, Gregor M, et al. Validation of the EuroQol questionnaire in patients with inflammatory bowel disease. Eur J Gastroenterol Hepatol 2002; 14:1205–1215.

Kosinski M, Keller SD, Ware JEJ, et al. The SF-36 Health Survey as a generic outcome measure in clinical trials of patients with osteoarthritis and rheumatoid arthritis: relative validity of scales in relation to clinical measures of arthritis severity. Med Care 1999; 37(suppl):39.

Lambert MJ. Psychotherapy outcome and quality improvement: introduction to the special section on patient-focused research. J Consult Clin Psychol 2001; 69:147–149.

Last JM. A Dictionary of Epidemiology. Oxford University Press, Oxford, 1995.

Lau J, Ioannidis JP, Schmid CH. Summing up evidence: one answer is not always enough. Lancet 1998; 351:123–127.

Law M, Baptiste S, McColl M, et al. The Canadian occupational performance measure: an outcome measure for occupational therapy. Can J Occup Ther 1990; 57:82–87.

Lee SJ, Earle CC, Weeks JC. Outcomes research in oncology: history, conceptual framework, and trends in the literature. J Natl Cancer Inst 2000; 92:195–204.

Leidy NK, Palmer C, Murray M, et al. Health-related quality of life assessment in euthymic and depressed patients with bipolar disorder: psychometric performance of four self-report measures. J Affect Disord 1998; 48:207–214.

Lindeboom R, Holman R, Dijkgraaf MG, et al. Scaling the sickness impact profile using item response theory: an exploration of linearity, adaptive use, and patient driven item weights. J Clin Epidemiol 2004; 57:66–74.

Lipsett PA, Swoboda SM, Campbell KA, et al. Sickness Impact Profile Score versus a Modified Short-Form survey for functional outcome assessment: acceptability, reliability, and validity in critically ill patients with prolonged intensive care unit stays. J Trauma 2000; 49:737–743.

Lohr KSAC. Assessing health status and quality-of-life instruments: attributes and review criteria. Qual Life Res 2002; 11:193–205.

Lueger RJ, Howard KI, Martinovich Z, et al. Assessing treatment progress of individual patients using expected treatment response models. J Consult Clin Psychol 2001; 69:150–158.

Luo N, Chew LH, Fong KY, et al. A comparison of the EuroQol-5D and the Health Utilities Index mark 3 in patients with rheumatic disease. J Rheumatol 2003a; 30:2268–2274.

Luo N, Chew LH, Fong KY, et al. Validity and reliability of the EQ-5D self-report questionnaire in Chinese-speaking patients with rheumatic diseases in Singapore. Ann Acad Med Singapore 2003b; 32:685–690.

Martin DP, Engelberg R, Agel J, et al. Comparison of the Musculoskeletal Function Assessment questionnaire with the Short Form-36, the Western Ontario and McMaster Universities Osteoarthritis Index, and the Sickness Impact Profile health-status measures. J Bone Joint Surg Am 1997; 79:1323–1335.

Marvel MK, Epstein RM, Flowers K, et al. Soliciting the patient's agenda: have we improved? JAMA 1999; 281:283–287.

McDowell I, Newell C, et al. Measuring Health. A Guide to Rating Scales and Questionnaires, 2nd edn. Oxford University Press, Oxford, 1996.

McGuirk B, King W, Govind J, et al. Safety, efficacy, and cost effectiveness of evidence-based guidelines for the management of acute low back pain in primary care. Spine 2001; 26:2615–2622.

McHorney CA. Ten recommendations for advancing patient-centered outcomes measurement for older persons. Ann Intern Med 2003; 139:403–409.

McHorney CA, Cohen AS. Equating health status measures with item response theory: illustrations with functional status items. Med Care 2000; 38:II43–II59.

McHorney CA, Ware JE, Raczek AE. The MOS 36-Item Short-Form Health Survey (SF-36): II. Psychometric and clinical tests of validity in measuring physical and mental health constructs. Med Care 1994; 31:247–263.

McPherson K, Wennberg JE, Hovind OB, et al. Small-area variations in the use of common surgical procedures: an international comparison of New England, England, and Norway. N Engl J Med 1982; 307:1310–1314.

McQuay HJ, Moore A. An Evidence-based Resource for Pain Relief. Oxford University Press, Oxford, 1998.

Mendelson DN, Goodman CS, Ahn R, et al. Outcomes and effectiveness research in the private sector. Health Aff (Millwood) 1998; 17:75–90.

Meyer-Rosberg K, Burckhardt CS, Huizar K, et al. A comparison of the SF-36 and Nottingham Health Profile in patients with chronic neuropathic pain. Eur J Pain 2001; 5:391–403.

Morishita L, Boult C, Ebbitt B, et al. Concurrent validity of administering the Geriatric Depression Scale and the physical functioning dimension of the SIP by telephone. J Am Geriatr Soc 1995; 43:680–683.

Mulrow CD, Lohr KN. Proof and policy from medical research evidence. J Health Politics Policy Law 2001; 26:249–266.

Nederhand MJ, Ijzerman MJ, Hermens HJ, et al. Predictive value of fear avoidance in developing chronic neck pain disability: consequences for clinical decision making. Arch Phys Med Rehabil 2004; 85:496–501.

Nunnally J. Psychometric Theory. McGraw-Hill, New York, 1978.

O'Boyle CA, McGee H, Hickey A, et al. Individual quality of life in patients undergoing hip replacement. Lancet 1992; 339:1088–1091.

Office of Technology Assessment. Identifying Health Technologies That Work: Searching for Evidence. US Congress, Washington, DC, 1994.

Oga T, Nishimura K, Tsukino M, et al. A comparison of the responsiveness of different generic health status measures in patients with asthma. Qual Life Res 2003; 12:555–563.

Osler W. Physic and physicians as depicted in Plato. In: Aequanimitas: With Other Addresses to Medical Students, Nurses and Practitioners of Medicine, 3rd edn. Blakiston Company, Philadelphia, PA, 1932: 45–71.

Parkerson GR Jr, Gehlbach SH, Wagner EH, et al. The Duke-UNC Health Profile: an adult health status instrument for primary care. Med Care 1981; 19:806–828.

Paterson C. Measuring outcomes in primary care: a patient generated measure, MYMOP, compared with the SF-36 health survey. Br Med J 1996; 312:1016–1020.

Patrick DL, Chiang YP. Measurement of health outcomes in treatment effectiveness evaluations: conceptual and methodological challenges. Med Care 2000; 38:II14–II25.

Perkins MR, Devlin NJ, Hansen P. The validity and reliability of EQ-5D health state valuations in a survey of Maori. Qual Life Res 2004; 13:271–274.

Pilote L, Tager IB. Outcomes research in the development and evaluation of practice guidelines. BMC Health Serv Res 2002; 2:7.

Pollard B, Johnston M. Problems with the sickness impact profile: a theoretically based analysis and a proposal for a new method of implementation and scoring. Soc Sci Med 2001; 52:921–934.

Post MW, Gerritsen J, Diederikst JP, et al. Measuring health status of people who are wheelchair-dependent: validity of the Sickness Impact Profile 68 and the Nottingham Health Profile. Disabil Rehabil 2001; 23:245–253.

Pransky G, Himmelstein J. Outcomes research, implications for occupational health. Am J Ind Med 1996; 29:573–583.

Prieto L, Alonso J, Ferrer M, et al. Are results of the SF-36 health survey and the Nottingham Health Profile similar? A comparison in COPD patients. Quality of Life in COPD Study Group. J Clin Epidemiol 1997; 50:463–473.

Read JL, Quinn RJ, Hoefer MA. Measuring overall health: an evaluation of three important approaches. J Chronic Dis 1987; 40(suppl 1):7S–26S.

Riddle DL, Stratford PW. Use of generic versus region-specific functional status measures on patients with cervical spine disorders. Phys Ther 1998; 78:951–963.

Rogers WH, Wittink H, Wagner A, et al. Assessing individual outcomes during outpatient multidisciplinary chronic pain treatment by means of an augmented SF-36. Pain Med 2000a; 1:44–54.

Rogers WH, Wittink HM, Ashburn MA, et al. Using the "TOPS," an outcomes instrument for multidisciplinary outpatient pain treatment. Pain Med 2000b; 1:55–67.

Roland M, Morris R. A study of the natural history of back pain: I. Development of a reliable and sensitive measure of disability in low-back pain. Spine 1983a; 8:141–144.

Roland M, Morris R. A study of the natural history of low-back pain: II. Development of guidelines for trials of treatment in primary care. Spine 1983b; 8:145–150.

Roper WL, Winkenwerder W, Hackbarth GM, et al. Effectiveness in health care. An initiative to evaluate and improve medical practice. N Engl J Med 1988; 319:1197–1202.

Rucker KS, Metzler HM, Kregel J. Standardization of chronic pain assessment: a multiperspective approach. Clin J Pain 1996; 12:94–110.

Ruta DA, Garratt AM, Leng M, et al. A new approach to the measurement of quality of life. The Patient-Generated Index. Med Care 1994; 32:1109–1126.

Ruta DA, Hurst NP, Kind P, et al. Measuring health status in British patients with rheumatoid arthritis: reliability, validity and responsiveness of the short form 36-item health survey (SF-36). Br J Rheumatol 1998; 37:425–436.

Sackett DL, Rosenberg WM, Gray JA, et al. Evidence Based Medicine: How to Practice and Teach EBM, 2nd edn. Churchill-Livingstone, New York, 1999.

Salkeld G, Cameron ID, Cumming RG, et al. Quality of life related to fear of falling and hip fracture in older women: a time trade off study. Br Med J 2000; 320:341–346.

Sanders C, Egger M, Donovan J, et al. Reporting on quality of life in randomised controlled trials: bibliographic study. Br Med J 1998; 317:1191–1194.

Sanders SH, Brena SF. Empirically derived chronic pain patient subgroups: the utility of multidimensional clustering to identify differential treatment effects. Pain 1993; 54:51–56.

Simon GE, Heiligenstein J, Revicki D, et al. Long-term outcomes of initial antidepressant drug choice in a "real world" randomized trial. Arch Fam Med 1999; 8:319–325.

Singh AC, Bilsbury CD. Measurement of subjective variables: the Discan method. Acta Psychiatr Scand Suppl 1989; 347:1–38.

Skevington SM, Carse MS, Williams AC. Validation of the WHOQOL-100: pain management improves quality of life for chronic pain patients. Clin J Pain 2001; 17:264–275.

Solomon GD. Evolution of the measurement of quality of life in migraine [review]. Neurology 1997; 48:S10–S15.

Stavem K, Jodalen H. Reliability and validity of the COOP/WONCA health status measure in patients with chronic obstructive pulmonary disease. Qual Life Res 2002; 11:527–533.

Stavem K. Reliability, validity and responsiveness of two multiattribute utility measures in patients with chronic obstructive pulmonary disease. Qual Life Res 1999; 8:45–54.

Stavem K, Bjornaes H, Lossius MI. Properties of the 15D and EQ-5D utility measures in a community sample of people with epilepsy. Epilepsy Res 2001; 44:179–189.

Stryer DB, Siegel JE, Rodgers AB. Outcomes research: priorities for an evolving field. Med Care 2004; 42:III1–III5.

Sullivan M, Ahlmen M, Bjelle A. Health status assessment in rheumatoid arthritis: I. Further work on the validity of the sickness impact profile. J Rheumatol 1990; 17:439–447.

Sullivan M, Ahlmen M, Bjelle A, et al. Health status assessment in rheumatoid arthritis: II. Evaluation of a modified Shorter Sickness Impact Profile. J Rheumatol 1993; 20:1500–1507.

Tanenbaum SJ. What physicians know. N Engl J Med 1993; 329:1268–1271.

Tarlov AR, Ware JEJ, Greenfield S, et al. The Medical Outcomes Study. An application of methods for monitoring the results of medical care. JAMA 1989; 262:925–930.

Tate R, Hodgkinson A, Veerabangsa A, et al. Measuring psychosocial recovery after traumatic brain injury: psychometric properties of a new scale. J Head Trauma Rehabil 1999; 14:543–557.

Taylor R, Kirby B, Burdon D, et al. The assessment of recovery in patients after myocardial infarction using three generic quality-of-life measures. J Cardiopulm Rehabil 1998; 18:139–144.

Testa MA, Simonson DC. Measuring quality of life in hypertensive patients with diabetes. Postgrad Med J 1988; 64(suppl 3):50–58.

Tidermark J, Bergstrom G, Svensson O, et al. Responsiveness of the EuroQol (EQ 5-D) and the SF-36 in elderly patients with displaced femoral neck fractures. Qual Life Res 2003; 12:1069–1079.

Tugwell P, Bombardier C, Buchanan WW, et al. The MACTAR Patient Preference Disability Questionnaire: an individualized functional priority approach for assessing improvement in physical disability in clinical trials in rheumatoid arthritis. J Rheumatol 1987: 14L446–14L451.

Turner-Bowker DM, Bayliss MS, Ware JE Jr, et al. Usefulness of the SF-8 Health Survey for comparing the impact of migraine and other conditions. Qual Life Res 2003; 12:1003–1012.

Uutela T, Hakala M, Kautiainen H. Validity of the Nottingham Health Profile in a Finnish out-patient population with rheumatoid arthritis. Rheumatology (Oxford) 2003; 42:841–845.

van Agt HM, Essink-Bot ML, Krabbe PF, et al. Test–retest reliability of health state valuations collected with the EuroQol questionnaire. Soc Sci Med 1994; 39:1537–1544.

Velozo CA, Kielhofner G, Lai JS. The use of Rasch analysis to produce scale-free measurement of functional ability. Am J Occup Ther 1999; 53:83–90.

Victora CG, Habicht JP, Bryce J. Evidence-based public health: moving beyond randomized trials. Am J Public Health 2004; 94:400–405.

Wagner AK, Gandek B, Aaronson NK, et al. Cross-cultural comparisons of the content of SF-36 translations across 10 countries: results from the IQOLA Project.

International Quality of Life Assessment. J Clin Epidemiol 1998; 51:925–932.

Ware JE Jr. Everyone into the "pools": a comment on the future of item banking. ISOQOL Newsletter 2003; 8:2.

Ware JE, Sherbourne CD. The MOS 36-item short-form health survey (SF-36): I. Conceptual framework and item selection. Med Care 1992; 30:473–483.

Ware JE Jr, Kosinski M, Keller SD. A 12-Item Short-Form Health Survey: construction of scales and preliminary tests of reliability and validity. Med Care 1996; 34:220–233.

Ware JE Jr, Bjorner JB, Kosinski M. Practical implications of item response theory and computerized adaptive testing: a brief summary of ongoing studies of widely used headache impact scales. Med Care 2000; 38:II73–II82.

Ware JE Jr, Kosinski M, Bjorner JB, et al. Applications of computerized adaptive testing (CAT) to the assessment of headache impact. Qual Life Res 2003; 12:935–952.

Weingarten SR, Henning JM, Badamgarav E, et al. Interventions used in disease management programmes for patients with chronic illness – which ones work? Meta-analysis of published reports. Br Med J 2002; 325:925.

Wells G, Boers M, Shea B, et al. Sensitivity to change of generic quality of life instruments in patients with rheumatoid arthritis: preliminary findings in the generic health OMERACT study. OMERACT/ILAR Task Force on Generic Quality of Life. Life Outcome Measures in Rheumatology. International League of Associations for Rheumatology. J Rheumatol 1999; 26:217–221.

Wells KB. Treatment research at the crossroads: the scientific interface of clinical trials and effectiveness research. Am J Psychiatry 1999; 156:5–10.

Wennberg J, Gittelsohn J. Small area variations in health care delivery. Science 1973; 182:1102–1108.

Wittink H, Turk DC, Carr DB, et al. Comparison of the redundancy, reliability, and responsiveness to change among SF-36, Oswestry Disability Index, and Multidimensional Pain Inventory. Clin J Pain 2004; 20:133–142.

Wittink HM, Carr DB. Evidence Based Medicine in Pain Management, 2003: www.Mdconsult.com Pain Medicine.

Wittink HM, Goudas LC, Strassels S, et al. Outcome measurements in pain medicine. In: Warfield CA, Bajwa ZH (eds), Principles and Practice of Pain Medicine. McGraw-Hill, New York, 2004.

World Health Organization. Constitution of the WHO, Basic Documents. WHO, Geneva, 1948.

Wright JG. Evaluating the outcome of treatment. Shouldn't we be asking patients if they are better? J Clin Epidemiol 2000; 53:549–553.

Wright JG, Rudicel S, Feinstein AR. Ask patients what they want. Evaluation of individual complaints before total hip replacement. J Bone Joint Surg Br 1994; 76:229–234.

Wu AW, Jacobson KL, Frick KD, et al. Validity and responsiveness of the euroqol as a measure of health-related quality of life in people enrolled in an AIDS clinical trial. Qual Life Res 2002; 11:273–282.

Zatzick D, Roy-Byrne P, Russo J, et al. A randomized effectiveness trial of stepped collaborative care for acutely injured trauma survivors. Arch Gen Psychiatry 2004; 61:498–506.

FURTHER READING

Agency for Health Care Policy and Research. Outcomes research. Fact sheet. AHRQ Publication No. 00-P011. AHCPR, Rockville, MD, 2000.

Agency for Health Care Policy and Research. Overview: Center for Outcomes and Effectiveness Research. AHCPR, Rockville, MD, 2003.

2

Choice of pain outcome measures from a clinimetric point of view

Henrica C.W. de Vet

INTRODUCTION

Clinimetrics means literally measurement of clinical phenomena. These phenomena include symptoms such as pain and swollen joints, the presence of diseases or disorders such as arthritis or radical lumbar syndrome, and health outcomes such as pain, disabilities and participation or quality of life. So clinimetrics is concerned with all health measurements with respect to diagnosis, prognosis and evaluation of treatment.

The term clinimetrics was introduced by Alvan Feinstein toward the end of the 20th century (Feinstein 1983). The quite new discipline of clinimetrics is related to the older disciplines of biometrics for measurements of biologic phenomena and psychometrics focused on the measurements of psychological phenomena. Within medicine the phenomena to be measured concern both biologic and psychological characteristics, and pain is a typical example of a construct at the intersection of both.

Biometrics, psychometrics and clinimetrics can be considered as methodologic disciplines. Clinimetrics is focused on the assessment of the quality of clinical measurements. A central issue in clinimetrics is to choose the most adequate measurement instrument for a specific purpose. If no adequate measurement instrument is found, a new one can be developed. Both the choice of an adequate measurement and the development of measurement instruments require the evaluation of the quality of the measurement instrument.

This chapter focuses on the role of clinimetrics in the choice of outcome measurements in pain research. I will first pay attention to some issues concerning the measurement of pain, followed by a description of clinimetric properties which determine the quality of a measurement instrument, resulting in a guideline about how to choose an appropriate measurement instrument.

SOME ISSUES IN PAIN MEASUREMENT

The measurement of pain is an excellent example for explaining some important issues and misunderstandings in clinimetrics.

The first issue concerns the scale of measurement. Questions frequently used in health sciences require only a "yes or no" response. Two answering options form a dichotomous scale. In other situations the response can be classified in more than two classes. If these classes have no logical order, for example in case of religions, it is called a nominal scale. A dichotomous scale is a special example of a nominal scale. If there are several classes and these do have a logical order, the scale is called an ordinal scale. Classifying pain in the classes "no pain," "mild pain," "moderate pain," "severe pain" and "unbearable pain" is an example of an ordinal scale. An interval scale has not only a logical order, but also a dimension. On an interval scale the distance between the numbers is known, which is not the case with an ordinal scale. It is unknown whether the "distance" between mild and moderate pain is the same as between severe and unbearable pain. An example of an interval scale is blood pressure, which is expressed in a number on a scale with the dimension of mmHg. The "distance" between 80 and 90 mmHg is the same as between 115 and 125 mmHg. Pain has long been measured on an ordinal scale. With the introduction of the Visual Analogue Scale (VAS), pain is measured on an interval scale. A horizontal line of 100 mm is drawn, with on the left side a mark for no pain at all (indicated with a 0) and on the right side the mark for the worst thinkable pain (indicated with 100). Patients are asked to indicate on this 100 mm line with a vertical arrow, for example, the intensity of their current pain. In case of severe pain the arrow will be more to the right side than in case of only mild pain. The pain can now be expressed in a number between 0 and 100. The scale of measurement determines the type of statistical analyses that can be performed. Both the amount of information and possibilities for analysis increases from nominal via ordinal to interval scales (Feinstein 1987; Streiner and Norman 1995).

The second issue in pain measurement concerns the choice between objective and subjective measurements. In subjective measurements the sense organs of patients or outcome assessors are involved. Pain is a typical example of a subjective measurement. A general misunderstanding is that objective measures are better than subjective ones. However, in the case of pain it is clear that asking the patient about the intensity of the current pain is more valid than measuring it indirectly via EMG recordings or another objective way. The example of measurement of pain on a VAS, which is an interval scale, also invalidates the conviction that objective measures are expressed in numbers and subjective measures are expressed in, at best, ordinal scales. The scale of measurement is therefore not related to the subjectiveness of the measurement.

The third issue concerns the definition of the construct being measured. Pain is not only defined by its intensity, but other aspects can be distinguished. The International Association for the Study of Pain Subcommittee on Taxonomy (IASP 1986) defined pain as "an unpleasant sensation and emotional experience associated with actual or potential tissue damage or described in terms of such damage." Melzack and Wall (1988) doubt whether a single definition of pain is possible. They remark that "The diversity of pain experiences explains why it has been impossible, so far, to achieve a satisfactory definition of pain. The word 'pain' represents a category of experiences, signifying a multitude of different, unique experiences having different causes, and characterized by different qualities varying along a number of sensory, affective and evaluative dimensions." Fordyce (1988) distinguishes nociceptive aspects, considered as input phenomena and described in physiologic terms as "mechanical, thermal, or chemical energy impinging on specialized nerve endings," and affective aspects, the suffering, which is an affective or emotional response to pain. These can be considered as output phenomena. Another aspect is pain behavior, which consists of "the things that people do when they suffer or are in pain." When one thinks about measuring pain, it is important to consider which aspect(s) of pain one wants information about.

CLINIMETRIC PROPERTIES

The quality of a measurement instrument is determined by its clinimetric properties. These clinimetric properties include the validity, reproducibility (that is reliability and agreement at test–retest), responsiveness and interpretability. These terms are described and explained in detail in handbooks on clinimetrics or health measurements (Feinstein 1987; McDowell and Newell 1987; Streiner and Norman 1995). Therefore I will only present a concise overview here.

Validity

The term *validity* means whether a measurement instrument indeed measures the entity or concept that it aims to measure; in other words how well an instrument does its job. Several different types of validity exist, depending on the way in which the validity can be assessed.

Criterion Validity

If a "gold standard" exists for the concept one wants to measure, the instrument under study can be compared with the gold standard. If the values obtained by the instruments agree with the gold standard to a large extent, the instrument has a high criterion validity. This is the most powerful form of validity.

Construct Validity

For many clinical phenomena no "gold standard" exists. This is also the case for pain. In the absence of an acceptable gold standard, construct validity is the next-best option. In that case, one measure of the construct "pain intensity" may be compared with another measure of pain intensity. To examine construct validity it is necessary to define hypotheses about how the scores on the instrument under study will correlate with the scores on other instruments. Confirmation of these hypotheses gives support to the validity of a measurement instrument. However, by absence of a gold standard, we are never sure that the level of pain that is measured is the "true" level of pain.

Content Validity

Content validity concerns judgment whether all important aspects or dimensions of the construct to be measured are covered by the instrument. A clear definition of the construct to be measured is a prerequisite.

Face Validity

Face validity implies an overall judgment of adequacy on the face of it, without necessarily paying close attention to the component parts. For example, to assess the intensity of the pain a VAS on which the intensity of the pain is scored has a high face validity.

Reproducibility

Reproducibility reflects whether the same answers are obtained by repeated measurements. This may be repeated measurements in time, or repeated measurements by different observers. In test–retest reproducibility two different concepts can be distinguished: agreement and reliability (de Vet et al. 2006).

Agreement

Represents lack of measurement error. It expresses how close the value of two different measurements is in absolute terms. Examples of parameters which express agreement is kappa for nominal or ordinal scales, and the Bland and Altman approach is a typical method to calculate and visualize the measurement error for interval scales (Bland and Altman 1986; de Vet et al. 2006).

Reliability

Represents the extent to which individuals can be distinguished from each other, despite measurement errors. Reliability is a relative measure. A reliability coefficient relates the variation due to measurement error to the variation between individuals within a population. In a heterogeneous population, the variation between individuals within a population is higher. Thus the reliability of a measurement instrument will be greater, given the same measurement error. Therefore individuals in a heterogeneous population are more easily distinguished from each other. In general, reliability parameters are important when the aim is to discriminate between individuals, and agreement parameters are important when one wants to detect changes in health status over time (Beaton et al. 2001; de Vet et al. 2006).

Responsiveness

Responsiveness is an important clinimetric parameter for measurement instruments which aim to measure change over time; for example, outcome measures in studies on the effects of treatment (Husted et al. 2000; Beaton et al. 2001; Terwee et al. 2003). In a short period of time, more than 30 different formulas have been developed to calculate responsiveness (Terwee et al. 2003). The most

important distinction is made between responsiveness measures which quantify the treatment effect (effect size), and measures that focus on the longitudinal construct validity by assessing the correlation of change scores with another measure (external standard) for change (Norman et al. 2001). This external standard can, for example, be the opinion of the patient or doctor about whether or not the health status has changed.

Interpretability

Interpretability of measurement is rarely mentioned as a clinimetric property. Interpretability concerns the meaning of a specific score on an instrument. What does a score of 10 on the McGill Pain Questionnaire mean? Is an improvement of 10 mm on a 100 mm VAS for pain intensity a clinically relevant improvement? Comparing scores on a new instrument with classifications or scores on well-known instruments facilitates the clinical interpretation of the new data.

CHOICE OF OUTCOME MEASURES

Choosing the outcome measures is an important step in the design of a study. It forms part of the research protocol in which the research question is formulated, the study population defined and relation with other measurements is described. In fact the research question determines to a large extent which measure of pain is the most appropriate.

The choice of the pain measurement depends on three questions (Figure 2.1):

1. What does one want to know about pain (which dimensions and which time frame)?
2. Why does one want to measure pain (goal of measurement)?
3. Which measurement instrument is the most appropriate?

WHAT DOES ONE WANT TO KNOW ABOUT PAIN?

With respect to the question about "what" we precisely define the aspects or dimensions of pain one wants to measure. Does one want to measure all dimensions of

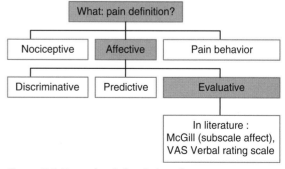

Figure 2.1 Example of the choice of measurement instruments for a study about the effect of coping strategies on affective pain.

pain, only the intensity, only the bothersomeness or the impact of pain on the daily activities of patients, pain behavior, or combinations of aspects?

Another important issue, which is sometimes overlooked, is the timeframe of the question. Does one want to have information about the current pain (after the inconvenience of the trip to the hospital), about the pain yesterday, about the average intensity of pain during last week, or about the worst pain during the last week? Or does one want to know the duration of severe pain periods?

WHY DOES ONE WANT TO MEASURE PAIN?

The "why" question is essential because a different purpose poses different requirements on the clinimetric properties (Guyatt et al. 1992). Although the measurement is always aimed to assess the health status, the measurement can serve different purposes. Purposes to be distinguished are discrimination, prediction or evaluation. If the measurement is aimed to discriminate between patients, for example to set a diagnosis, one needs a measurement instrument that has good discriminative power. If the objective of a measurement instrument is to predict the prognosis of patients, one needs a predictive instrument. Measurements that are aimed to evaluate change over time or effects of treatments are called evaluative measurement instruments.

I will give a few examples of the different requirements for the different instruments (Guyatt et al. 1992). Instruments that are used to evaluate change over time should be very responsive. This means that they should be able to detect small changes, but at the same time stay stable, if the health status of the patient does not change over time. Items that cannot be influenced or cannot change should not be included in an evaluative measurement instrument. For example, if patients with low back pain are only moderately impaired at the start of treatment on the Roland Disability Questionnaire (i.e., they are able to perform most activities included in the questionnaire) their potential to improve is low. Only items that they cannot perform are eligible to improve by treatment. For that reason a patient-specific measurement instrument is usually more responsive than a disease-specific instrument (Beurskens et al. 1999). In the case of a patient-specific measurement instrument one asks the patient beforehand to choose the activity that is most important for them, that cannot be avoided and patients have much difficulty in performing because of back pain. So patients choose an activity that is very relevant for them and there is much room for improvement.

Variables that are not sensitive for change can be usefully included in discriminative and predictive instruments. For example age or success of previous treatment are variables that cannot be influenced. If a diagnostic test is composed on the basis of demographical and clinical characteristics, the age of the patient may be important for distinguishing between patients with knee arthrosis and arthritis. And information on success of previous treatments may be a very important predictor of the success of the current treatment. As said in evaluative measurement instruments, stable items have no place.

WHICH MEASUREMENT IS MOST ADEQUATE TO SERVE THE PURPOSE?

After having answered the previous questions, one has to choose between the available measurement instruments. First one has to search in the literature for adequate instruments. An additional strategy is to ask experts in the field. Only if it is certain that there is no adequate instrument one may start thinking about developing a new instrument.

In some areas overviews of available measures exist. For example, for pain Von Korff et al. (2000) and Sim and Waterfield (1997) present inventories of existing measurements. In some areas researchers have reached consensus on a core set of measurement instruments to assess the effects of treatment. For low back pain a core set of outcome measures was defined by a panel of experts (Deyo et al. 1998) (see Chapter 17). In other words, there is consensus among researchers that when evaluating the effects of treatment of low back pain at least five measurement instruments should be used, which can be supplemented with other ones if the researchers choose to do so. Also rheumatologists reached consensus on a core set of measures to evaluate treatment in patients with rheumatoid arthritis (Boers et al. 1994). It is recommendable to reach consensus for other diseases as well, as such core sets make results from different studies more comparable.

A new development is the recent appearance of systematic reviews of clinimetric properties of measurement instruments (Coons et al. 2000; Michener and Leggin 2001). Michener and Leggin (2001) published a review of questionnaires used for the assessment of functional limitation and disability of the shoulder. Coons et al. (2000) examined the clinimetric properties of 7 broadly used general Health Related Quality of Life (HR-QOL) scales. They compared the clinimetric properties and described which instruments are applicable to evaluate the effect of treatments. These systematic reviews not only provide an overview of the available instruments, but they also show the clinimetric properties, such as the reproducibility and the responsiveness, and provide a basis for the choice of the most adequate measurement instrument. Systematic reviews of available measurement instruments should precede the decision to develop a new measurement instrument, analogous to the need for a systematic review of available trials in a specific field before one decides to design a new trial (de Vet et al. 2003).

If the literature search does not yield measurement instruments, experts in the field should be asked. However, in most fields there is an abundance of instruments. For example Feinstein (1987) reported already 230 instruments to measure mobility. The decision to develop a new measurement instrument must be avoided as much as possible. It takes years to develop an instrument, and after the development it should of course be evaluated on its clinimetric properties, in order to show that it measures what it aims to measure.

CONCLUSION

Clinimetrics is focused on the assessment of the quality of clinical measurements. A central issue in clinimetrics is to choose the most adequate measurement instrument for a specific purpose. The quality of a measurement instrument is determined by its clinimetric properties. These clinimetric properties include the validity, reproducibility (that is, reliability and agreement at test–retest), responsiveness and interpretability. The guideline before starting research is that the aim of the pain measurements has to be well considered. With respect to the measurements this includes at least the questions of "what one wants to measure" and "for which purpose."

REFERENCES

Beaton DE, Bombardier C, Katz JN, et al. A taxonomy for responsiveness. J Clin Epidemiol 2001; 54:1204–1217.

Beurskens AJHM, de Vet HCW, Köke AJA, et al. A patient specific approach for measuring functional status in low back pain. J Manipul Physiol Ther 1999; 22:144–148.

Bland JM, Altman DG. Statistical methods for assessing agreement between two methods of clinical measurement. Lancet 1986; 1(8476):307–310.

Boers M, Tugwell P, Felson DT, et al. World Health Organization and International League of Associations for Rheumatology core endpoints for symptom modifying antirheumatic drugs in rheumatoid arthritis clinical trials. J Rheumatol 1994; 41(suppl):86–89.

Coons SJ, Rao S, Keininger DL, et al. A comparative review of generic quality of life instruments. Pharmacoeconomics 2000; 17:13–35.

de Vet HC, Terwee CB, Knol DL, Bouter LM. When to use agreement versus reliability measures. J Clin Epidemiol. 2006; 59:1033–1039.

de Vet HCW, Beurskens AJHM, Bezemer PD, et al. Reproducibility and responsiveness of evaluative outcome measures. Theoretical considerations illustrated by an empirical example. Int J Health Technology Assess Health Care 2001; 17:479–487.

de Vet HCW, Terwee CB, Bouter LM. Current challenges in clinimetrics. J Clin Epidemiol 2003; 56(12):1137–1141.

Deyo RA, Battie AJ, Beurskens AJ, et al. Outcome measures for low back pain. A proposal for standardized use. Spine 1998; 23:2003–2013.

Feinstein AR. An additional basic science for clinical medicine: IV. The development of clinimetrics. Ann Intern Med 1983; 99:843–848.

Feinstein AR. Clinimetrics. Yale University Press, New Haven, CT, 1987.

Fordyce WE. Pain and suffering. A reappraisal. Am Psychologist 1988.

Guyatt GH, Kirschner B, Jaeschke R. Measuring health status: what are the necessary measurement properties? J Clin Epidemiol 1992; 45:1341–1345.

Husted JA, Cook RJ, Farewell VT, et al. Methods for assessing responsiveness: a critical review and recommendations. J Clin Epidemiol 2000; 53:459–468.

IASP. Classification of chronic pain: descriptions of chronic pain syndromes and definitions of pain terms. Pain 1986; 27(suppl):S1–S225.

McDowell I, Newell C. Measuring Health: A Guide to Rating Scales and Questionnaires. Oxford University Press, New York, 1987.

Melzack R, Wall PD. The Challenge of Pain. 3rd edn, Penguin Books, Harmondsworth, 1988.

Michener LA, Leggin BG. A review of self-report scales for the assessment of functional limitation and disability of the shoulder. J Hand Ther 2001; 14:68–76.

Norman GR, Gwadry Sridhar F, Guyatt G, et al. Relation of distribution- and anchor-based approaches in interpretation of changes in health related quality of life. Med Care 2001; 39:1039–1047.

Sim J, Waterfield J. Validity, reliability and responsiveness in the assessment of pain. Physiother Theory Pract 1997; 13:23–37.

Streiner DL, Norman GR. Health Measurement Scales. A Practical Guide to Their Development and Use. 2nd edn, Oxford University Press, Oxford, 1995.

Terwee CB, Dekker FW, Wiersinga WM, et al. On assessing responsiveness of health related quality of life instruments: guidelines for instrument evaluation. Qual Life Res 2003; 12(4):349–362.

Von Korff M, Jensen MP, Karoly P. Assessing global pain severity by self-report in clinical and health services research. Spine 2000; 24:3140–3151.

Qualitative research with people who live with chronic illness and pain

Debbie Kralik • Tina Koch • Kay Price

INTRODUCTION

A chronic illness qualitative research program that has been in progress since 1996 has focused on understanding the experience of long-term illness and how people can learn to incorporate the symptoms and consequences of illness into their lives. A primary healthcare philosophy has underpinned this research program which has been undertaken in a community health practice setting. The philosophy guiding this research program has been researching *with* people; hence the principles of primary healthcare (PHC) and participatory action research (PAR) have provided the theoretical framework.

We have researched *with* both men and women who have diverse chronic conditions. Pain appears to be a constant companion in the lives of some people. We have come to understand that health workers may be the expert in clinical matters, but the person with the illness is the expert in his or her own life. Prescriptions for treatment may have little impact unless an understanding of the social and cultural context of a person's life is gained. Qualitative research is a mode of research that may lead us to a greater appreciation of the complexity of living with chronic pain.

In this chapter we focus on ways people with chronic illness express and experience pain and how qualitative research can facilitate our understandings of their experiences. Our aim is to reveal the possibilities of qualitative research as an approach that may give voice to people who may be silent or have been silenced by objectivist research practices. Rather than focus on the cause or treatment of pain, we show the way we have used qualitative research to provide context to the lives lived with pain and the meanings ascribed to the experience of pain.

The aims of this chapter are to trace the development and share the findings of our research with men and women who live with pain, and to explore the ways that qualitative research can inform our understandings of the experience of living with long term and persistent pain.

To achieve this, we will begin by introducing the chronic illness experience research program of which these studies with people who live with pain have been a part, and then explicate the participatory action research methodology we have utilized extensively to harness qualitative research findings. We will share our current theorizing and work in progress and explore contributions from the wider qualitative research literature.

CHRONIC ILLNESS EXPERIENCE RESEARCH PROGRAM

During the past few years our chronic illness experience research program has been consolidated by collaboratively researching with more than 300 men and women who were living in the community with adult-onset chronic illness (Koch and Kelly 1999a,b; Koch et al. 1999, 2000a,b, 2001, 2002b; Koch and Kralik 2001; Kralik et al. 2001a,b,c; Eastwood et al. 2002; Kralik 2002). Recruitment of participants has crossed diverse medical diagnoses and relied upon the participant's own construct of living with the consequences and symptoms of chronic illness (Kralik 2000; Kralik et al. 2001c). We have researched with people who have multiple and complex diagnoses including cancers, Crohn's disease, multiple sclerosis, fibromyalgia, asthma, arthritis, schizophrenia, HIV and diabetes. Findings have revealed that symptoms such as fatigue and pain, and the consequences of illness such as changes to self-identity, relationships and employment, are often experiences that are shared by people across these medical diagnostic category groups. When we have researched with people who have a specific medical diagnosis it has been because it has been the focus of the funding body (such as MS Australia, Diabetes Australia). We will share the emerging constructs based on theorizing and experience from a broad range of projects and across chronic illness experiences.

EMERGING CONSTRUCTS

Our research program has been informed by people's storied accounts of their experiences of learning to live with a diverse range of chronic illness and conditions. A major construct of transition in illness has emerged which people have described as convoluted movement between states that we have called Extraordinariness and Ordinariness (Kralik 2000, 2002).

Extraordinariness was manifested when people were first confronted by the changes to their sense of well-being that are imposed by an illness or condition; they experience turmoil and difficulty in coming to terms with the intrusion of illness. They may experience an assault to the "taken-for-granted-ness" of their everyday lives, in addition to dealing with the impact of the physical manifestations of illness. Profound disruption, isolation, powerlessness and loss accompany the impact of chronic illness. One participant described her world as "laying like shattered glass" at her feet when illness intruded. Illness becomes a focal point and there may be a perceived lack of control over the seemingly constant disruption to every facet of their lives as completing common daily routines becomes difficult. Physical changes and sensations may exacerbate a feeling of being betrayed by their bodies.

Most people have experienced a powerful sense of loss exacerbated by the inability to continue work in paid employment, changes to sexual feelings which may result in modification to sexual practices, shifts in relationships, the inability to parent effectively, loss of spontaneity in life, and loss of control over both their lives and bodies. Self-absorption may dominate their perspective on life; however, our research has revealed that the process of focusing on, thinking through and turning over these thoughts, feelings and responses may provide the impetus for the passage to Ordinariness.

People have experienced Ordinariness when they have learnt ways to manage and incorporate the constant change imposed by chronic illness into their daily life. We have found that people who are in supportive relationships may experience a smoother transition toward Ordinariness because acknowledgment by others assists in the reconstruction of self-identity (Koch et al. 2002a). Through reflection on their experiences and responses to illness they develop an altered perception of self that has enabled them to reclaim control. Illness becomes an ordinary part of life. Actively making choices to reshape their lives provides an important sense of progress. Feelings of being betrayed by their body are replaced with a desire to nurture it. People in Ordinariness develop a sense of mastery over, and responsibility for, their responses to illness. Through the day-to-day experience of living with illness, they learn that maintaining themselves in Ordinariness means incorporating the consequences of living with chronic illness into their lives. In these ways, a sense of order is created.

The literature that has focused on transition when experiencing chronic illness is sparse. Publications are predominantly attributed to nurses (Chick and Meleis 1986; Cantanzaro 1990; Loveys 1990; Meleis and Trangenstein 1994; Schumacher and Meleis 1994; Meleis et al. 2000; Kralik 2002). Loveys (1990) identified transition as a state of being "at-risk" of progressive illness when people are living with chronic illness. Cantanzaro (1990) focused on transition as the impact on living with a partner, parenting and working. Transition has been identified as both a result of and results in change to lives, health, relationships and environments (Meleis et al. 2000). Several authors have concurred that transitional experiences are complex and multidimensional (Chick and Meleis 1986; Meleis and Trangenstein 1994; Schumacher and Meleis 1994; Meleis et al. 2000; Kralik 2002).

The transition between Extraordinariness and Ordinariness is a convoluted process embedded in and impacted upon by the context of life. Our recent research has aimed to explicate this complex transition and, to achieve this, each of our research projects has been a building block towards new understandings of chronic illness experience.

LITERATURE REVIEW

Before presenting the conceptual threads identified within the literature related to qualitative research and chronic pain and their influence on our research, the search strategy or the way in which references have been identified will be outlined.

LITERATURE SEARCH STRATEGY

The types of references obtained for the review were primarily journal articles from a diverse range of journals, books and book chapters, and several theses. CINAHL and Medline databases provided the majority of these references.

The CINAHL database was selected because it provided access to a comprehensive range of English language nursing journals in addition to publications from various allied health disciplines. The database covers the literature from 1982 onwards and it is updated monthly. The search strategy for CINAHL was very basic as it retrieved an acceptable results set that was very specific. The initial search statement was the phrase "chronic pain" which was mapped to subject headings – a result set of 2369 references was obtained. A second search statement for the word "qualitative" was also mapped to subject headings. Two headings were selected: "qualitative validity" and "qualitative studies" – a result set of 12,857 references was obtained. These two result sets were then combined to obtain a result set of 49 references containing both search statements. The result set was then limited to research papers and English language papers only, and hence a final result set of 43 references was achieved. The result set was exported into an EndNote library.

Medline was the other primary database used and was selected because it covers the medical and biomedical literature in the areas of allied health, biological and physical sciences, humanities and information science as they relate to medicine and healthcare, communication disorders, population biology and reproductive biology. Medline's coverage of the literature dates from 1966. The search statements used in the CINAHL database were again used here in a slightly different format due the different nature of the database. The first search statement entered was "Aged/ or Pain, Intractable/ or Chronic Disease/ or Adult/ or Pain/ or Pain Measurement/ or Middle Aged/" resulting in a result set of 3,537,893 references. The second search statement entered was "qualitative research" with a result set of 1280 references. Combining the two sets gave a result set of 622 references. Limiting to "English language and systematic reviews" provided a final result set of 18 references that were also exported into an EndNote library.

The above search statements were also used (with variations according to the requirements of individual databases) in the following databases: AUSThealth, Cochrane library, Health business fulltext elite, Blackwell Synergy, Science Direct and Wiley InterScience, with varying results. Where possible the full text of

the references was obtained electronically from the following databases: Health business fulltext elite, Blackwell Synergy, ingenta, Science Direct, Wiley InterScience and Academic Search Elite. Papers identified will be woven into the review of the literature and the discussion section of the chapter.

The references identified by the search strategy detailed above were reviewed to ensure their relevance; many were ineligible because they were not research based. Those remaining were read to explicate research designs and findings.

WHAT IS CHRONIC PAIN?

The literature reveals that a definition of chronic pain remains elusive because the phenomenon is multidimensional lying at the intersection between biology, culture and life world. The modern understanding of pain takes into account emotional, psychological, sociopolitical and existential aspects of pain as well as physiologic, anatomical factors. A view that appears increasingly common in biomedical literature for health workers is that chronic pain will continue to be difficult to define, understand and treat (Livingston 1998). Loeser (2002, p. 9) wrote:

The complex nature of chronic pain, related to tissue damage, injury to the nervous system, affective state, and interactions with the environment, will long delay its resolution into manageable components that can be targeted by pharmacological, psychological, or physical interventions... There are so many arguments about the nature of chronic pain that it is naïve to think that more science will resolve them.

Nevertheless science has attempted to resolve them. The complexity of chronic pain means that understandings, and/or the functioning status of the biological body, and/or the social context in which a person lives, works and plays impacts upon a person's life (Padilla et al. 1990; Bowman 1994; Rhodes et al. 1999; Subramaniam et al. 1999; Cook and Hassenkamp 2000; Carter et al. 2002; Davis et al. 2002; Sallfors et al. 2002; Steihaug et al. 2002; Howden et al. 2003).

When pain becomes part of daily living it may interrupt normalcy and life itself becomes unpredictable (Martin 1989; Seers and Friedli 1996; Kelley and Clifford 1997; Carson and Mitchell 1998; Soderberg et al. 1999; Hallberg and Carlsson 2000; Thomas 2000; Dudgeon et al. 2002; Ohmen et al. 2003; Smith 2003). If people are able to develop agency and a sense of control over their lives, they may be better able to cope with pain (Bates and Rankin-Hill 1994; Culver and Kell 1995; Hallberg and Carlsson 1998; Smith and Friedemann 1999; Hellstrom 2001; Werner et al. 2003).

Cultural differences have also been recognized in understandings of chronic pain and how people may receive care from health workers (Kodiath and Kodiath 1992, 1995; Bates et al. 1997; Dickson and Kim 2003; Roberts et al. 2003) and how culture impacts upon the relationship between providers and people with chronic pain (Bates et al. 1997). Health worker attitudes and preferences have been found to influence the chronic pain care provided to both older and younger people (Carter 2002; Blomqvist 2003). People who were perceived by health workers as exaggerating pain evoked frustration in workers while people who were perceived as enduring their pain evoked satisfaction (Blomqvist 2003). Pain has been perceived as being reinterpreted and mistranslated through health workers' own paradigms of understanding (Carter 2002). People with chronic pain have reported being disbelieved, judged and labeled as dysfunctional, which has further compounded the turmoil in their lives created by chronic pain (Carter 2002). People living with chronic pain face obstacles when dealing with health professionals and the healthcare system primarily because health worker perceptions may influence pain relieving treatment and activities that are offered (Walker 1989, 1994; Grace 1995; De Souza and Frank 2000; Lansbury 2000; McHugh and Thoms 2001; Paulson et al. 2001; Augello 2002; Blomqvist and Edberg 2002; Carter 2002; Steihaug and Malterud 2002; Blomqvist 2003; Neville-Jan 2003; Lillrank 2003).

What has been de-emphasized in this brief review is the way that the researchers have given pain meaning. Indeed, while a definition of chronic pain was generally included in the introduction of an article, there was minimal critique of the implications this definition had on research design, methods of data collection and analysis, and presentation of research findings.

Qualitative methodologies

In relation to the research approach on which findings were based, many authors only stated that they had used interviews and/or focus groups when generating data. This assumes that authors believed that by using these methods they were "doing" qualitative research. We contend that using interviews or focus groups to generate qualitative data does not translate into "doing" qualitative research. Other researchers had been guided by the principles of phenomenology or grounded theory when exploring the experience of chronic pain with participants. There exist established processes within those approaches that speak to both rigor and legitimacy, so the findings generated by these approaches resonate with our research. Sometimes the qualitative approach used can have therapeutic benefits for participants. Kelley and Clifford (1997) used narrative approaches with people living with chronic pain. The findings suggested that the narrative approach assisted people to find their own strengths and means of coping with pain and helped them find

identities beyond that of being a "patient." It is important, however, for the qualitative researcher not to lose sight of the ethical, political and very real consequences of their research. Having this sight in our vision at all times is paramount to our efforts as we acknowledge that qualitative research to participants is not just about doing a research project or producing a report but, for them, it is life (Ohmen et al. 2003).

What is important to us whilst researching is to ensure that women and men who are participants are not silenced or that we conceal their presence (sense of self) in any way. How this has been achieved is outlined in the next section.

METHODOLOGY

Our research program has been shaped by a collaborative research approach and guided by participatory action research (PAR) and PHC principles. Firstly, it is important to articulate the PHC philosophy driving our research agenda. We are researchers and nurses working in the community, hence we have embraced PHC principles (equity, social justice, working *with* people and health promotion) to guide our research and nursing practice. A key aspect of this PHC philosophy has been researching *with* people, hence our use of PAR. PAR has provided a democratic approach that is equitable and liberating because participants construct meaning during the process of research. The PAR process embraces principles of participation, reflection, empowerment and emancipation with the creation of positive social change for the participants being the predominant driving force.

Since Lewin's seminal work in the 1940s, action research has emerged as a critique of traditional approaches in social science (Reason and Bradbury 2001). Rather than making causal links between predictor and dependent variables based on data from past events, this research approach aims to understand past events and also to explore ongoing dynamics of human interactions in the present and further prepare for future intentions through joint organizing with all stakeholders. The inquiry commences with everyday experiences of people living with chronic illness and their development of living knowledge. When people narrate their stories, they hear their life anew through hearing and prompts made by the others (Aranda 2001). The narrative process creates the possibility to "reconstitute and repair ruptures between body, self and world by linking-up and interpreting different aspects of biography in order to realign present and past and self with society" (Williams 1984). When possible, participants are co-researchers, and we collaboratively decide on action and what can be done to "make" or shape the future. PAR principles enable a potentially democratic process that is equitable and liberating as participants construct meaning or make sense of their experiences whilst researching. The PAR principles that have guided our research have been: a recognition of power relationships, recognition of the value of "the lived experience" of people and the empowerment of people through the process of constructing and using their own knowledge (Reason 1994). These principles appeal to participants because a sense of unity is promoted, and a "safe" environment created where individual constructions and interpretations can be compared and contrasted, thus facilitating negotiated action.

The cyclical processes inherent in PAR promote reflection and reconstruction of experiences that can lead to the enhancement of people's lives, either at an individual or community level, or both (Koch and Kralik 2001). Participants have been encouraged to systematically investigate their problems and issues, formulate experiential accounts of their situations, and to devise action plans to deal with the problems at hand. Incorporating grassroots initiatives with change-oriented strategies, we have found that a PAR approach has maximized people's involvement in knowledge building on behalf of their own development (Koch and Kralik 2001; Koch et al. 2002b). Guided by PAR principles, we have identified three useful data generation strategies: one-to-one in-depth interviews, PAR group meetings and PAR groups utilizing electronic mail (email). The research described in this chapter is the findings from the third data generation strategy, but we will explicate all data generation strategies below. We are concurrently working with both men and women who live with chronic illness in the effort to describe transition (Australian Research Council Discovery Grant 2003–2005) and PAR using email correspondence has been the methodology selected. A website provides more detailed information about the background to the research (http://www.unisa.edu.au/nur/arc_project/).

STORY TELLING

Rich data have been generated through one-to-one in-depth interviews. Initially we invite the participant to tell their story in their own words. Further questions have been shaped by Stringer's (1999) application of PAR drawing out three central components; look, think and act. *Looking* means gathering information, defining and describing the situation. *Thinking* refers to exploring, analyzing, interpreting and explaining. Thinking is stimulated as participants ask "What is happening here?" and "Why are things as they are?" Finally, for the *action* component, participants are asked what is important to them in terms of living with a chronic illness and to consider ways they may be able to enact their desires. Not all questions have been asked in the same interview sitting; however, each conversation builds on the previous, as the look, think and act process is actualized. Feedback is provided before another

interview is commenced. Interviews are audio recorded, transcribed verbatim and analyzed using established analysis guidelines.

PAR GROUPS

There are a range of PAR methodologies and focus group approaches; however, we have used Stringer's (1999) work to guide our research practice. Stringer's PAR approach favors consensual and participatory procedures that enable the participants to set the agenda for discussion, to prioritize issues they wish to discuss and devise plans to deal with the problems at hand. Meetings have been held weekly or fortnightly, and up to ten meetings are held with a group of between six to twelve research participants that may last between two and three hours. The time of the meetings and the setting has been mutually agreed upon. Data analysis occurs systematically and collaboratively. Conversations are audio recorded with participant consent. In addition, a person with excellent speed and accurate typing skills processes the PAR group conversations verbatim. This has meant that we have immediate access to data for concurrent analysis. Ideas are extracted and discussed by the research team before the next PAR meeting. Analysis has followed pre-established guidelines. At the subsequent PAR meetings the findings from concurrent analysis is fed back to participants for reflection, discussion and validation before we move on. Hence our findings are shaped collaboratively.

PARTICIPATORY ACTION AND ELECTRONIC DATA GENERATION

The aim of the project in progress was to further unpack the evolving transition theory, but in a way that would enable access into the private space of a human being over a longer period of time. We wanted to avoid the "snapshot" of chronic illness experience that can be captured during face to face interviews or focus group conversations. The intention of the research was to "capture" the ways people who live with illness incorporate the symptoms and consequences into their daily lives, and we perceived this would be best achieved through regular, reflective contact over a period of time. Email seemed the answer because people could remain in the comfort of their homes, communicate at a time that suited them, discuss issues as they arose in their lives, and have the opportunity to communicate with others who were also learning to live well with illness.

Once approval for the study was obtained from a University Human Research Ethics Committee, consent was obtained from participants and we had conducted a pilot group, we convened an email discussion group for men and a group for women. The reason we separated the groups by gender was because our previous research had revealed that the experience of illness may be impacted upon by the social constructions of gender.

The research team (the three authors) are involved in communication exchange with participants for a period of 21 months, engaging in daily email conversations using mailing list software, thereby creating building blocks of text that, when analyzed, will further explicate the experience of incorporating a long term illness into daily life. We have developed a website that provides more detailed information about the background to the research (http://www.unisa.edu.au/nur/arc_project/).

THE ROLE OF THE FACILITATOR

In addition to "managing" group dynamics, facilitation of an online discussion group demands participation from the researcher. To keep a group progressing and discussion interesting, the facilitator must post messages to maintain a presence, but also to facilitate discussion that will generate data to meet the aims of the research. In this research we again use the process of "look, think and act" to facilitate collaborative inquiry from Stringer's (1999) participatory action. The facilitator's thoughtful response to the group is based on asking what is going on here (looking), reflecting before responding (think) and what can be said (act) that will further the discussion in exploring the nature of transition. This process promotes conversation beyond social chat and problem identification toward taking action in their lives. People want to make connections with others, and to participate in interesting and relevant discussion. A discussion list needs to be engaging to maintain participant interest, so an email from the researcher that furthers the conversations within the group is considered to be good hosting, facilitating and participation all at once. Garry wrote: "interesting as you are making me think and analyze my current situation."

The time taken to read and write email responses allows the opportunity for reflection of every contribution sent and received by both participants and researchers. One other advantage is that the research team has immediate access to research text rather than waiting for transcription.

What constitutes "good" facilitation has been the subject of discussions by the research team at a monthly meeting. The facilitator maintains a reflective journal of her experiences, and together with the research team examines dialogue data critically. In the effort to make the research process transparent we ask the question, what is going on whilst researching? (Koch 1998). In so doing the role of the facilitator is made obvious, and the team can discuss implications on the research findings.

TESTING THE ASSUMPTIONS

We have outlined three data generation strategies but we alert the reader that "doing" interpretive research is not an easy option. Our understanding is that researchers give accounts which are framed within a specific story telling tradition, often described as a paradigm. Paradigms are tentative philosophical structures for incorporating a package of beliefs about the nature of reality, the nature of knowledge and how one can conduct a research inquiry.

The paradigm that frames our research program is that research is an interactive process shaped by personal history, biography, gender, social class, race and ethnicity between all stakeholders including researchers and participants. As researchers we hold a position that incorporates our own prejudices, values and interests. Like Code (1991) who wrote, "knowledge is neither value-free nor value-neutral; the processes that produce it are themselves value-laden; and these values are open to evaluation." We bring this position to the research endeavor. These prejudices, values and interests cannot be bracketed out; rather they are articulated in the effort to make our position visible. We are constantly aware that interpretations may privilege any number of different positions and therefore scrutinize our research process in order to make our position apparent and to reveal the way in which our values are operating. We also test the assumptions underpinning most research practice and so in this inquiry we test the assumptions when pain is discussed. It should not be assumed that everyone appropriates the same meaning to the experience of pain.

WHAT CONSTITUTES A LEGITIMATE RESEARCH PRODUCT?

Researchers in interpretive traditions are often called journalists or soft scientists. Story telling work may be described as unscientific, full of bias or entirely personal. The writer's place (the fusion of researcher and researched) in the text is often challenged. Stories are criticized for not being generalizable. Writers of stories can be accused of making it up. There appears to be no agreed upon method for ensuring rigor. In the effort to satisfy demand for rigor within story-telling traditions, researchers in the 1980s struggled to apply criteria from quantitative research to qualitative work (Koch and Harrington 1998; Bailey 1999). During the late 1980s researchers adapted the parallel criteria *credibility*, *transferability* and *dependability* for assessing qualitative work based on the work by Lincoln and Guba (1985) and Koch (1994). These are just some of the possibilities for enhancing the rigor of the research product. Even during the 1990s much of the vast literature surrounding rigor was concerned with "rule governed approaches" (Healy 1996).

Our position at the time of writing is one that emphasizes reflexivity, which is when researchers turn a critical gaze towards themselves. Reflexivity is a challenging endeavor because it requires the researcher to identify and interrogate personal and professional practices (Finlay and

Gough 2003). There is an acknowledgment that interpretation exists in a complex matrix of alternative representations and "derives its critical power and insight from this awareness" (Marcus 1994). The focus is upon reflexive awareness of the historical connections that already link it to its subject matter; such representations become an integral part of fieldwork. We closely examine and record the way in which our own values are operating. Our awareness provides the context for our decision making and the mapping of the routes we take when engaged in the process of research. The research process we claim should be transparent, so that the reader can determine whether the text created is credible.

Credibility is enhanced when the text is multivoiced and multiple points of view are presented. Diversity and commonality are celebrated alongside each other. A story, when well told, resonates in a person's life. A good story asks us to pause, reflect and even change the way we understand. The most desirable outcome of our research is a new or better informed understanding. When we embark on sharing the findings of our research we strive to make our writing accessible to both parties: those who live with illness and pain and health workers. We start with enabling communication between people.

ENABLING COMMUNICATION BETWEEN PEOPLE

Learning to live with chronic pain can be facilitated by connecting with others, which is important for a sense of validation and affirmation (Steihaug et al. 2002). People in areas where groups are unavailable may go to great lengths to connect with others, by corresponding with groups on the internet or starting groups of their own.

In the email project, participants across metropolitan and rural Australia communicate on a regular basis, making connections, sharing and validating experiences. Joan wrote: "...the Internet is a wonderful resource if used for the right reasons, this group proves that." Heather commented:

illness is a very isolating and lonely affair. You can get very depressed thinking about all the things you can't do or go to and cancelled outings are even worse. You feel you are the only one whose is governed by health considerations. It really helps that there are people out there like this group who understand. Family members try to understand but only those whose lives are dictated by their health can really empathize.

How are emotions communicated online? During our everyday communications we create our identities accordingly and present what we want others to know about us and how we feel. Emotional cues and reactions are missing in an online situation but the use of emoticons provides an indication of how participants are feeling. The use of emoticons such as smiley faces or abbreviations such as lol (laughing out loud) have proved popular amongst participants for conveying the emotion and context surrounding their writings.

Many participants have spoken of previous face to face experiences where they have felt shunned by others, not believed, or have been judged. Often people with multiple and complex medical diagnoses (or their symptoms elude medical diagnosis) feel that they do not fit into a support group situation which has been defined by medical diagnosis (i.e., a group for people who have multiple sclerosis, diabetes or arthritis). Jemma wrote:

I find that joining online groups such as this that nobody knows you in person, you can be yourself. Nobody judges you because you are not the same as everyone else. The common ground here is chronic illness and I have found that those with chronic illness really understand what you are going through. Even my husband finds it difficult to understand. He does not seem to comprehend that I battle daily with pain all day and often during the night. Just because I don't complain about it constantly he thinks that for that moment I am fine. You don't feel so isolated as I have found that when I have joined groups in the real world (lol) that often there is somebody in the group who will tell you that she is worse than you are. I joined an arthritis group and they were all in gophers at the time. I didn't get mine until later. One girl told me how bad she was and then proceeded to ask what I was doing there when I didn't seem to limp or show any signs of arthritis!! I saw her later at [a shopping center] walking around without her gopher and I was in mine.

Many participants may not actually attend or communicate in a face to face group or interview but would participate in an online forum because no traveling is required, and if mobility, pain or continence are an issue, turning on the computer may seem an easier option. Cindy wrote:

I'm feeling really ill today and unable to go out. Sometimes I fear that I won't be able to do what I need to do, that I will be alone with this illness. Does anyone else have these fears?

Holly said:

I feel so comfortable with this group that it would be easy not to go out much and get all my socializing this way. I know that is the reality for some people...but I think it is important for me to try getting out when possible. My family are very happy that I receive such support from this group.

Creating research participation possibilities for people for whom mobility and/or pain are concerns is an issue. Through the use of email discussion groups, geographic location is no longer a problem. Reflective conversation is promoted rather than spontaneous conversation in a face to face group conversation. People can contribute in their own time and remain largely anonymous. Holly said, "...if I have a sleepless night with thoughts rushing around my head, I can send them in the middle of the night without disturbing anyone."

FINDINGS

This section reveals the findings of an ongoing study that investigated the experiences of 35 women and 17 men living with chronic illness. "Pain" data generated over 18 months have been isolated from interactive dialogue between participants and the facilitator. A storyline has developed as several themes have emerged:

- Daily life cannot be taken for granted
- Being silenced
- The consequences of communicating pain
- Failure of language to describe chronic pain experience
- Pain is the background noise
- Learning to live with chronic pain
- Understanding what is possible each day is part of learning
- What is important to people living with chronic pain?
- Self-care.

DAILY LIFE CANNOT BE TAKEN FOR GRANTED

Chronic pain destroys people's taken for granted assumptions about the world. "We who have pain on a daily basis have lost what others take for granted...the comfort and ease of a pain free body. I often try to remember how that felt." Ultimately pain introduces people to an unsettling world where time has stopped:

Since there is no treatment for me, I live very often, by the minute or even by the second. Every day must be taken one at a time, and even every hour.

The time before pain intervened in their lives can be almost inconceivable, or recedes in people's memory like a faded dream. For people with chronic pain, suffering becomes interspersed with enduring.

Apart from the [name of pain medication], which eased the pain a lot but gave me bad side effects, I have only been completely free of jaw pain once in the last twenty years or so. I was given an injection of pethidine for a very bad migraine. It did nothing for the migraine and made every nerve in my body twitch, but it took away the jaw pain for a while. I remember thinking this is how it should feel all the

time. Now I know what I'm missing. I do tend to think of my pain as separate from me. It seems to have a life of its own and almost rules my life. Whether I go out or do a particular task on any given day is determined by how much pain I have.

BEING SILENCED

Chronic pain is a place where, gradually, almost without noticing, people may find themselves alone. Chronic pain penetrates the sense of self, it lives deeply within people, often unseen to the outside world. "I live in silence... I can't keep 'whingeing' about it so I have to keep it to myself. Nobody wants to hear about my problems, do they?" The person living with chronic pain belongs to a world that no one else can entirely share or comprehend. "You can't begin to imagine what chronic pain is until you've experienced it yourself." People with chronic pain learn protective behaviors, one of which is to retreat into isolation.

I think that the worst part of living with pain is that it is very isolating – as others have said, there is little point in telling people about it, as they don't understand. In my case, I look forward to the day where my children are old enough to understand that chronic pain can put people in a "snappy" mood, and can't be explained to young children – I have tried, numerous times!

Dealing with the consequences of living with pain was described by Lois:

My family have no concept – my mother relates chronic pain to the ache that she gets in her hip when the weather changes...it lasts about a day for her, and doesn't require any pain relief. She doesn't understand when I say "No, I can't do that today – I'm too sore," so I usually come up with another excuse rather than get the "Humph" down the phone.

One person's pain was described as "screaming" and the consequences were withdrawing from others which led to isolation:

The screaming pain enforces a sort of isolation from others because they are not experiencing the pain and it is better to rest or "lay low."

THE CONSEQUENCES OF COMMUNICATING PAIN

We may better grasp the dilemmas confronting people with chronic pain – especially their sense of dislocation from others – if we consider the ways in which our culture teaches us to confront pain with silence.

People with chronic pain soon discover that their complaints often exhaust, frustrate and perhaps alienate family and friends and health workers: "I don't complain about my pain all the time but I do need sympathy when it is so bad I can't stand it anymore... I also think because mine is ongoing and I never get a let up I find it difficult to accept." Pain can encourage an inward focus that may make it difficult to nurture the needs or experiences of others. Gazes of suspicion from health workers can silence cries for help, particularly when in the absence of a biomedical explanation for the pain.

Chronic pain has a stigma attached to it because often the public can't see any outward signs that you are disabled. With most of the above it's inside me. There are flare ups when the disease is rampant then periods of a lull, then another flare up for no reason or perhaps overdoing something that day and regretting it. With the fibromyalgia, one of the symptoms is irritable bowel syndrome and when there is a flare up of this. Days of constant diarrhoea for no medical reason, or days of pain...

People may experience suspicion and judgment from health workers when their claims of pain are perceived to be exaggerated.

...there were the various doctors with different attitudes to deal with during this time. From the ones who regard anyone using opiate analgesics as a druggie, like the pain clinic registrar who forced me to stop taking Endone (10 mg tds) for months (which others at same clinic had put me on) by refusing to writing the script and sending me out the door (one of the worst weekends of my life, cramps, vomiting etc) to GPs and even a pharmacist who refused to fill a legally filled in prescription from my GP and confiscated it!

FAILURE OF LANGUAGE TO DESCRIBE CHRONIC PAIN EXPERIENCE

People often experience first hand the failure of words in the face of prolonged suffering with pain. When trying to describe pain to a doctor, their language runs dry as the experience of pain escapes articulation.

It is a vulnerable position to be in because the pain specialist kept looking at me to see if I would say the wrong thing and he would promptly say I was a druggie or whatever they are. I took the left over [medication] back to him in case he could give them to someone as a trial. I had to try and not look too pleased when he suggested I take this drug because it was stronger than any other medication I had been on. I was just glad to be given a chance to find a drug that would help the pain.

Some have found mutual language to communicate pain severity by using pain scales.

I have come across a pain scale written by someone and posted to the internet that I found helpful. I have always been asked what my pain levels are on scale 1 to 10 but nobody could define what the levels were except for vague responses. This scale goes from 0 = no pain to 5 = can be ignored for 30 minutes if busy, to 10 = totally non functional. This has helped me because I always undervalued my pain levels as I have been to 10 a number of times, and considered my normal levels at 3s. But in this scale I vary between 7 and 10 every day after I take pain killers.

However, indicating a pain level has not always been helpful:

When I am asked to give a level to my pain...this must be defined to the patient and not be a hairy fairy pluck a number from the air thing that it currently is. It needs a consistent scale used by all health people.

It is mostly acute pain that we learn about during our early lives and we can be unprepared for pain that becomes a constant companion.

Short-term pain is different to long term pain. Psychologically the loss of hope and the need to "just get on with life" is a big change. The problem is that just "getting on with life" is near impossible due to a lot of reasons, the main one being flare ups. But for me another major problem is continuing, worsening health which makes it impossible to guess what I can and can't do with much clarity.

PAIN IS THE BACKGROUND NOISE

Several participants confirm that pain is ever present.

Ever present pain becomes a background noise to your every moment of life. You can often lose conscious awareness of it during "good" times, but you never become fully unaware of it. You know it is there and it wears away at you reducing your ability to cope with normal life occurrences, and worse it makes the times when high level pain flares up even harder to cope with. It can become soul crushing leaving little space for you to exist. I am not talking about slight aches and pains but consistently high levels of pain that cannot be ignored for any length of time.

No one teaches us what to do with pain that never stops but only wavers in intensity.

Yes, pain is like a screaming banshee and pain management is a difficult technique because I believe it is somewhat different for each individual. I've never really known what to do about degrees of pain.

I have developed a fairly high tolerance to pain in my face, but not in other areas necessarily. It leads me on to say that GPs need to learn how to deal with pain management for patients, in particular those with chronic illnesses where the patient has so much to contend with every day.

Whilst those communicating pain are silenced in the effort not to be dismissed by those around them, the actual pain experienced is not silent, as it screamed:

I'm in the throes of a psoriatic arthritis flare and despite some days off work last week and only working some hours per day this week, the pain isn't silent and I wonder if I have gained a better understanding of why some people self mutilate...that piercing, burning, volcanic chaos could spew over into anything...the pain of a "flare" is so different from the chronic, daily pain which degrades and devalues...and it is so tiring balancing resisting the force of the volcano and the persisting of people.

Then I thought a bit more and decided that the every day pain of ordinary arthritis was a pain to put up with but the gut wrenching scream of the flareup was the silent one and an isolating one because, as others have said, it's the pain the outside world doesn't see often. We suffer in silence. We shut ourselves off from society. It's not a pretty sight.

LEARNING TO LIVE WITH CHRONIC PAIN

People learn nevertheless as the pain experience is forced upon them and desperation for relief of pain becomes a way of life.

And managing and coping skills and techniques are different for all of us, like medication. The trick is to find the one that does it for you. As I am about to try my third lot of pain inhibitors I am very aware of the sometimes experimental nature of managing problems. I am about to embark on a course of Baclofen. If it doesn't work there are more we can try.

Making sense of pain and the best way to deal with it occupies many moments of the day:

Pain every waking moment which medications often fail to help. Pain can often take a hold of you like a drug addiction you think, eat and sleep pain. Never going away. It tears away at your life, often destroying you if you let it. You can turn it around and try to do things that will help lessen the pain.

Entering a drug trial is more likely to be a decision born out of desperation:

I'm about to undertake another drug trial. The current one [second one we've tried] does absolutely nothing

for the pain. All it does is make me sleep better than I have for years. So I have to get off this one and try the next on the list. If it's like the previous two it will be a good month before I build up to the correct dose and another month before we can tell if it is "the one." Trying not to get frustrated and defeated. It's just that this has been going on for almost twelve months! When I consider that the pain has been with me in some form or other for over thirty years I get it all in perspective.

However, hope is always in the background:

I am hopeful that something else is around the corner failing that I just learn to live with the never ending pain especially in the lower back.

Pain appears to drain off that which gives the world vividness, color, coherence and value. The blankness of pain may be its most intrusive attribute.

I don't dwell on the pain, and use sedentary, mental activities as my "distraction"...but sometimes I'm just sick of being sick and not being able to really enjoy myself like a healthy person... I just wish I could sit and enjoy something without the bombardment of the pain...sit and enjoy a sunrise 100% (not 70% with the pain taking away 30% of the enjoyment). As you can see, I'm not asking to be able to climb Mt Everest, just to be able to SIT and enjoy something with no interruptions from the pain. Even for 10 seconds.

People may seek answers to the existential question of "why me?" to try to make sense of their changed body and the chaos that has intruded into their lives. Logic and understanding of life with pain can seem insurmountable but, for some, a process of moving through the pain experience occurs.

First off its the "why me?" stage. Life's not fair. A negative response, then depression. Then learning to accept that you can no longer live a pain free life. Learning to accept that you can no longer work. Learning to adapt and to realize your limitations on what you can do and can't do.

I do get upset about my pain and suffering, although as time goes by and I really come to accept it all, I am developing better coping skills.

Books and media resources can also be important for people seeking validation and knowledge from the experiences of others. Validation and affirmation from others can chip away at the sense of aloneness that often accompanies chronic pain as people enduring chronic pain can be reminded of their unique strengths and qualities.

My huge disappointment that there is no chronic pain community group or association where I can meet up with others, see a psychologist, etc. Why do they have cancer, heart, arthritis, etc., organizations…but nothing for those experiencing chronic pain?

Distraction from pain can be achieved at times when pain can be pushed into the background of conscious thought.

I try to read and I sit here at my computer, sometimes talk on the phone (although no-one wants to hear from me when I'm too miserable!) I also do some housework, which is surprisingly beneficial.

How do I distract my self from pain, by literally saying "I will not look at it now" and purposefully putting it to the back of my mind? This often takes some time, which finally resorts in my taking analgesics but I try very hard, mentally, to do as much as I can, to block what I don't like. I find that pain, no matter how severe or slight, never fully leaves but if I am able to control it, my life is enriched.

Finding other things to do may give temporary relief:

I find that sometimes doing something interesting helps me forget the pain but there are times when every part of my face, indeed my whole head, just hurts. On these really bad days nothing I can do makes it any easier and I just have to endure it. Hence my willingness to undergo all this trying of pain-inhibitors.

On a fairly good day I forget about the pain if I can keep occupied. I find even physical tasks like housework help with this. I also try to keep my brain active. On those days when the pain is really bad it "shouts" through every distraction and sleep is the only way to blot it out [if I can manage to sleep].

The good days with lessened pain are often treated with suspicion, as the person knows that bad days will follow. Often there is judgment about the value of the activity. Sometimes it is perceived to be "worth it" to push the boundaries of chronic pain.

I agree about the pain being worth it if you have achieved something in the process. I also think it is better to live a little, even if it costs me a day or two in bed. Boredom is a real hazard and can make me feel much worse. I also try to keep the memory of the really bad spell when I did virtually nothing except sleep and cry. I know whatever I am going thru is nothing compared to that episode and I never want to be there again or submit the family to that ordeal.

UNDERSTANDING WHAT IS POSSIBLE EACH DAY IS PART OF LEARNING

The unpredictability of pain brings with it the constant companion of uncertainty: "…each day is different, yet after a while they're 'all the same'…muddled together."

I always know its not going to last so I make the best of the good days when they appear. And yes, on a good day I can move mountains (lol) even if the pain is still there. I do feel a lot of it is psychological that is to say that if we are happy and in a positive frame of mind that our pain doesn't seem so bad but it is often hard to keep this way of thinking when you are in constant chronic pain. Then boom we are feeling flat and then the pain rears its ugly head again. But then again some days I feel positive etc. and the pain is so high I wonder if I can go on. So it's not to say that we don't have pain just that if we can manage our pain better and try and nurture it, we can keep it at bay.

Pain confiscates the opportunity to make choices in daily life. Recognizing choice is important for feeling a sense of control over the chaos that pain creates in life.

One can always learn more and I still can get caught out with wanting the quick fix solution or become tired and fatigued and lose sight of what choices I have to make things better for myself.

Life becomes characterized by trial and error and a process of learning the boundaries created by chronic pain. Patterns of daily living are created that incorporate pain as people make peace with uncertainty, incorporate self-monitoring into their lives, develop validating relationships with others and find voice to advocate for themselves.

After a couple of years then it's "why not me?" This continuous pain you would not wish on someone else. You begin to learn to live with the pain and the best way to do this is to pace yourself in what you do during the day. Never again doing general housework in one day. Each day has a different job or a couple of jobs depending on the pain level.

One participant described that living with constant pain meant dealing with children, so that they can come to terms with their mother not being able to do the things she used to do with them. Shifts in parenting may be one significant consequence of a life with chronic pain, but the consequences also spread further to impact on others. "My husband now does the vacuuming and heavy chores. I do the dusting, dishes and he helps." It also meant that the husband has to come to terms with his wife not being able to participate sexually if she is in constant pain. "This can be overcome if both parties work through it. We found it better for us in the morning where my pain would be through the roof by night. We worked at what was best for my pain."

The experience of ever-present pain can spiral and entwine with other symptoms, particularly fatigue. When chronic pain and fatigue become entwined powerlessness and depression may be close behind.

> I've been thinking about how fatigue and pain go together. If I am in pain of any sort I also feel fatigued and the worse the pain the more fatigue I experience. I have also noticed how introverted I become when I am in pain. At my worst I am so focused on my pain that I can hardly think about anything else. Hence my wish to get some pain relief and my willingness to struggle through all these drugs in the hope of getting one which gives me some relief without unacceptable side effects.

There was some agreement as participants conversed that fatigue and pain are intimately tied together:

> Yes pain and fatigue do go together. I was first introduced to this idea by an occupational therapist at the MS society. It's a bit like the chicken and the egg...they are so closely related. I find when I do too much and get fatigued my pain increases. Similarly to you I find a day of bad pain leaves me feeling fatigued. These days I find myself making a conscious attempt to avoid fatigue and the suffering that comes with it. I can also relate to the withdrawing that comes with pain. . . . but I reckon when I allow myself to focus inward I feel worse. It's like the pain takes over. It works better for me to distract myself even if it's a struggle in the beginning. I usually force myself to do something I find pleasurable or go out and interact at some level. But each person's pain is unique, as is the challenge of dealing with it.

Reflecting on past pain experiences can pave a smoother way for people learning strategies for self-care that may be tried in the future.

> Journaling is an incredible way of finding ourselves in the life we are leading, reading them back, gives us insights into our actions and thoughts, we may remember the confusion of the time and find the stream that brought us out of that place, leaving a trail we may use again if we ever return to on a visit.

WHAT IS IMPORTANT TO PEOPLE LIVING WITH CHRONIC PAIN?

It is common that people want their experiences of pain to be acknowledged:

> I'd like to be given respect by health professionals, family and friends. I'd like doctors to be educated as to what it really is like living with constant, chronic pain. There are those of us who are genuine and in constant pain and we need to be regarded with respect because appointments take a lot out of us getting to and from and because of this how pain levels are pretty high and we can't take much more of this attitude.

What is important to people living with chronic pain? Understanding and support from health workers and others are central for facilitating effective self-care. Recognition and acknowledgment of "just how hard it is" to live with ever present pain. People with chronic pain desire health workers to go further than simply to focus on the symptoms and progression of disease, but also to incorporate the impact of the illness and the meaning within the person's life. Respect for the context of the person becomes central to the relationship between health worker and client.

> Being treated with respect by medical professionals. Being treated as an equal in decision making about my treatment. Being shown consideration for my limitations without being fussed over by family and friends.

Moral codes or judgmental attitudes imposed by health workers were not received as helpful:

> we are not just slack, or lazy, or wimps who expect everyone to do things for them, but people in a difficult situation trying to make the best of their lives, to be as productive as they can be and to have the physical ability to maintain social relationships and whatever else is entailed in feeling some self-worth. Can remember once dragging myself around the supermarket, leaning on the trolley to support myself, drenched in sweat from the pain and seeing a GP who had just refused to give me a script because she thought it "inappropriate at my age, etc., to be taking such strong meds" (codral forte at the time) flitting about from one aisle to the next in her lunch-hour and thinking, "if you could just feel that I'm experiencing for five minutes, you'd soon change your tune."

> Excuse me if I lack focus in appointments but sometimes it's impossible to concentrate. The fact that we may ask questions – be patient and give us answers if you can. It's our future, after all. We have a right to our own opinions. You tell us to exercise. Fine but I won't do it if I can't. Maybe you should delve deeper as to WHY I can't.

> I'm now on regular medication which has given me my life back. I can do so much more than I used to, have a great pain specialist whom I only need to see if the

dose needs increasing, which it hasn't in over five years, and a great GP who writes my scripts and with whom I can talk about anything.

SELF-CARE

People have come to understand what is needed for self-care. Recovering a valued life is important and becomes a focus.

I have found that I need to set myself goals to be accomplished, as I am able. Any task is broken into small bight size chunks that I can hopefully complete within a reasonable space of time. I do not set time limits on completion. Having these goals gives me some purpose to living, and this is necessary. Personally I am too stubborn to roll over and stare at the walls all day so I must keep active, albeit physically or mentally, doing or planning. I now consider having rests or sleeps during the day as an activity with a purpose. I realize this may sound odd but if I do not rest/sleep then I become non functional later in the day.

Acknowledgment that self-care is a process that fluctuates and shifts over time is important.

Pain killers, or any medication, has always been a last resort for me. Even now I try to put off taking pain meds until absolutely necessary. My datum for necessary is much different now to what it was 20 years ago, now if I cannot move without severe impairment to function I say "necessary."

Every movement must be controlled or I can suffer. I have to take care not to bump against anything as even the slightest touch can be painful, like typing at this keyboard. Reflex actions have to be avoided. I have days when clothing on my body is painful, ok in summer but winter gets hard. This control requires a lot of concentration and another reason for rests and sleeps during the day.

What do people want health workers to know about what it is like to live on a long-term basis with chronic pain? One participant said "if only some of the medical professions would realize what they put us through."

On one return to the clinic I saw a new registrar and he asked me about the exercises, so I showed him. He said sit down, you obviously haven't been doing them! He then wrote out my endone script but did not get a telephone approval for the authority script. I pointed out that the pharmacy could not fill it without the authority number. He refused to budge. His whole attitude seemed to be that I was a fat white female who wasn't prepared to help herself so he wasn't

going to help. Of course when I took the script to the chemist he couldn't fill it, which left me withdrawing from 60mg endone tds cold turkey. Needless to say I never went back to that pain clinic. Should have made a formal complaint, but was too sick to do so.

Further advice to health workers:

Never give "off pat" responses. If there is little that can be done, say so. Too often I have been told that 90% of people get better. I have been too often within that 10%, and when that 10% occurs multiple times health workers lose credibility. Another example is the "rest and exercise" and most people recover. In my case, and others with similar, cannot do much positive exercise and treatment is really trial and error by the patient.

Listen to what we say and respect our expertise. When the patient says "I am trying this or that" listen, and don't wave off these as they won't work. When you live with pain long enough you have to test alternative methods to the mainstream medical methods. Sometimes they work, and I do not refer to quack cures, but every day things like vitamin and mineral supplements.

It is important that health workers reaffirm their support:

I asked my doctor to be there for me and ready to see me, hear me at my most vulnerable negative down times. To check in on my safety and to give me information and things to check out. I was choosing him and not my family and friends, because they can't get it when they think I look so well, and am being me. They also get exhausted by it and we have other things to do together.

There has been an emerging tolerance and acceptance of alternative or complementary therapies. Acupuncture, Reiki, relaxation training, visualization and aromatherapy have received increasing attention.

I have looked to many different alternative therapies for ms. I reckon the most important part for me is that it usually gives me a feeling of taking some control over my health. The medical system often leaves me feeling as if I have no control in management of my health. That sense of doing something for my health rather than being done to is important in my wellbeing. Another thought I have about alternative healing is that I believe really it should not be considered alternative but mainstream, and accessible to all of us and I think "alternative" healing/therapies tap into each individual's power to heal which I think orthodox medicine tends to separate and alienate us from. "They" have taken away or at least not encouraged and supported our own innate ability to heal ourselves in relationship with others, and instead bottled it up, and sold it back to us.

DISCUSSION

The quest for this chapter was to deepen our understanding of living with long-term pain and to answer the question, what could health workers do better to understand the ways people self-care when enduring chronic pain?

UNDERSTANDING

The understandings that have been brought forward from the perspective of the person living with chronic pain build on work of previous authors (Carson and Mitchell 1998; Thomas 2000; Dudgeon et al. 2002; Ohmen et al. 2003). It was found that pain adversely affected many dimensions of people's lives. The adverse effect pain has on family and friends became evident, exemplifying that the experience of pain affects not only that person but also a much wider circle of people. For people living with chronic pain a consequence of not wishing to burden others with "whingeing" about pain can lead to a feeling of being silenced and socially isolated. Some people are less isolated if they live in supportive relationships (Koch et al. 2002a). Smith (2003) supported our finding that supportive relationships are important. Exploring family relationships and intimacy of women experiencing chronic pain from the perspective of women and their family members, Smith (2003) concluded that chronic pain affects important basic relationships and both emotional and physical intimacy.

The way in which pain affected many dimensions of a participant's life and emphasized the complex and multidimensional nature of pain, pain became a plural phenomenon as it included everything that was associated with pain. Pain was rarely a single experience and often episodes of pain were not alike. It further supported findings that looking for a cause, getting information, being believed and getting the pain legitimated are all vital factors for people with chronic pain. Personal and social meanings of chronic pain include how it may disrupt an individual's past history, anticipated life course, family and community, and a sense of self and identity (Koch et al. 2002a; King and Cathers 2003; Ohmen et al. 2003; Smith 2003). Pain can be in the present, emerging from the past or anticipated with dread in the future. Each assault of pain is a threat to a sense of self.

Carson and Mitchell (1998) explored with 17 people the experience of living with persistent pain and described three themes arising from their analysis: forbearance surfaces with the drain of persistent anguish; isolating retreats coexist with comforting engagements;

and hope for relief clarifies priorities for daily living. Their conclusion could well be ours, as they also challenge health workers to begin focusing on the person who lives with pain as the messenger of how to endure.

Finding a language to describe pain was discussed by participants. Screaming pain was a term not previously heard but resonated with many as a descriptor of their agony. Likewise, Thomas (2000) undertook a study, where 13 people with chronic pain described their lived experiences, described pain as an unremitting torment by a force or monster that cannot be tamed. A study by De Souza and Frank (2000) explored subjective pain experience of people with chronic back pain. Language used was a descriptor of the quality of their pain. Interestingly the use of simile was common to emphasize both what the pain was, and what it was not. A loss of words in trying to describe pain was evident. Authors were keen to point out that whilst these people provided graphic and in-depth descriptions of their pain experience, these bore little resemblance to commonly used assessment tools. In other words, the appropriateness of existing pain measuring instruments was challenged.

Whilst we have privileged the perspective of those living with pain, gaining the insider's view is an increasingly legitimate way to proceed with research. A good example is the work undertaken by Dudgeon et al. (2002). These authors obtained the insider's view about disability-related pain. Participants described pain as a part of daily living that influenced many lifestyle decisions. They characterized pain as plural, meaning that it has multiple locations, distinctive descriptions and different implications. They also were concerned about pain being a mystery, having unclear causes and consequences. Typically they described pain as a personal venture, with little or dissatisfying communication about pain with family, friends or healthcare providers.

WHAT CAN HEALTH PROFESSIONALS DO?

On a day-to-day basis the person living with pain is in charge of his or her own health. Of course healthcare professionals are important but it is estimated that between 95 and 99% of chronic illness care is given by the person who has the illness (Kralik and Koch 2004). Nevertheless, it is important to communicate to health professionals what people living with pain want. Building on this observation, our research with participants living with chronic illness shows that conversational threads have emerged about the way in which people live with pain and how they consider their conversations about pain are listened to or heard by health professionals.

Healthcare professionals can offer people living with pain much in helping them come to terms with the way in which pain has affected both themselves and their lives. It is understood that healthcare professionals and family members may question the authenticity of participants' pain. Participants sometimes felt they had to "prove" their pain, and were undermined by doubt over whether or not their pain was "real." If health professionals transmitted this doubt to a partner or spouse, then this can have inevitable stigmatizing consequences. Lillrank (2003) in a study about back pain and the resolution of diagnostic uncertainty considered 30 Finnish women's written narratives about the process of having back pain diagnosed. The women's common story was the stigmatizing experience when doctors did not take pain seriously. Instead, doctors' neglectful attitudes became part of the prolonged problem. As for our participants, to be taken seriously as a person was considered to be the greatest relief.

People with chronic pain have reported feeling not heard. Our findings have been revealed in the work of others (Seers and Friedli 1996; Paulson et al. 2001; Carter 2002; Dewar and White 2003). Having others believe the pain is real was crucial to many participants. Carter (2002) explored the experience of chronic pain in childhood. Children and families experienced numerous encounters with health professionals during their "quest for a diagnosis" for chronic pain. During these clinical encounters families reported feeling judged, disbelieved and labeled as difficult. The families described situations in which their accounts of pain were reinterpreted through a variety of professional lenses, and the children felt that their voices were muted or ignored.

When those living with pain are not "heard" the consequence may be that people are prevented from dealing with the situation. This notion was found by Henriksson (1995) who gained an understanding of the person's perspective of living with chronic pain and noted that the women (40 people with fibromyalgia) felt rejected, misunderstood and disbelieved. The relief participants felt when they could talk about their pain to someone who was interested is highlighted in our findings and current literature. The need to be heard and believed is a common finding.

As for our participants, using metaphorical expressions to make the pain visible was recorded by Paulson et al. (2001) who researched with men's descriptions of their experience of fibromyalgia-type pain. Once more the request by these authors was to listen intently to each man's narrative and learn to interpret the descriptions of their experience of long-term pain. This request was viewed as essential for the health professionals when offering support and relief to men with pain. Care and treatment provided by staff should be based on people's needs rather than on health professional's attitudes and preferences (Blomqvist and Edberg 2002).

People have difficulty quantifying pain intensity and articulating or describing pain (De Souza and Frank 2000) and therefore seek greater validation of their

lived experience of chronic pain. Talking to people with pain about what their pain means to them would seem crucial in helping them come to terms with their pain, and improve their quality of life despite the pain. This is the challenge for healthcare professionals.

SELF-CARE

Participants were keen to talk about ways they could self-care. Activity surrounding self-care was proudly conveyed. In other words, finding even temporary relief of pain was a reward and easily shared among the group. Many activities were suggested and there is a copious literature to support these self-help strategies. This is not to undermine their value, but rather show that the person themselves is central in making decisions about self-care. We have termed taking control for decisions as self-agency (Koch et al. 2004). One of the papers supporting self-care was Taylor's (2001) study with participants living with arthritis and pain. As with our participants, self-care was conveyed as the ways people enabled capacity and participation in their daily lives. People described many self-care activities including how they managed mornings, did housework, cooked meals, exercised, acknowledged feelings, minimized pain and dealt with depression. This was quite a list; however, what was important was that self-care had meaning within the context of people's lives rather than prescriptive treatment offered by health workers.

Life with a chronic condition such as pain certainly cannot be taken for granted; every move needs to be planned (Kralik et al. 2004). Bullington and Nordemar (2003) shared our understanding of self-care. Seeking order out of chaos was the main metaphor used in their study to describe the path from the seeking of medical help to successful rehabilitation. Interestingly, the role of flexibility and creativity in the healing process was vital toward rehabilitation. However, the kind of clinical encounter conducive for the journey from chaos to the creation of new meaning was paramount. Oftentimes the person living with pain "self-cares," nevertheless the quality of the clinical encounter should not be underestimated.

There is a need for further study on healthcare professional–participant communication in terms of quality clinical encounters. Dewar and White (2003) supported our participants' experiences of having difficulty finding accessible, effective and acceptable care. Many participants perceived their family physician or other healthcare providers as not adequately meeting their healthcare needs.

Ways in which health professionals may be able to assist people who live with pain are to listen attentively and work closely with them to build capacity. Instead of identifying problems, let us work with people's strengths. Our study in progress describing transition aims to describe not only what is involved in moving on with life despite one's condition, but also ways in which we, as healthcare professionals, can assist in this transitional process. It may be relevant to explore with our participants their protective behaviors. Interestingly the work of King and Cathers (2003) described protective processes in the lives of people with chronic disabilities. The major protective factors were social support, traits such as perseverance and determination, and spiritual beliefs. These findings echo our transition thesis. Authors identified three new protective processes: replacing a loss with a gain (transcending), recognizing new things about oneself (self-understanding) and making decisions about relinquishing something in life (accommodating). We concord with these authors that ways in which people draw sense and meaning in life have important implications for service delivery.

REFLECTIONS

Paterson (2003) highlighted some of the difficulties and limitations encountered when researchers attempt to define the experience of living with chronic illness through the lens of a single perspective. As discussed, a particular way of thinking has informed how we have undertaken this study. In this way of thinking we position a person who speaks or writes of pain as a conscious being. When attempts are made to understand pain as a human event or experience, it is through language that this event/experience may be transformed into meaning. It has been important to explore the way in which people "make sense" of pain.

It has been proposed that pain is an experience in search of interpretation and/or diagnosis. The question "what or why do I have this pain?" is most likely to be the reason people visit health professionals. We have heard that making sense of pain and the best way to deal with it occupies many moments of the day. Let us follow this through from a person experiencing pain and who seeks an interpretation of the event from health professionals. Most likely the health worker operates within a scientific-medical way of thinking or, as some say, the biomedical model; the search for discovery will often follow a clinical decision-making path informed by knowledge gained through science. When the person presents, a cause will be attempted to be identified (measurements may be sought) so that a diagnosis can be made. What will then generally follow is a treatment plan that can also measure the outcomes or judge if a cure has or has not been found. Health workers may hold beliefs regarding the clinical characteristics of people with chronic pain, and those they consider to be "good" to treat, whilst they challenge people who were "difficult" to treat (Daykin and Richardson 2004). Further, biomedical-oriented pain beliefs may influence the clinical reasoning processes of health workers including the explanations they give to the people (Daykin and Richardson 2004).

People have expressed concern about chronic pain being a mystery, having unclear causes and consequences (Dudgeon et al. 2002), and seek to determine the cause of the pain so as to bring about cure. This way of thinking about interpreting/diagnosing pain can lead to difficulties if health professionals can find no cause or cure. How can this pain be given meaning (or be believed) if it has no cause? Does this become a meaningless pain? Does pain become meaningless in terms of the limits placed on an individual to know pain or in ways of knowing how to give pain meaning?

The search for meaning then becomes the journey. This journey is likely to be undertaken by researchers and those living with pain. Livingston (1998, p. 1) wrote:

Everyone knows or thinks he [sic] knows what the word "pain" means, yet authorities have never been able to agree on how to define it... The main obstacle to such investigations is that pain is neither objective nor any single entity. Many different kinds of pain arise in both normal and abnormal states of mind and body. Each pain represents a unique, subjective sensory experience that can be described only by the conscious human being who is experiencing it.

If we cannot agree what constitutes pain, what are we to do? Madjar (1998) argued that pain needs a voice and that this must be the voice of the person who is experiencing pain. Madjar (1998, p. 40) wrote "because bodily pain resists objectification in language, this contributes to its unsharebility." In other words, pain actively destroys language; in order to gain control over pain it is necessary to give it voice so that its verbal expression serves as a prelude to the shared project of reducing pain. However, if pain is an experience in search of interpretation then this search may not only be that of the person experiencing pain but of researchers and clinicians as well. If pain means different things to different people, it is also important for researchers to appreciate how their own values and meanings may influence the ways in which they generate data.

The following quote by Hooks (1990, pp. 151–2) challenges researchers who utilize interviews as a way of seeking people to talk about pain, to think about how they give authority to the person who speaks:

No need to hear your voice when I can talk about you better than you can speak about yourself. No need to hear your voice. Only tell me about your pain. I want to know your story. And then I will tell it back to you in a new way. Tell it back to you in such a way that it has become mine, my own... I am still the author, authority.

If pain means different things to different people, it is critical to our role as researchers to ensure that what we write does not frame the lives of participants and what they talk about, only within the definitions of chronic pain that have been offered by the biomedical paradigm. We have attempted to make our work transparent through creating a multi voiced text. Numerous voices, using fictional names, are represented in the storied accounts. We have privileged the voices of people that live with chronic pain.

We may have dealt with Hook's criticism that the researcher's voice should not override the participant's voice; however, we need to reexamine how an event termed pain is framed or how it is given meaning by us. Why is it that pain can be categorized as chronic? Is this a product of a scientific-medical way of thinking about pain as actual or potential tissue damage? In saying this we are not discounting this way of thinking; however, our point is that if pain means different things to different people, then researchers need to challenge the perspective and the way that chronic pain is talked about. How chronic pain as an event is made visible through research so that all persons involved in the research are referring to the same event cannot be taken for granted.

We contend that it is important for researchers to appreciate and explore how framing of chronic pain can discipline the actions of researchers and participants and that through research findings actions and perceptions may be reshaped.

CONCLUSION

Qualitative research approaches have enabled contextual understandings to emerge about what life is like when living with chronic pain. Chronic pain destroys assumptions that people take for granted: "every day must be taken one at a time, and even every hour." Pain becomes a constant companion. Pain becomes the background noise in daily life. Whilst those communicating pain are silenced in the effort not to be dismissed by those around them, the actual pain experienced is not silent, it often "screams." Pain drains everything that gives the world vividness, color, coherence and value. The experience of ever-present pain can spiral into other symptoms such as fatigue and depression.

Being silenced is experienced because "nobody wants to hear about my problems" and means the person living with pain is often isolated. Not complaining is adaptive and protective behavior as people with chronic pain discover that "whingeing" often exhausts, frustrates and perhaps alienates family, friends and health workers. People may experience suspicion and judgment from health workers when their claims of pain are perceived to be exaggerated. When trying to describe pain to a health professional, language runs dry as the experience of pain escapes articulation. Some have found mutual language to communicate pain severity by using pain scales.

Nevertheless people learn as the pain experience is forced upon them and desperation for relief of pain becomes a way of life. Making sense of pain and the best way to deal with it occupies many moments of the day. Distraction from pain can be achieved at times when pain can be pushed into the background of conscious thought. Patterns of daily living are created that incorporate pain as people make peace with uncertainty, incorporate self-monitoring into their lives, develop validating relationships with others and find voice to advocate for themselves.

People want their experiences of pain to be acknowledged. They want recognition and acknowledgment of "just how hard it is" to live with ever-present pain. Validation and affirmation from others can chip away at the sense of aloneness that often accompanies chronic pain as people enduring chronic pain can be reminded of their unique strengths and qualities. Understanding and support from health workers and others are central for facilitating effective self-care of persistent pain.

REFERENCES

Aranda S. From individual to groups: use of narratives in a participatory research process. J Adv Nurs 2001; 33(6):791–797.

Augello JDB. Workers with Chronic Pain: Recovery and Reintegration. University of Utah, Salt Lake City, 2002:170.

Bailey L. Refracted selves? A study of changes in self-identity in the transition to motherhood. Sociology 1999; 33(2):335–352.

Bates MS, Rankin-Hill L. Control, culture and chronic pain. Soc Sci Med 1994; 39(5):629–645.

Bates MS, Rankin-Hill L, Sanchez-Ayendez M. The effects of the cultural context of health care on treatment of and response to chronic pain and illness. Soc Sci Med 1997; 45(9):1433–1447.

Blomqvist K. Older people in persistent pain: nursing and paramedical staff perceptions and pain management. J Adv Nurs 2003; 41(6):575–584.

Blomqvist K, Edberg A. Living with persistent pain: experiences of older people receiving home care. J Adv Nurs 2002; 40(3):297–306.

Bowman JM. Reactions to chronic low back pain. Issues Mental Health Nurs 1994; 15(4):445–453.

Bullington J, Nordemar R. Meaning out of chaos: a way to understand chronic pain. Scand J of Caring Sci 2003; 17(4):325–331.

Cantanzaro M. Transitions in midlife adults with long-term illness. Holistic Nurse Practitioner 1990; 4(3):65–73.

Carson MG, Mitchell GJ. The experience of living with persistent pain. J Adv Nurs 1998; 28(6):1242–1248.

Carter B. Chronic pain in childhood and the medical encounter: professional ventriloquism and hidden voices. Qualitative Health Res 2002; 12(1):28–41.

Carter B, Lambrenos K, Thursfield J. A pain workshop: an approach to eliciting the views of young people with chronic pain. J Clin Nurs 2002; 11(6):753–762.

Chick N, Meleis AI. Transitions: a nursing concern. In: Chinn PL (ed). Nursing Research Methodology: Issues and Implementation, Aspen, Rockville, MD, 1986:237–257.

Code L. What Can She Know? Feminist Theory and the Construction of Knowledge. Cornell University Press, Ithaca, NY, 1991.

Cook FM, Hassenkamp A. Active rehabilitation for chronic low back pain: the patient's perspective. Physiotherapy 2000; 86(2):61–68.

Culver MD, Kell MJ. Assessment. Working with chronic pain patients: spirituality as part of the treatment protocol. Am J Pain Manage 1995; 5(2):55–61.

Davis GC, Hiemenz ML, White TL. Barriers to managing chronic pain of older adults with arthritis. J Nurs Scholarship 2002; 34(2):121–126.

Daykin AR, Richardson B. Physiotherapists' pain beliefs and their influence on the management of patients with chronic low back pain. Spine 2004; 29(7):783–795.

De Souza LH, Frank AO. Subjective pain experience of people with chronic back pain. Physiother Res Int 2000; 5(4):207–219.

Dewar A, White M. Using nominal group technique to assess chronic pain, patients' perceived challenges and needs in a community health region. Health Expect 2003; 6(1):44–52.

Dickson GL, Kim JI. Reconstructing a meaning of pain: older Korean American women's experiences with the pain of osteoarthritis. Qualitative Health Res 2003; 13(5):675–688.

Dudgeon BJ, Gerrard BC, Jensen MP, et al. Physical disability and the experience of chronic pain. Arch Phys Med Rehabil 2002; 83(2):229–235.

Eastwood S, Kralik D, Koch T. Compromising and containing: self-management strategies used by men and women who live with multiple sclerosis and urinary incontinence. Australian J Holistic Nurs 2002; 9(1):33–43.

Finlay L, Gough B. Reflexivity: A Practical Guide for Researchers in Health and Social Sciences. Blackwell, Oxford, 2003.

Grace VM. Problems women patients experience in the medical encounter for chronic pelvic pain: a New Zealand study. Health Care Women Int 1995; 16(6):509–519.

Hallberg LR, Carlsson SG. Psychosocial vulnerability and maintaining forces related to fibromyalgia: in-depth interviews with twenty-two female patients. Scand J Caring Sci 1998; 12(2):95–103.

Hallberg LR, Carlsson SG. Coping with fibromyalgia: a qualitative study. Scand J Caring Sci 2000; 14(1):29–36.

Healy P. Situated rationality and hermeneutic understanding: a Gadamerian approach to rationality. Int Philos Quart 1996; 2:142.

Hellstrom C. Affecting the future: chronic pain and perceived agency in a clinical setting. Time and Society 2001; 10(1):77–92.

Henriksson CM. Living with continuous muscular pain: patient perspectives: II. Strategies for daily life. Scand J Caring Sci 1995; 9(2):7–86.

Hooks B. Yearning: Race, Gender and Cultural Politics. South End, Boston, MA, 1990.

Howden S, Jones D, Martin D, et al. Employment and chronic non-cancer pain: insights into work retention and loss. Work 2003; 20(3):199–204.

Kelley P, Clifford P. Coping with chronic pain: assessing narrative approaches. Social Work 1997; 42(3):266–277.

King G, Cathers T. Turning points and protective processes in the lives of people with chronic disabilities. Qualitative Health Res 2003; 13(2):184–206.

Koch T. Establishing rigour in qualitative research: the decision trail. J Adv Nurs 1994; 19:976–986.

Koch T. Story telling: is it really research? J Adv Nurs 1998; 28(6):1182–1190.

Koch T, Harrington A. Reconceptualizing rigour: the case for reflexivity. J Adv Nurs 1998; 28(4):882–890.

Koch T, Kelly S. Identifying strategies for managing urinary incontinence with women who have multiple sclerosis. J Clin Nurs 1999a; 8:550–559.

Koch T, Kelly S. Understanding what is important for women who live with multiple sclerosis. Australian J Holistic Nurs 1999b; 6(1):14–24.

Koch T, Kralik D. Chronic illness: reflections on a community-based action research programme. J Adv Nurs 2001; 36(1):23–31.

Koch T, Kralik D, Sonnack D. Women living with type two diabetes: the intrusion of illness. J Clin Nurs 1999; 8(6):712–722.

Koch T, Kralik D, Kelly S. We just don't talk about it: men living with urinary incontinence and multiple sclerosis. Int J Nurs Pract 2000a; 6:253–260.

Koch T, Kralik D, Taylor J. Men living with diabetes: minimising the intrusiveness of the disease. J Clin Nurs 2000b; 9:247–254.

Koch T, Kralik D, Eastwood S, et al. Breaking the silence: women living with multiple sclerosis and urinary incontinence. Int J Nurs Pract 2001; 7:16–23.

Koch T, Kralik D, Eastwood S. Constructions of sexuality for women living with multiple sclerosis. J Adv Nurs 2002a; 39(2):137–145.

Koch T, Selim P, Kralik D. Enhancing lives through the development of a community-based participatory action research programme. J Clin Nurs 2002b; 11:109–117.

Koch T, Jenkin P, Kralik D. Chronic illness self-management: locating the "self." J Adv Nurs 2004; 48(5):484–492.

Kodiath MF, Kodiath A. A comparative study of patients with chronic pain in India and the United States. Clin Nurs Res 1992; 1(3):278–291.

Kodiath MF, Kodiath A. A comparative study of patients who experience chronic malignant pain in India and the United States. Cancer Nursing 1995; 18(3):189–196.

Kralik D. The quest for Ordinariness; midlife women living through chronic illness. School of Nursing, Faculty of Health Sciences, Flinders University of South Australia, Adelaide, 2000:489.

Kralik D. The quest for ordinariness: transition experienced by midlife women living with chronic illness. J Adv Nurs 2002; 39(2):146–154.

Kralik D, Koch T. What do people with chronic illness want from district nurses? Pursuit of Excellence 2004:28.

Kralik D, Brown M, Koch T. Women's experiences of "being diagnosed" with a long-term illness. J Adv Nurs 2001a; 33(5):594–602.

Kralik D, Koch T, Telford K. Constructions of sexuality for midlife women living with chronic illness. J Adv Nurs 2001b; 35(2):180–187.

Kralik D, Koch T, Webb C. The domination of chronic illness research by biomedical interests. Australian J Holistic Nurs 2001c; 8(2):4–12.

Kralik D, Koch T, Price K, et al. Chronic illness self-management: taking action to create order. J Clin Nurs 2004; 13(2):259–267.

Lansbury G. Chronic pain management: a qualitative study of elderly people's preferred coping strategies and barriers to management. Disabil Rehabil 2000; 22(1/2):2–14.

Lillrank A. Back pain and the resolution of diagnostic uncertainty in illness narratives. Social Science Med 2003; 57(6):1045–1054.

Lincoln YM, Guba E. Naturalistic Inquiry. Sage Publications, California, 1985.

Livingston WK. Pain and Suffering. IASP Press, Seattle, WA, 1998.

Loeser JD. The future: will pain be abolished or just pain management specialists? Pain Clin Updates 2002; 8(6):1–4.

Loveys B. Transitions in chronic illness: the at-risk role. Holistic Nurs Pract 1990; 4:45–64.

Madjar I. Giving Comfort and Inflicting Pain. Qual Institute Press, Edmonton, 1998.

Marcus GE. What comes (just) after "post"? The case of ethnography. In: Denzin N, Lincoln Y (eds). Handbook of Qualitative Research. Sage Publications, London, 1994:563–574.

Martin JA. The Meaning of Chronic Low Back Pain: A Phenomenological Study. University of Alabama at Birmingham, 1989: DSN 111.

McHugh G, Thoms G. Patient satisfaction with chronic pain management. Nurs Stand 2001; 15(51):33–38.

Meleis AI, Trangenstein PA. Facilitating transitions: redefinition of the nursing mission. Nurs Outlook 1994; 42(6):255–259.

Meleis AI, Sawyer LM, Im E-O, et al. Experiencing transitions: an emerging middle-range theory. Adv Nurs Sci 2000; 23(1):12–28.

Neville-Jan A. Encounters in a world of pain: an autoethnography. Am J Occupat Ther 2003; 57(1):88–98.

Ohmen M, Soderberg S, Lundman B. Hovering between suffering and enduring: the meaning of living with serious chronic illness. Qualitative Health Res 2003; 13(4):528–542.

Padilla GV, Ferrell B, Grant MM, et al. Defining the content domain of quality of life for cancer patients with pain. Cancer Nursing 1990; 13(2):108–115.

Paterson B. The koala has claws: application of the shifting perspectives model in research of chronic illness. Qualitative Health Res 2003; 13(7):987–994.

Paulson M, Danielson E, Larsson K, et al. Men's descriptions of their experience of nonmalignant pain of fibromyalgia type. Scand J Caring Sci 2001; 15(1):54–59.

Reason P. Chapter 20. In: Handbook of Qualitative Research. Sage Publications, London, 1994:324–339.

Reason P, Bradbury H. Handbook of Action Research. Sage Publications, London, 2001.

Rhodes LC, McPhillips–Tangum CA, Markham C, et al. The power of the visible: the meaning of diagnostic tests in chronic back pain. Social Sci Med 1999; 48(9): 1189–1203.

Roberts G, Kent B, Prys D, et al. Describing chronic pain: towards bilingual practice. Int J Nurs Stud 2003; 40(8):889–902.

Sallfors C, Fasth A, Hallberg LR. Oscillating between hope and despair: a qualitative study. Child: Care, Health Devel 2002; 28(6):495–505.

Schumacher KL, Meleis AI. Transitions: a central concept in nursing. J Nurs Scholarship 1994; 26(2):119–127.

Seers K, Friedli K. The patients' experiences of their chronic non-malignant pain. J Adv Nurs 1996; 24(6):1160–1168.

Smith AA. Intimacy and family relationships of women with chronic pain. Pain Manage Nurs 2003; 4(3):134–142.

Smith AA, Friedemann M. Perceived family dynamics of persons with chronic pain. J Adv Nurs 1999; 30(3):543–551.

Soderberg S, Lundman B, Norberg A. Struggling for dignity: the meaning of women's experiences of living with fibromyalgia. Qualitative Health Res 1999; 9(5):575–587.

Steihaug S, Malterud K. Recognition and reciprocity in encounters with women with chronic muscular pain. Scand J Primary Health Care 2002; 20(3):151–156.

Steihaug S, Ahlsen B, Malterud K. "I am allowed to be myself": women with chronic muscular pain being recognized. Scand J Public Health 2002; 30(4):281–287.

Stringer E. Action Research: A Handbook for Practitioners. Sage, Thousand Oaks, CA, 1999.

Subramaniam V, Stewart MW, Smith JF. The development and impact of a chronic pain support group: a qualitative and quantitative study. J Pain Sympt Manag 1999; 17(5):376–383.

Taylor B. Promoting self-help strategies by sharing the lived experience of arthritis. Contemp Nurse 2001; 10(1/2):117–125.

Thomas SP. A phenomenological study of chronic pain [including commentary by Johnson M with author response]. Western J Nurs Res 2000; 22(6):683–705.

Walker JM. The Management of Elderly Patients With Pain: A Community Nursing Perspective, Council for National Academic Awards, 1989:434.

Walker JM. Caring for elderly people with persistent pain in the community: a qualitative perspective on the attitudes of patients and nurses. Health Social Care Community 1994; 2(4):221–228.

Werner A, Steihaug S, Malterud K. Encountering the continuing challenges for women with chronic pain: recovery through recognition. Qualitative Health Res 2003; 13(4):491–509.

Williams G. The genesis of chronic illness: narrative re-construction. Sociol Health Illness 1984; 6:175–200.

4

Measuring patient treatment preferences

Liana Fraenkel • Dick R. Wittink

INTRODUCTION

In this chapter we discuss the role of patients as active participants in medical decision-making. Patients are becoming increasingly informed about medical illnesses and potential treatment options. Yet they often do not have an opportunity to be actively involved in the consideration of alternative treatments. Physicians are trained to diagnose illnesses and to decide which treatment is best, given the diagnosis. For acute diseases, such an approach is appropriate. However, for chronic diseases such as arthritis, asthma and diabetes, it seems critical that patients are actively involved in the management of their disease. Adherence with the recommended treatment is likely to be a positive function of the extent to which the patient is consulted about the selection between medically acceptable options.

If one considers the increases in medical liability insurance premiums, the pressure by various parties on physicians to reduce the time they spend with patients, and the lack of training physicians receive in learning patients' unique perspectives, physicians should be interested in support systems that efficiently capture patients' perspectives. We also contend that greater involvement of patients in the decision-making process pertaining to management of their diseases will increase patient satisfaction and adherence. In addition, patient involvement should improve health outcomes. Furthermore, recent studies have shown that involving patients in medical decision-making may result in fewer invasive procedures, thus reducing direct costs for certain diseases.

The assessment of patient preferences has similarities with the assessment of customer preferences for commercial products or services. Such assessments have been extensively studied and used in the fields of psychology, economics and marketing. In market research, a common approach for determining customer interests in modifications of existing products and services is conjoint analysis, an approach that derives from mathematical psychology (Luce and Tukey 1964). Consulting companies, market research firms and manufacturers have been heavy users of this approach to predict market interest for new products that represent modifications in product and/or service characteristics. We review the use of this approach in assessing patient preferences for alternative treatments of a given disease with specific examples, and we suggest how it can be applied to pain treatment.

PATIENT INVOLVEMENT

The nature of medical care is changing. The paternalistic model, in which physicians unilaterally decide which treatment of a disease is best for each patient, is gradually being replaced by an approach in which patients have an active role in healthcare decisions. In addition to adhering to the principles of informed consent and patient autonomy, greater patient involvement may improve health outcomes. For example, adherence to complex regimens in the treatment of diabetes is greater if patients are active participants in treatment planning.

To be sure, situations differ in the relevance of shared decision-making. For example, there are situations in which there is a single superior therapy and relatively little risk, such as treatment of community acquired pneumonia in an otherwise healthy host or care of a young patient with an uncomplicated closed fracture. In these cases decision-making is relatively straightforward, and patient participation is limited to providing consent for the appropriate therapy. However, for millions of Americans with chronic illnesses, appropriate and medically feasible treatment options vary in the route of administration, expected benefits, risks (side effects) and costs. It seems obvious that patients should have the opportunity to be actively involved in decisions that affect their health outcomes, unless they prefer to assign this responsibility to someone else.

The idea of active patient participation in medical decision-making related to chronic diseases is based on several arguments. First, alternative treatments differ on dimensions that are outside the physician's domain. For example, only a patient with knee arthritis can judge whether she or he is willing to accept the risk of stomach upset, and in some cases stomach ulceration, for a modest decrease in the level of pain.

Second, involving patients in medical decision-making is desirable if patients want to be informed about available alternatives. Physicians often worry that describing a long list of side effects will increase patient anxiety. The results of many studies show, however, that the vast majority of patients want to be fully informed of all available alternatives and their associated risks, even if they do not want to participate in actual decision-making. Indeed, quite a few patients examine the documents that accompany medicines provided by the pharmacist and/or search the internet for additional information. Therefore, despite physicians' concerns regarding the negative consequences of lengthy discussions of possible risks, patients' needs for full disclosure obligate healthcare professionals to ensure that their patients are well-informed.

Third, although studies show that patients vary in their interests to participate (with younger patients, on average, preferring a more active role while older adults tend to prefer a more passive role), involving all patients to some extent is essential in order for physicians to make the best treatment decision for each patient. For example, consider someone who was recently diagnosed with early prostate cancer. A physician could not properly decide between careful monitoring, radiation and surgery as options without knowing how this person evaluates differences in specific risks relative to differences in expected benefits.

Despite these arguments, one might claim that for complex decisions physicians should simply incorporate their own values when they make treatment decisions. In that case, in any given practice all patients with a given disease would be treated alike in the absence of other medically relevant aspects. Imputing a physician's own values into the decision-making process would be acceptable if physicians and patients generally valued conflicting tradeoffs in the same manner. However, studies in various disciplines show that physicians' and patients' priorities differ substantially.

We do not propose that patients actually make decisions. Rather, we advocate that patients are invited to express their *preferences* for alternative combinations of treatment modes, efficacy, side effects and costs. Based on an individual patient's preferences relevant to a specific disease, available treatments might be ranked in terms of fit for that patient at a particular time. This assessment of patient preferences is not to be done by having a patient compare, say, four alternative treatments defined on, say, twelve dimensions. Rather, the idea is to ask patients to consider specific tradeoffs between alternatives defined on two dimensions, ceteris paribus. For example, for a patient diagnosed with lupus nephritis, two of the dimensions are efficacy and alopecia. The patient could be asked to indicate her preference for one treatment defined as 95% of all patients taking the medication having working kidneys after 10 years but 25% having hair loss and another treatment for which 60% will have working kidneys after 10 years and 0% hair loss. A physician naturally would choose the first treatment since hair loss is inconsequential relative to kidney failure. But if the patient worries about hair loss and does not take the medication, the patient will face consequences that can be more severe than if they would receive the preferred treatment.

Despite physicians' best intentions, there are many reasons why shared decision-making is infrequently applied in clinical practice. The reasons include difficulties associated with communicating probabilistic information, the sheer quantity of information and the limited amount of time physicians have per patient visit. At the same time, physicians are concerned about the increasing frequency with which patients demand specific treatments based on advertisements. After the US Food and Drug Administration (FDA) eliminated some restrictions on advertising of prescription drugs in 1997, DTC advertising expenditures reached almost $3 billion in 2002. To encourage informed shared decision-making, tools are needed to elicit patient preferences systematically and without bias. Ideally patients consider the tradeoffs between conflicting considerations in a neutral setting. The implications (e.g., a rank order of treatment options for a given patient's disease) could be the basis for a discussion between the physician and the patient prior to a prescription being written.

MEASUREMENT OF PREFERENCES

Patient preferences are often measured with one of the following three approaches: standard gamble, time tradeoff and rating scale. These methods suffer from well-known limitations including poor inter-method agreement, susceptibility to biases and the difficulty associated with the standard gamble and time tradeoff tasks (e.g., Llewellyn-Thomas et al. 1984, 1995; Llewellyn-Thomas 1996). We advocate conjoint analysis because it is easy to use, reliable and valid (e.g., Johnson 1987; Wittink and Cattin 1989; Green and Srinivasan 1990). It has been used for the assessment of patient preferences for healthcare (Ryan 2000; Fraenkel et al. 2001), for patient priorities in the relationship with physicians (Vick and Scott 1998; Scott and Vick 1999), and for patient healthcare services and treatment alternatives (Ryan and Hughes 1997; Singh et al. 1998).

Conjoint analysis derives from conjoint measurement (Luce and Tukey 1964). Conjoint *measurement* is concerned with, among other things, the conditions under which metric output is obtainable from nonmetric input. Conjoint *analysis* represents the practical application of this idea. It seeks to obtain a quantified expression (value system or utility function) of the tradeoffs an individual makes between conflicting considerations such as efficacy and side effects. Such a value system results from a respondent's answers to questions about the desirability of hypothetical representations of product characteristics. The researcher chooses the characteristics to be manipulated (so that the objects to be evaluated satisfy statistical criteria for experimentation *and* realism), and the number of objects to be evaluated (sufficiently large for each respondent to have a unique value system). This still leaves the question whether answers to hypothetical questions are predictive of marketplace behavior. There is a substantial body of literature that shows positive evidence (e.g., Wittink and Bergestuen 2001). However, it should be noted that respondents must be motivated to provide meaningful answers and must be informed about the relevance of product characteristics manipulated.

Once a value system is obtained for a patient, relevant to the treatment of a given disease, it is then possible to predict which of the available and medically acceptable treatments best fits that patient at a given time. Alternatively, the output could consist of the two most suitable treatments or even a predicted rank order of all treatments. With computerized data collection and analysis approaches, a patient can obtain this information after answering a modest number of questions. The patient would then share the result with a physician who can formulate a treatment plan based on the patient's values. Note that patients should be given an opportunity to restate their preferences periodically. For example, a patient with type I diabetes might initially prefer to use multiple injections over an insulin pump. Once the patient has come to terms with the diagnosis, they may prefer the pump due to its convenience. The point is not that we know how patients' preferences will change over time but that it is important to allow for changes in patients' considerations of conflicting aspects, even if the available treatments do not change.

We briefly examine two applications. The first one involves lupus nephritis, a disease for which treatment options have distinct risk–benefit ratios. For this disease, drug toxicity may have a profound influence on quality of life. Under these conditions, patients should be actively involved in the treatment decisions. We used Adaptive Conjoint Analysis (ACA), a process that collects and analyzes preferences with an interactive computer program (Johnson 1987). The method is adaptive in that it uses an individual's answers to initial questions (self-explicated data) to generate respondent-specific paired comparisons that involve tradeoffs between conflicting considerations (conjoint data). ACA's design allows a large number of attributes (dimensions) to be included without information overload. For example, part of the exercise is that respondents are asked to indicate intensity of preference for one option over another, each one defined on just two attributes, ceteris paribus. One option might be superior in efficacy, the other could be superior in a specific side effect. By presenting multiple questions in this way, a respondent gets to reflect on tradeoffs in all aspects. It ensures that respondents evaluate all attributes on which treatment options may differ, and it facilitates the conduct of simulations that show how patients' predicted choices change if the characteristics of one or more treatment options change.

We show a description of the nine attributes in the lupus nephritis application in Table 4.1. Except for the first one, all attributes represent side effects. We created two or three alternative levels for each of the attributes to represent known or estimated variation across alternative treatments. In the simulations we focused on cyclophosphamide and azathioprine. The specific attribute levels that apply to these two treatments are shown in Table 4.2. It is clear from this table that cyclophosphamide is superior in efficacy and oral ulcers but inferior on alopecia, zoster, infertility and cystitis.

Table 4.1 Description of attributes for lupus nephritis

1. Benefit of medication. The number of people with functioning kidneys after 10 years. For example after 10 years, 95 out of 100 people on the medication will have functioning kidneys and the other 5 will be on dialysis

2. Nausea and vomiting. The nausea and vomiting usually occur only around the time when the medication is taken. These symptoms can almost always be controlled with medications. The nausea and/or vomiting go away if the dose of the medication is lowered or if necessary when the medication is stopped

3. Hair loss. The hair will slowly grow back when the medication is stopped

4. Mouth sores. Canker sores that go away if the dose of the medication is lowered or if necessary when the medication is stopped

5. Blistering rash. Painful blisters that usually occur in a patch on one side of the body. The rash goes away in a week to 10 days

6. Infection. These are serious infections like blood, joint or lung infections. Patients with these infections need to be admitted to the hospital for treatment with intravenous antibiotics for one to two weeks. Most people get better. Rarely, when severe, this type of infection can be life threatening

7. Premature menopause and infertility. The medication can cause permanent damage to the ovaries, which leads to premature menopause. This means one will stop having periods (permanently) and one will not be able to become pregnant

8. Bleeding from the bladder. The medication can irritate the lining of the bladder and cause bleeding. This problem almost always gets better just by stopping the medication, but sometimes patients have to be admitted to the hospital for intravenous treatment. Bleeding from the bladder can almost always be prevented by drinking a lot of water

9. Cancer. The medication can increase the risk of developing cancer. Tumors occur only in a small number of patients. The tumors that doctors watch for are of the bladder, cervix and lymph nodes

Reprinted with permission from Fraenkel L, Bodardus S, Wittink DR. Understanding patient preferences for the treatment of lupus nephritis with adaptive conjoint analysis. Med Care 2001; 39(11):1203–1216.

The respondents were 103 women with lupus in three community rheumatology practices. All participants completed the conjoint task in 14 ± 5 minutes. We show patient utilities (value systems) in Table 4.3. The results show that efficacy and risk of infection have the greatest impact on preferences, on average, for all women ($N = 65$) regardless of their desire for more children. Impact is indicated by the magnitude of the largest average utility values for an attribute (since the smallest for each attribute is zero). Thus, for the group wanting more children, efficacy (max $= 122$) is closely followed by infection (max $= 119$). For the group not wanting more children, efficacy is also very important (max $= 139$), followed by infection (max $= 113$). In the simulation, premenopausal women wanting more children were predicted to choose cyclophosphamide less often than their counterparts, as expected (Table 4.4). This holds for all situations considered in the simulations. For more detail see Fraenkel et al. (2001).

A second application focuses on rheumatoid arthritis and allows for a comparison of patient preferences with medical guidelines (Fraenkel et al. 2004). We restricted our study to disease-modifying antirheumatic drugs (DMARDs), specifically the traditional treatments

methotrexate and gold, and new treatments leflunomide and etanercept. We used sixteen attributes, characterized as route of administration, amount of physician experience, three efficacy components, ten adverse effects and cost (see Table 4.5). We show the specific levels of the attributes that pertain to the treatment options in Table 4.6. We find that while current medical guidelines recommend methotrexate as the initial DMARD of choice, 95% of the respondents are predicted to choose etanercept over the other options. This percentage decreases if the co-pay for etanercept increases but it remains very high (see Table 4.7). Thus, patient preferences differ strongly from medical practice to the extent that physicians adhere to medical guidelines (see Fraenkel et al. 2004 for more details).

For an application to pain management, one could consider a variety of treatments covering a broad spectrum that includes psychotherapy, yoga, massage therapy, acupuncture, physical therapy, ergonometry, pills and anesthesiology. This breadth of treatment options is typically not meaningful to cover in a single conjoint application for several reasons. One is that most patients only actively consider a subset of the options. Another is that the great variety in the nature of

Table 4.2 Base-case attribute levels for lupus nephritis treatments

Attribute	Level	Assigned value for cyclophosphamide	Assigned value for azathioprine
Efficacy	After 10 years, 95% have kidneys that work/5% need dialysis	X	
	After 10 years, 80% have kidneys that work/5% need dialysis		
	After 10 years, 60% have kidneys that work/5% need dialysis		X
Infection	0% get a serious infection		
	10% get a serious infection	X	X
	30% get a serious infection		
Cancer	0% get cancer		
	1/1000 get cancer	X	X
Alopecia	0% get hair loss		X
	25% get hair loss	X	
	50% get hair loss		
Zoster	0% get a blistering rash		
	10% get a blistering rash		X
	25% get a blistering rash	X	
Infertility	0% become infertile/enopausal		X
	25% become infertile/menopausal	X	
	50% become infertile/menopausal		
Nausea	0% get nausea and vomiting		
	10% get nausea and vomiting	X	X
	30% get nausea and vomiting		
Cystitis	0% get bleeding from the bladder		X
	1/1000 get bleeding from the bladder	X	
Oral ulcers	0% get painful mouth sores	X	
	5% get painful mouth ulcers		X

Reprinted with permission from Fraenkel L, Bodardus S, Wittink DR. Understanding patient preferences for the treatment of lupus nephritis with adaptive conjoint analysis. Med Care 2001; 39(11):1203–1216.

treatments makes it virtually impossible to define a set of attributes that is common to all options. In practice, one either focuses on a meaningful subset of the options or one has to create a supra-exercise that allows the subset to be respondent-specific.

For our discussion, assume an application that is restricted to pharmaceutical products such as topical creams (e.g., capsaicin), analgesics (e.g., acetaminophen), traditional nonselective nonsteroidal anti-inflammatory drugs (e.g., ibuprofen) and selective cyclooxygenase 2 inhibitors (e.g., celecoxib). Relevant attributes could be the following:

- route of administration (topical versus pills);
- form (tablet, capsule, liquid);
- dosage schedule (1–4 times daily);
- onset of action (30–60 minutes);
- relieves inflammation (proportion of people who benefit, e.g., in 0 to 75% of patients);
- relieves stiffness (0 to 75% of patients);

Table 4.3 Patient utilities (mean ± SD) for lupus nephritis attribute levels

Attribute	Level	Premenopausal women wanting more children (N = 25)	Premenopausal women not wanting more children (N = 40)
Efficacy	After 10 years, 95% have kidneys that work/5% need dialysis	122±30	139±33
	After 10 years, 80% have kidneys that work/20% need dialysis	69±25	74±29
	After 10 years, 60% have kidneys that work/40% need dialysis	0	0
Infection	0% get a serious infection	119±27	113±35
	10% get a serious infection	65±23	62±29
	30% get a serious infection	0	0
Cancer	0% get cancer	74±34	76±33
	1/1000 get cancer	0	0
Alopecia	0% get hair loss	70±30	64±36
	25% get hair loss	32±26	39±23
	50% get hair loss	3±8	2±5
Zoster	0% get a blistering rash	55±24	56±30
	10% get a blistering rash	27±21	31±26
	25% get a blistering rash	5±11	5±12
Premature ovarian failure	0% become infertile/menopausal	87±44	47±39
	25% become infertile/menopausal	40±26	29±25
	50% become infertile/menopausal	2±11	10±17
Nausea	0% get nausea and vomiting	44±27	57±27
	10% get nausea and vomiting	21±21	28±26
	30% get nausea and vomiting	5±11	7±14
Cystitis	0% get bleeding from the bladder	29±20	33±27
	1/1000 get bleeding from the bladder	1±4	2±6
Oral ulcers	0% get painful mouth sores	24±18	26±20
	5% get painful mouth ulcers	4±13	1±4

Reprinted with permission from Fraenkel L, Bodardus S, Wittink DR. Understanding patient preferences for the treatment of lupus nephritis with adaptive conjoint analysis. Med Care 2001; 39(11):1203–1216.

- causes tiredness (0 to 10%);
- causes dizziness (0 to 10%);
- causes stomach pain or nausea (0 to 10%);
- availability (prescription or over the counter); and
- out-of-pocket monthly cost ($5–$15; maximum of $15 assumes that all are insured).

The use of these attributes and levels in a conjoint exercise allows patients to consider the tradeoffs between components of mode of treatment, efficacy, adverse effects, availability and cost (co-pay). Note that brand name is not used as an attribute so as not to allow brand preferences that result from advertising to

Table 4.4 Percent of patients predicted to choose cyclophosphamide with varying probabilities of renal survival, infection, and cancer

Attributes for base-case	Change from base-case	Premenopausal women (%) Wanting more children (N = 25)	Not wanting more children (N = 40)	Postmenopausal women (%)
Base-case*	—	56	80	82
Cyclophosphamide's renal survival advantage over azathioprine = 35%	Cyclophosphamide's renal survival advantage decreased to 25%	28	58	61
	Cyclophosphamide's renal survival advantage decreased to 20%	24	43	61
Infection risk for both drugs = 10%	Cyclophosphamide's risk of infection increased to 20%	36	65	66
	Cyclophosphamide's risk of infection increased to 30%	20	45	55
Cancer risk for both drugs = 1/1000	Azathioprine's risk of cancer decreased by 25%	44	70	66
	Azathioprine's risk of cancer decreased by 50%	28	60	58
Cyclophosphamide's risk of premature ovarian failure = 25%, no risk of premature ovarian failure due to azathioprine	Cyclophosphamide's risk of premature ovarian failure increased to 50%	28	70	74
	Cyclophosphamide's risk of premature ovarian failure decreased to 12.5%	64	90	87
	No risk of premature ovarian failure	88	90	90

*Levels for the base-case are depicted in Table 4.2.

Table 4.5 Description of attributes for DMARDs

Route of administration:
  One pill taken once a day in the morning
  Subcutaneous injection. An injection given right under the skin, like an insulin injection. You can give it yourself or have someone else do it. It can be given at home or in a clinic
  Intramuscular injection. An injection given into the muscle (usually your upper arm or buttock), like the flu vaccine. It is given by a nurse in a clinic

Experience. This refers to the amount of experience doctors have with the medication

Time for the medication to start working. You can use other medications like anti-inflammatories (celebrex, naprosyn, ibuprofen) or prednisone until the new medication starts working

Benefit of medication:
  Better means that you feel much more energetic and less achy since taking the medication
  Some of your joints still bother you, but you are in much less pain than you were before starting the medication
  You are able to perform all your daily activities like shopping and housework on most days with little if any difficulty
  You are able to engage in leisure activities with your friends on most days with little if any difficulty

Bone damage. This refers to the number of people who develop new or more bone damage on x-rays after 1 year. The bone damage can be seen on x-rays only

Injection site reaction. This refers to a red itchy localized rash at the site of the injection. These usually stop happening after a few weeks

Itchy rash. The rash can be treated with medications and creams to stop the itch. The rash goes away in a few weeks after the dose of the medication is lowered or if necessary when the medication is stopped

Mouth sores. The arthritis medication can cause painful mouth sores. The sores feel like canker sores. The sores can be treated with a gel or a mouth rinse. The sores go away when the dose of the medication is lowered or if necessary when the medication is stopped

Hair thinning. The medication can cause some hair thinning. Your hair will grow back after the dose of the medication is lowered or if necessary when the medication is stopped

Nausea/vomiting. The arthritis medication can cause mild or moderate nausea and vomiting (you sometimes feel a little queasy and vomit about once a day). The nausea and vomiting go away after the dose of the medication is lowered or if necessary when the medication is stopped

Diarrhea. The arthritis medication can cause moderate diarrhea (you have occasional stomach cramps and have watery bowel movements about 2 to 3 times per day). The diarrhea goes away after the dose of the medication is lowered or if necessary when the medication is stopped

Cancer. Theoretical risk of cancer means that because the medication affects the immune system it has the potential to increase cancer risk with long-term use. An increased risk has not been shown in studies of this drug, but the studies have followed patients for less than 5 years. If the medication does turn out to increase the risk of cancer after long-term use, the risk might be 1/1000

Kidney damage. The medication can cause reversible damage to the kidneys. This type of kidney damage does not usually cause any symptoms, but some patients can develop swelling in their legs. The kidneys recover once the medication is stopped

Liver damage. The arthritis medication can cause liver damage. People with liver damage may become tired, weak, and lose their appetite. Many patients do not get other symptoms, but in some, the liver damage gets worse, and can cause yellow skin, intense itching and bloating of the stomach

Lung damage. The arthritis medication can cause lung problems that cause a dry cough, shortness of breath and fever. Patients with this side effect need to be admitted to hospital for treatment with oxygen and intravenous medications (steroids by vein). Treatment takes an average of two weeks

Costs. Cost refers to your co-pay (that is your out-of-pocket costs) per month

Reproduced with permission from Fraenkel L, Bogardus ST, Concato J, et al. Patient preferences for treatment of rheumatoid arthritis. Ann Rheum Dis 2004; 63(11):1372–1378.

Table 4.6 Base-case scenario with four DMARDs

Characteristic	Methotrexate	Gold	Leflunomide	Etanercept
Route of administration	PO	IM	PO	SC
Physician experience	>20 years	>20 years	New	New
Onset of action	4 weeks	8 weeks	4 weeks	2 weeks
Percent who benefit	60%	60%	60%	75%
Percent without new bone erosions	60%	60%	60%	75%
Injection site reaction	0	0	0	40%
Rash	10%	40%	10%	0
Oral ulcers	10%	10%	10%	0
Alopecia	10%	0	10%	0
Nausea	10%	0	10%	0
Diarrhea	10%	0	20%	0
Cancer	0	0	0	1/1000
Renal toxicity	0	1/100	0	0
Hepatic toxicity	1/1000	0	1/1000	0
Pneumonitis	1/100	1/1000	0	0
Co-pay	$5.00	$5.00	$5.00	$5.00

Table 4.7 Predicted DMARD choices

	Percent of patients predicted to choose a specific option			
Scenario	Methotrexate	Gold	Leflunomide	Etanercept
Base case	1.7 ± 1.2	2.5 ± 1.4	0.8 ± 0.8	95.0 ± 2.0
All equally effective	4.2 ± 1.8	7.5 ± 2.4	0	94.2 ± 2.1
All equally effective, co-pay of etanercept increased to $30.00	6.7 ± 2.3	14.2 ± 3.2	6.7 ± 2.3	72.5 ± 4.1
All equally effective, co-pay of etanercept increased to $30.00, risk of methotrexate pneumonitis decreased to 0.1%	14.2 ± 3.8	10.0 ± 2.7	0.8 ± 0.8	75.0 ± 4.0

Reproduced with permission from Fraenkel L, Bogardus ST, Concato J, et al. Patient preferences for treatment of rheumatoid arthritis. Ann Rheum Dis 2004; 63(11):1372–1378.

play a role. Including brand names would pose multiple problems. For example, the preference for one brand name over another is often at least partly based on characteristics that are already included as separate attributes. Even if this could be avoided, brand preferences would be based on emotional reactions to advertisements or claims made by relatives or friends, and their relevance to treatment effects is unclear.

IMPLEMENTATION

These advances in preference and value assessment provide the option for patients to explore the tradeoffs between treatment modes, frequency, efficacy, side effects and cost, and to have their preferences with respect to conflicting considerations be known to the physician. If this option were available in physicians' waiting rooms or over the internet, patients could spend about 15 minutes answering tradeoff questions relevant to treatment options for a given disease before they meet the physician. With educational plug-ins, patients could also learn more about relevant characteristics of the disease and potential treatments. If databases are also available with complete information, constantly updated, on all alternative treatments for each chronic disease, the diffusion of new treatment options would be vastly accelerated compared with the current situation. Importantly, the technology exists for relevant parties to obtain a quantified representation uniquely for each individual patient's treatment preferences so that available treatment options for a given disease can be rank ordered based on that patient's value system. And these rank orders can be appropriately modified over time based on both changes in the available treatments and changes in a patient's preferences.

Since all individuals are subject to biases in judgments, such a system will also improve the quality of treatment decisions. With a current and constantly updated database that includes all treatments and the best available evidence on all relevant aspects, fully informed decisions can be made. Computer programs capable of eliciting individual patient preferences and providing the predicted choices to the patients will allow the medical decision-making process to be more complete and efficient than is currently possible.

CONCLUSION

Given the rapid changes in medical technology and the vast array of new study results, it is critical that patients have easy access to relevant developments. With complete and fully updated information on all treatment alternatives in a database, it is possible to use each individual patient's assessments of tradeoffs to predict preferences (choices) for alternative treatments defined on the aspects on which differences exist. If physicians can efficiently learn how individual patients make tradeoffs between conflicting considerations of competing options, they will be better equipped to make recommendations concordant with individual patient values and priorities. The result is that treatment decisions will be closer to optimal, and with more involvement by patients, adherence to recommended treatments will increase. Patients will benefit from treatment decisions that closely match their tradeoffs between conflicting considerations. And as patients' perspectives change

over time, they have the opportunity to have their value systems reassessed. This is especially important given that the experience with chronic diseases influences how patients assess the tradeoffs between conflicting considerations.

REFERENCES

Fraenkel L, Bogardus S, Wittink DR. Understanding patient preferences for the treatment of lupus nephritis with adaptive conjoint analysis. Med Care 2001; 39:1203–1216.

Fraenkel L, Bogardus ST, Concato J, et al. Patient preferences for treatment of rheumatoid arthritis. Ann Rheumatoid Dis 2004; 63:1372–1378.

Green PE, Srinivasan V. Conjoint analysis in marketing research: new developments and directions. J Marketing 1990; 54:3–19.

Johnson RM. Adaptive conjoint analysis. In: Sawtooth Software Conference Proceedings, Sawtooth Software, Ketchum, ID, 1987:253–265.

Llewellyn-Thomas HA. Health state descriptions: purposes, issues, a proposal. Med Care 1996; 34(suppl 12): DS109–DS118.

Llewellyn-Thomas HA, Sutherland HJ, Hogg SA, et al. Linear analogue self-assessment of voice quality in laryngeal cancer. J Chronic Dis 1984; 37:917–924.

Llewellyn-Thomas HA, Thiel EC, Sem FW, et al. Presenting clinical trial information: a comparison of methods. Patient Educ Counsel 1995; 25:97–107.

Luce RD, Tukey JW. Simultaneous conjoint measurement: a new type of fundamental measurement. J Math Psychol 1964; 1:1–27.

Ryan M, Farrar S. Using conjoint analysis to elicit preferences for health care. Br Med J 2000; 3(320):1530–1533.

Ryan M, Hughes J. Using conjoint analysis to assess women's preferences for miscarriage management. Health Econ 1997; 6:261–273.

Scott A, Vick S. Patients, doctors, and contracts: an application of principal-agent theory to the doctor–patient relationship. Scot J Political Econ 1999; 46:111–134.

Singh JL, Cutler M, Shin JB, et al. Medical decision-making and the patient: understanding preference patterns for growth hormone therapy using conjoint analysis. Med Care 1998; 36(suppl 8):AS31–AS45.

Vick S, Scott A. Agency in health care. Examining patients' preferences for attributes of the doctor–patient relationship. J Health Econ 1998; 17:587–605.

Wittink DR, Cattin P. Commercial use on conjoint analysis: an update. J Marketing 1989; 53(3):91–96.

Wittink DR, Trond Bergestuen T. Forecasting with conjoint analysis. In: Scott Armstrong J (ed). Forecasting Principles Handbook. Kluwer, Boston, 2001:147–167.

5

Pain assessment in clinical trials

Mark P. Jensen

INTRODUCTION

Clinical trials of pain treatment are essential for identifying and estimating the effectiveness of interventions that might provide pain relief. In order for the results of such trials to be deemed valid, the measures used should have proven reliability and validity. This chapter reviews the evidence concerning the psychometric properties of self-report measures of pain, including those that assess pain intensity, pain relief, and pain quality.

In the first section of the chapter, and for each pain dimension covered, the review includes a brief description of the measure(s), a review of the available evidence concerning its validity and reliability, and a summary of its strengths and weaknesses. The second section discusses specific recommendations concerning the assessment of each outcome dimension, based on the results of the review presented in the first section.

REVIEW OF PAIN MEASURES

RATINGS OF PAIN INTENSITY

Single-item ratings of pain intensity are the most commonly used measures in pain research and clinical settings. The three most commonly used pain intensity scales are the Visual Analogue Scale, Numerical Rating Scale, and Verbal Rating Scale. Table 5.1 summarizes the strengths and weaknesses of these three types of pain intensity rating scales.

Visual Analogue Scale of pain intensity

A Visual Analogue Scale of pain intensity (VAS-I) consists of a line, usually 100 mm long, with each end of the line labeled with descriptors representing the extremes of pain intensity (e.g., "no pain," "extreme pain"). Respondents place a mark on the line that represents his or her pain intensity level, and the distance measured from the "no pain" end to the mark (possible range = 0–100 mm) is that person's VAS pain score.

The VAS-I has consistently demonstrated sensitivity to changes in pain associated with treatment or time (e.g., Joyce et al. 1975; Stambaugh and Sarajian 1981; Seymour 1982; Turner 1982; Anderson et al. 1991; Sandouk et al. 1991; Moore et al. 1994; Ingham et al. 1996; Tannock et al. 1996; Talmi et al. 1997;

Table 5.1 The strengths and weaknesses of three measures of pain intensity

Scale	Strengths	Weaknesses
Visual Analogue Scale	Many ("infinite") response categories Average (group) scores can be treated as ratio data Good evidence for validity	Extra step in scoring the paper-and-pencil version can take more time and adds an additional source of error Some people, especially older people, have difficulty using VASs
Numerical Rating Scale	Easy to administer Many response categories if NRS-101 chosen; adequate number of response categories if 0–10 NRS is chosen Easy to score Good evidence for validity Compliance with measurement task is high	Average (group) scores cannot necessarily be treated as ratio data
Verbal Rating Scale	Easy to administer Easy to score Good evidence for validity Compliance with measurement task is high May approximate ratio scaling if CMM methods (or scores developed from CMM methods) are used	Can be difficult for persons with limited vocabulary Relatively few response categories compared to the VAS or NRS If scored using the ranking method, the scores do not necessarily have ratio qualities People forced to choose one word, even if no word on the scale adequately describes their pain intensity

Holland et al. 1998; Frost et al. 2000; Manfredi et al. 2000; Mercandante et al. 2000; Zeppetella 2000; Lundeberg et al. 2001; Rice et al. 2001; Barton et al. 2002; Jensen et al. 2002; Steiner et al. 2003; Birbara et al. 2003; Meier et al. 2003; Joshi et al. 2004), and usually shows strong associations with other pain intensity ratings (e.g., Kremer et al. 1981; Seymour 1982; Walsh and Leber 1983; Ahles et al. 1984; Ekblom and Hansson 1988; Littman et al. 1985; Jensen et al. 1986; Wilkie et al. 1990; Gaston-Johansson et al. 1992; Grossman et al. 1992; Soh and Ang 1992; Paice and Cohen, 1997; Sze et al. 1998; Ramer et al. 1999; Chang et al. 2000; Klepstad et al. 2000; Freeman et al. 2001; Good et al. 2001; Singer et al. 2001). VAS measures of pain intensity have been shown to be distinct from VAS measures of pain unpleasantness, supporting the discriminative validity of both (Price et al. 1987).

The scores from VAS-Is appear to have the qualities of ratio data for groups of people (Price and Harkins 1987; Price et al. 1983). This means that differences in pain intensity (for groups, not necessarily for individuals) as measured by VASs represent good estimates of actual differences in magnitude, on average. For example, a significant change in average pain intensity from 60mm to 30mm on a VAS computed from a group of individuals would indicate that perceived pain intensity was halved in this sample of patients.

Test–retest reliability of the VAS-I has been examined in a number of studies, with time periods ranging

from five minutes ($r = 0.95$; Grossman et al. 1992) to one week ($r = 0.75$; Chang et al. 2000; $r = 0.85$, Fischer et al. 1999). These reliability coefficients are almost always very high (see also Padilla et al. 1983; Hollen et al. 1993; Roach et al. 1997; Bergh et al. 2000; Good et al. 2001; Lundeberg et al. 2001; Gallagher et al. 2002), and only very rarely drop below .70 (e.g., Love et al. (1989) reported VAS-I test–retest reliability coefficients as .77 for current pain but only .49 for "worst" pain and .57 for "best" pain over the course of several days).

Three studies have examined the amount of change in VAS scores that can be considered meaningful. One study asked 61 patients with complex regional pain syndrome, type 1, to rate their current pain intensity on a 10cm VAS three times per day for four days before treatment with spinal cord stimulation (Forouzanfar et al. 2003). These same measures were repeated at 6-, 12-, and 24-month follow-ups, as was a 7-point categorical scale of global treatment effect. Percent change (in VAS scores) associated with "a little improved" were 30, 26, and 31% for the 6-, 12-, and 24-month follow-up points, respectively. The average percent changes associated with "much improved" were 71, 63, and 58%, respectively. The authors also classified patients as "successful" or "unsuccessful" (defined as reporting that their pain was "much improved" versus reporting that their pain was only "a little improved" or lower), and found that a cutoff of a 50% or more decrease had the best balance of accuracy, sensitivity, and specificity in identifying patients who were classified as treatment successes. In a separate study, Jensen and colleagues (Jensen et al. 2003) reanalyzed data from two clinical trials examining the effects of a treatment on postoperative pain. Patients undergoing knee surgery and laparotomy were administered a 100 mm VAS-I before and then on 16 occasions after (within a 24-hour period) receiving one of three study medications (ketorolac, morphine, or placebo) during the postoperative period. A 5-point categorical scale of pain relief (none, a little, some, a lot, complete) was also administered at the post-treatment assessments. The percent changes in pain associated with each relief rating were –11% and –13% (no relief), 18% and 13% (a little relief), 36% and 41% (some relief), 64% and 66% (a lot of relief), and 99% and 100% (complete relief) for the knee surgery and laparotomy patients, respectively. The absolute 100 mm VAS change scores associated with these levels of relief were −7 mm and −7 mm (no relief), 13 mm and 9 mm (a little relief), 20 mm and 27 mm (some relief), 44 mm and 44 mm (a lot of relief), and 62 mm and 67 mm (complete relief) for the knee surgery and laparotomy patients, respectively. Jensen and colleagues also found that the amount of change needed for a change in pain to be deemed as meaningful varied as a function of pretreatment pain; the higher the pain at pretreatment, the more change needed for that change to be deemed as meaningful; this biasing effect was less for percent change than it was for absolute change (Jensen et al. 2003). In a third study, Hägg and colleagues (2003) identified the absolute VAS change scores associated with global ratings of improvement in 289 patients enrolled in a randomized controlled trial of fusion surgery for chronic low back pain two years following treatment. "Much better" was associated with a difference score 43 mm, "better" with 21 mm, "unchanged" with 3 mm, and "worse" with −6 mm. They also found that higher pretreatment pain levels required larger absolute changes in VAS ratings for these changes to be deemed meaningful. Taken together, these findings suggest that absolute VAS decreases in the range 20–27 mm and percent VAS decreases in the range 26–41% might be considered meaningful by most patients, and that absolute decreases of 43 mm to 44 mm and percent decreases in the range 58–71% might be considered substantial by most patients. These percent and absolute change scores are very similar to those found for 0–10 scales (see review below).

One potential strength of VAS-I measures over other measures of pain intensity is the high number of response categories of VASs. Because they are usually measured in millimeters, a 100 mm VAS can be considered as having 101 response levels. This high number of response categories makes the VAS potentially more sensitive to changes in pain intensity than measures with fewer numbers of response categories. Of course, there is an upper limit to the number of response categories necessary to fully characterize different levels of perceived pain intensity, and 101 may be well beyond that limit. For example, laboratory research indicates that people are able to identify, on average, about 21 noticeable differences between weak and intolerable experimental pain (Hardy et al. 1952). Based on this alone, measures with more than 21 response levels are not likely to be any more sensitive than measures that have 21 response levels.

One way to empirically determine whether different measures are more, or less, sensitive to changes in pain is to administer the measures before and after a pain treatment, and determine whether there is a difference between measures in their ability to detect changes in pain. In such research, responsivity to changes in pain can be operationalized as a statistic that reflects the effect size for detecting a change in pain (e.g., pretreatment to post-treatment) or a difference between treatment and control conditions. Relevant statistics include the t-statistic, the F-statistic, the p-value associated with these statistics, or some measure of change divided by a measure of variance (e.g., lambda). Larger t- and F-statistics and smaller p- or lambda values indicate greater sensitivity.

Using this strategy, Wallenstein (1991) performed a reanalysis of 11 randomized controlled trials (RCTs) of analgesics for cancer (2 RCTs) and postoperative (9 RCTs) pain. Ten of these studies included both a VAS-I and VRS-I (Verbal Rating Scale of pain intensity; see below) measure of pain. The VAS-I was more responsive than the VRS-I in six of these studies, and the VRS-I was more responsive than the VAS-I in the remaining four studies. Littman and colleagues (Littman et al. 1985) similarly performed a reanalysis of 23 RCTs of analgesics for postoperative, cancer, acute trauma, or renal or urethral colic pain (total number of subjects 1330). They found that three scales (VRS-I, VAS-I, and a VRS of pain relief) were similarly responsive, although the relief ratings tended to show slightly greater responsivity than VAS-I difference scores did, and VAS-I difference scores showed slightly greater responsivity than VRS-4 difference scores did.

Other researchers have also found VASs are slightly more responsive (Holland et al. 1998; Stockler et al. 1998; Bellamy et al. 1999; Frost et al. 2000; Graff-Radford et al. 2000; Bone et al. 2002) than other measures of pain intensity for detecting changes in pain. However, some studies have shown VAS-Is to be slightly less responsive (Moore et al. 1994; Jenkinson et al. 1995; Magnusson et al. 1995; Bolton et al. 1998; Jensen et al. 1998) or essentially equivalent in responsivity (Stambaugh and Sarajian 1981; Kucuk et al. 2001; Jensen et al. 2002) to other pain measures. In one study, a VAS-I was equivalent in responsivity to a NRS-I, but both were more sensitive than a 4-point VRS-I

(Breivik et al. 2000). In short, studies comparing VAS-Is to other pain intensity measures (in particular VRS-Is and Numerical Rating Scales of pain intensity, or NRS-Is) suggest that the VAS-I is not consistently more, or less, responsive (i.e., valid for detecting changes in pain or treatment effects) than other existing measures.

Although VAS-Is appear to be about as responsive to changes in pain as other pain intensity measures are, there is evidence that VASs may be more difficult than other pain ratings for patients to understand and complete. For example, Bruera and colleagues (1991) found that 16% of 101 palliative care patients were unable to complete a VAS-I, even with nurse assistance, and that this number increased to 84% as disease progressed. Littman and colleagues (1985), who performed the reanalysis of 23 RCTs cited above, also reported on the frequency of missing data in these clinical trials. Of the 167 subjects in these studies who had missing data, 93 (56%) were missing data on all scales (VAS-I, VRS-I, VRS-Relief). However, most of the rest (63, or 44%) were missing data only for the VAS-I.

Kremer and colleagues (1981) examined the failure rates of and preferences for a VAS-I, a 0–100 NRS-I, and a 5-point VRS-I among 50 patients seen at a pain clinic. They found that the VAS had the highest failure rate (11%), and that the failure rates for the 0–100 NRS (2%) and VRS (0%) were very low. The mean age of the persons unable to complete the VAS (73.3 years) was significantly higher than those who were able to complete this measure (54.4 years). In this study, the VRS was the scale most preferred (by 59% of the patients), followed by the 0–100 NRS (25%); the VAS was least preferred by the patients (16%). Gagliese and Melzack (1997) also found that the failure rate of a VAS-I was much higher among the elderly (60–79 years; 30% failure rate) than among middle-aged participants (46–59 years, 19%), while young participants had no problem with the measure (27–45 years, 0%).

Mostly replicating the findings of Kremer and colleagues (1981), Paice and Cohen (1997) compared the preference and failure rates of a VAS-I, 0–10 NRS-I, and 5-point VRS-I in 50 patients with cancer-related pain. While 10 (20%) of their subjects were unable to complete the VAS, all were able to complete the VRS and NRS. Moreover, mean opioid intake was significantly higher for subjects unable to complete the VAS than for those who were able to complete this measure. They found that half (50%) of the patients preferred the 0–10 NRS, but that many (28%) also preferred the VRS over the other scales. Only six (12%) of the subjects preferred the VAS over the other scales.

Shannon and colleagues (1995) administered the McGill Pain Questionnaire (MPQ; see below), three VAS scales (of pain intensity, pain relief, and mood), a VRS of pain intensity, and a Face Scale to 63 inpatients with cancer. Again, the VAS scales evidenced the highest failure rate, with 89% able to complete the VRS, 84% the MPQ, 81% the Face Scale, and 75% the VAS scales. Soh and Ang (1992) asked 79 patients with various cancer diagnoses to complete a VAS-I and a VRS-I. Although they did not report specific failure rates, they did comment that the VAS was more difficult to explain to patients than the VRS was. Sze and colleagues (1998) administered a VAS-I and a 0–10 NRS-I to 95 patients with various cancer diagnoses. Again, the failure rate for the VAS-I (14%) was higher than for the NRS-I (3%). Stahmer and colleagues (1998) also found the failure rate for a VAS-I (15%) to be much higher than that for a NRS-I (0%) in a sample of hospitalized patients with pain. On the other hand, Tannock and colleagues (1996) found a 6-point VRS-I and a VAS-I to have similar failure rates (8% and 11%, respectively) in a sample of 136 men with prostate cancer. Clearly, although patients do not always have difficulty using pain rating scales, when they do have difficulty with pain measures, they tend to have more difficulty with the VAS than with other measures, including NRSs and VRSs.

Numerical Rating Scale of pain intensity

A Numerical Rating Scale of pain intensity (NRS-I) consists of a range of numbers (usually 0–10, but sometimes 0–20, 0–100, or other ranges). Respondents are told that the lowest number represents "no pain" and the highest number represents an extreme level of pain (e.g., "pain as intense as you can imagine"). They are asked to write down, circle, or state the single number that best represents their level of pain intensity, and the number they select is their pain intensity score.

Although traditionally NRS-I measures have been used less often than VAS-I or VRS-I (Verbal Rating Scales of pain intensity; see below) measures, an increasing number of researchers have been using NRS-Is to test for treatment effects in pain clinical trials. The findings of the research that has been performed support the validity and reliability of NRS scales, and indicates that their psychometric properties are very similar to those of VAS measures. For example, NRS-I scales tend to show strong associations with other pain rating scales (Kremer et al. 1981; Seymour 1982; Jensen et al. 1986; Ekblom and Hansson 1988; Jensen et al. 1989; Wilkie et al. 1990; Paice and Cohen 1997; Sze et al. 1998; Singer et al. 2001). NRS-Is have also shown to be sensitive to changes (increases) in pain associated with treatments often associated with short-term increases in pain (e.g., radiotherapy for cancer, Trotti et al. 1998; physical therapy, Smith et al. 1998), and to decreases associated with pain treatment (e.g., Chesney and Shelton 1976; Stenn et al. 1979; Keefe et al. 1981; Turner 1982; Paice and Cohen 1997; Backonja et al. 1998; Bolton and Wilkinson 1998; Farrar et al. 1998; Rowbotham et al. 1998; Grond et al. 1999; Holzheimer et al. 1999; Jensen et al. 1999; Leksowski 2001; Wilkie et al. 2000; Eisenbert et al. 2001; Lundeberg et al. 2001; Meuser et al. 2001; Rice et al. 2001; Palangio et al. 2002; Gammaitoni et al. 2003).

NRS-Is have demonstrated criterion-related validity through their significant and positive associations with analgesic medication use (Daut et al. 1983), perceived need to contact healthcare providers (Sandbloom et al. 2001), pain interference (Daut et al. 1983; Owen et al. 2000), dyspnea (Smith et al. 2001), and a number of additional specific symptoms sometimes associated with painful conditions, such as nausea, dry mouth, lack of appetite, fatigue, and constipation (Chang et al. 2000), and negative associations with treatment satisfaction (Lin 2000) and measures of global quality of life (Wang et al. 1999; Chang et al. 2000; Owen et al. 2000; Poulos et al. 2001; Sandbloom et al. 2001).

Further support for the validity of 0–10 NRS-Is comes from Portenoy and colleagues (1999), who found that the responses to this scale showed an appropriate dose-response to treatment with oral transmucosal fentanyl citrate. In another study, a 0–10 NRS-I completed on one occasion predicted subsequent decreases in functioning among 93 persons with various cancer diagnoses (Dodd et al. 2001). However, average NRS-I scale scores may not have ratio qualities (Price et al. 1994), especially when compared to VASs, which do appear to have ratio qualities when averaged across a number of people.

De Wit and colleagues (1999b) showed that 86% of a sample of 156 patients with various cancer diagnoses was able to complete 2 months' worth of daily diaries that included a 0–10 NRS. They found that patient ratings of average pain provided during interviews every two weeks showed strong associations with actual diary averages (r values ranged from 0.80 to 0.91), which provides some support for the validity of retrospective ratings of average pain. However, patient retrospective ratings tended to be higher by about 0.5 on the 0–10 scale, on average, than their actual average pain intensity was (as calculated from the diaries), calling into question the accuracy of retrospective rating of past pain using 0–10 NRSs.

Two studies found that a NRS-I had a very high degree of test–retest stability over a several-minute period ($r = 0.82$, Bergh et al. 2000; $r = 0.91$, Lundeberg et al. 2001). Another study found that very good stability for NRS-I ratings of worst pain ($r = 0.93$) and average pain ($r = 0.78$), but not for current pain ($r = 0.59$), over about a 2-day period (Daut et al. 1983). The coefficients were much lower (0.34, 0.24, and 0.22) when the time period was extended to about 91 days (Daut et al. 1983), although a high degree of stability in pain intensity ratings would not necessarily be expected over a 3-month period, since pain can change from one moment to the next.

Farrar and colleagues (2000) performed a study that provides important information concerning the meaning of change in pain as defined by a 0–10 NRS. They operationalized a meaningful change in pain as that level of change that is associated with a patient *not* requesting a rescue dose as part of a titration phase of a clinical trial. They found that an absolute change of 2 points (out of 10) and a percent change of 33% in the 0–10 NRS showed the optimal sensitivity and specificity for detecting a meaningful change in pain in a sample of 130 patients with various cancer diagnoses. In another study, Farrar and colleagues (2001) performed a study using data from 2724 patients with various chronic pain diagnoses (including diabetic neuropathy, postherpetic neuralgia, chronic low back pain, fibromyalgia, and osteoarthritis) who participated in trials of the effects of pregabalin on pain. In this study, patient ratings of improvement (using a standard 7-point patient global impression of change rating; PGIC) were the standard to which intensity change scores were compared. They found a consistent relationship between change in a 0–10 NRS and the PGIC rating across diagnostic groups. On average, a change of about 30% was associated with a PGIC rating of "much improved" and an average decrease of about 50% was associated with a PGIC rating of "very much improved." Also, and consistent with the findings using 0–10 NRS-Is, reviewed above, subjects with higher baseline pain levels required greater decreases in raw score pain ratings for those changes to be deemed clinically important. This biasing effect of pretreatment pain level did not occur with percent change, however. In a third study, Farrar and colleagues (2003) identified 33% as the 0–10 NRS change score cutoff that was best able to discriminate episodes of pain for which a rescue medication was not needed from episodes of pain for which a rescue medication was requested in a clinical trial of oral transmucosal fentanyl citrate versus immediate release morphine sulfate for breakthrough cancer pain.

Cepeda and colleagues (2003) asked 700 patients who had undergone a surgery to rate their pain intensity before and every 10 minutes after receiving intravenous opioids. Following treatment, they were also asked to rate their level of pain improvement using a 5-point categorical scale. The percent change associated with patient ratings of minimal, much, and very much improvement were 20, 35, and 45%. As a group, these findings on the clinical importance of changes in 0–10 NRS-Is indicate that percent change in the 30–35% range might safely be considered to indicate a meaningful change in pain. Interestingly, this range of percent change is remarkably similar to that found for VAS-I scales (26–41%), reported above.

Also consistent with studies on VAS-I measures, research sometimes finds NRS-Is to be a little more responsive to changes in pain than other measures (Jensen et al. 1998; Du Pen et al. 1999; Eisenberg et al. 2001), sometimes a little less responsive (Portenoy et al. 1999), and sometimes to show essentially the same level of responsivity (Bolton et al. 1998; Ekblom and Hansson 1988). One study, cited above, found an 11-point NRS-I to be about as responsive as a VAS-I, and both of these to be more responsive than a 4-point VRS-I (Breivik et al. 2000). In short, if a treatment has a significant effect on pain, the evidence indicates that the NRS-I (or VAS-I or VRS-I, for that matter) is about as likely as other measures of pain intensity to detect the effect of the treatment.

On the other hand, NRS-Is tend to be preferred over VASs by patients (Williams et al. 2000). Interestingly, among possible ranges of NRS, a 0–10 range is most preferred (by 54% of respondents), followed by a 0–100 range (16%), followed by 0–20 (1%; Williams et al. 2000), in a sample of patients with chronic pain. Twenty-nine percent of the respondents in this study did not have a preference for one pain measure over the others. In another study, there appeared to be a slight preference for a NRS-I over a VRS-I in a sample of English-speaking patients seeking care in an emergency room (59% preferred the NRS-I and 41% preferred the VRS-I; Puntillo and Neighbor 1997). However, among the Spanish-speaking patients, there was a tendency for the VRS-I (55%) to be preferred over the NRS-I (45%). But these differences in preference rates were not statistically significant for either sample (Puntillo and Neighbor 1997).

Cognitive impairment may interfere with the comprehension and use of pain rating scales, although it may impact the use of some scales more than others. Radbruch and colleagues (Radbruch et al. 2000) administered a Mini Mental Status Examination (MMSE) to 108 patients with advanced cancer in a palliative care unit, and also attempted to administer the Brief Pain Inventory (Cleeland and Ryan 1994) intensity and interference items (all 0–10 NRSs) to these patients. If the patients were unable to complete the BPI items, they were asked to scale the intensity of their pain on a 4-point VRS (none, mild, moderate, severe). If they were unable to use the 4-point VRS, they were simply asked to confirm the presence or absence of pain (i.e., a 2-point VRS-I) along with other symptoms. Radbruch and colleagues found that only 75% of these patients with advanced cancer were able to complete the 0–10 intensity items, and 62% the 0–10 interference items. Moreover, the number of missing responses for the BPI intensity items ($r = -0.64$) and interference items ($r = -0.47$) were both associated significantly with the MMSE score, indicating that a patient's degree of cognitive impairment impacts his or her ability to respond appropriately to 0–10 NRS scales. However, many of the patients unable to complete the BPI 0–10 NRS items were able to complete a 4-point VRS of pain

intensity, and all of the patients, even those who could not rate their pain using a 4-point VRS, were able to report on the presence or absence of pain.

Verbal Rating Scale of pain intensity

Verbal Rating Scales of pain intensity (VRS-I), also known as categorical scales, consist of a list of descriptors or phrases (e.g., "none," "some," "moderate," "severe") that represent varying degrees of pain intensity. Each word or phrase has a number associated with it (e.g., "none" = 0, "severe" = 3). Respondents are asked to select the single word or phrase that best represents his or her pain level, and the respondent's score is the number associated with the word chosen. In the pain literature, the number of descriptors in VRS-Is can range from 4 (e.g., Seymour 1982) to as many as 15 (e.g., Gracely et al. 1978; and this latter scale would have 16 descriptors if "no pain" were added to it).

Like VAS-Is and NRS-Is, VRS-Is demonstrate responsivity to changes in pain with treatment (Fox and Melzack 1976; Rybstein-Blinchik 1979; Stambaugh and Sarajian 1981; Tannock et al. 1989; Bergman et al. 1992; Stelian et al. 1992; Bergman et al. 1994; Murphy et al. 1994; Ellershaw et al. 1995; Ingham et al. 1996; Tannock et al. 1996; Hammerlid et al. 1997; Bolton and Wilkinson 1998; Farrar et al. 1998; Rogers et al. 1998a; Portenoy et al. 1999; Molenaar et al. 2001; Doyle et al. 2002; Jensen et al. 2002; Kubitzek et al. 2003), and show strong associations with other measures of pain intensity (Kremer et al. 1981; Walsh and Leber 1983; Littman et al. 1985; Jensen et al. 1986; Fishman et al. 1987; Ekblom and Hansson 1988; Paice and Cohen 1997; Rogers et al. 1998b; Klepstad et al. 2000). Concerning test–retest stability, one study found the VRS-I to be adequately stable over a matter of minutes (kappa = 0.71; Ellershaw et al. 1995), and a second found the VRS-I to demonstrate relatively low stability ($r = 0.55$; Sneeuw et al. 1997) over a 1-week period.

Although VRSs are usually scored by using a rank method (e.g., scoring "no pain" as 0, "mild pain" as 1, "moderate pain" as 2, etc.), this scoring method has been criticized because it assumes equal intervals between the intensity descriptors, even though it is extremely unlikely that equal perceptual intervals exist. This characteristic of rank-scoring procedures can pose several problems when one is interpreting VRS data given that, rank scoring does not allow for adequate interpretations of the magnitude of any differences found. For example, a change from 3 to 2 (on a 4-point VRS) might represent a 10% decrease in perceived pain or a 50% change, depending on the perceived interval represented by the words on the list. In addition, some investigators have raised the objection that ranked data should not be analyzed with the more common (and usually more powerful) parametric statistics. However, it has become increasingly recognized that most parametric techniques (such as analysis of variance and the t-test) are still valid when used with data that do not necessarily represent equal-interval values, especially if the number of categories on the scale is five or more (Cicchetti et al. 1985; Philip 1990; Rasmussen 1989; see also Baker et al. 1966).

Cross-modality matching procedures have been used as a means of transforming VRS ratings to scale scores that are more likely to have ratio properties, that is, to scores with equivalent intervals (Gracely et al. 1978a,b; Price et al. 2001). The matching procedure involves asking each patient to indicate the severity that each word represents in reference to one or more other modalities (such as the loudness of a tone, the length of a line, or handgrip force). The rating that the patient gives to a particular word (or the average of several, if the patient rates each word more than once) is then used as the score for that word for that patient. Because the modalities used by patients to match pain descriptors can themselves be indexed using ratio scales, the numbers or scores derived from such a procedure are believed likely to have ratio properties and to reflect actual perceived differences in magnitudes.

There are two major limitations of cross-modality matching procedures. First, the procedure is time consuming and can be tedious, both of which can adversely affect patient compliance (Ahles et al. 1984). One way to address this problem is to assign standardized scores for each word based on data from groups of previously tested individuals (see Gracely et al. 1978a; Tursky et al. 1982; Urban et al. 1984 for standardized scores for specific words). Second, most of the standardized scores have been developed using nonpatients in response to experimental pain. There is evidence that chronic pain patients may rate the intensity of pain words differently than do patients with acute (i.e., postoperative) pain (Wallenstein et al. 1980). Even within diagnostic subgroups, the score given to a word by one patient has been shown to vary from that given by other patients, indicating that standardized scores for VRS adjectives may be less reliable than originally hoped (Urban et al. 1984).

Moreover, VRS-I scores obtained through cross-modality procedures may correlate so highly with those obtained by using the ranking method that they contain essentially the same degree of useful information (Hall 1981; Levine and De Simone 1991). Similarly, VRS-I scores created by either of the two methods show the same patterns of associations to other pain measures, again suggesting that the information contained in the scores derived from the two methods are comparable (Jensen et al. 1989). Therefore, until strong evidence emerges to support the validity and utility of cross-modality matching procedures or scores over ranked scores, it probably makes sense to use the simpler ranking method when relationships between pain intensity and other factors are examined. The more

sophisticated cross-modality matching procedures might be considered when ratio-like scaling is required (i.e., when one needs to know the specific magnitude of differences in pain ratings across time or between groups).

The strengths of VRS-Is include the ease with which they can be administered and scored, provided that scores are calculated using the ranking method or from data developed from previous cross-modality matching experiments. Because they are generally easy to comprehend, compliance rates for VRS-Is are as good and often better than those for other measures of pain intensity (Jensen et al. 1986, 1989). For example, in the study cited above on compliance rates, many of the patients with advanced cancer in a palliative care unit who were unable to complete 0–10 NRSs were able to complete a simple 4-point VRS (Radbruch et al. 2000). VRS-Is are also often preferred as much (Puntillo and Neighbor 1997) or even more than NRS-Is (Kremer et al. 1981).

One weakness of VRSs is that patients need to read over, or be familiar with, the entire list of pain adjectives before they can select the one that most closely describes their pain. For longer lists (e.g., 15 or more items), this requirement can make the task time consuming, and the clinician or researcher cannot be assured that the patient or subject adequately reviewed the entire list of adjectives. Also, because VRS-Is require patients to select from a finite number of descriptors, patients may be unable to find one that accurately describes their perceived pain intensity (Joyce et al. 1975). Among illiterate patients, VRSs are less reliable than other pain intensity measures (Ferraz et al. 1990). When differences are found in the relative sensitivity of scales for detecting treatment effects, VRS-Is tend not to fare as well as VAS-Is or NRS-Is (e.g., Breivik et al. 2000). Finally, a clinician or researcher using a Verbal Rating Scale must select a scoring procedure; and, as already discussed, each scoring method has its drawbacks. Possibly because of the relative weaknesses of VRSs, and the availability of other measures of pain intensity, VRSs are being used less often as primary outcome measures than they have previously in pain treatment outcome research.

Other single-item measures of pain intensity

Single-item measures other than VAS-Is, NRS-Is, and VRS-Is are used much less often to assess pain intensity in pain research. Measures that have been used include Mechanical Visual Analogue Scales, Graphic Rating Scales, Face Scales, and various combination scales.

A Mechanical Visual Analogue Scale of pain intensity (M-VAS-I) is very similar to the VAS-I, except that instead of making a pencil or pen mark on a line on a paper, the respondent moves a slider between the two extremes of pain on a plastic or cardboard scale.

The scale administrator then looks on the back of the scale and directly reads the distance that the slider was moved from a ruler printed on the back of the measure. M-VAS-Is are very strongly associated with VAS-Is ($r = 0.99$, Grossman et al. 1992; $r = 0.77$, Ramer et al. 1999) and other pain intensity ratings (Geddes et al. 1990; Ramer et al. 1999). They are also highly reliable over a 5-minute period ($r = 0.95$, Grossman et al. 1992). In short, they appear to share many of the properties of VAS-Is.

Graphic Rating Scales of pain intensity (GRS-I) are also similar to VAS-Is. The primary difference is that GRS-Is add specific markers along the VAS continuum with labels associated with each marker. For example, a GRS-I used by Greenwald and colleagues (1987) consisted of a 100 mm line with the numbers 1 through 5 evenly spaced along the line, and descriptors ("no pain," "slight pain," "moderate pain," "very bad pain," "pain as bad as can be") below each number. Depending on the specific instructions, respondents to GRSs might circle the number or descriptor or make a mark on the line (using the numbers or descriptors as guidelines) that best represents their pain intensity. McMillan and colleagues (1988) showed that a 0–10 GRS was sensitive to decreases in pain that occurred when a pain monitoring system in an inpatient cancer treatment center was established. Ekblom and Hansson (1988) found that a GRS-I showed a similar sensitivity to change in pain with treatment as did a VAS-I and NRS-I.

Face Scales of pain intensity present the respondent with drawings of facial expressions representing increasing levels of pain intensity and suffering. Respondents select the single drawing that best represents their pain level, and their score is the number (rank order) of the expression chosen. Although Face Scales were originally developed, and have been primarily used, for assessing pediatric pain, Face Scales have also been used to assess pain intensity in adults. Evidence supports the ability of Face Scales to detect changes in pain with treatment (Bellamy et al. 1999). Two studies found the Face Scale to show strong associations with a VAS-I in two separate samples of patients with pain (e.g., $r = 0.82$, Ramer et al. 1999;

$r = 0.92$, Freeman et al. 2001), and Shannon et al. (1995) found that about 81% of their sample with various cancer diagnoses were able to complete the Face Scale (compared with 75% who were able to complete a VAS-I and 89% a VRS-I). These preliminary studies suggest that Face Scales could potentially be valid as measures of pain intensity. However, Ramer and colleagues (1999) commented that some of the male patients in their study were uncomfortable with rating their pain at the highest level using the Face Scale because the expression representing the most severe level of pain had tears on the face of the drawing. This raises the possibility that the Face Scale (or at least one that includes tears) may underestimate pain intensity in some patients with severe pain.

Finally, different components of pain intensity measures can be combined into single scales (e.g., combine numbers with descriptors making a NRS/VRS-I: see Grossman et al. 1992; Campbell et al. 2000; Maunsell et al. 2000; or a diagram with descriptors: see Sneeuw et al. 1999; Sneeuw et al. 1997). The evidence from studies looking at NRS/VRS-Is suggests that they, too, are valid as measures of pain intensity, as shown by their strong associations with other measures of pain intensity (Grossman et al. 1992), association with analgesic use, pain interference, and measures of global quality of life (Maunsell et al. 2000), and association with treatment history and concern about cancer (Campbell et al. 2000).

MEASURES OF PAIN RELIEF

Whereas pain intensity ratings ask patients to rate the intensity of felt pain, pain relief ratings ask patients to rate how much "relief" from pain they have experienced, usually in reference to a specific treatment or intervention. Table 5.2 lists and summarizes the primary findings of this review concerning the assessment of pain relief in clinical trials.

Relief ratings have been shown to be sensitive to the effects of treatment (VAS relief ratings: Wallenstein 1991; Shannon et al. 1995; Manfredi et al. 2000; VRS relief ratings: Stambaugh and Saragian 1981; Littman et al. 1985; Wallenstein 1991; Farrar et al. 1998; Barton

Table 5.2 Summary of the primary research findings on measures of pain relief

Relatively little research has compared VAS, NRS, and VRS pain relief measures to each other
Pain relief measures are sensitive (sometimes more so than pain intensity measures) to the effects of pain treatments

Measures of pain relief are statistically distinct from measures of pain intensity:
    Pain relief is sometimes endorsed even when pain changes little or worsens
    Perceived pain relief is more strongly associated with treatment satisfaction than with change in pain intensity

VAS = Visual Analogue Scale; NRS = Numerical Rating Scale; VRS = Verbal Rating Scale.

et al. 2002; Steiner et al. 2003; Kubitzek et al. 2003; Lynch et al. 2003; 0–100% relief rating: Gammaitoni et al. 2003; Hwang et al. 2003). Also, in one study, relief ratings were strongly and negatively associated with pain intensity ratings (VAS relief rating, Fishman et al. 1987). However, in two other studies, the associations between pain relief and pain intensity measures were weak (VAS rating, Ramer et al. 1999; NRS rating, Daut and Cleeland 1982).

Pain relief ratings may be somewhat more sensitive to changes in pain associated with treatment when compared to pain intensity change scores in some situations (Ohnhaus and Adler 1975; Littman et al. 1985; Wallenstein 1999; Fischer et al. 1999). However, the differences in sensitivity are rarely large. Also, some studies have found relief ratings to be less sensitive (Hwang et al. 2003), and some about as sensitive (Ekblom and Hansson 1988; Jensen et al. 2002), as pain intensity change scores. Thus, the use of relief ratings over pain intensity change scores will not usually result in substantial increases in ability to detect treatment effects.

Supporting the validity of relief ratings as indicants of change in pain intensity, some studies have shown positive associations between pain intensity change scores and relief ratings (VAS, Angst et al. 1999; NRS, De Conno et al. 1994). Interestingly, however, the association between pain relief and change in pain intensity is not always strong, so ratings of these two constructs (pre- to post-treatment change in pain, pain relief) appear to measure related but also distinct constructs (Haas et al. 2002). For example, Angst and colleagues (1999) found that when pain intensity and pain relief were assessed 10, 20, and 30 minutes following an infusion (pain intensity was also assessed pre-infusion), pain relief ratings tended to increase as pain intensity decreased. However, for many patients, pain relief ratings remained above 0 (indicating at least some relief) even when pain intensity returned to pre-infusion levels (see also Dalton et al. 1988). Similarly, Jensen and colleagues (2002) found that the strength of the association between pain relief and change in pain ratings decreased as time since pretreatment increased (see also Feine et al. 1998). In this study, the correlation coefficients between pain relief and pain intensity change scores were 0.75 and 0.80 in two samples of post-operative patients 15 minutes following treatment, but dropped to between 0.56 and 0.65 by 24 hours after treatment. Moreover, a close examination of their data indicated that there was always a subset of patients who reported that they experienced some pain relief even when pain was higher post-treatment relative to pretreatment levels (Jensen et al. 2002).

Further support for the distinction between pain relief and pain intensity change scores was found by Fischer and colleagues (1999), who reported that perceived pain relief was more strongly associated with satisfaction with treatment than was actual change in pain intensity (change in pain intensity ratings). Consistent with this finding, De Wit and colleagues (1999a) demonstrated the distinction between a VRS rating of pain relief from a measure of pain intensity by performing a factor analysis of pain intensity ratings, a VRS rating of pain relief, and other measures. They found that the pain relief rating loaded with measures of treatment satisfaction and perceived adequacy of analgesia, but not with the pain intensity ratings. In short, the data strongly support the conclusion that perceived pain relief and change in pain intensity are related but also distinct dimensions of pain.

Farrar and colleagues' (2000) findings concerning the meaningfulness of change in pain as measured by a change in a 0–10 NRS were described above. These investigators also identified the specific rating of relief (using a 5-point VRS-R scale: none, slight, moderate, lots, complete) best associated with a meaningful change in pain. They found that a rating of "moderate" relief best represented meaningful change to the participants with cancer pain in their study, supporting this rating as a reasonable treatment outcome goal if relief ratings are included as an outcome measure in a clinical trial.

MEASURES OF THE QUALITATIVE AND AFFECTIVE COMPONENTS OF PAIN

Pain has many sensory and affective qualities in addition to its intensity component. The most common measure of these aspects of pain is the McGill Pain Questionnaire, but the short-form McGill Pain Questionnaire and single-item ratings have also been used, and there are a number of new measures of pain quality designed to assess neuropathic pain, specifically: the Neuropathic Pain Scale (and associated Pain Quality Assessment Scale), the Leeds Assessment of Neuropathic Signs and Symptoms Pain Scale, the Neuropathic Pain Questionnaire, and the Neuropathic Pain Symptom Inventory. Table 5.3 lists and summarizes the primary findings of this review concerning the assessment of pain quality (including pain affect) in clinical trials. A summary of the primary pain assessment recommendations is provided in Table 5.4.

McGill Pain Questionnaire (MPQ)

The MPQ consists of 78 pain descriptors classified into 20 categories of pain that can be scored to assess four major dimensions of pain: sensory, affective, evaluative, and miscellaneous pain, as well as a total pain severity score ("Pain Rating Index" or "PRI" MPQ scores represent the sum of the ranked values of descriptors selected within each pain dimension and "Number of Words Chosen" or "NWC" MPQ scores represent the total number of words selected within each pain dimension; Melzack 1975). Data support the conclusion that the MPQ qualitative scale scores assess

Table 5.3 Summary of the primary research findings on measures of pain qualities (including pain affect)

Measures of pain quality and affect used relatively infrequently in pain clinical trials
Evidence supports the validity of the MPQ, SF-MPQ and NPS as outcome measures
The MPQ and SF-MPQ scale scores appear to be less sensitive than measures of pain intensity to changes in pain
Use of MPQ and SF-MPQ scale scores obscures the specific qualities of pain
Evidence supports the NPS items for identifying the effects of pain treatments on specific pain qualities
The NPS and NPSI lack content validity for assessing all of the most common neuropathic pain qualities; while there is some overlap in content, there are also pain qualities assessed that are unique to each measure
The PQAS appears to have adequate content validity for assessing both neuropathic and non-neuropathic pain; however, there are not data yet available for the PQAS items that do not overlap with the NPS items
The LANSS, LANSS-S, NPQ, and NPQ-SF are able to distinguish neuropathic from non-neuropathic pain; the LANSS appears to be more accurate than the other measures
Data regarding the validity of single-item measures of pain affect are limited and mixed

MPQ = McGill Pain Questionnaire; SF-MPQ = short-form McGill Pain Questionnaire; NPS = Neuropathic Pain Scale; NPSI = Neuropathic Pain Symptom Inventory; PQAS = Pain Quality Assessment Scale; LANSS = Leeds Assessment of Neuropathic Symptoms and Signs Pain Scale; LANSS-S = Leeds Assessment of Neuropathic Symptoms and Signs Pain Scale – short form; NPQ = Neuropathic Pain Questionnaire; NPQ-SF = Neuropathic Pain Questionnaire – short form.

something other than pain intensity. For example, Chung and colleagues (2001) found very weak associations between a pain intensity rating and both the total MPQ-NWC ($r = -0.09$) and total MPQ-PRI ($r = 0.00$). Other investigators have found stronger associations between MPQ scale scores and pain intensity ratings (Graham et al. 1980, r values up to 0.40, lowest r-value not specified; Ahles et al. 1984, r ranged from 0.49 to 0.57; Wilkie et al. 1992, r up to 0.58, lowest r-value not specified; Zalon 1999, r between 0.33 and 0.76). While these associations are usually positive, indicating that the MPQ scales and pain intensity usually assess related dimensions, they are not strong enough to support the conclusion that MPQ scales and pain intensity rating scales assess the same thing.

Further evidence for a distinction between the MPQ scale scores and pain intensity ratings was found by De Conno and colleagues (1994). They performed two factor analyses using a VAS-I, a NRS-I, a VRS-I, the MPQ-PRI score, and a composite measure of the frequency of five different qualities of pain obtained at two different points in time in 53 patients with various cancer diagnoses. A single factor emerged from each factor analysis, with the three pain intensity measures loading most strongly on this factor (factor loadings ranged from 0.79 to 0.92), and the MPQ-PRI showing a weak loading in one analysis (0.39; but it showed a stronger loading in the second analysis, 0.72). Similarly, a factor analysis of change scores in these measures from one time point to the next, plus a 5-point rating of pain relief, resulted in a single factor with the pain intensity change scores showing stronger loadings (range = 0.80 to 0.83) and the MPQ-PRI

score showing a weaker loading (0.47) on this factor (De Conno et al. 1994).

The MPQ scales have been found to be positively associated with analgesic medication use (Ahles et al. 1983), illness conviction (Dalton et al. 1988), and reported quality of life (Schipper et al. 1984). Also, the MPQ scales have shown expected responsivity to the effects of pain treatments (Briggs 1996; Burchiel et al. 1996; Eija et al. 1996; Nikolajsen et al. 1996; Pozehl et al. 1995; Tannock et al. 1989; Tesfaye et al. 1996; Plesh et al. 2000; Naeser et al. 2002; Lynch et al. 2003), supporting the validity of the MPQ scales as measures of pain. Support for the validity of the MPQ-Affective scale to assess the affective component of pain, specifically, was reported by Ahles and colleagues (1983), who found that this scale was more strongly associated with measures of psychological distress that with measures of pain intensity. Also, Kremer and colleagues (1982) reported that cancer patients with low pain intensity report a greater affective component of their pain on the MPQ-Affective scale than patients with low back pain do, consistent with the hypothesis that cancer pain may have a greater affective associations (e.g., be more worrisome and cause more fear) than low back pain.

Responses to the MPQ have also been found to discriminate between different pain diagnoses. For example, in an early study, Dubuisson and Melzack (1976) found that patients with each of eight types of pain (e.g., menstrual pain, toothache, cancer pain) used different words from the MPQ to describe their pain experience. Subsequent investigators have found that the MPQ scales and/or items can discriminate between

Table 5.4 Pain assessment recommendations

Pain intensity

In most trials, a measure of pain intensity is the appropriate primary outcome dimension

The 0–10 NRS-I appears to have the most strengths and fewest weaknesses of pain intensity measures

VRS-4-I (none, mild, moderate, severe) may be a useful secondary measure

Pain relief

Should be considered as a secondary outcome measure in pain clinical trials

No strong evidence to support one type of pain relief measure (VAS-R, NRS-R, VRS-R) over the others, although concerns raised about VAS-I may encourage investigators to select a NRS-R (e.g., 0 = none; 10 = complete) or VRS-R (e.g., none, a little, some, a lot, complete relief) over a VAS-R for this purpose

The VRS-R may be more useful than the VAS-R or NRS-R, because the use of specific categorical descriptors may help patients distinguish the VRS-R from VAS or NRS measures of pain intensity

Qualitative aspects of pain (including affective quality[ies])

Should be considered as secondary outcome measure(s) in pain clinical trials

Measures that can be scored to identify changes in specific pain qualities (e.g., SF-MPQ, PQAS, NPS, NPSI) can be used to determine if treatments affect some pain qualities more than others. Such information may be used to identify the patients for whom the treatments may be most effective, and also may ultimately be useful for identifying the mechanism(s) of treatment efficacy

The 20-item PQAS appears to be the most content valid of the pain quality scales that assess specific pain qualities and casts a "wider net" than the other available measures

If assessment burden is a significant issue, the 15-item SF-MPQ should be considered when assessing non-neuropathic pain conditions, and the 10-item NPS or 12-item NPSI when assessing neuropathic pain

The LANSS (both the clinician-administered and self-administered versions) appears to be the most useful measure available for distinguishing neuropathic from non-neuropathic pain. This measure might be improved further by adding other items that assess pain qualities also shown to differentiate between pain types

Single-item measures (VAS-A, NRS-A, VRS-A) may provide a useful summary measure of pain affect if a measure of pain affect is needed and a multiple-item measure is not practical. If a single-item measure is chosen, the VRS-A may be more effective than VAS-A or NRS-A for helping subjects distinguish between pain affect and intensity

The MPQ or SF-MPQ affective scale scores should be considered over single-item ratings if a measure of pain affect is needed; they probably tap into the complex (and multidimensional) construct of pain affect more effectively than single-item ratings do

NRS-I = Numerical Rating Scale of pain intensity; VRS-4-I = 4-item Verbal Rating Scale (categorical scale) of pain intensity; VAS-R = Visual Analogue Scale of pain relief; NRS-R = Numerical Rating Scale of pain relief; VRS-R = Verbal Rating Scale (categorical scale) of pain relief; SF-MPQ = short-form McGill Pain Questionnaire; PQAS = Pain Quality Assessment Scale; NPS = Neuropathic Pain Scale; NPSI = Neuropathic Pain Symptom Inventory; NPQ = Neuropathic Pain Questionnaire; LANSS = Leeds Assessment of Neuropathic Symptoms and Signs Pain Scale; MPQ = McGill Pain Questionnaire; VAS-A = Visual Analogue Scale of pain affect; NRS-A = Numerical Rating Scale of pain affect; VRS-A = Verbal Rating Scale of pain affect.

patients whose pain can be ascribed to physical causes from patients whose pain had no detectable physical cause (Leavitt and Garron 1980; Perry et al. 1988, 1991), patients who carried a diagnosis of trigeminal neuralgia from patients who carried a diagnosis of atypical facial pain (Melzack et al. 1986), patients with leg pain caused by diabetic neuropathy from patients with leg pain from other origins (Masson et al. 1989), patients with cluster headache from patients with other (migraine and mixed) headache (Jerome et al. 1988),

patients with temporal mandibular joint-related pain from patients with myogenous facial pain (Mongini and Italiano 2001), and patients with nociceptive from patients with neuropathic pain (Wilke et al. 2001). However, the MPQ descriptors have not been universally successful in distinguishing patients with different types of pain problems (Seymour et al. 1983).

Several studies have examined the reliability of the MPQ. In studies with patients with cancer pain, studies have found that responses to the MPQ are generally consistent over the time span of several days (Graham et al. 1980; Love et al. 1989; Walsh and Leber 1983). In a study with patients with low back pain, Love and colleagues (Love et al. 1989) found adequate test–retest stability for the MPQ scale scores (Total: $r = 0.83$; Sensory: $r = 0.76$; Affective: $r = 0.78$) over the course of several days. Concerning utility, one study found the MPQ to be difficult for many persons with terminal cancer receiving palliative care to use (Talmi et al. 1997). However, a second study found that 84% of a sample of patients with cancer were able to complete the MPQ (Shannon et al. 1995).

Despite some evidence that the MPQ scales are responsive to the effects of pain treatments, when differences are found in the sensitivity of MPQ scales compared to the more simple pain intensity ratings, the MPQ scales tend to be less able to detect changes in pain than the intensity ratings are (Jenkinson et al. 1995; Bellamy et al. 1999; Graff-Radford 2000). Interestingly, however, the failure rate of the MPQ (among the elderly) is higher for the traditional VAS measure (30%) than for the MPQ (13%) (although the failure rate for a simple 6-point VRS was even less among the elderly in this sample: 9%) (Gagliese and Melzack 1997).

Short-Form McGill Pain Questionnaire (SF-MPQ)

The SF-MPQ consists of a subset of 15 descriptors from the MPQ drawn from the sensory and affective categories (Melzack 1987). Responses to the 15 SF-MPQ items can be scored to form a total SF-MPQ score as well as both Sensory and Affective SF-MPQ subscale scores.

While not a great deal of research has been performed with the SF-MPQ, the research that has been performed is promising. The SF-MPQ Sensory, Affective, and Total scores are strongly associated with the original MPQ scales (Dudgeon et al. 1993; Melzack 1987). Also, preliminary data suggest that the SF-MPQ items, like the items from the original MPQ, may be useful in discriminating patients with different types of pain problems from one another (Melzack 1987), although they may not appear to be useful for distinguishing between different types or etiologies of spinal cord injury-related pain (Putzke et al. 2002).

In one study, the internal consistency (Cronbach's alpha) of the SF-MPQ items was shown to be excellent in a sample of persons with cancer pain (0.91; Hollen et al. 1994a). However, in a sample of patients with post-operative pain, the internal consistency of the total scale score (0.72 for describing current pain and 0.85 for describing pain in the past 24 hours) and the subscales (Sensory: 0.64 for current pain and 0.81 for pain in the past 24 hours; Affective: 0.41 for current pain and 0.63 for pain in the past 24 hours) were diminished. Also, the two SF-MPQ subscales were strongly associated with one another, suggesting the possibility that they may tap into a similar underlying construct (Hollen et al. 1994b).

The SF-MPQ Total and scale scores have also been shown to be sensitive to the effects of pain treatments (Serrao et al. 1992; King et al. 1993; Fowlow et al. 1995; Thomas et al. 1995; Backonja et al. 1998; Rowbotham et al. 1998; Rice et al. 2001), but like the MPQ, the SF-MPQ scales do not appear to be as sensitive to the effects of pain treatments as more traditional single-item pain intensity rating scales (Stelian et al. 1992; Frost et al. 2000; but see Harden et al. 1991 for a study in which the SF-MPQ was about as sensitive as a VAS-I for detecting a treatment effect).

Neuropathic Pain Scale and Pain Quality Assessment Scale

The Neuropathic Pain Scale (NPS) was developed to assess the pain qualities most common to neuropathic pain conditions (Galer and Jensen 1997). This measure sought to retain an ability to assess the multiple components and qualities of neuropathic pain, while also maintaining brevity to minimize assessment burden. Also, by assessing and scoring each of 10 pain domains specifically (and not necessarily combining the items into composite scale scores), it was hoped that the NPS could be used to identify profiles of pain qualities associated with different neuropathic pain diagnoses and also to identify the specific effects of pain treatments on different pain qualities. To the extent that different pain descriptors reflect different underlying pain mechanisms, a measure such as the NPS might also be useful for diagnosing pain conditions by pain mechanism and not just by pain site ("low back pain") or condition ("cancer pain").

The 10 NPS items include two global ratings (pain intensity and pain unpleasantness) and eight descriptors. The descriptors ask patients to rate six specific pain qualities (sharp, hot, dull, cold, sensitive, itchy) and two pain locations (deep, surface). Respondents are asked to rate the intensity or severity of each pain descriptor on 0–10 scales, with 0 = "No _____" (for intense, deep, and surface pain) or "Not _____" (for unpleasant, sharp, hot, dull, cold, sensitive, and itchy) for the other pain qualities, and 10 = "The most _____ sensation imaginable" (e.g., "intense pain," "sharp," etc.). The NPS also includes a single item that allows respondents to describe the temporal pattern of their pain (background pain with occasional flare-ups, single constant pain, or intermittent pain).

Preliminary evidence supports the validity of the NPS for assessing neuropathic pain. For example, the items are sensitive to treatments known to impact neuropathic pain (Galer and Jensen 1997), and the associations among the items tend to be weak to moderate, supporting their discriminant validity (Galer and

Jensen 1997). The NPS items are also able to discriminate among patients with different neuropathic pain conditions (Galer and Jensen 1997; Carter et al. 1998; Galer et al. 2000).

Moreover, preliminary evidence suggests that different treatments might impact the NPS items differentially, supporting the potential use of the NPS as means to determine a profile effect for specific treatments. For example, in one study, intravenous adenosine had a significant effect on the NPS intensity, unpleasantness, hot, sensitive, and itchy items, but not on the other NPS items, relative to placebo, in a sample of patients with neuropathic pain (Lynch et al. 2003). In a different study, controlled-release oxycodone was effective for reducing both the NPS intensity and unpleasantness global ratings as well as sharp, hot, dull, and deep pain sensations, relative to placebo, in a sample of patients with diabetic neuropathy (Jensen et al. 2002). In this study, oxycodone did not show a significant effect on cold, itchy, or surface pain, relative to placebo. In a third study, gabapentin was only effective for reducing the global rating of pain intensity, relative to placebo, and showed nonsignificant trends for reducing hot pain ($p = 0.065$) and pain unpleasantness ($p = 0.094$) in a small sample ($N = 7$) of patients with spinal cord injury and chronic pain. These preliminary studies suggest the potential of the NPS for identifying patients who might benefit most from specific treatments; for example, patients reporting hot, dull, and deep pains may be most likely to benefit from oxycodone, while patients reporting high levels of hot, sensitive, and itchy pain may be more likely to benefit from intravenous adenosine.

Although the NPS was originally designed to be scored to create a "profile" of sensation severity across the different pain quality domains, it is possible to combine the item responses into specific composite scores. Galer and colleagues (2002), for example, created four different NPS composite scores when examining the effects of a lidocaine patch in a sample of patients with post-herpetic neuralgia: an average of all 10 items (NPS10), an average of the eight descriptors excluding the global ratings of pain intensity and unpleasantness (NPS8), an average of the eight items that do not reflect allodynia (i.e., excluding the "sensitive" and "surface" items; NPS NA), and an average of four items thought to reflect peripheral pain mechanisms ("dull," "deep," "sharp," and "burning" items; NPS4). Interestingly, although the individual NPS items (including the global pain intensity item) did not show significant treatment effects in this study, the composite scores all showed significant treatment effects, relative to placebo. The NPS4 was similarly shown to be responsive to the effects of an oxycodone/acetaminophen formulation, relative to placebo, in a sample of patients with low back pain

(Gammaitoni et al. 2003). However, data concerning the relative sensitivity of the other NPS scale scores and items were not reported in this latter study.

Despite data that support the validity of the NPS for assessing neuropathic pain, it has some drawbacks. First, there are some pain qualities associated with neuropathic pain that were not included in the original NPS items. These include electric, tingling (or "pins and needles") and numb sensations (Boureau et al. 1990; Bennett 2001; Wilkie et al. 2001; Krause and Backonja 2003). These items should be added to the NPS. In addition, limiting a measure to only pain qualities common to neuropathic pain conditions limits the ability of that measure to assess pain qualities in other pain conditions, and also, perhaps to help differentiate neuropathic from non-neuropathic pain conditions. Thus, the NPS would also be improved if it included pain qualities common to other pain conditions, such as a number of the pain quality domains included in the MPQ-SF that are not on the NPS (e.g., tender, shooting, cramping, throbbing, aching, and heavy). A number of these additional pain qualities have traditionally thought to be primarily associated with nociceptive pain, although data suggest that this may only be the case for the descriptor "heavy" (Boureau et al. 1990; Wilkie et al. 2001). The descriptors "tender," "throbbing," and "aching" may in fact be more common among patients with neuropathic than nociceptive pain (Wilkie et al. 2001). In any case, the content validity of the NPS for assessing both neuropathic and non-neuropathic pain would be expanded considerably by the inclusion of items that assess these additional pain qualities.

An expanded NPS was therefore recently created that included not only the original 10 NPS descriptors, but also an additional 10 descriptors common to neuropathic and also to non-neuropathic pain conditions. The NPS temporal pain pattern item was also revised slighty to more clearly differentiate between three primary temporal patterns of pain: intermittent (i.e., variable pain with some pain-free periods), variable (variable pain without pain-free periods), and stable (i.e., constant pain with little variation) pain. Because the new measure might be useful for describing the pain qualities of persons with both neuropathic and non-neuropathic pain, the word "neuropathic" was removed from the title. The new measure is called the *Pain Quality Assessment Scale (PQAS)* and is presented in Appendix 5.1. The 10 NPS items within this scale already have preliminary support for their validity as measures of neuropathic pain. Psychometric data are now being collected using the PQAS in samples of patients with both neuropathic and non-neuropathic pain to further validate the original NPS items, as well as to obtain validity data concerning the additional items that make up the PQAS.

Leeds Assessment of Neuropathic Symptoms and Signs (LANSS) Pain Scale

The Leeds Assessment of Neuropathic Symptoms and Signs (LANSS) Pain Scale was designed to help distinguish neuropathic from nociceptive pain (Bennett 2001). It has two components: a pain questionnaire and a sensory testing component. The pain questionnaire consists of five items that ask respondents to indicate, yes or no, if their pain could be described as: (1) "strange, unpleasant sensations...like pricking, tingling, pins and needles...;" (2) "[making]...the skin in the painful area look different from normal...like mottled...;" (3) "[making]...the affected skin abnormally sensitive to touch...;" (4) "[coming]...on suddenly and in bursts for no apparent reason...like electric shocks, jumping and bursting...;" (5) "[feeling]...as if the skin temperature in the painful area has changed abnormally...like hot and burning..." The sensory testing component asks a clinician to test for allodynia (by lightly stroking a nonpainful and the painful area with cotton wool) and to test to altered pin-prick threshold (by comparing the patient response to a 23 gauge needle mounted inside of a syringe barrel placed gently on the skin in a nonpainful and then in the pain area). Each response is weighted, and the weights of all positive responses are summed to create a total score, with a score of less than 12 indicating an unlikelihood that neuropathic mechanisms are contributing to the patient's pain, and a score of 12 or greater indicating that neuropathic mechanisms are likely to be contributing to the patient's pain.

Initial validation comparing samples of patients with neuropathic versus nociceptive pain indicated a very high rate of accurate classification (85%) with high degrees of both sensitivity (83%) and specificity (87%; Bennett 2001). These rates were replicated in a cross-validation sample, with 82% correct identification, 85% sensitivity, and 80% specificity (Bennett 2001). Support for the reliability of the LANSS items was evidenced by a high rate of agreement between clinicians administering the scale for the overall classification (kappa = 0.65) as well as for the scale items (kappas range 0.60 to 0.88). Internal consistency of the LANSS scale was also high (Cronbach's alpha = 0.74) (Bennett 2001).

Additional support for the validity of the LANSS comes from a study that sought to discriminate patients with neuropathic from patients with non-neuropathic cancer pain (Potter et al. 2003). In this study, clinicians classified the type of pain in 25 patients with cancer, and the LANSS showed a correct classification rate of 85% (sensitivity 79%; specificity 100%). The 5-item questionnaire component of the LANSS also had excellent sensitivity (86%) and specificity (91%). These investigators reported that the LANSS only took about five minutes to complete, and that the "procedure was acceptable to all patients" in their study.

The LANSS also shows some promise for discriminating among patients with different diagnoses. Martinez-Lavin and colleagues (2003) found that, although samples of patients with fibromyalgia and rheumatoid arthritis did not differ significantly on 0–10 ratings of pain intensity or fatigue, there were very large (and statistically significant) differences between the two samples in the frequency with which they endorsed dysesthesia ("...strange, unpleasant sensation...," FM = 95%; RA = 30%), evoked pain ("...abnormally sensitive to touch...," 95% versus 35%), paroxysmal sensations ("...come on suddenly...," 90% versus 15%), and hot pain (90% versus 20%). No significant differences were found between the two conditions in the LANSS autonomic dysfunction question, with both samples reporting relatively low frequency endorsement of this item (35% versus 10%).

One potential drawback to the LANSS, which might limit its use in some clinical and research settings, is that it requires a trained clinician to administer. However, a self-report version of the LANSS (S-LANSS) has been developed (see Appendix 5.2). In one study, and using a cut-off score of 12 or more to indicate neuropathic pain, the S-LANSS was able to correctly classify 75% of 200 patients as having neuropathic versus nociceptive pain (with 74% sensitivity and 76% specificity rates; Bennett et al. 2004). In addition, each of the S-LANSS items was significantly related to pain type (neuropathic versus nociceptive), confirming the contribution of each to the overall score and discriminant ability of the S-LANSS. Finally, the internal consistency of the S-LANSS (Cronbach's alpha = 0.76) supports the reliability of the measure, and the conclusion that the S-LANSS items tap into the same underlying dimension. These psychometric properties were found to be even better if the LANSS-S was administered in the presence of a research nurse, who could describe the measure and answer any questions that were raised. Correct classification with the LANSS-S administered with the assistance of a clinician was 80%, with a sensitivity and specificity of 80% each, although the optimum cutoff point for the assisted LANSS-S was 10 instead of 12. Internal consistency (Cronbach's alpha) of the assisted LANSS-S was 0.81.

Neuropathic Pain Questionnaire

Like the LANSS, the Neuropathic Pain Questionnaire (NPQ) was developed to help distinguish neuropathic from non-neuropathic pain (Krause and Backonja 2003). The 12 items of the NPQ were selected from an initial list of 32 based on their ability to discriminate between a group of patients with neuropathic pain and a group of patients with non-neuropathic pain (diagnosed by chart review) and include the following descriptor domains: burning pain, overly sensitive to touch, shooting pain, numbness, electric pain, tingling pain, squeezing pain, freezing pain, pain unpleasantness, overwhelming pain, increased pain due to touch, and increased pain due to weather changes. Respondents are asked to rate the severity of each pain domain on a 0–100 numerical scale. The responses are weighted based on the results of a discriminant function analysis from the development sample, and patients are then classified as presenting with neuropathic (final weighted score greater than 0) or non-neuropathic pain (final weighted score equal to or less than 0). Preliminary support for the discriminant validity of the NPQ items was evidenced by the finding that the original discriminant function analyses correctly classified 76% (75% sensitivity and 78% specificity) of subjects into neuropathic and non-neuropathic pain groups (Krause and Backonja 2003). There was a slight reduction in the accuracy of classification in a cross-validation (hold-out) sample, with the NPQ evidencing a 67% sensitivity, 74% specificity, and 71% overall accuracy (Krause and Backonja 2003).

In an analysis using the original NPQ development sample, Backonja and Krause (2003) sought to identify the minimum number of NPQ items that would discriminate neuropathic from non-neuropathic pain conditions without a significant loss of predictive accuracy. Three items emerged from their analysis (tingling pain, numbness, and increased pain due to touch) that were used in a short-form version of the NPQ (NPQ-SF). The total predictive accuracy of these three items in the original sample was 73%, with a sensitivity of 64% and a specificity of 79%. Backonja and Krause (2003) pointed out that these three items cover the primary sensory domains of neuropathic pain; that is, positive sensory phenomenon (allodynia), negative sensory phenomenon (numbness), and phenomenon suggestive of dysesthesia ("tingling pain"). However, the accuracy of classification of NPQ-SF has not yet been cross-validated.

Neuropathic Pain Symptom Inventory

The Neuropathic Pain Symptom Inventory (NPSI; Bouhassira et al. 2004) was developed to achieve the same goals as the NPS: to assess the pain qualities most common in persons with neuropathic pain. The 12 items of the NPSI were selected from an original item set of 18 to assess four global domains of neuropathic pain (spontaneous ongoing pain, spontaneous paroxysmal pain, evoked pain, and paresthesias/dysesthesia). Respondents rate the severity or intensity of each pain domain on 0–10 numerical rating scales. Two items also assess the temporal qualities of pain (number of hours of spontaneous pain in the past 24 hours, number of paroxysms during the last 24 hours).

Bouhassira and colleagues (2004) provide support for the reliability and validity of the NPSI items. Short-term (three hours) and long-term (one month) test–retest stability of the items was very high, as

measured by intra-class correlation coefficients (short-term: range 0.87–0.98; long-term: 0.78–0.98). A factor analysis of the sensory (i.e., excluding the temporal) items yielded five factors that seemed to reflect evoked pain, pressive (or deep) pain, paroxysmal pain, abnormal sensations, and burning pain. Validity for the evoked pain items was evidenced through their significant associations (r range 0.66–0.73) with related clinician scores of pain evoked by brushing, pressure, and cold stimuli. Overall, the findings provide strong preliminary support for the psychometric properties of the NPSI.

Assessing pain affect with single-item rating scales

Both the MPQ and SF-MPQ include scales that assess the affective component of pain. In addition to these multiple-item measures of pain affect, several investigators have advocated the use of single-item rating scales to assess the affective dimension of pain. Assessment of pain affect, or pain unpleasantness, is supported by the evidence that the affective component of pain is conceptually and empirically distinct from pain intensity (Turskey 1976; Gracely et al. 1978a,b; Melzack and Wall 1983; Jensen et al. 1989, 1991), although it is important to remember that pain affect is not completely independent from pain intensity (Fernandez and Turk 1992; Gracely 1992). Whereas pain intensity may be defined as the magnitude of the pain (how much a person hurts), pain affect may be defined as the emotional arousal, or distress, caused by pain. The most common single-item measures of pain affect have been VASs (VAS-A), VRSs (VRS-A), and NRS-As.

VASs of pain affect are very similar to VASs of pain intensity. Only the end-point descriptors are different. Examples of the extremes used in VAS-affect scales are "not bad at all" and "the most unpleasant feeling possible for me" (Price et al. 1987). There is evidence that supports the validity of VAS affect measures. Studies have shown that they are more sensitive than VAS intensity measures to treatments that should influence pain affect more than pain intensity (Price et al. 1980, 1987; Price 1984). Also, as with VASs of pain intensity, VAS-As appear to have the qualities of ratio scales (Price et al. 1983; Price and Harkins 1987). VAS-As are also sensitive to treatment effects (Price et al. 1985, 1986; Price and Barber 1987).

Price and colleagues (Price et al. 1987) examined the ability of a VAS of pain intensity and pain affect to distinguish between different diagnostic groups. They found that a sample of patients with cancer (and patients with low back pain and causalgia) showed a significantly larger difference between the intensity and unpleasantness ratings than patients with upper back pain, myofascial pain, labor pain, or orofacial pain did. This further supports the distinction between the affective and intensity components of pain, and the ability of the VAS to assess each pain component separately. However, patients may not always be able to distinguish between the sensory and affective components of pain (Turk et al. 1985; Williams et al. 2000), and the association between measures of each pain dimension may be so strong that in many situations they may appear to be measuring the same thing (Turk et al. 1985; Good et al. 2001).

Other weaknesses of VAS-affect measures are likely to be similar to those of VAS-intensity measures. Most of the research using these measures has been conducted with young or middle-aged subjects. The utility of such measures in geriatric populations has not yet been examined; it may be that older people have difficulty with VAS-A scales as they do with VAS-I scales. Because VAS-A measures are single-item scales, they may also be less reliable and less valid for examining the full spectrum of affective responses relative to multiple-item measures, such as the Affective subscale of the MPQ or SF-MPQ. Also, there is limited research comparing VAS-A measures to other measures of pain affect. A single experiment suggests that a VAS-A may be less able than a VRS-A (see below) to discriminate between pain intensity and pain affect (Duncan et al. 1989), perhaps because words are so often used to describe emotional reaction, whereas VASs (and NRSs) may pull for more of the intensity (magnitude) component of the pain experience.

NRS measures of pain affect (NRS-As) are uncommon in the pain research literature; only two studies that report data concerning the psychometric properties of NRS-As were identified. Spiegel and colleagues (Spiegel et al. 1983) administered a 0–10 NRS of pain intensity and a 0–10 NRS of pain suffering to 86 women with breast cancer. They found that the two NRS scales were very strongly associated with one another ($r = 0.81$). They also found that the NRS of pain affect was significantly associated with measures of maladaptive coping, emotional distress, and use of analgesics. Smith and colleagues (Smith et al. 1998) also administered 0–10 scales of pain intensity and pain affect (0 = "not unpleasant at all," 10 = "as unpleasant as you can imagine"), to 32 patients with various cancer diagnoses, and found that physical therapy increased the intensity rating but not the unpleasantness rating of pain. Such a finding supports the distinction between pain intensity and pain unpleasantness, even though measures of these two dimensions of pain may be strongly associated with one another (Gracely 1992).

Similar to VRS-Is, affect VRSs (VRS-As) consist of adjectives describing increasing amounts of discomfort and suffering. Respondents select a single word from the list that best describes the degree of unpleasantness of their pain. Like VRS-I measures, VRS-A scales may be scored in three ways: (a) the ranking method, (b) the cross-modality matching method, or (c) the

standardized score method (using scores developed from cross-modality matching procedures with a standardization group). The advantages and disadvantages of these methods have already been discussed with respect to VRSs of pain intensity, and the same cautions are offered here. That is, the simpler ranking method is recommended if the investigator wishes to examine the relation between pain intensity and other constructs, and the use of standardized scores developed from cross-modality matching procedures if the investigator requires a measure more likely to have ratio properties.

Evidence for the validity of VRS-As is mixed. On the positive side, VRS-As appear to be more sensitive than measures of pain intensity to treatments designed to impact the emotional component of pain (Gracely et al. 1978a,b, 1979; Heft et al. 1984; Fernandez and Turk 1994). In another study, a VRS-A was only moderately associated with a VAS-I, which itself was strongly associated with a NRS-I (Ahles et al. 1984). This finding provides additional support for a distinction between pain intensity and pain affect, and supports the validity of a VRS-A for assessing pain affect.

On the other hand, several other factor analytic and correlational investigations among patients with chronic pain, patients with postoperative pain, and laboratory volunteers indicate that, like VAS-As, VRS-As are not always distinct from measures of pain intensity (Jensen and Karoly 1987; Jensen et al. 1989; Levine and De Simone 1991; Gaston-Johansson et al. 1992). This pattern of overlap between similar measures of pain intensity and affect may have something to do with the relatively low level of reliability of single-item measures. Alternatively, a lack of independence among measures of these two dimensions may reflect the simple fact that they are not completely independent; in most if not all situations, some degree of pain intensity is necessary for someone to experience pain affect, and pain affect should increase as pain intensity increases (more intense pain is usually more bothersome). Pain intensity and pain affect may be conceptually distinct, but often closely related to one another in the same way that height and weight are distinct by being closely associated with each other (Gracely 1992). Another drawback to VRS-A affect is that they force respondents to choose only one descriptor, even when none of the available descriptors (or more than one of the available descriptors) captures their affective response to pain.

RECOMMENDATIONS FOR ASSESSING PAIN IN CLINICAL TRIALS

The results of this review summarize evidence concerning the validity and reliability of both established and more recent pain measures. The findings support the multidimensional nature of pain, and provide varying degrees of support for the validity and reliability of measures of pain intensity, pain relief, and pain quality (including affective qualities of pain). The findings also provide guidance for researchers and clinicians concerning which measures may have the most utility.

MEASURING PAIN INTENSITY

There are several conclusions that may be drawn from the findings of the research on the psychometric properties of pain intensity measures. First, and most importantly, each of the commonly used ratings of pain intensity, including the VAS-I, the NRS-I, and the VRS-I, appears adequately valid and reliable as measures of pain intensity among the many different samples of persons with pain. Other pain intensity rating scales (e.g., Mechanical Visual Analogue Scales, Graphic Rating Scales) are used less often, but the research that has been performed using these measures generally supports their validity as well. Moreover, no one scale consistently shows greater responsivity than any other in their ability to detect changes associated with pain treatment. For both VAS-I and 0–10 NRS-I scales, changes (decreases) between about 30 and 35% appear to indicate a meaningful change in pain to patients across patient populations.

While reliability is an important issue for pain intensity measures, as it is for any measure, reliability can be difficult to determine for single-item measures of pain. Internal consistency, one of the most common measures of reliability, cannot be computed from single-item rating scales. Also, test–retest stability coefficients for measures of pain may not always reflect reliability, since pain can, and often does, change from one moment to the next. Such changes in pain can reduce the test–retest coefficient even for pain measures that are highly reliable. However, when examined, the single-item measures of pain intensity appear to have adequate test–retest stability (often, but not always, greater than 0.80) over short periods of time.

While assessing the reliability of pain measures poses challenges, assessing the validity of pain measures for detecting change associated with treatment is relatively straightforward. Measures that show expected (and statistically significant) decreases following pain treatments known to be effective can be judged to be valid for detecting changes in pain in pain clinical trials. Thankfully, the findings from the studies reviewed support the validity of all commonly used ratings of pain intensity for this purpose.

However, there do appear to be consistent and important differences between VRS-Is, NRS-Is, and VAS-Is in terms of their failure rates and in patient preference. VAS-Is usually show higher failure rates than NRS-Is and VRS-Is, and NRS-Is tend (when differences are found) to show slightly greater failure rates than VRS-Is. Similarly, VRS-Is and NRS-Is tend to be preferred over VAS-Is by patients. Higher failure rates with VAS-Is have been shown to be associated with greater age and amount of opioid intake, and mental impairment has been shown to be associated with inability to complete 0–10 NRS ratings of pain intensity. Many patients unable to complete 0–10 NRS-Is appear to be able to complete 4-point VRS-Is, however.

As a group, these findings suggest that the VAS-I rating is not the best choice for assessing pain intensity in clinical trials, especially among patients who are elderly or who may be using opioid medications. NRS-Is, on the other hand, appear to be well tolerated by most patients, and appear to be at least as responsive and valid as the more traditional VAS-I rating scales. However, if the population is expected to include patients with significant cognitive impairment, a simple 4-point VRS-I (e.g., no, mild, moderate, severe pain) may be the best choice as the primary outcome measure in a pain clinical trial. Also, even if a 0–10 NRS-I is selected as the measure of choice in a particular clinical trial (or even as the primary outcome measure in a trial), investigators should consider including a VRS-I as a secondary measure to help describe the effects of the pain treatment in terms of changes in these descriptors (e.g., the percentages of study participants in each condition who described their pain as decreasing from one level, such as severe, to a lower level, such as moderate), to help ensure fewer failure rates in pain assessment if there are any study participants who have difficulty with the NRS-I measure, and to be able to compare findings across studies that also include a VRS-I as one of the outcome measures.

MEASURING PAIN RELIEF

On the surface, many clinicians or researchers might assume that a rating of pain relief following a treatment represents, or should represent, the same thing as a pretreatment to post-treatment decrease in pain intensity. If this were true, then asking patients to rate pain relief following a pain treatment could be used as an alternative to assessing change in pain intensity pretreatment to post-treatment. However, even though relief ratings are responsive to the effects of pain treatment, pain relief ratings are not always strongly associated with pre- to post-treatment changes in pain intensity ratings. Moreover, some patients rate themselves as having experienced "relief" even when post-treatment pain returns to, or even becomes higher than, pretreatment levels. These findings suggest that pain relief ratings should not be interpreted to represent the same thing as pretreatment to post-treatment changes in pain (Jensen et al. 2002). Supporting the use of pain relief as a secondary outcome measure, however, there is evidence that perceived pain relief may be more meaningful to patients than actual change in pain (Fischer et al. 1999). Also, pain relief measures are sometimes more sensitive to the effects of pain treatment than pain intensity change scores are.

Regarding the selection of pain relief rating scales, the available evidence does not clearly support the use of any one type of relief rating (e.g., VRS, NRS, or VAS) over any other. However, practical considerations might suggest that a VRS of pain relief (e.g., "no relief," "slight relief," "moderate relief," "lots of relief," "complete relief") may help limit the chances that patients will confuse the relief rating with pain intensity ratings, since NRS and VAS pain intensity measures can look very similar to NRS and VAS measures of pain relief.

MEASURING THE QUALITATIVE ASPECTS OF PAIN

Pain is known to have qualities in addition to its intensity. It can be experienced as hot, cold, tingly, deep, dull, worrisome, or any one (or more) of many other qualities. Measures of the qualitative and affective components of pain may be used to more fully describe a patient's pain experience. Such measures could also potentially contribute to improved evaluation and treatment of pain. Given the likelihood that some pain treatments will be found to impact some pain qualities more than others, inclusion of pain quality measures in clinical trials might help determine the specific qualities of pain that would most benefit from each pain treatment that is evaluated (Galer and Jensen 1997). Moreover, to the extent that a treatment might impact a relatively small subset of pain qualities, ratings of specific pain qualities may be more responsive to the effects of some treatments than ratings of global pain intensity are. If so, then systematic use of pain quality measures in clinical analgesia trials may help identify effective treatments that might otherwise have been determined to have little effect on pain.

There are several measures of pain quality to choose from, and each has its strengths and weaknesses. If an investigator wishes to assess the three pain quality domains that form the basis of the MPQ (that is, to assess global sensory, affective, and evaluative domains), then the MPQ should be used. As reviewed above, the MPQ has been the measure most often used to assess the qualitative aspects of pain in pain research. Discriminative validity of the MPQ is evidenced by the moderately strong associations between the MPQ scale scores and measures of pain intensity. These associations are strong enough to indicate that the MPQ scores assess pain, but also not so strong to suggest that MPQ scores assess only pain intensity. The findings also show that the MPQ scales are associated with measures of quality of life, and are sensitive to the effects of pain treatment. Evidence supports the validity of the MPQ-Affective subscale, in particular, for assessing pain-related distress, given the stronger associations of this scale with measures of psychological distress than with measures of pain intensity, and the relatively high scores on the MPQ-Affective scale among persons with cancer pain compared with persons with low back pain.

However, the MPQ is a relatively lengthy measure (listing 78 descriptors), and many of the descriptors may not be appropriate or needed in many groups of patients with pain. In addition, despite the possibility that certain pain qualities may be more strongly affected by a particular analgesic or pain treatment than others, more often than not the MPQ scale scores are less responsive to the effects of pain treatments than simple single-item measures of pain intensity are. This may be due to the fact that the MPQ scale scores represent composites of a large variety of pain qualities – some of which might be affected by an intervention and others which might not be affected. The inclusion of so many pain qualities into single scales may therefore weaken the ability to detect treatment effects.

The Short-Form MPQ has some strengths that may make it more practical than the MPQ to use in pain clinical trials. First, it includes only 15 descriptors instead of 78, markedly reducing the assessment burden on subjects. In addition, it retains descriptors from two of the MPQ primary categories (sensory and affective), making it possible to assess these global dimensions of pain quality. Finally, unlike the MPQ, which requires patients to select no more than a single word from each of 20 word lists (even if more than one word describes their pain), respondents to the SF-MPQ are allowed to rate the severity of each pain descriptor on a 0–3 scale. This allows for scoring and analysis of each unique pain descriptor.

However, like the MPQ scales, the SF-MPQ scales have not demonstrated greater sensitivity to the effects of pain treatments than simple pain intensity rating scales. Moreover, to date, the SF-MPQ has not been used to determine whether pain treatments affect some pain qualities (i.e., the specific MPQ descriptors) and not others. Also, although the SF-MPQ total scale score has been found to have adequate to excellent internal consistency, the SF-MPQ-Sensory and SF-MPQ-Affective scales evidence less reliability. The SF-MPQ also does not include a number of descriptors that have been linked to neuropathic pain conditions (such as "cold pain" and words that describe allodynia) making the SF-MPQ less practical than other measures for assessing the qualities of neuropathic pain. Finally, unlike other measures, the SF-MPQ items have not yet been demonstrated to be useful for detecting different patterns of changes in individual pain quality items associated with specific pain treatments. Thus, at this point, the SF-MPQ might be most useful when researchers are looking for a brief and valid measure that provides scores of the sensory and affective dimensions of pain similar to those provided by the original MPQ.

The PQAS (see Appendix 5.1) was designed specifically as a measure of pain qualities that can be used for assessing both nociceptive and non-nociceptive pain. It has a number of strengths that make it suitable for this purpose. First, it has content validity. That is, the items include the majority of pain qualities assessed by measures of both neuropathic pain (as assessed, for example, by the NPS, NPQ, LANSS, and NPSI) and nociceptive pain (as assessed, for example, by the SF-MPQ). No other measure, except perhaps the original MPQ, assesses as many core pain qualities. However, unlike the PQAS, the MPQ cannot be scored to assess the intensity or severity of each descriptor. Also, although a number of measures of neuropathic pain exist (e.g., NPS, NPQ, NPSI), these other measures do not include all of the pain qualities that appear to be central to the experience of neuropathic pain. For example, the NPS does not assess electrical and tingling sensations. The NPQ does not include dull, cold, throbbing, aching, heavy, tender, or itchy descriptors, even though some of these sensations are common in patients with neuropathic pain, and all have been shown to discriminate between patients with neuropathic and non-neuropathic pain (Boureau et al. 1990; Wilkie et al. 2001). The NPSI similarly lacks descriptors that have been shown to be common in neuropathic pain and/or to differentiate pain types (dull, cold, throbbing, aching, itchy, numb). The high degree of content validity of the PQAS makes it more useful than these other measures for detecting changes in specific pain qualities caused by different treatments. A second strength of the PQAS is that it includes the NPS items, as well as the NPS format. The 0–10 response format is easy for most patients to use and understand, and also provides for an adequate number of response levels to help gauge the effects of pain treatment on each quality domain. Also, and as reviewed above, the NPS items that are included in the PQAS have demonstrated responsivity to analgesic treatment, and studies have shown that these items can help describe the specific effects of different treatments on different pain qualities.

One weakness of the PQAS relative to other measures is its length (20 descriptors), which can produce an unacceptable assessment burden in some situations. Also, there is not yet research on the validity of the additional 10 (non-NPS) items as used in the context of the PQAS. It is possible that future research may show that some of these additional items are of minimal use for detecting changes in pain, for describing different pain conditions, or for identifying pain treatment profiles. Similarly, future research may identify even more pain qualities or domains that should be assessed in clinical trials not yet included in the PQAS or in the other measures described here. In the meantime, however, the PQAS appears to be an excellent choice when a global, and content valid, measure of neuropathic or non-neuropathic pain qualities is needed.

If there is a need for a more brief measure of neuropathic pain qualities, specifically, then there are six options to choose from: the NPS (Galer and Jensen 1997), the LANSS and LANSS-S (Bennett 2001; Appendix 5.2), the NPQ and NPQ-SF (Krause and Backonja 2003; Backonja and Krause 2003), and the NPSI (Bouhassira et al. 2004). For the most part, the available evidence supports the validity of each of these measures, and no single one of these has emerged as the single best measure to use in all situations. However, enough differences exist between the measures, and the data that support them so far, to allow for some preliminary recommendations.

Concerning the assessment of the multiple components of pain for the purpose of detecting changes in specific neuropathic pain qualities with treatment, there appear to be two viable choices at this point: the NPS and the NPSI (the LANSS and the NPQ were designed to discriminate neuropathic from non-neuropathic pain; these two measures are described below). Because the format of the two scales is so similar (each asks respondents to rate each pain quality using a 0–10 scale), the decision regarding which one to use depends for the most part on their content. Both assess sharp/stabbing pain, hot/burning pain, and allodynia. However, the NPS (and not the NPSI) includes global measures of pain intensity and unpleasantness, as well as items that assess the specific qualities of dull, cold, itchy, and deep pain. On the other hand, electrical, tingling, and pressure sensations are assessed by the NPSI and not by the NPS.

Because of the differences in content between the measures, selecting either over the other would mean that some pain qualities that are common in neuropathic pain might not be assessed. For example, the effects of intravenous adenosine on itchy pain (Lynch et al. 2003), and the effects of oxycodone on dull and deep pain (Jensen et al. 2002), would have been missed if the NPSI had been used as an outcome measure in these studies instead of the NPS. Similarly, these treatments might have affected electric, tingling, or pressure pain sensations; yet these effects, had they been there, could not have been detected because the NPS was used instead of the NPSI. Given that the format of the two measures is so similar, it would make the most sense to simply add the three descriptors from the NPSI that are missing from the NPS to the NPS (or add the four NPS descriptors that are missing from the NPSI to the NPSI), to provide for a more thorough assessment of neuropathic pain. Alternatively, researchers might wish to again consider the use of the PQAS, which includes items that assess the pain qualities covered in both the NPS and NPSI, among others.

Four measures of neuropathic pain have been designed to discriminate neuropathic from non-neuropathic pain: the LANSS, LANSS-S, NPQ, and

NPQ-SF. Of these measures, the LANSS and (if a self-report measure is needed) the LANSS-S appear to be more successful than the NPQ or the NPQ-SF for this purpose for several reasons. First, at this point in time, there are more data supporting the LANSS and LANSS-S than for the NPQ or NPQ-SF. Second, the accuracy rates (including both sensitivity and specificity rates) tend to be higher for the LANSS and LANSS-S than for the NPQ or NPQ-SF. Finally, the 7-item LANSS and LANSS-S are somewhat briefer than the 12-item NPQ, making the former more appealing in situations where assessment burden is an issue. Although the 3-item NPQ-SF is briefer still, its relatively low accuracy rate (especially its low sensitivity rate of 64%) would suggest that it has limited utility for identifying neuropathic pain in some settings. However, additional research comparing these measures (and even perhaps combining the best items or domains from all existing scales to create a new, even more sensitive and specific tool) is needed before firm conclusions can be drawn concerning their relative strengths and weaknesses.

There is limited research on the reliability and validity of single-item measures of pain affect, and the research that has been performed is mixed. On one hand, such measures have been found to respond more than measures of pain intensity to treatments that should influence pain affect more than pain intensity. On the other hand, in some samples, single-item ratings of pain affect and pain intensity are often so closely related that they seem to measure the same dimension (i.e., pain severity). Until more research is performed that helps identify the specific settings where such measures may be most useful, there does not appear to be a compelling reason to include single-item measures of pain affect in all clinical trials. If a measure of the affective response to pain is needed, then the MPQ or SF-MPQ affective items would likely be more useful, given that they may better reflect the multidimensional characteristics of emotional responses to pain.

CONCLUSION

A great deal of research has been performed that provides data concerning the psychometric properties of pain measures. The findings from this research support and confirm the multidimensional nature of pain. The results also support validity of a number of measures, especially the most commonly used measures of pain intensity. Measures of other dimensions of pain, such as pain relief and the temporal and qualitative aspects of pain, are less often used and studied. Yet measures of these and other pain dimensions may prove to be invaluable for assessing pain and the efficacy of pain treatment. Future research that develops, refines, and evaluates such measures will provide important information that investigators and clinicians may then use to select specific scales for their research and clinical work. By increasing knowledge about and options for pain assessment, investigators will ultimately contribute to a better understanding and alleviation of pain.

REFERENCES

Ahles TA, Ruckdeschel JC, Blanchard JB. Cancer-related pain: assessment with visual analogue scales. J Psychosom Res 1984; 28:21–124.

Anderson PE, Cohen JI, Everts JC, et al. Intrathecal narcotics for relief of pain from head and neck cancer. Arch Otolaring Head Neck Surg 1991; 1117:1277–1280.

Angst MS, Brose WG, Dyck JB. The relationship between the Visual Ancological Pain Intensity and Pain Relief Scale changes during analgesic studies in chronic pain patients. Anesthesiology 1999; 91:34–41.

Backonja M, Krause SJ. Neuropathic Pain Questionnaire – Short Form. Clin J Pain 2003; 19:315–316.

Backonja M, Beydoun A, Edwards KR, et al. Gabapentin for the treatment of painful neuropathy in patients with diabetes mellitus. JAMA 1998; 280:1831–1836.

Baker BO, Hardyck CD, Petrinovich LF. Weak measurement vs strong statistics: an empirical critique of S. S. Stevens' prescriptions on statistics. Educat Psychol Meas 1966; 26:291–309.

Barton SF, Langeland FF, Snabes MC, et al. Efficacy and safety of intravenous parecoxib sodium in relieving acute postoperative pain following gynecologic laparotomy surgery. Anesthesiology 2002; 97:306–314.

Bellamy N, Campbell J, Syrotuik J. Comparative study of self-rating pain scale in osteoarthritis patients. Curr Med Res Opin 1999; 15:113–119.

Bennett M. The LANSS Pain Scale: the Leeds assessment of neuropathic symptoms and signs. Pain 2001; 92:147–157.

Bennett MI, Smith BH, Torrance N, et al. Validation of the LANSS pain scale as a self-report questionnaire. Poster presented at the IASP special interest group meeting on neuropathic pain: Neuropathic Pain: Changing Paradigms in Diagnosis and Treatment, Madrid, Spain, 2004.

Bergh B, Sjöströrom B, Odén A, et al. An application of pain rating scales in geriatric patients. Aging Clin Exp Res 2000; 12:380–387.

Bergman B, Sullivan M, Sörenson S. Quality of life during chemotherapy for small cell lung cancer. Acta Oncol 1992; 31:19–28.

Bergman B, Aaronson N, Ahmedzai S, et al. The EORTC QLQ-LC13: a modular supplement to the EORTC Core Quality Of Life Questionnaire (QLQ-30) for use in lung cancer clinical trials. Eur J Cancer 1994; 30:635–642.

Birbara CA, Puopolo AD, Munoz DR, et al. Treatment of chronic low back pain with etoricoxib, a new cyclo-oxygenase-2 selective inhibitor: improvement in pain and disability: a randomized, placebo-controlled, 3-month trial. J Pain 2003; 4:307–315.

Bolton JE, Wilkinson RC. Responsiveness of pain scales: a comparison of three pain intensity measures in chiropractic patients. J. Manipulative Physiop Ther 1998; 21:1–7.

Bone M, Critchley P, Buggy DJ. Gabapentin in postamputation phantom limb pain: a randomized, double-blind, placebo-controlled, cross-over study. Pain 2002; 27:481–486.

Bouhassira D, Attal N, Fermanian J, et al. Development and validation of the Neuropathic Pain Symptom Inventory. Pain 2004; 108:248–257.

Boureau F, Doubrere JF, Luu M. Study of verbal description in neuropathic pain. Pain 1990; 42:145–152.

Breivik EK, Björnsson GA, Skovlund E. A comparison of pain ratings scales by sampling from clinical trial data. Clin J Pain 2000; 16:22–28.

Briggs M. Surgical wound pain: a trial of two treatments. J Wound Care 1996; 5:456–460.

Bruera E, Kuehn N, Miller M, et al. The Edmonton Symptom Assessment System (ESAS): a simple method for the assessment of palliative care patients. J Palliat Care 1991; 1:6–9.

Burchiel KJ, Anderson VC, Brown FD, et al. Prospective, multicenter study of spinal cord stimulation for relief of chronic back and extremity pain. Spine 1996; 21:2786–2794.

Campbell BH, Marbella A, Layde PM. Quality of life and recurrence concern in survivors of head and neck cancer. Laryngoscope 2000; 110:895–906.

Carter GT, Jensen MP, Galer BS, et al. Neuropathic pain in Charcot-Marie-Tooth disease. Arch Phys Med Rehabil 1998; 79:1560–1564.

Cepeda MS, Africano JM, Polo R, et al. What decline in pain intensity is meaningful to patients with acute pain? Pain 2003; 105:151–157.

Chang VT, Hwang SS, Feuerman M. Validation of the Edmonton Symptom Assessment Scale. Cancer 2000; 88:2164–2171.

Chesney MA, Shelton JL. A comparison of muscle relaxation and electromyogram biofeedback treatments for muscle contraction headache. J Behavior Ther Exper Psych 1976; 7:221–225.

Cicchetti DV, Showalter D, Tyrer PJ. The effect of number of rating scale categories on levels of interrater reliability: a Monte Carlo investigation. Appl Psych Meas 1985; 9:31–36.

Cleeland CS, Ryan KM. Pain assessment: global use of the Brief Pain Inventory. Ann Acad Med 1994; 23:129–138.

Dalton JA, Toomey T, Workman MR. Pain relief for cancer patients. Can Nurs 1988; 11:322–328.

Daut RL, Cleeland CS, Flannery RC. Development of the Wisconsin Brief Pain Questionnaire to assess pain in cancer and other diseases. Pain 1983; 17:197–210.

De Conno F, Caraceni A, Gamba A, et al. Pain measurement in cancer patients: a comparison of six methods. Pain 1994; 57:161–166.

de Wit R, van Dam F, Abu-Saad HH, et al. Empirical comparison of commonly used measures to evaluate pain treatment in cancer patients with chronic pain. J Clin Oncol 1999a; 17:1280–1287.

de Wit R, van Dam F, Hanneman M, et al. Evaluation of the use of a pain diary in chronic cancer pain patients at home. Pain 1999b; 79:89–99.

Dodd MJ, Miaskowski C, Paul SM. Symptom clusters and their effect on the functional status of patients with cancer. Oncol Nurs Forum 2001; 8:465–470.

Doyle G, Jayawardena S, Ashraf E, et al. Efficacy and tolerability of nonprescription ibuprofen versus celecoxib for dental pain. J Clin Pharmacol 2002; 42:912–919.

Dubuisson D, Melzack R. Classification of clinical pain descriptors by multiple group discriminant function analysis. Exper Neurol 1976; 51:480–487.

Dudgeon D, Ranbertas RF, Rosenthal S. The short-form McGill Pain Questionnaire in chronic cancer pain. J Pain Sympt Manage 1993; 8:191–195.

Duncan GH, Bushnell MC, Lavigne GJ. Comparison of verbal and visual analogue scales for measuring the intensity and unpleasantness of experimental pain. Pain 1989; 37:295–303.

Du Pen SL, Du Pen AR, Polissar N, et al. Implementing guidelines for cancer pain management: results of a randomized controlled clinical trial. J Clin Oncol 1999; 17L:361–370.

Eija K, Tasmuth T, Pertti NJ. Amitriptyline effectively relieves neuropathic pain following treatment of breast cancer. Pain 1996; 4:293–302.

Eisenberg E, Lurie Y, Daoud D, et al. Lamotrigine reduces painful diabetic neuropathy: a randomized controlled study. Neurology 2001; 57:505–509.

Ekblom A, Hansson P. Pain intensity measurements in patients with acute pain receiving afferent stimulation. J Neuro Neurosurg Psych 1988; 51:481–486.

Ellershow J, Peat SJ, Boys LC. Assessing the effectiveness of a hospital palliative care team. Palliat Med 1995; 9:145–152.

Farrar JT, Cleary J, Rauck R, et al. Oral transmucosal fentanyl cirate: randomized, double-blinded, placebo-controlled trial for treatment of breakthrough pain in cancer patients. J Natl Cancer Inst 1998; 90:611–616.

Farrar JT, Portenoy RK, Berlin JA. Defining the clinically important difference in pain outcome measures. Pain 2000; 88:287–294.

Farrar JT, Young JP, LaMoreaux L, et al. Clinical importance of changes in chronic pain intensity measures on an 11-point numerical rating scale. Pain 2001; 94:149–158.

Farrar JT, Berlin JA, Strom BL. Clinically important changes in acute pain outcome measures: a validation study. J Pain Sympt Manage 2003; 25:406–411.

Feine JS, Lavigne GJ, Thuan Dao TT, et al. Memories of chronic pain and perceptions of relief. Pain 1998; 77:137–141.

Fernandez E, Turk DC. Demand characteristics underlying differential ratings of sensory versus affective components of pain. J Behav Med 1994; 17:375–390.

Fischer D, Stewart AL, Bloch DA, et al. Capturing the patient's view of change as a clinical outcome measure. JAMA 1999; 282:1157–1162.

Fishman B, Pasternak S, Wallenstein SL, et al. The Memorial Pain Assessment Card: a valid instrument for the evaluation of cancer pain. Cancer 1987; 60:1151–1158.

Forouzanfar T, Weber WEJ, Kemler M, et al. What is a meaningful pain reduction in patients with Complex Regional Pain Syndrome Type I? Clin J Pain 2003; 19:281–285

Fowlow B, Price P, Fung T. Ambulation after sheath removal: a comparison of 6 and 8 hours of bedrest after sheath removal in patients following a PTCA procedure. Heart Lung 1995; 24:28–37.

Fox EJ, Melzack R. Transcutaneous electrical stimulation and acupuncture: comparison of treatment for low-back pain. Pain 1976; 2:141–148.

Freeman K, Smyth C, Dallam L, et al. Pain measurement scales: a comparison of the vision analogue and faces rating scales in measuring pressure ulcer pain. J WOCN 2001; 28:290–296.

Frost S, Grossfeld S, Kirkley A, et al. The efficacy of femoral nerve block in pain reduction for outpatient hamstring anterior cruciate ligament reconstruction: a double-blind, prospective, randomized trial. Arthroscopy 2000; 16:243–248.

Gagliese L, Melzack R. Age differences in the quality of chronic pain: a preliminary study. Pain Res Manage 1997; 2:157–162.

Galer BS, Jensen MP. Development and preliminary validation of a pain measure specific to neuropathic pain: the Neuropathic Pain Scale. Neurology 1997; 48:332–338.

Galer BS, Henderson J, Perander J, et al. Course of symptoms and quality of life measurement in complex regional pain syndrome: a pilot survey. J Pain Sympt Manage 2000; 20:286–292.

Galer BS, Jensen MP, Ma T, et al. The lidocaine patch 5% effectively treats all neuropathic pain qualities: results of a randomized, double-blind, vehicle-controlled, 3-week efficacy study with use of the Neuropathic Pain Scale. Clin J Pain 2002; 18:297–301.

Gallagher EJ, Bijur PE, Latimer C, et al. Reliability and validity of a visual analog scale for acute abdominal pain in the ED. Am J Emerg Med 2002; 20:287–290.

Gammaitoni AR, Galer BS, Lacouture P, et al. Effectiveness and safety of new oxycodone/acetaminophen formulations with reduced acetaminophen for the treatment of low back pain. Pain Med 2003; 4:21–30.

Gaston-Johansson F, Franco T, Zimmerman L. Pain and psychological distress in patients undergoing autologous bone marrow transplantation. Oncol Nurs Forum 1992; 19:41–48.

Geddes D, Dones L, Hill E, et al. Quality of life during chemotherapy for small cell lung cancer: assessment and use of a daily diary card in a randomized trial. Eur J Cancer 1990; 26:484–492.

Good M, Stiller C, Zauszniewski JA, et al. Sensation and distress of pain scales: reliability, validity, and sensitivity. J Nurs Measure 2001; 9:219–238.

Gracely RH. Evaluation of multi-dimensional pain scales. Pain 1992; 48:297–300.

Gracely RH, McGrath P, Dubner R. Ratio scales of sensory and affective verbal pain descriptors. Pain 1978a; 5:5–18.

Gracely RH, McGrath P, Dubner R. Validity and sensitivity of ratio scales of sensory and affective verbal pain descriptors: manipulation of affect by diazepam. Pain 1978b; 5:19–29.

Gracely RH, Dubner R, McGrath PA. Narcotic analgesia: fentanyl reduces the intensity but not the unpleasantness of painful tooth pulp sensations. Science 1979; 203:1261–1263.

Graff-Radford SB, Shaw LR, Naliboff BN. Amitriptyline and fluphenazine in the treatment of postherpetic neuralgia. Clin J Pain 2000; 16:188–192.

Graham C, Bond S, Gerkovich M. Use of the McGill Pain Questionnaire in the assessment of cancer pain: reliability and consistency. Pain 1980; 8:377–387.

Greenwald H, Bonica J, Bergner M. The prevalence of pain in four cancers. Cancer 1987; 60:2563–2569.

Grond S, Radbruch L, Meuser T, et al. Assessment and treatment of neuropathic cancer pain following WHO guidelines. Pain 1999; 79:15–20.

Grossman S, Sheidler V, McGuire D, et al. A comparison of the Hopkins Pain Rating instrument with Standard Visual Analogue and Verbal Descriptor scales in patients with cancer pain. J Pain Sympt Manage 1992; 7:196–203.

Haas M, Nyendo J, Aickin M. One year trend in pain and disability relief recall in acute pain and chronic ambulatory low back pain patients. Pain 2002; 95:83–91.

Hägg O, Fritzell P, Nordwall A. The clinical importance of changes in outcome scores after treatment for low back pain. Eur Spine J 2003; 12:12–20.

Hall W. On ratio scales of sensory and affective verbal pain descriptors. Pain 1981; 4:101–107.

Hardy JD, Wolff HG, Goodell H. Pain Sensations and Reactions. Williams & Wilkins, Baltimore, MD, 1952.

Hammerlid E, Bjordal K, Ahlner-Elmqvist M, et al. Prospective, longitudinal quality-of-life study of patients with head and neck cancer: a feasibility study including the EORTC QLQ-C30. Otolaring Head Neck Surg 1997; 116:666–673.

Harden RN, Carter TD, Gilman CS, et al. Ketorolac in acute headache management. Headache 1991; 31:463–464.

Holland J, Romano S, Heiligenstein J, et al. A controlled trial of fluoxetine and desipramine in depressed women with advanced cancer. Psycho-Oncol 1998; 7:291–300.

Hollen P, Gralla R, Kris M, et al. Quality of life assessment in individuals with lung cancer: Testing the Lung Cancer Symptom scale (LCSS). Eur J Cancer 1993; 29(suppl 1): S51–S58.

Hollen P, Gralla R, Kris M, et al. Quality of life during clinical trials: conceptual model for the Lung Cancer Symptom Scale (LCSS). Sup Care Cancer 1994a; 2:213–222.

Hollen P, Gralla R, Kris M, et al. Measurement of quality of life in patients with lung cancer in multicenter trials of new therapies. Cancer 1994b; 73:2087–2098.

Holzheimer A, McMillan SC, Weitzner M. Improving pain outcomes of hospice patients with cancer. Oncol Nurs Forum 1999; 26:1499–1504.

Hwang SS, Chang VT, Kasimis B. Cancer breakthrough pain characteristics and responses to treatment at a VA medical center. Pain 2003; 101:55–64.

Ingham J, Seidman A, Yao T-J, et al. An exploratory study of frequent pain measurement in a cancer clinical trial. Qual Life Res 1996; 5:503–507.

Jenkinson C, Carrol D, Egerton M, et al. Comparison of the sensitivity to change of long and short from pain measures. Qual Life Res 1995; 4:353–357.

Jensen MP, Karoly P. Assessing the subjective experience of pain: what do the scale scores of the McGill Pain Questionnaire measure? Poster presented at the eighth annual scientific sessions of the Society of Behavioral Medicine, Washington, DC, 1987.

Jensen MP, Karoly P, Braver S. The measurement of clinical pain intensity: a comparison of six methods. Pain 1986; 27:117–126.

Jensen MP, Karoly P, O'Riordan EF, et al. The subjective experience of acute pain: an assessment of the utility of 10 indices. Clin J Pain 1989; 5:153–159.

Jensen MP, Miller L, Fisher LD. Assessment of pain during medical procedures: a comparison of three scales. Clin J Pain 1998; 14:343–349.

Jensen MP, Turner JA, Romano JM, et al. Comparative reliability and validity of chronic pain intensity measures. Pain 1999; 83:157–162.

Joshi GP, Viscusi ER, Gan TJ, et al. Effective treatment of laparoscopic cholecystectomy pain with intravenous followed by oral COX-2 specific inhibitor. Ambul Anesthes 2004; 98:336–342.

Joyce CRB, Zutshi DW, Hrubes V, et al. Comparison of fixed interval and visual analogue scales for rating chronic pain. Eur J Clin Pharm 1975; 8:415–420.

Keefe FJ, Schapira B, Williams RB, et al. EMG-assisted relaxation training in the management of chronic low back pain. Am J Clin Biofeedback 1981; 4:93–103.

King RB. Topical aspirin in chloroform and the relief of pain due to herpes zoster and postherpetic neuralgia. Arch Neurol 1993; 50:1046–1053.

Klepstad P, Borchgrevink PC, Kaasa S. Effects on cancer patients' health-related quality of life after the start of morphine therapy. J Pain Sympt Manage 2000; 20:19–26.

Krause SJ, Backonja MM. Development of a neuropathic pain questionnaire. Clin J Pain 2003; 19:306–314.

Kremer EF, Atkinson JH Jr, Ignelzi RJ. Measurement of pain: patient preference does not confound measurement. Pain 1981; 10:241–248.

Kremer EF, Atkinson JH Jr, Ignelzi RJ. Pain measurement: the affective dimensional measure of the McGill Pain Questionnaire with a cancer pain population. Pain 1982; 12:153–163.

Kubitzek F, Ziegler G, Gold MS, et al. Analgesic efficacy of low-dose Diclofenac versus paracetamol and placebo in postoperative dental pain. J Orofac Pain 2003; 17:237–244.

Kucuk O, Fisher E, Moinpour CM, et al. Phase II trial of bicalutamide in patients with advanced prostate cancer in whom conventional hormonal therapy failed: a southwest oncology group study (SWOG 9235). Urology 2001; 58:53–58.

Leavitt F, Garron DC. Validity of a back pain classification scale for detecting psychological disturbance as measured by the MMPI. J Clin Psych 1980; 36:186–189.

Leksowski K. Thoracoscopic splanchnicectomy for control of intractable pain due to advanced pancreatic cancer. Surg Endosc 2001; 15:129–131.

Levine FM, De Simone LL. The effects of experimenter gender on pain report in male and female subjects. Pain 1991; 44:69–72.

Lin CC. Applying the Am Pain Society QA standards to evaluate the quality of pain management among surgical, oncology, and hospice inpatients in Taiwan. Pain 2000; 87:43–49.

Littman GS, Walker BR, Schneider BE. Reassessment of verbal and visual analog ratings in analgesic studies. Clin Pharm Therap 1985; 38:16–23.

Love A, Leboeuf C, Crisp TC. Chiropractic chronic low back pain sufferers and self-report assessment methods: I. A reliability study of the visual analogue scale, the pain drawing and the McGill Pain Questionnaire. J Manipulative Physiol Ther 1989; 12:21–25.

Lundeberg T, Lund I, Dahlin L, et al. Reliability and responsiveness of three different pain assessments. J Rehabil Med 2001; 33:279–283.

Lynch ME, Clark AJ, Sawynok J. Intravenous adenosine alleviates neuropathic pain: a double blind placebo controlled crossover trial using an enriched enrolment design. Pain 2003; 103:111–117.

Magnusson T, List T, Helkimo M. Self-assessment of pain and discomfort in patients with temporomandibular disorders: a comparison of five different scales with respect to their precision and sensitivity as well as their capacity to register memory of pain and discomfort. J Oral Rehabil 1995; 22:549–556.

Manfredi PL, Chandler S, Pigazzi A, et al. Outcome of cancer pain consultations. Cancer 2000; 89:920–924.

Martinez-Lavin M, López S, Medina M, et al. Use of the Leeds Assessment of Neuropathic Symptoms and Signs Questionnaire in patients with fibromyalgia. Semin Arth Rheum 2003; 32:407–411.

Masson EA, Hunt L, Gem JM, et al. A novel approach to the diagnosis and assessment of sympathetic diabetic neuropathy. Pain 1989; 38:25–28.

Maunsell E, Allard P, Dorval M, et al. A brief pain diary for ambulatory patients with advanced cancer. Cancer 2000; 88:2387–2397.

Melzack R. The McGill Pain Questionnaire: major properties and scoring methods. Pain 1975; 1:277–299.

Melzack R. The short-form McGill Pain Questionnaire. Pain 1987; 30:191–197.

Melzack R, Terrence C, Fromm G, et al. Trigeminal neuralgia and atypical facial pain: use of the McGill Pain Questionnaire for discrimination and diagnosis. Pain 1986; 27:297–302.

Meuser T, Pietruck C, Radbruch L, et al. Symptoms during cancer pain treatment following WHO guidelines: a longitudinal follow-up study of symptom prevalence, severity and etiology. Pain 2001; 93:247–257.

Molenaar S, Sprangers MA, Rutgers EJ, et al. Decision support for patients with early-stage breast cancer: effects of an interactive breast cancer CDROM on treatment decision, satisfaction, and quality of life. J Clin Oncol 2001; 19:1676–1687.

Mongini F, Italiano M. TMJ disorders and myogenic facial pain: a discriminative analysis using the McGill Pain Questionnaire. Pain 2001; 91:323–330.

Moore MJ, Osoba D, Murphy K, et al. Use of palliative end points to evaluate the effects of mitoxantrone and low-dose prednisone in patients with hormonally resistant prostate cancer. J Clin Oncol 1994; 12:689–694.

Nikolajsen L, Hansen CL, Nielsen J, et al. The effect of ketamine on phantom pain: a central neuropathic disorder maintained by peripheral input. Pain 1996; 67:69–77.

Ohnhaus JE, Adler R. Methodological problems in the measurement of pain: a comparison between the verbal rating scale and the visual analogue scale. Pain 1975; 1:379–384.

Owen JE, Klapow JC, Casebeer L. Evaluating the relationship between pain presentation and health-related quality of life in outpatients with metastatic or recurrent neoplastic disease. Qual Life Res 2000; 9:855–863.

Padilla GV, Presant C, Grant MM, et al. Quality of life index for patients with cancer. Res Nurs Health 1983; 6:117–126.

Paice J, Cohen F. Validity of a verbally administered numeric rating scale to measure cancer pain intensity. Cancer Nurs 1997; 20:88–93.

Palangio M, Northfelt DW, Portenoy RK, et al. Dose conversion and titration with a novel once-daily, OROS osmotic technology, extended-release hydromorphone formulation in the treatment of chronic malignant or nonmalignant pain. J Pain Sympt Manage 2002; 23:355–368.

Perry F, Heller PH, Levine JD. Differing correlations between pain measures in syndromes with or without explicable organic pathology. Pain 1988; 34:185–189.

Perry F, Helle PH, Levine JD. A possible indicator of functional pain: poor pain scale correlation. Pain 1991; 46:191–193.

Philip BK. Parametric statistics for evaluation of the visual analog scale. Anesth Analg 1990; 71:710.

Plesh O, Curtis D, Levine J, et al. Amitriptyline treatment of chronic pain in patients with temporomandibular disorders. J Oral Rehabil 2000; 27:834–841.

Potter J, Higginson IJ, Scadding JW, et al. Identifying neuropathic pain in patients with head and neck cancer: use of the Leeds Assessment of Neuropathic Symptoms and Signs Scale. J Roy Soc Med 2003; 96:379–383.

Portenoy RK, Payne R, Coluzzi P, et al. Oral transmucosal fentanyl citrate (OTFC) for the treatment of breakthrough pain in cancer patients: a controlled dose titration study. Pain 1999; 79:303–312.

Poulos AR, Gertz MA, Pankratz VS, et al. Pain, mood disturbance, and quality of life in patients with multiple myeloma. Oncol Nurs Forum 2001; 28:1163–1171.

Pozehl B, Barnason S, Zimmerman L, et al. Pain in the postoperative coronary artery bypass graft patient. Clin Nurs Res 1995; 4:208–222.

Price DD. Roles of psychophysics, neuroscience, and experimental analysis in the study of pain. In: Kruger L, Liebeskind JK (eds). Advances in Pain Research and Therapy, vol 6. Raven Press, New York, 1984: 341–355.

Price DD, Barber J. An analysis of factors that contribute to the efficacy of hypnotic analgesia. J Abnormal Psych 1987; 96:46–51.

Price DD, Harkins SW. Combined use of experimental pain and visual analogue scales in providing standardized measurement of clinical pain. Clin J Pain 1987; 3:1–8.

Price DD, Barrell JJ, Gracely RH. A psychophysical analysis of experiential factors that selectively influence the affective dimension of pain. Pain 1980; 8:137–149.

Price DD, McGrath PA, Rafii A, et al. The validation of visual analogue scales as ratio scale measures for chronic and experimental pain. Pain 1983; 17:45–56.

Price DD, Von der Gruen A, Miller J, et al. A psychophysical analysis of morphine analgesia. Pain 1985; 22:261–269.

Price DD, Harkins SW, Rafii A, et al. A simultaneous comparison of fentanyl's analgesic effects on experimental and clinical pain. Pain 1986; 24:197–203.

Price DD, Harkins SW, Baker C. Sensory-affective relationships among different types of clinical and experimental pain. Pain 1987; 28:297–307.

Price DD, Bush FM, Long S, et al. A comparison of pain measurement characteristics of mechanical visual analogue and simple numerical rating scales. Pain 1994; 56:217–226.

Price DD, Riley JL III, Wade JB. Psychophysical approaches to measurement of the dimensions and stages of pain. In: Turk DC, Melzack R (eds). Handbook of Pain Assessment, 2nd edn. Guildford Press, New York, 2001: 53–75.

Puntillo KA, Neighbor ML. Two methods of assessing pain intensity in English-speaking and Spanish-speaking emergency department patients. J Emerg Nurs 1997; 23:597–601.

Putzke JD, Richards JS, Hicken BL, et al. Pain classification following spinal cord injury: the utility of verbal descriptors. Spinal Cord 2002; 40:118–127.

Radbruch L, Sabatowski R, Loick G, et al. Cognitive impairment and its influence on pain and symptom assessment in a palliative care unit: development of a Minimal Documentation System. Palliat Med 2000; 14:266–276.

Ramer L, Richardson JL, Zichi Cohen M, et al. Multimeasure pain assessment in an ethnically diverse group of patients with cancer. J Trans Nurs 1999; 10:94–101.

Rasmussen JL. Analysis of Likert-Scale data: a reinterpretation of Gregoire and Driver. Psychol Bull 1989; 105:167–170.

Rice ASC, Maton S. Postherpetic Neuralgia Study Group. Gabapentin in postherpetic neuralgia: a randomized, double-blind, placebo controlled study. Pain 2001; 94:215–224.

Roach KE, Brown MD, Dunigan KM, et al. Test–retest reliability of patient reports of low back pain. JOSPT 1997; 26:253–259.

Rogers SN, Humphris G, Lowe D, et al. The impact of surgery for oral cancer on quality of life as measured by the Medical Outcome Short Form 36. Oral Oncol 1998a; 34:171–179.

Rogers SN, Lowe D, Brown JS, et al. A comparison between the University of Washington Head and Neck Disease-Specific Measure and the Medical Short Form 36, EORTC QOQ-C33 and EORTC Head and Neck 35. Oral Oncol 1998b; 34:361–372.

Rowbotham M, Harden N, Stacey B, et al. Gabapentin for the treatment of postherpetic neuralgia. JAMA 1998; 280:1837–1842.

Rybstein-Blinchik E. Effects of different cognitive strategies on chronic pain experience. J Behav Med 1979; 2:93–101.

Sandblom G, Carlsson P, Sigsjo P, et al. Pain and health-related quality of life in a geographically defined population of men with prostate cancer. Br J Cancer 2001; 85:497–503.

Sandouk P, Serrie A, Urtizberea M, et al. Morphine pharmacokinetics and pain assessment in patients with terminal cancer. Clin Pharmacol Ther 1991; 49:442–448.

Schipper H, Clinch J, McMurray A, et al. Measuring the quality of life of cancer patients: the functional living index-cancer: development and validation. J Clin Oncol 1984; 2:472–483.

Serrao JM, Marks RL, Morley SJ, et al. Intrathecal midazolam for the treatment of chronic mechanical low back pain: a controlled comparison with epidural steroid in a pilot study. Pain 1992; 48:5–12.

Seymour RA. The use of pain scales in assessing the efficacy of analgesics in post-operative dental pain. Eur J Clin Pharm 1982; 23:441–444.

Seymour RA, Charlton JE, Phillips ME. An evaluation of dental pain using visual analogue scales and the McGill Pain Questionnaire. J Oral Maxillofac Surg 1983; 41:643–648.

Shannon MM, Ryan MA, D'Agostino N, et al. Assessment of pain in advanced cancer patients. J Pain Sympt Manage 1995; 10:274–278.

Singer AJ, Kowalska A, Thode HC. Ability of patients to accurately recall the severity of acute painful events. Acad Emerg Med 2001; 8:292–295.

Smith EL, Hann DM, Ahles TA, et al. Dyspnea, anxiety, body consciousness, and quality of life in patients with lung cancer. J Pain Sympt Manage 2001; 21:323–329.

Smith WB, Gracely RH, Safer MA. The meaning of pain: cancer patients' rating and recall of pain intensity and affect. Pain 1998; 78:123–129.

Sneeuw KCA, Aaronson NK, Osoba D, et al. The use of significant others as proxy raters of the quality of life of patients with brain cancer. Med Care 1997; 35:490–506.

Sneeuw KCA, Aaronson NK, Spranger MAG, et al. Evaluating the quality of life of cancer patients: assessments by patients, significant others, physicians and nurses. Br J Cancer 1999; 81:87–94.

Stahmer SA, Shofer FS, Marino A, et al. Do quantitative changes in pain intensity correlate with pain relief and satisfaction? Acad Emerg Med 1998; 5:851–857

Steiner TJ, Lange R, Mvoelker. Aspirin in episodic tension-type headache: placebo-controlled dose ranging comparison with paracetamol. Cephalagia 2003; 23:59–66.

Stelian J, Gil I, Habot B, et al. Improvement of pain and disability in elderly patients with degenerative osteoarthritis of the knee treated with narrow-band light therapy. J Am Geriat Soc 1992; 40:23–26.

Stenn PG, Mothersill KJ, Brooke RI. Biofeedback and a cognitive behavioral approach to treatment of myofascial pain dysfunction syndrome. Behav Ther 1979; 10:29–36.

Stockler MR, Osoba D, Goodwin P, et al. Responsiveness to change in health-related quality of life in a randomized clinical trial: a comparison of the Prostate Cancer Specific Quality of Life Instrument (PROSQOLI) with analogous scales from the EORTC QLQ-C30 and a trial specific module. J Clin Epidemiol 1998; 51:137–145.

Sze FK, Chung TK, Wong E, et al. Pain in Chinese cancer patients under palliative care. Palliat Med 1998; 12:271–277.

Talmi YP, Waller A, Bercovici M, et al. Pain experienced by patients with terminal head and neck carcinoma. Cancer 1997; 80:1117–1123.

Tannock I, Gospodarowicz M, Meakin W, et al. Treatment of metastatic prostatic cancer with low-dose prednisone. Evaluation of pain and quality of life as pragmatic indices of response. J Clin Oncol 1989; 7:590–597.

Tannock IF, Osoba D, Stockler MR, et al. Chemotherapy with mitoxantrone plus prednosone or prednisone alone for symptomatic hormone-resistant prostate cancer: a Canadian randomized trial with palliative end points. J Clin Oncol 1996; 14:1756–1764.

Tesfaye S, Watt J, Benbow SJ, et al. Electrical spinal-cord stimulation for painful diabetic peripheral neuropathy. Lancet 1996; 348:1698–1701.

Thomas V, Heath M, Rose D, et al. Psychological characteristics and the effectiveness of patient-controlled analgesia. Br J Anaesth 1995; 74:271–276.

Trotti A, Johnson DJ, Gwede C, et al. Development of a head and neck companion module for the quality of life-radiation therapy instrument (QOL-RTI). Int J Rad Oncol Biol Phys 1998; 42:257–261.

Turk DC, Rudy TE, Salovey P. The McGill Pain Questionnaire reconsidered: confirming the factor structure and examining appropriate uses. Pain 1985; 21:385–397.

Turner JA. Comparison of group progressive-relaxation training and cognitive-behavioral group therapy for chronic low back pain. J Cons Clin Psych 1982; 50:757–765.

Tursky B, Jamner LD, Friedman R. The pain perception profile: a psychophysiological approach to the assessment of pain report. Behav Ther 1982; 13:376–394.

Wallenstein SL. The VAS relief scale and other analgesic measures. Adv Pain Res Ther 1991; 18:97–103.

Wallenstein SL, Heidrich G III, Kaiko R, et al. Clinical evaluation of mild analgesics: the measurement of clinical pain. Br J Clin Pharm 1980; 10:319S–327S.

Walsh TD, Leber B. Measurement of chronic pain: visual analog scales and McGill Melzack pain questionnaire compared. Adv Pain Res Ther 1983; 5:897–899.

Wang XS, Cleeland CS, Mendoza TR, et al. The effect of pain severity on health-related quality of life. Cancer 1999; 86:1848–1855.

Wilkie D, Lovejoy N, Dodd M, et al. Cancer pain intensity measurement: concurrent validity of three tools – Finger dynamometer, Pain Intensity Number Scale, Visual Analogue Scale. Hosp J 1990; 6:1–13.

Wilkie DJ, Keefe FJ, Dodd MJ, et al. Behavior of patients with lung cancer: description and associations with oncologic and pain variables. Pain 1992; 51:231–240.

Wilkie DJ, Kampbell J, Cutshall S, et al. Effects of massage on pain intensity, analgesics and quality of life in patients with cancer pain: a pilot study of a randomized clinical trial conducted within hospice care delivery. Hosp J 2000; 15:31–53.

Wilkie DJ, Huang HY, Reilly N, et al. Nociceptive and neuropathic pain in patients with lung cancer. J Pain Sympt Manage 2001; 22:899–910.

Williams ACD, Oakley Davies HT, Chadury Y. Simple pain rating scales hide complex idiosyncratic meanings. Pain 2000; 85:457–463.

Zalon ML. Comparison of pain measures in surgical patients. J Nurs Meas 1999; 7:135–152.

Zeppetella G. An assessment of the safety, efficacy, and acceptability of intranasal fentanyl citrate in the management of cancer-related breakthrough pain: a pilot study. J Pain Sympt Manage 2000; 20:253–258.

FURTHER READING

Ahles TA, Blanchard JB, Ruckdeschel JC. The multidimensional nature of cancer-related pain. Pain 1982; 17:277–288.

Bolton J. Accuracy of recall of usual pain intensity in back pain patients. Pain 1999; 83:533–539.

Cronbach LJ. Essentials of Psychological Testing. Harper and Row, New York, 1970.

Everts B, Karlson B, Währborg AN-J, et al. Pain recollection after chest pain of cardiac origin. Cardiology 1999; 2:115–120.

Frisbie JH, Aguilera EJ. Chronic pain after spinal cord injury: an expedient diagnostic approach. Paraplegia 1990; 28:460–465.

Heft MW, Gracely RH, Dubner R. Nitrous oxide analgesia: a psychophysical evaluation using verbal descriptor scaling. J Dent Res 1982; 63:129–132.

Jensen MP, McFarland C. Increasing the reliability and validity of pain intensity measurement in chronic pain patients. Pain 1993; 55:195–203.

Jensen MP, Turner LR, Turner JA, et al. The use of multiple-item scales for pain intensity measurement in chronic pain patients. Pain 1996; 67:35–40.

Jensen MP, Smith DG, Ehde DM, et al. Pain site and the effects of amputation pain: further clarification of the meaning of mild, moderate, and severe pain. Pain 2001; 91:317–322.

Jensen MP, Chen C, Brugger AM. Postsurgical pain outcome assessment. Pain 2002a; 99:101–109.

Jensen MP, Richards P, Dhanda R. The effect of controlled-release oxycodone on neuropathic pain sensations. Poster presented at the 21st Annual Meeting of the American Pain Society, Baltimore, MD, 2002b.

Meier T, Wasner G, Faust M, et al. Efficacy of lidocaine patch 5% in the treatment of focal peripheral neuropathic pain syndromes: a randomized, double-blind, placebo-controlled study. Pain 2002; 106:151–158.

Naesern MA, Hahnn K-AK, Liebermann BE. Carpal tunnel syndrome pain treated with low-level laser and microamperes transcutaneous electric nerve stimulation: a controlled study. Arch Phys Med Rehabil 2002; 83:978–988.

Radwanski M. Self-medicating practices for managing chronic pain after spinal cord injury. Rehabil Nurs 1992; 17:312–317.

Serlin RC, Mendoza TR, Nakamura Y, et al. When is cancer pain mild, moderate or severe? Grading pain severity by its interference with function. Pain 1995; 61:277–284.

Siddall PJ, Loeser JD. Pain following spinal cord injury. Spinal Cord 2001; 39:63–73.

Soh G, Ang HG. Comparison of two pain rating scale among Chinese cancer patients. Chin Med J 1997; 105:953–956.

Turner JA, Cardenas DD. Chronic pain problems in individuals with spinal cord injuries. Semin Clin Neuropsychiat 1999; 4:186–194.

Urban BJ, Keefe FJ, France RD. A study of psychophysical scaling in chronic pain patients. Pain 1995; 20:157–168.

Widerström-Naga EG, Felipe-Cuervo E, Yezierski RP. Relationships among clinical characteristics of chronic pain after spinal cord injury. Arch Phys Med Rehabil 2001; 82:1191–1197.

5.1

Pain quality assessment scale (PQAS)

Instructions: There are different aspects and types of pain that patients experience and that we are interested in measuring. Pain can feel sharp, hot, cold, dull, and achy. Some pains may feel like they are very superficial (at skin level), or they may feel like they are from deep inside the body. Pain can also be described as unpleasant.

The Pain Quality Assessment Scale helps us measure these and other different aspects of your pain. For one patient, a pain might feel extremely hot and burning, but not at all dull, while another patient may not experience any burning pain, but feel like their pain is very dull and achy. Therefore, we expect you to rate very high on some of the scales below and very low on others.

Please use the 19 rating scales below to rate how much of each different pain quality and type you may or may not have felt *OVER THE PAST WEEK, ON AVERAGE.*

Place an "X" through the number that best describes your pain. For example:

0	1	2	3	4	5	✗	7	8	9	10

1. Please use the scale below to tell us how **intense** your pain has been over the past week, on average.

No pain | 0 | 1 | 2 | 3 | 4 | 5 | 6 | 7 | 8 | 9 | 10 | The most **intense** imaginable

2. Please use the scale below to tell us how **sharp** your pain has felt over the past week. Words used to describe sharp feelings include *"like a knife," "like a spike,"* or *"piercing."*

Not sharp | 0 | 1 | 2 | 3 | 4 | 5 | 6 | 7 | 8 | 9 | 10 | The most **sharp** sensation imaginable ("like a knife")

3. Please use the scale below to tell us how **hot** your pain has felt over the past week. Words used to describe very hot pain include *"burning"* and *"on fire."*

Not hot | 0 | 1 | 2 | 3 | 4 | 5 | 6 | 7 | 8 | 9 | 10 | The most **hot** sensation imaginable ("burning")

4. Please use the scale below to tell us how **dull** your pain has felt over the past week.

Not dull | 0 | 1 | 2 | 3 | 4 | 5 | 6 | 7 | 8 | 9 | 10 | The most **dull** sensation imaginable

5. Please use the scale below to tell us how **cold** your pain has felt over the past week. Words used to describe very cold pain include *"like ice"* and *"freezing."*

Not cold | 0 | 1 | 2 | 3 | 4 | 5 | 6 | 7 | 8 | 9 | 10 | The most **cold** sensation imaginable ("freezing")

6. Please use the scale below to tell us how **sensitive** your skin has been to light touch or clothing rubbing against it over the past week. Words used to describe sensitive skin include *"like sunburned skin"* and *"raw skin."*

Not sensitive | 0 | 1 | 2 | 3 | 4 | 5 | 6 | 7 | 8 | 9 | 10 | The most **sensitive** sensation imaginable ("raw skin")

7. Please use the scale below to tell us how **tender** your pain is when something has pressed against it over the past week. Another word used to describe tender pain is *"like a bruise."*

Not tender | 0 | 1 | 2 | 3 | 4 | 5 | 6 | 7 | 8 | 9 | 10 | The most **tender** sensation imaginable ("like a bruise")

8. Please use the scale below to tell us how **itchy** your pain has felt over the past week. Words used to describe itchy pain include *"like poison ivy"* and *"like a mosquito bite."*

Not itchy | 0 | 1 | 2 | 3 | 4 | 5 | 6 | 7 | 8 | 9 | 10 | The most **itchy** sensation imaginable ("like poison ivy")

9. Please use the scale below to tell us how much your pain has felt like it has been **shooting** over the past week. Another word used to describe shooting pain is *"zapping."*

Not shooting | 0 | 1 | 2 | 3 | 4 | 5 | 6 | 7 | 8 | 9 | 10 | The most **shooting** sensation imaginable ("zapping")

10. Please use the scale below to tell us how **numb** your pain has felt over the past week. A phrase that can be used to describe numb pain is *"like it is asleep."*

Not numb | 0 | 1 | 2 | 3 | 4 | 5 | 6 | 7 | 8 | 9 | 10 | The most **numb** sensation imaginable ("like it is asleep")

11. Please use the scale below to tell us how much your pain sensations have felt **electrical** over the past week. Words used to describe electrical pain include *"shocks,"* *"lightning,"* and *"sparking."*

Not electrical | 0 | 1 | 2 | 3 | 4 | 5 | 6 | 7 | 8 | 9 | 10 | The most **electrical** sensation imaginable ("shocks")

12. Please use the scale below to tell us how **tingling** your pain has felt over the past week. Words used to describe tingling pain include *"like pins and needles"* and *"prickling."*

Not tingling | 0 | 1 | 2 | 3 | 4 | 5 | 6 | 7 | 8 | 9 | 10 | The most **tingling** sensation imaginable ("like pins and needles")

13. Please use the scale below to tell us how **cramping** your pain has felt over the past week. Words used to describe cramping pain include *"squeezing"* and *"tight."*

Not cramping | 0 | 1 | 2 | 3 | 4 | 5 | 6 | 7 | 8 | 9 | 10 | The most **cramping** sensation imaginable ("squeezing")

14. Please use the scale below to tell us how **radiating** your pain has felt over the past week. Another word used to describe radiating pain is *"spreading."*

Not radiating | 0 | 1 | 2 | 3 | 4 | 5 | 6 | 7 | 8 | 9 | 10 | The most **radiating** sensation imaginable ("spreading")

15. Please use the scale below to tell us how **throbbing** your pain has felt over the past week. Another word used to describe throbbing pain is *"pounding."*

Not throbbing | 0 | 1 | 2 | 3 | 4 | 5 | 6 | 7 | 8 | 9 | 10 | The most **throbbing** sensation imaginable ("pounding")

16. Please use the scale below to tell us how **aching** your pain has felt over the past week. Another word used to describe aching pain is *"like a toothache."*

Not aching | 0 | 1 | 2 | 3 | 4 | 5 | 6 | 7 | 8 | 9 | 10 | The most **aching** sensation imaginable ("like a toothache")

17. Please use the scale below to tell us how **heavy** your pain has felt over the past week. Other words used to describe heavy pain are *"pressure"* and *"weighted down."*

Not heavy | 0 | 1 | 2 | 3 | 4 | 5 | 6 | 7 | 8 | 9 | 10 | The most **heavy** sensation imaginable ("weighted down")

18. Now that you have told us the different types of pain sensations you have felt, we want you to tell us overall how **unpleasant** your pain has been to you over the past week. Words used to describe very unpleasant pain include *"annoying," "bothersome," "miserable,"* and *"intolerable."* Remember, pain can have a low intensity but still feel extremely unpleasant, and some kinds of pain can have a high intensity but be very tolerable. With this scale, please tell us how **unpleasant** your pain feels.

Not unpleasant | 0 | 1 | 2 | 3 | 4 | 5 | 6 | 7 | 8 | 9 | 10 | The most **unpleasant** sensation imaginable ("intolerable")

19. Finally, we want you to give us an estimate of the severity of your *deep* versus *surface* pain over the past week. We want you to rate each location of pain separately. We realize that it can be difficult to make these estimates, and most likely it will be a "best guess," but please give us your best estimate.

HOW INTENSE IS YOUR *DEEP* PAIN?

No pain | 0 | 1 | 2 | 3 | 4 | 5 | 6 | 7 | 8 | 9 | 10 | The most **intense deep** pain sensation imaginable

HOW INTENSE IS YOUR *SURFACE* PAIN?

No pain | 0 | 1 | 2 | 3 | 4 | 5 | 6 | 7 | 8 | 9 | 10 | The most **intense surface** pain sensation imaginable

20. Pain can also have different time qualities. For some people, the pain "comes and goes" and so they have some moments that are completely without pain. This is called **intermittent** pain. Others are never pain free, but their pain types and pain severity can vary from one moment to the next. This is called **variable** pain. For these people, the increases can be severe, so that they feel they have moments of very intense pain ("breakthrough" pain), but at other times they can feel lower levels of pain ("background" pain). Still, they are never pain free. Other people have pain that really does not change that much from one moment to another. This is called **stable** pain. Which of the following best describes the time pattern of your pain? (Please select only one.)

( ) I have **intermittent** pain (I feel pain sometimes but I am pain-free at other times).
( ) I have **variable** pain ("background" pain all the time, but also moments of more pain, or even severe "breakthrough" pain or varying types of pain).
( ) I have **stable** pain (constant pain that does not change very much from one moment to another, and no pain-free periods).

5.2

Leeds assessment of neuropathic symptoms and signs – self-report (S-LANSS)

Please answer the questions below about how your pain has felt over the past week.

1. In the area where you have pain, do you also have "pins and needles," tingling or prickling sensations?
   (a) NO – I don't get these sensations
   (b) YES – I get these sensations often

2. Does the painful area change color (look mottled or more red) when the pain is particularly bad?
   (a) NO – the pain does not affect the color of my skin
   (b) YES – I have noticed that the pain does make my skin look different from normal

3. Does your pain make the affected skin abnormally sensitive to touch? Getting unpleasant sensations or pain when lightly stroking the skin might describe this.
   (a) NO – the pain does not make my skin in that area abnormally sensitive to touch
   (b) YES – my skin in that area is particularly sensitive to touch

4. Does your pain come on suddenly and in bursts for no apparent reason when you are completely still? Words like "electric shocks," "jumping" and "bursting" might describe this.
   (a) NO – my pain doesn't really feel like this
   (b) YES – I get these sensations often

5. In the area where you have pain, does your skin feel unusually hot like a burning pain?
   (a) NO – I don't have burning pain
   (b) YES – I get burning pain often

6. Gently *rub* the painful area with your index finger and then rub a non-painful area (for example, an area of skin further away or on the opposite side from the painful area). How does this rubbing feel in the painful area?
   (a) The painful area feels no different from the non-painful area
   (b) I feel discomfort, like pins and needles, tingling or burning in the painful area that is different from the non-painful area

7. Gently *press* on the painful area with your finger tip then gently press in the same way onto a non-painful area (the same non-painful area that you chose in the last question). How does this feel in the painful area?
   (a) The painful area does not feel different from the non-painful area
   (b) I feel numbness or tenderness in the painful area that is different from the non-painful area

SHORT FORM MCGILL PAIN QUESTIONNAIRE AND PAIN DIAGRAM

See Melzack R. The Short Form McGill Pain Questionnaire. Pain 1987; 30:191–197.

Date:_____ Name:_____

Check the column to indicate the level of your pain for each word, or leave blank if it does not apply to you.

	Mild 1	*Moderate 2*	*Severe 3*
1 Throbbing			
2 Shooting			
3 Stabbing			
4 Sharp			
5 Cramping			
6 Gnawing			
7 Hot–burning			
8 Aching			
9 Heavy			
10 Tender			
11 Splitting			
12 Tiring–exhausting			
13 Sickening			
14 Fearful			
15 Cruel–punishing			

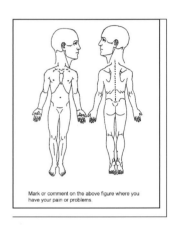

Mark or comment on the above figure where you have your pain or problems.

Indicate on this line how bad your pain is – at the left end of line means no pain at all, at right end means worst pain possible.

No Pain _____ Worst Possible Pain

Score:

S-PRI (Sensory Pain Rating Index)	(questions 1–11)	max score = 33
A-PRI (Affective Pain Rating Index)	(questions 12–15)	max score = 12
T-PRI (Total Pain Rating Index)	(questions 1–15)	max score = 45
PPI-VAS (Present Pain Intensity-Visual Analog Scale)		max score = 10

Placebo effects in clinical pain trials

Ron C. Kupers • Hans Rasmussen

I think and imagine now,
That all who stand before me know
Have oft heard of my wondrous fame,
And understand my glorious name –
The Italian doctor Dulcamara,
And my wonderful renown
Is known through all the world
I am the greatest, wondrous benefactor.
I sell the Magic Pain Extractor,
an admirable mixture
Which cures every sort of toothache,
And ne'er was known to fail.
This cures the apoplectical,
the asthmathical,
the paralytical, the diuretical,
deafness too
All evils are at once upset
By this new and fashionable mode

Donizetti, *L'Elisir D'Amore* (Act I, scene V)

INTRODUCTION

THE PLACEBO EFFECT: FROM AN UNPOPULAR TO A TRENDY TOPIC

In 1991, Patrick Wall wrote an editorial in the journal *Pain* with the provocative title: "The placebo effect: an unpopular topic." Indeed, until the mid-1990s, basic scientists had devoted little attention to the placebo effect as a legitimate topic for fundamental research (Wall 1991). The placebo effect was largely considered a mere nuisance variable: a disconcerting effect in clinical studies that had to be controlled for in order to distill genuine treatment effects from the totality of observed effects (Evans 1985). The placebo effect was widely recognized as a clinical reality but was dismissed from further scientific consideration (White 1985). This situation has changed dramatically in recent years and the scientific interest in the placebo effect has increased at a tremendous pace. In this respect, the results of a Medline search on the number of articles including placebo as a keyword is highly revealing. Whereas placebo was mentioned only 250 times in the scientific literature between 1969 and 1973, this number rose to 10,019 in the period 1983–1987 and to an astonishing 23,693 citations in the period 1999–2003. Today it is generally believed that the placebo effect is a powerful and common phenomenon that forms an integral part of any medical and non-medical therapy (Turner et al. 1994). While the placebo effect seems to have been taken seriously by the scientific community in general, the number of studies actually investigating its underlying mechanisms nonetheless represents only a minute fraction of the entirety of the placebo literature.

THE UBIQUITOUS PLACEBO

The placebo response is a common phenomenon that is observed in a wide variety of conditions. It has been described for mood disorders, pain, Parkinson's disease, common cold, dysmenorrhea, insomnia, asthma, hypertension, angina pectoris, and other diverse complaints. Although the main emphasis in this chapter will be on placebo analgesia, we will also provide a brief summary of some of the recent findings of the placebo response in Parkinson's disease and depression.

Placebo analgesia is the best-studied form of the placebo responses (Evans 1985). In placebo analgesia, the administration of an inert substance, presented to the patient as a painkiller, produces an analgesic response. The nature of pain lends itself well to the provoking of placebo responses. The subjective experience of pain is largely shaped by one's beliefs, expectations and past experiences. Nowadays, there is abundant evidence that there is no linear relationship between the incoming sensory input and the resulting pain sensation. External stimuli undergo a complex modulation by cognitive, attentional, motivational and affective processes at the spinal and supraspinal level. Hypnosis-induced analgesia (Rainville et al. 1997; Faymonville et al. 2000), emergency analgesia (Wall 1979) and placebo analgesia (Amanzio and Benedetti 1997; Benedetti et al. 1999; Petrovic et al. 2002; Price and Fields 1997; Wager et al. 2004) are typical examples of how these higher processes are capable of modulating the impact of incoming sensory stimuli. Recent studies have shown that classical conditioning (Voudouris et al. 1990; Suchman and Ader 1992), expectancy (Montgomery and Kirsch 1997; Price et al. 1999) and motivation for pain relief (Benson and Friedman 1996; Harrington 1997) are likely to form important components of the placebo analgesic effect. Thus, insight into the mechanisms mediating placebo analgesia should furnish us valuable information about the interaction between psychological and physiologic processes. More specifically, a better insight may lead to improved understanding of the brain's endogenous pain modulatory networks and the way they can be triggered by external cues. This knowledge may ultimately be applied therapeutically for the relief of pain. A better understanding of how psychological manipulations of a placebo administration produce biologic changes could shed light on and refine factors that are effective in general pain management (Moerman 2002b; Soerensen and Price 2002). If we establish the experimental factors necessary and sufficient for the placebo response, we can use specific placebo treatments to alter human physiologic and pathophysiologic processes. This strategy would have a beneficial effect on the negative consequences of chronic pain such as reduced immune response and depression (Liebeskind 1991; Price 1999).

If we follow the principle that any treatment which provides benefit to the patient ought to be incorporated into clinical practice (de la Fuente-Fernandez and Stoessel 2002), we should not ask "how can we avoid the placebo effect?" but rather "how can we use it better?" (Benson and Friedman 1996; Moerman 2002b; Oh 1994). If we succeed in achieving this, we are on the way to replace the term *placebo* with designated procedural variables and specific laws of behavior making the unknown known (White et al. 1985). On a theoretical level, an exploration of the interaction between the psychological and physiologic processes evoking the placebo effect may contribute to the interdisciplinary understanding of the placebo effect within a single theoretical framework. Empirically, this approach might bring about more progressive procedures to measure and validate placebo effects in particular, and pain management in general (Soerensen and Price 2002).

A BRIEF HISTORICAL ACCOUNT OF THE MODERN HISTORY OF THE PLACEBO EFFECT

The word placebo is derived from Latin, meaning "I shall please." Until the term became introduced in modern medicine, placebos were considered equivalent to quackery. Amusing examples of this perception can be found in music and theatre plays such as Donizetti's *L'Elisir D'Amore* and Molière's *La Maladie Imaginaire* or *Monsieur de Pourceaugnac*. We can distinguish three phases in the modern history of the placebo effect. During the first phase (pre-World War II), placebos were seen as morally acceptable and innocent management tools without curative or symptomatic consequences. They were often used as diagnostic tools to separate imaginary "psychological symptoms" from real medical problems. A positive placebo response was considered as a strong indication that the patient was hysterical or that the apparent disease or symptom was not real. The emphasis was clearly on the response of the single subject. This situation changed dramatically after World War II when the placebo became strongly associated with the double-blind randomized control trial. Until then, the evaluation of new therapies was strongly dependent on the personal opinions and preferences expressed by recognized leaders in the field. In other words, clinical impressions and poorly controlled evidence played a major role in the assessment of a drug or therapy. With the enormous expansion of biomedical research after World War II, efforts were undertaken to impose more scientific rigor in clinical research through the use of blind assessment, random assignment of subjects to an experimental or control condition, and the use of statistics (Kaptchuk 1998). Thus, the randomized controlled trial (RCT) was born. Two persons who were very instrumental in this second placebo phase are Harry Gold from Cornell University, considered as the inventor of the double-blind RCT, and Henry Beecher of the Harvard Medical School. The need for blind assessment created the necessity for a control condition which was, of necessity, often a placebo. As a consequence, the emphasis shifted away from how an individual reacted to a placebo towards the response of the group to a placebo. Placebo became a tool that allowed for the objective and unbiased evaluation of new therapies. However, there was a delay of several more decades before a real interest in the portrayal and the understanding of the placebo effect would arise. This brings us to the third phase of the modern history of the placebo. Starting in the 1980s, we see for the first time a genuine interest in the placebo phenomenon itself. Rather than uncritically showcasing its huge potential and power, a more critical attitude and more rigorous methodology succeeded in portraying the power of placebo more accurately. Soon it became evident that much of what had originally been considered as placebo was actually due to factors such as regression to the mean and natural course of the disease (see below). This more critical attitude towards placebo recently culminated in a meta-analysis study concluding that placebos are lacking any power (see further). At the same time, the first papers appeared that tried to explain the mechanisms underlying the placebo response. The combination of intelligent behavioral paradigms and brain imaging techniques have led in the past decade to great progress in our understanding of the biopsychosocial mechanisms involved in the placebo effect. Another factor that came to influence greatly placebo research was the imposition of the principle of informed consent at the beginning of the 1970s. If the patient is told that he or she will receive *either* a real therapy *or* a placebo, there will naturally be speculation about the condition to which he has been assigned. This situation is very artificial and far from the natural daily clinical setting where high expectations of relief are offered to the patient. Knowledge that one has a chance of receiving placebo may introduce uncertainty and ambivalence on the part of the subject, leading to a reduction in the magnitudes of both the response to placebo and the active drug. We will discuss this issue at length in the section on placebo study designs.

A DEFINITION

IS IT POSSIBLE TO DEFINE PLACEBO?

There has been a strong tendency in biomedical research to stay on one side of the border between psychology and medicine. The biomedical paradigm is based on the assumption that disease and treatment belong solely to the domain of molecular biology, pharmacology and physiology. Accordingly, successful treatment is accomplished through changes in the underlying pathophysiology (Roth 2003). It follows that within the biomedical tradition there is no room left for the effects of the mental state. As such, a way to dismiss the placebo phenomenon has been to employ the double-blind procedure, and merely dismiss placebo effects as methodologic noise (Macedo 2003). Consequently, placebo became synonymous with the administration of an inert substance as part of a double-blind RCT procedure. This is, however, not the same as acknowledging that placebos are without effect. The placebo is inert, but not devoid of effect. A broader perspective holds that since the placebo is inert in itself, its effects are due to nonspecific factors (Kirsh 1997). Here it is stressed that the placebo should be seen in a broader context. What elicits the placebo effect is not the inert substance but the entire context in which it is administered (Harrington 1997; Benedetti 2002).

It is difficult or maybe even impossible to define the placebo and the placebo effect in a coherent and logical manner (Grünbaum 1985; Götzsche 1994; Hrobjartsoson 1996; Moerman and Jonas 2002). This becomes obvious when looking at classical definitions of the placebo. For instance, Shapiro (1964) defined placebo as: "any therapeutic procedure (or that component of any therapeutic procedure) which is given deliberately to have an effect, or unknowingly, and has an effect on a symptom, syndrome, disease, or patient but which is objectively without specific activity for the condition being treated. The placebo effect is defined by the changes produced by placebos." Consequently, the placebo is described as being: "without specific activity for the condition being treated." Putting this phrase in place of the word itself, it then reads: "The placebo effect is defined as the changes produced by things without specific activity for the condition being treated," a statement that does not make any sense. Since placebos are inert, they do not cause the placebo effect. If they in fact were active, they would not be inert. The definition can be criticized for confusing coincidence with cause (Moerman 2002) such that the placebo effect becomes a contradiction in itself (Kienle and Kienle 1997). Because of the difficulty to provide a clear definition of placebo, some authors have suggested the abandonment of the entire concept of placebo (Götzsche 1994; Moerman and Jonas 2002). It has been proposed to rename placebo effects as "meaning responses," by which is meant the physiologic and psychological effects of meaning in the origins or treatment of illness (Moerman and Jonas 2002). Meaning responses following the administration of inert or sham treatment can be labeled "placebo effect" when they are desirable and "nocebo effect" when they are undesirable. This definition excludes several elements that are often included in the conceptualization of the placebo effect such as natural history of disease and regression to the mean (see further). This definition also has the advantage of avoiding the use of the term "nonspecific" effects.

Ideally, a definition should be accurate enough to clearly demarcate the phenomenon but still be open enough to include a range of possible empirical hypotheses about causative mechanisms (Brody 2000). From the above definition it follows that the number of placebos can be infinite. People have indeed inflated the concept of placebo enormously to include nearly every imaginable biologic, psychological, or social interaction. This is misleading since it implies that there are nebulous influences in treatment that mysteriously may alter behavior (Kazdin 1980). Consequently, placebo seems like a problematic territory for science that seeks to pinpoint and separate cause and effect. This might account for the fact that placebo has

been often looked upon as a nuisance variable within a biologic reductionistic model.

Placebo effects have in common with other unexplained phenomena that they lack an adequate theory and empirical procedures to explore the subject. They are, however, open for scientific inquiry (White et al. 1985). The crucial question is "which interdisciplinary model is most capable of specifying the nonspecifics, making the unknown known?" Employing a purely biomedical framework to explore the placebo effect as defined above would fall frustratingly short. Ultimately, we are interested in the link between psychological and physiologic processes. A biomedical framework embraces the view that complex phenomena should be explained from purely biologic processes. The possibility that non-biologic (behavioral and psychosocial) factors impinge upon biologic processes is rejected in this model. In this chapter, we propose a biopsychosocial approach to the placebo phenomenon (Engel 1977; Roth 2003).

It is problematic that many of the contemporary definitions hold the implausible claim that the placebo effect is brought about by the placebo agent per se, independent of its perception (Richardson 1994; Vase et al. 2002). The concept that a placebo must lack any specific properties is dubious since the placebo effect can be very specific. For example, placebos can have opposite effects on heart rate, or blood pressure, depending on whether they are given as tranquilizers or as stimulants (de la Fuente-Fernandez and Stoessel 2002). Consequently, Price and colleagues define the placebo effect as "the reduction in a symptom as a result of factors related to a subject's/patient's perception of the therapeutic intervention" (Vase et al. 2002).

This chapter deals mostly on pain and placebo analgesia. Pain is a subjective multidimensional experience with a sensory, affective, and cognitive dimension (Mersky and Bogduk 1994). Consequently, we will use the following working definition of placebo analgesia: "the reduction in pain intensity and/or unpleasantness as a result of factors related to a subject's perception of the therapeutic intervention." This definition tends to satisfy the demands raised by Brody (2000). It demarcates the phenomenon of placebo to the realm of the psychology of the subject and his social context but is still open enough to include a range of possible empirical hypotheses about cause and mechanisms. Furthermore, this definition distinguishes between the placebo as an agent and the placebo effect as related to the subject's perception of the placebo. The present definition guides but does not excessively restrict the explorative field of a biopsychosocial perspective.

PLACEBO AND NONSPECIFIC EFFECTS

When looking at the results of the placebo effect, we are struck by some of the high reported success rates. Whereas Beecher reported an average placebo response rate of 35%, a more recent study mentioned placebo response rates ranging between 42 and 100% (Turner et al. 1994). These astonishingly high rates are in sharp contrast with the results of a recent meta-analysis, which concluded that placebos lack major clinical effects (Hrobjartsson and Götzsche 2001). This meta-analysis only included studies that also used a no-treatment group. The conclusions of this study have been heavily criticized because of methodologic errors (Kaptchuk 2001; Kupers 2001; Miller 2001). This brings us, however, to confront the common confusion between nonspecific treatment effects and placebo effects. Nonspecific treatment effects refers to all kinds of effects that are attributable to factors other than the specific pharmacologic, surgical or other specific effect of an intervention. This is a very broad category of processes including natural course of the disease, regression to the mean, routine medical care, associated regimens such as diet, rest, relaxation, the doctor–patient relationship, etc. The significance of natural course of the disease and regression to the mean are explained in more detail below.

Natural course

It is argued above that the lack of a natural history group biased the conclusion of Beecher's classical review paper (1955) of the placebo effect. Some symptoms resolve spontaneously over time and do not require any particular intervention. A prototypical example is a common cold. Therefore, if a natural history group is lacking, the normal course of the disease or symptom may be overlooked and mistakenly attributed to a placebo effect. This leads to a misinterpretation of the cause–effect relationship (Benedetti et al. 2003a). For example, Thomas (1974) studied 3848 patients presenting at general practitioners' consultations. In 1656 patients (43%), no clear diagnosis could be made and patients were asked to return if symptoms did not improve. Of these, 72% did not return whereas the remaining returned with the same or another complaint. If a placebo had been given to these patients during their first visit, this would have led to the false conclusion that more than 70% of the patients improved due to placebo. Thus, a placebo effect can be demonstrated only when there is control for the natural history. This can be accomplished by having a no-treated control group or a control group on a waiting list. Another implication of this result is that it is very difficult or sometimes impossible to assess the placebo effect in an individual patient since there is no possibility to find out how the patient would have evolved spontaneously. Price (1999) therefore distinguishes between the placebo analgesic effect and the placebo analgesic response. The former refers to the mean reduction in pain in a group of subjects administered a placebo treatment, whereas the latter refers

to the reduction in pain in a single subject given a placebo.

Regression to the mean

Closely linked to natural course of the disease is the phenomenon of regression to the mean. Like the former issue, regression to the mean is often overlooked, although it may explain a considerable amount of variance that is normally attributed to placebo or treatment effects (McDonald et al. 1983). Regression to the mean describes a statistical tendency of extreme data measures to move closer to their central tendency when they are re-assessed at a later time-point. Chronic pain largely fluctuates over time and, in many chronic pain patients, periods of severe pain intersperse with periods of less or minimal pain (Price 1999). Since individuals tend to seek clinical assessment and treatment when their pain and discomfort becomes unbearable (extreme value), what is most likely to happen is a natural improvement since many acute and some chronic pains resolve spontaneously and do not need a special intervention. This "improvement" is erroneously interpreted as a treatment or placebo effect, depending on whether an active therapy or a placebo was administered (Davis 2002; Fava et al. 2003).

PLACEBO ANALGESIA

Beecher (1955) was the first to review the clinical and experimental literature on placebo and to consider placebo as a subject worthy of scientific study. He reviewed 15 clinical studies covering 1082 patients suffering a variety of conditions including postoperative pain, angina pectoris, anxiety and the common cold. On average, symptoms were satisfactorily relieved in 35% of the patients. Shapiro (1960) reported a similar success rate. At an early stage of placebo research, it became clear that placebo analgesic responses are much more pronounced for clinical pain than for experimentally-induced pain (Lasagna et al. 1954). Whereas placebos seemed to lead to satisfactory pain relief in about 30 to 40% of patients suffering clinical forms of pain, they reduced experimental pain in only 3% of the subjects. One of the possible reasons for these low placebo rates may be that early experimental placebo studies used radiant heat and brief electric shock as pain stimuli. For example, two studies employing brief experimental pain stimuli (five-second heat stimuli applied to the skin and one-second electrical stimuli applied to the tooth pulp) failed to reveal a placebo effect (Price and Fields 1997). There seemed to be not only a significant difference in the placebo response rates for clinical and experimental pain but also in the magnitude of the placebo effect. Whereas Beecher used 50% pain reduction as a criterion for a significant placebo analgesic effect, most experimental pain studies report placebo analgesic effects that are much smaller in amplitude, varying mostly between 0.5 and 1 point reductions on a 10-point visual analogue (VAS) pain scale (Voudouris et al. 1990; Wager et al. 2004). We studied placebo responses in a patient with chronic pain following failed back surgery (Figure 6.1A). The average pain rating in the weeks preceding placebo administration was 7 on a 10-point VAS rating scale, indicating severe pain. Pain ratings dropped to values between 0 and 2 following placebo (epidural saline delivered by means of a programmable controlled analgesia (PCA) pump). The placebo effect persisted over the 50 days during which the patient was followed. During this period, we interrupted the PCA pump on two separate days. During these "placebo holidays,"

the pain returned to pre-placebo levels, indicating that the observed effect was not due to regression to the mean or natural history of the disease (Kupers et al. 2007). This raises the following question: what makes clinical pain more susceptible to placebo effects? Is it because in chronic pain, expectancy, desire and motivation for pain relief are more pronounced? Or is it because of differences in the neurobiology of acute and chronic pain (Kupers et al. 2004)?

Notwithstanding these findings, recent studies by the group of Benedetti (Benedetti et al. 1999; Amanzio and Benedetti 1999) have shown that relatively powerful experimental placebo effects can be obtained (see Vase et al. 2002 for a meta-analysis). These authors introduced two important changes in the experimental

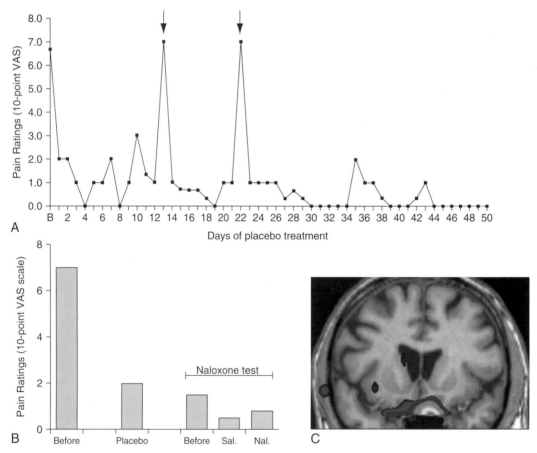

Figure 6.1 A. Time course of the placebo response in a patient with pain following failed back surgery. Before placebo was started, the average pain rating was around 7 on a 10-point VAS scale. The patient's pain was significantly reduced by placebo (epidural saline) during the 50 days the patient was followed. On two occasions, indicated by the arrows, the placebo administration was stopped and the original pain reappeared. This indicates that natural course of the disease or regression to the mean are unlikely to explain this patient's pain improvement. The data also indicate that placebo analgesia can last over extended periods. B. Effect of naloxone on the placebo response in a patient suffering from chronic pain. Naloxone (10 mg, i.v.) or saline were administered in a double-blind manner in a patient with placebo analgesia. The left bar (before) shows average pain ratings before placebo. Patient's average pain ratings during the 30 days of placebo administration dropped significantly (placebo). Naloxone did not abolish the placebo response in this patient. C. Prefrontal activation in a patient with phantom limb pain that responded positively to a placebo.

design of placebo studies. First, unlike in the majority of the experimental studies that used short-lasting pain stimuli, they used a tonic pain stimulus lasting more than 10 minutes. This may more aptly mimic clinical forms of pain and may consequently lead to a higher desire for pain relief. Second, they introduced drug-conditioning procedures to boost the placebo response. Subjects were first tested for baseline pain responsiveness to ischemic pain (Tourniquet test). Next, they were given a genuine analgesic drug for two consecutive days while they were submitted to the same pain test. On day four, the genuine drug was replaced by a placebo without informing the participants and pain responsiveness was tested again. Placebo responses were significantly higher in the group that had been submitted to pharmacologic conditioning than in a control group without conditioning.

PAIN AND TOP-DOWN MODULATION

Before trying to explain the neurobiology of placebo analgesia we will give a brief overview of the neurobiology of pain and what is known about the endogenous modulation of pain.

In 1965, Melzack and Wall proposed the "gate control" theory, according to which activation in large myelinated fibers is capable of inhibiting nociceptive information. This model struck against the contemporary belief that pain processing is a hard-wired process, mediated exclusively by pain-dedicated pathways. The consequences of this theory can hardly be overestimated. In essence, it was the first clear formulation of the fact that the body has its own built-in pain-modulatory mechanisms. A few years later, Melzack and Casey described their theory about the multidimensional processing of pain. This theory added a rostral (cerebral) extension to the gate control, which had previously focused on activity in the spinal cord dorsal horn. According to Melzack and Casey (1968), pain is a complex multidimensional experience comprising sensory-discriminative, motivational-affective and cognitive-evaluative components. For the first time, the concepts of cognition and emotion were introduced to a field that, until then, had belonged exclusively to the domain of sensory physiologists. Nowadays, most pain researchers accept the idea that pain is a complex multidimensional experience that involves both a sensory analysis of the painful stimulus and accompanying emotions and thoughts. Over the years, a number of assumptions have been added to Melzack and Casey's scheme. A first assumption is that the sensory and affective components are independent dimensions that can be measured separately (Gracely et al. 1978; Price and Harkins 1992). A second assumption is that distinct anatomical pathways are involved in the sensory and affective pain dimension (Albe-Fessard et al. 1985; Bushnell and

Duncan 1989; Price 1988). The sensory component of pain would involve the somatosensory thalamus and its projections to the primary and secondary somatosensory cortices and insula. The affective component on the other hand would involve the medial thalamus and its projections to the anterior cingulate and prefrontal cortices. Recent neuroimaging studies have endeavored to yield evidence for the selective activation of brain areas involved in the sensory-discriminative or affective dimension of pain (Rainville et al. 1997; Hofbauer et al. 2001) by using hypnotic suggestion specifically targeted at activating either system. While, according to the model by Melzack and Casey, cognitive and affective processing is performed in parallel with sensory processing, Price (2000) proposes a serial two-stage model in which the emotional component is the result of the interaction between a hard-wired sensory input and contextual processes. Price's theory views pain perception as a self-contained process simply driven by a reliable sensory process. However, cognitive expectations directly influence the operation of the sensory system. Wall (1999) therefore argued for a unified system that is permanently modified by experience. Nociceptive processing is not something purely dictated by the sensory characteristics of the stimulus but results from the interaction between the latter and the state of the nervous system at that particular time. The state of the nervous system depends both on past experiences and on the cognitive and emotional processes of the organism at the time of sensory input. A series of elegant animal studies by Dubner and co-workers in the 1980s provide strong experimental support for this view (Dubner et al. 1981; Duncan et al. 1987). The authors trained monkeys to discriminate between noxious thermal stimuli of different temperatures applied to the face during the recording of neuronal activity in medullary dorsal horn neurons. The onset of the noxious stimuli was announced to the animal by a light signal preceding the noxious stimulus by a variable time. In naïve monkeys, neuronal activity in the dorsal horn was limited to the actual period of the application of the nociceptive stimulus. However, in monkeys that had been trained for several months in the discrimination task, dorsal horn cells already started responding to the warning signal that preceded the noxious stimulus. In other words, the light stimulus had become a conditioned stimulus following repetitive pairings with the unconditioned (noxious) stimulus and now produced a conditioned response in the dorsal horn. This was the first example of top-down modulation at such an early (spinal) stage of pain processing. This finding may be of fundamental importance for the understanding of some forms of top-down modulation of pain in humans such as is observed in placebo analgesia. Other types of top-down modulation of pain exist that do not need such extensive learning procedures. For example, the attentional and emotional state of the subject can profoundly modify the responses to pain. Bushnell and colleagues (1985) showed that selective attention towards a sensory stimulus decreases its detection latency. This effect of selective attention was more pronounced for painful than for nonpainful stimuli. A series of recent neuroimaging studies in humans investigated cerebral mechanisms involved in this top-down modulation (Peyron et al. 1998; Petrovic et al. 2000; Bantick et al. 2002; Tracey et al. 2002; Lorenz et al. 2003; Valet et al. 2004). These studies have shown that prefrontal cortical areas such as the anterior cingulate cortex and the dorsolateral and orbitofrontal cortices play an important role in the endogenous modulation of pain and that they exert their influence at least in part through increased connectivity with the periaqueductal gray (PAG) of the mesencephalon.

There is ample evidence that the modulation of nociception is mediated by the midbrain PAG and the rostral ventromedial medulla (RVM) (Fields and Basbaum 1999). The RVM contains antinociceptive descending pathways targeting the spinal and trigeminal dorsal horn (Urban and Smith 1994; Hudson et al. 2000). Although there are no known direct descending projections from the PAG to the spinal cord, it has been hypothesized that the analgesic effects of PAG are mediated through relays in the RVM and the dorsolateral pontine tegmentum (DLPT). The PAG and RVM function as a unit exerting global control over pain transmission neurons in the dorsal horn. Opioids injected into the PAG and RVM produce analgesia (Urban and Smith 1994; Price and Fields 1997; McGaraughty et al. 2003). This analgesic effect can be blocked by administration of the opioid antagonist naloxone into the same area, which suggests a specific action at opioid receptors (Wang and Wessendorf 2002). Regions of the frontal lobe and the amygdala project via the hypothalamus and also directly to the PAG (An et al. 1998; Ongur et al. 1998).

BIOPSYCHOSOCIAL MECHANISMS OF PLACEBO ANALGESIA

It is interesting to note that many of the ascending pain pathways terminate in cortical and subcortical areas which are also at the origin of pain modulatory systems (Burstein et al. 1987; Bernard et al. 1996; Helmstetter et al. 1998; Fields and Basbaum 1999; Price 1999). These areas also play a major role in threat-elicited defensive behavior, learning and memory. This observation raises the following important questions in relation to placebo analgesia: (1) which cognitive and environmental circumstances are able to trigger these pain inhibitory mechanisms? and (2) once they are triggered, how do they produce their analgesic effect?

Animal studies over the past three decades have shed some light on the answers to these questions.

Activation of the endogenous pain modulatory circuits requires specific extrinsic environmental cues or conditions (Price 1999). Watkins and Mayer (1982) demonstrated that severe physical or psychological stressors (inescapable footshock, whole body rotation) are capable of inducing robust non analgesic responses. Some, but not all, of these environmentally-induced analgesic responses are blocked by the opioid antagonist naloxone, suggesting that non opioid systems must be involved in addition to the endogenous opioid system. Even more interestingly with respect to placebo analgesia, when the animals are later placed in the apparatus where they had been submitted to the noxious stimulation, analgesia was induced. In other words, the environmentally induced analgesic response is prone to classical conditioning (Hayes et al. 1978; Price 1999). These experimental findings may be of great relevance to placebo analgesia in humans. Cues associated with previous pain relief may become effective for evoking endogenous analgesic mechanisms because they were previously associated with an effective treatment (Price 1999). Furthermore, the findings call for the formulation of a pain theory that incorporates cognitive expectations and the state of the nervous system at the time of nociceptive processing.

In the following text, we will provide some classes of explanation of the placebo response. We start with a discussion of the potential contribution of conditioning and expectancy and desire for pain relief (psychosocial level). Next we will discuss the potential role of opioids and other neurotransmitters and discuss some recent brain imaging findings that have explored the cerebral correlates of the placebo response (biologic level).

PSYCHOSOCIAL LEVEL

Conditioning

One of the main theories of placebo analgesia is that it is mediated by classical (Pavlovian) conditioning. In the original classical conditioning paradigm, an unconditioned stimulus (UCS) (food) produces an unconditioned response (UCR) (salivation). Following repeated pairings of the UCS with a neutral stimulus (e.g., a tone), the neutral stimulus may become a conditioned stimulus (CS) capable of eliciting the salivation response previously elicited by the UCS, the odor of food. This process is called the conditioned response (CR) (Hergenhahn 1988), which can be considered a stimulus-substitution model because the new stimulus replaces the older one. The model states that the repeated exposure to a CS paired with an UCS is a necessary and sufficient condition for a CR to occur. Furthermore, the model states that there is no requirement for a conscious association between the CS and UCS (Kirsch 1997; Price 1999).

In the context of placebo analgesia, active agents that reduce pain act as UCS and the inert vehicles and settings in which they are delivered (pills, syringes, the medical setting, etc.) act as CS. It follows that medical treatments act as acquisition phases or conditioning trials where vehicles and active agents are paired. Repeated pairings enable the CS to produce therapeutic effects as CR (Wickramasekera 1980; Kirsch 1997; Montgomery and Kirsch 1997). Voudouris and colleagues (1985, 1989, 1990) were among the first to provide empirical evidence in support of the classical conditioning hypothesis of placebo analgesia, using experimentally induced pain in a laboratory setting. In brief, subjects first underwent a baseline testing without drug administration in order to assess baseline pain thresholds. Next, a placebo was administered and the subjects were told that it was a powerful painkiller. At the same time, unknown to the participants, the intensity of the painful stimulus was significantly reduced, leading to lower pain ratings. Following this conditioning trial, another placebo was administered and the test was repeated again but this time with the stimulus reset to the original intensity (placebo testing). It was found that subjects in whom conditioning had taken place showed significantly lower pain ratings during the testing phase compared to subjects in whom no conditioning had taken place. These results show that analgesic placebo behavior (CR) can be conditioned by pairing a decreased painful stimulation (UCS) with a placebo (CS) (Voudouris et al. 1989). Benedetti and co-workers went one step further and introduced another novel aspect in placebo design, pharmacologic conditioning. As in the Voudouris approach, subjects first underwent baseline assessment of pain sensitivity. In a next step, they were given a genuine analgesic drug, e.g. morphine, or a nonsteroidal anti-inflammatory drug such as ketorolac. As a result, pain tolerance levels increased significantly. Next, the active drug was replaced by a placebo but subjects were not informed of this change. Compared to a classical setup in which subjects are given a placebo with only the verbal instruction of pain relief, placebo responses were significantly stronger following pharmacologic conditioning (Amanzio and Benedetti 1999).

Further evidence for a role of conditioning in the placebo response comes from studies showing that prior treatment with analgesic drugs increases the analgesic effect of a subsequently administered placebo (Batterman and Lower 1968). This finding is in accordance with the prediction of the conditioning model that the use of active ingredients (UCS) should produce stronger placebo effects than the use of neutral ingredients (CS) because a regular UCS–CS association enhances the CR (Price and Fields 1997; Price 1999). In other words, the strength of a CR correlates with the strength of the UCR (Rescorla 1988). A study by Laska and Sunshine (1973) further supports and

expands this hypothesis. These authors reported a linear "dose–response-relationship" between the amplitude of the analgesic response produced by the conditioning drug and the amplitude of the ensuing placebo response. Placebos that were administered after a powerful analgesic were more powerful than placebos that were administered after a mild analgesic. Likewise, Price and colleagues (1999) showed that a placebo is more potent when given following a drug than when given following an earlier placebo. Taken together, these results provide evidence for the involvement of conditioning in placebo analgesia (Roth 2003). Further support for a role of classical conditioning is provided by a vast number of animal studies on conditioned pharmacologic responses. These studies have provided ample evidence that animals with a history of having received active drugs are likely to show behavioral responses similar to those evoked by the drug itself when a placebo is administered in a drug-associated context (Siegel 1985).

Not all researchers agree with the purported role of classical conditioning in placebo analgesia (see also next session on the role of expectancy). For instance, Kirsch (1997) has made some observations that challenge the classical conditioning paradigm. He argued that conditioning trials with tranquilizers have an inverse effect rather than the predicted strengthening of the placebo effect. Furthermore, placebo effects are sometimes not in accordance with the pharmacologic property of the active conditioning drug, but seem to be dependent upon context and suggestion. In addition, placebo effects occasionally fail to extinguish (i.e., decline after cessation of pairing with the UCS) and are sometimes stronger than the effects of the active drug (Price and Fields 1997). However, Price (1999) argues that these exceptions may be peculiar to a certain kind of study. For example, except for the lack of extinction, the Laska and Sunshine (1973) study fulfills all criteria of classical conditioning. Nevertheless, the observation that the pairing of a CS with an UCS sometimes did not lead to associative learning seems to challenge the original stimulus-substitution model of classical conditioning. This disparity is observed when the information value of the CS as a predictor of the UCS is masked. For example, if the UCS occurs frequently and the CS does not, the effect of the pairing between the two is poor (Montgomery and Kirsch 1997).

Expectancy

Some of the above considerations have led to the adoption of an informational (cognitive) view of classical conditioning in order to explain better the placebo effect. According to Brewer (1974) and Rescorla (1988), the traditional conceptualization of classical conditioning as a low-level physiologic process, where the control of a response is switched between two stimuli, is deemed inadequate. Instead, one should properly view conditioning as learning that is brought about from the exposure to environmental relations among events, allowing the individual to form a representation of the structure of the world. According to this view, conditioning produces expectancies that certain events will follow other events. Conditioning depends on the information that the CS provides about the UCS (Rescorla 1988). The UCR is seen as the anticipatory response preparing the organism for the occurrence of the anticipated UCS. In accordance with our working definition of the placebo analgesic effect, we argue that in order for a stimulus to serve as a UCS, it has to be *perceived*; what is perceived is the active drug's *effect*. Essentially what is learned is that drugs produce specific effects; consequently, conditioning is one way to obtain response expectancies. This implies that the drug response becomes the UCS rather than the UCR. It follows that the placebo effect is dependent on the strength of an individual's expectancies and not on how these expectancies have been formed (Kirsch 1997; Montgomery and Kirsch 1997).

Wall (1991) argued that conditioning and expectancy might represent two separate dimensions of a common process. It is likely that each mechanism can be applied to explain placebo analgesia under different experimental conditions (Roth 2003). Some recent studies have been designed to dissociate expectancy from conditioning in order to test their relative contributions to placebo analgesia. One such attempt was carried out by Montgomery and Kirsch (1997). These authors basically replicated the studies of Voudouris and co-workers (1985, 1989), but they also included an "informed pairing" group in which subjects were informed about the lowering of the stimulation intensity during conditioning trials. The rationale was that if the conditioning effect is a direct result of CS–UCS pairings, then the act of informing the subjects about the manipulations should not abolish it. If, however, the conditioning effect is mediated by expectancy, a pain reduction in the informed pairing group should not be expected. In line with previous findings, a placebo response was present in the uninformed group. In sharp contrast with earlier studies, subjects in the informed group had a lower expectancy of analgesia such that no placebo analgesic effect was observed. Furthermore, when the uninformed subjects' expectancy scores were taken into account, the conditioning effect became nonsignificant, indicating that the relation between conditioning trials and the development of placebo analgesia was mediated by expectancy (see also Price et al. 1999). Moreover, in contrast with predictions from the classical conditioning theory, a series of ten extinction trials showed an unexpected enhancement (instead of abolishment) of the placebo analgesic effect (Montgomery and Kirsch 1997; Roth 2003).

Benedetti and colleagues (2003b) further clarified the distinct roles of expectancy and conditioning in the placebo effect. They used the same approach of pharmacologic conditioning as in their earlier study (see above), but they added an extra condition in which subjects received the verbal suggestion that the drug was an hyperalgesic substance and would *increase* the pain. If the placebo response were a mere result of conditioning, the placebo response should also occur in the condition where subjects were told that they were receiving a pain-enhancing drug. The investigators tested placebo responses for pain, movement velocity in Parkinson's disease (not further discussed here) and endocrine hormone (cortisol and growth hormone) secretion. The results showed that after preconditioning with the analgesic ketorolac, no placebo effect occurred if a prior suggestion of hyperalgesia had been given. In contrast, hormone secretion following conditioning was not influenced by suggestions of decreased hormone secretion. From these results it can be concluded that conditioning mediates the placebo effect when an unconscious physiologic function such as hormonal secretion is involved. However, even though a conditioning procedure has taken place, the placebo effect is mediated by expectancy when conscious physiologic processes like pain and motor performance are involved. In other words, the placebo effect is learned at an unconscious or a conscious level depending on the system involved (in this case hormone secretion versus pain).

The above findings clearly indicate that expectancy of a therapeutic effect may profoundly affect the occurrence of a placebo response. Not only expectancy from the part of patients or subjects enrolled in a study but also expectancy from the treating physician or experimenter may influence the placebo response. An elegant demonstration of this comes from a study by Gracely and colleagues (1985). Sixty patients were enrolled in a double-blind placebo controlled study of the effect of fentanyl in postoperative pain following dental extraction. Patients were informed that they might receive fentanyl, placebo, or the opioid antagonist naloxone. The physicians administering the drugs knew that whereas some patients would receive either placebo or naloxone, others would receive any of the three drugs. The results showed that the response to the placebo drug was higher when physicians believed that patients had a chance to receive the real drug. The two placebo groups differed only in the clinician's knowledge of possible treatment allocation. This knowledge may have led to subtle changes in behavior that influenced the patient's responsiveness to treatment. Along the same lines, Beecher (1961) compared the effect of investigator enthusiasm on the outcome of internal mammary artery ligation for treatment of angina and gastroenterostomy for treatment of duodenal ulcer. These surgical interventions were at that time believed to be genuine effective therapies, but later turned out to be completely useless. When the results were compared according to the level of investigator enthusiasm, it turned out that investigators who believed in the merits of the therapy had "success" rates that were close to double the success rates of the skeptics. This phenomenon may also explain why the results of new therapies are often higher than when the effect of the same therapy is reassessed in follow-up studies. A potential new therapy for a disease or symptomatic treatment is apt to considerable enthusiasm on the part of the investigator, which may influence the patient's response to the intervention, be it a drug, surgical, psychological, or other intervention (Moerman 2002b).

BIOLOGIC LEVEL

Endogenous opioids

The question whether placebo analgesia is mediated by the release of endogenous opioids has long divided the research community. Levine and colleagues (1978) provided the first demonstration that opioids are involved in the placebo response by showing that the opioid antagonist naloxone is able to block placebo analgesia. This finding was important for two reasons. First, it showed that endogenous opioids may mediate the placebo response; second, it was the first neurobiologic legitimation for the unpopular topic of placebo. The study lent placebo analgesia a biologic underpinning and initiated a series of studies, most of which confirmed Levine's findings (Amanzio and Benedetti 1997, 1999; Benedetti et al. 1999). However, Gracely et al. (1983) reported that placebo analgesia can occur without the involvement of endogenous opioids. Likewise, Grevert et al. (1983) showed that placebo analgesia was only partly blocked by naloxone. We recently also studied the involvement of the endogenous opioid system in two patients suffering from chronic low back pain (Kupers et al. 2007). Both patients showed a profound and long-lasting placebo response to spinal saline infusions. Naloxone and saline were administered in a double-blind manner to test whether the placebo response was mediated by endogenous opioids. Naloxone (10 mg) failed to block the placebo response in both patients, suggesting that the placebo response in these patients was not mediated by the endogenous opioid system (Figure 6.1B). In order to understand better the conditions that produce naloxone-reversible and naloxone-insensitive placebo effects, Amanzio and Benedetti (1999) evoked different types of placebo analgesic effects by using cognitive expectation cues, drug-conditioning or a combination of both. Their aim was to dissect placebo analgesia into opioid and non-opioid parts and determine their relation with expectancy and conditioning. The drug conditioning trials were carried out with either morphine (opioid

agonist) or ketorolac (nonsteroidal anti-inflammatory drug). Morphine conditioning without expectation cues (verbal suggestion of pain relief) generated a naloxone-reversible placebo effect. Morphine conditioning together with expectation cues produced a naloxone-reversible placebo effect that was larger than that observed following morphine conditioning alone. This large placebo effect was the result of both expectancy and conditioning and was entirely naloxone reversible. When conditioning was performed with the non-opioid ketorolac, the resulting placebo effect was not antagonised by naloxone. In contrast, ketorolac conditioning together with expectancy cues resulted in a placebo effect that was partially blocked by naloxone (Amanzio and Benedetti 1999). Expectancy cues presented alone generated a small placebo effect that was completely blocked by naloxone, indicating that an expectancy manipulation produces a placebo effect that is mediated by the endogenous opioid system. In conclusion, Amanzio and Benedetti (1999) provided evidence that there exist different types of placebo responses, some of which are completely or partially blocked by naloxone and others that are naloxone insensitive. The demonstration that placebo analgesia can be dissected into opioid and non-opioid components, depending on the procedure used to evoke the placebo effect, may resolve the old controversy of the role of opioids in placebo analgesia. Results of the study indicate that cognitive factors and conditioning are differently balanced in relation to placebo analgesia, activating either the opioid or non-opioid system. Whereas expectation triggers the endogenous opioid system, conditioning procedures may activate either opioid or non-opioid systems. When conditioning is carried out with opioids, placebo analgesia is likely to be mediated via opioid receptors. If, on the other hand, conditioning is brought about by means of non-opioid drugs, non-opioid systems are likely to be involved (Amanzio and Benedetti 1999; de Pascalis 2002).

A subsequent study by the same group (Benedetti et al. 1999) further elaborated on how endogenous opioids are activated by expectancy cues. In this study, specific expectancies of analgesia were directed towards different body parts. In brief, a noxious stimulus (an intracutaneous injection of capsaicin which is the pungent ingredient in chilli peppers) was simultaneously applied to four different body areas (arms and legs, left and right). A placebo cream was applied to one of the stimulated body parts and the subjects were informed that the cream was an analgesic (induction of expectations). The expectancy of an analgesic effect was exclusively directed towards the site where the placebo had been applied. The results showed a placebo analgesic effect that was restricted to the treated site and that was completely abolished by a hidden injection of naloxone. These data show that a spatially directed expectancy of a therapeutic effect produces a placebo response that is somatotopically restricted to the body site that was the target of expectation. They further suggest that placebo-activated endorphins act only on the expected target of action and not on the entire body. It can thus be hypothesized that a cognitive component in the form of spatial attention or spatial directed expectation plays a pivotal role in the activation of specific opioid systems (Benedetti et al. 1999; Price 1999).

The findings discussed above imply that the activation of the pain modulatory circuitry, including the PAG and the RVM, is triggered by psychological factors. Fields and co-workers already emphasized the role of expectation, arousal and attention in the modulation by the PAG and RVM (Fields and Price 1997). Furthermore, Soper and Melzack (1982) gave evidence that the PAG is functionally and somatotopically organized. In particular, they found that stimulation of different sites of the PAG produced an analgesic effect in different cutaneous areas. In other words, the spatially directed effect may be explained by the somatotopical organization of the PAG. Because the pain-modulatory circuitry is influenced by opioids, it can be hypothesized that the endogenous opioid system has a role in organizing the activity of PAG and RVM (Benedetti et al. 1999). We will discuss this possibility in greater detail in the section on supraspinal structures involved in the placebo response.

Dopamine

From the above discussion it already became clear that, although the opioid system may play an important role in the placebo response, it is not the only neurotransmitter system involved. Another candidate is dopamine. Evidence for a purported role of the dopamine system in the placebo response comes from a series of brain imaging studies in patients with Parkinson's disease (PD). These studies showed that the placebo response in PD is associated with a significant release of dopamine in the striatum (see section on PD below for more details). Interestingly, the biochemical responses following a placebo were as powerful as those produced by the active drug apomorphine. A tempting conclusion is therefore that there exist at least two types of placebo analgesic effects: one type that is mediated by opioids and that is implicated in pain conditions and another type that is mediated by dopamine and can be evoked in PD. However, it is also possible that a common mechanism mediates the placebo effect observed in different conditions. First, placebo responses have most frequently been described within the context of pain, depression and PD (de la Fuente-Fernandez 2002a,b); second, pain and depression are often co-morbid (Magni 1987; Dworkin and Gitlin 1991; Blackburn-Munro et al. 2001); finally, both pain and depression are frequently present in PD (Ford 1998; Factor et al. 2000). It could therefore be

hypothesized that the placebo effect in these conditions is mediated by a common change in neurotransmitter transmission, for which a likely candidate is dopamine, given its key role in the pathophysiology of PD.

There are several reasons why dopamine could also have a potential role in mediating placebo analgesic effects. Animal, behavioral, and neurophysiologic studies provide considerable evidence for a role of forebrain dopaminergic systems in pain and analgesia. They have shown that a number of dopamine agonists, including cocaine, amphetamine, and methylphenidate, have analgesic actions, particularly in pain tests that involve supraspinal function (Dennis and Melzack 1983; Pertovaara et al. 1988; Lin et al. 1989). Electrophysiologic studies have revealed dopamine modulation of nociceptive activity in the medial and lateral thalamus of rats (Shyu et al. 1992), and neurons responding to noxious stimuli have been identified in the dopamine-rich basal ganglia (Romo et al. 1989; Chudler et al. 1993, 1995). The injection of dopamine agonists and antagonists into the rat striatum alters nociceptive behavior (independent of motor deficits), indicating that forebrain dopamine systems are important in pain modulation (Burkey et al. 1999; Gear et al. 1999; Magnusson et al. 2000). Data from brain imaging studies in humans showed increases of cerebral blood flow in the basal ganglia during pain (Coghill et al. 1994; Idarola et al. 1998; Becerra et al. 2001; Casey et al. 2001; Zubieta et al. 2001), further supporting a role of forebrain dopamine systems in pain modulation. A recent PET study demonstrated a correlation between baseline D2 dopamine receptor binding and the response to a painful stimulus, suggesting a role of dopamine in endogenous pain modulation (Hagelberg et al. 2002). Clinical reports showed that dopaminergic agonists reduce pain associated with a variety of chronic pain conditions such as metastatic bone pain (Dickey et al. 1972; Nixon 1975), pain related to PD (Battista et al. 1973; Ford 1998; Factor et al. 2000), herpes zoster (Kernbaum et al. 1981) and thalamic pain (Miley et al. 1978). Conversely, pain associated with withdrawal from levodopa in PD patients has also been described (Riley et al. 1993). Finally, patients with several clinical syndromes in which dopamine neurotransmission may be perturbed (e.g. schizophrenia, PD and Huntington's disease) have altered pain perception (see Chudler and Dong 1995 for a review). The dopamine mesocortical system has also been reported to be involved in affect and mood. For example, imaging studies have suggested decreased striatal dopamine transmission associated with depression (Ebert et al. 1996; Shah et al. 1997). One could therefore hypothesize that dopamine may be particularly important for affective aspects of pain processing.

In a recent PET study, Zubieta et al. (2001) used $[^{11}C]$ carfentanil to study the function of the supraspinal opioid receptor system in healthy human subjects during painful stimulation. In the light of the in vivo competition model, sustained pain appeared to induce the regional release of endogenous opioids interacting with mu-opioid receptors in a number of cortical and subcortical brain regions, such as the thalamus, the amygdala and the anterior cingulate cortex. The activation of the mu-opioid receptor system was associated with reductions in the sensory and affective ratings of the pain experience. Interestingly, [^{11}C]carfentanil binding was also altered in the nucleus accumbens, a subcortical complex that belongs to the ventral part of the basal ganglia and has a high concentration of dopamine receptors. In view of the known interactions between the dopamine and opioid systems, this finding indirectly suggests a role for the dopaminergic system in endogenous pain control. It has been argued earlier that expectancy of a therapeutic effect is an integral part of the placebo response; those subjects who believe in the efficacy of a treatment are most likely to show a placebo effect. There is ample evidence that expectancy of reward is mediated by dopamine transmission (Schultz 1998; de la Fuente-Fernandez et al. 2002a,b; O'Doherty et al. 2002). The ventral striatum, including the nucleus accumbens and ventral putamen, belong to the limbic corticostriatal loop which includes the amygdala, hippocampus, and orbitofrontal and cingulate cortices. These structures are involved in emotional behavior and reward processing (Bolam et al. 2000). Furthermore, midbrain dopamine neurons are activated by primary rewards and reward-predicting stimuli. Since there is structural, electrophysiologic and biochemical evidence for dopamine–opioid interactions in the brain (Sesack and Pickel 1992; Hagelberg et al. 2002), we hypothesize that the activation of dopaminergic systems is involved in the placebo analgesic effect in general. There is indeed recent evidence from PET studies that prediction of a therapeutic effect releases dopamine in the brain, as measured by the D2-D3 dopamine tracer [11C]raclopride (Boileau et al., 2006). More specifically, placebo analgesia could be the result of dopamine–opioid interconnections. The limbic and prefrontal cortex and the amygdala, which are all under dopaminergic control, can modulate opioid release in the PAG. There are reciprocal connections between the ventral tegmental area, the source of dopaminergic projections to the nucleus accumbens, and the PAG. It is thus possible that dopamine release could mediate placebo analgesia by controlling opioid release through the PAG (de la Fuente-Fernandez et al. 2002b; de la Fuente-Fernandez and Stoessel 2002).

Cortical network involved in placebo analgesia

Brain imaging studies over the past decade have greatly advanced our understanding of the mechanisms underlying placebo analgesia. Their contribution has been twofold. First, these results showed that the pain relief reported following a placebo is associated with a concomitant decrease of brain activity in pain-related areas such as thalamus, insula and anterior cingulate cortex. This is important in view of the discussion whether

reported pain reductions following placebos represent genuine analgesic effects or mere compliance with experimental instructions. Second, these studies pointed out a number of brain structures that may be at the origin of the placebo effect. Among these figure importantly the dorsolateral and orbital prefrontal cortex, the anterior cingulate cortex and the midbrain. Interestingly, the dorsolateral prefrontal cortex has also been proposed to be an important structure in the endogenous modulation of pathologic pain (Lorenz et al. 2003).

The first brain imaging study that investigated the mechanisms of placebo analgesia was carried out by Ingvar's group at the Karolinska institute. Using PET, Petrovic and colleagues (2002) scanned a group of healthy volunteers following the administration of a short acting opioid (remifentanil), placebo or no drugs. Subjects were scanned during nonpainful and painful tonic heat stimulation of the dorsum of the left hand. Pain ratings following placebo administration were significantly lower than when no drugs were given. The placebo response was associated with a significant increase in regional cerebral blood flow (rCBF) in the orbitofrontal and anterior cingulate cortices, areas in which rCBF was also reliably activated by the opioid remifentanil. When the results were analyzed separately for the high and low placebo responders, it was found that only in the high placebo responders was CBF increased in the rostral ACC (rACC) during remifentanil analgesia. This suggests that there exists a relationship between how effectively opioids activate the rACC and how well subjects respond to placebo during pain. This further implies that placebo responders have a more efficient opioid system. A regression analysis of the PET data showed that in the pain–opioid condition, rCBF in the rACC covaried with activity in an area near the PAG and the pons. In the pain–placebo condition, a significant covariation was observed between rCBF in the rACC and the pons and, at a subsignificant level, between activity in rACC and PAG. No covariation between these areas was observed in the pain-only condition. The correlation between rCBF in rACC and PAG/pons indicates that higher cortical areas may take control over descending pain modulatory systems during opioid and placebo analgesia. As mentioned before, cognitive factors such as expectation and desire for pain relief contribute significantly to the occurrence of the placebo response. The ACC and lateral orbitofrontal cortex may play an important role in this cognitive modulation of pain via their projections to the PAG, an area involved in descending inhibitory control of pain.

Wager and colleagues (2004) used fMRI to study the brain mechanisms mediating the placebo response. In two separate experiments, they addressed the following questions: (1) which pain-responsive areas of the brain show reduced activity following a placebo? and (2) which areas in the brain show increased activity following the administration of a placebo? The previous PET study was designed to answer the second question and it did not address the first one. To increase the likelihood of the occurrence of a placebo response, the authors used a conditioning procedure. In brief, subjects were first submitted to a painful electrical shock. Next, a placebo cream was applied after the subjects were told that the cream was a powerful local analgesic. Subjects received another electric shock, but the intensity of the shock was secretly reduced in the placebo condition, to create high expectations of pain relief during the placebo challenge. In the third (test) phase, subjects were tested again with the original shock intensity and the placebo cream. With respect to the first question, placebo significantly reduced the blood oxygenation level-dependent (BOLD) response in the rostral anterior cingulate cortex, contralateral insula and thalamus, areas that are part of the so-called pain-matrix (Peyron et al. 2000). In order to answer the second question, they looked at the BOLD response in the anticipation period of pain. The authors found that the BOLD signal in the dorsolateral and orbitofrontal cortices and midbrain periaqueductal gray was significantly increased during placebo compared to a control condition. In addition, the increased activity in these regions was correlated with the placebo-induced reductions in pain-evoked activity in thalamus, insula and anterior cingulate cortex. The increased BOLD response in the prefrontal cortex is in line with the hypothesis that brain areas involved in generating and mediating expectation contribute to placebo analgesia. A recent study by Lieberman and co-workers (2004) investigated placebo responses in patients with irritable bowel syndrome. They also found evidence for an important role of the prefrontal cortex in placebo analgesia. In contrast with the results of Wager and Petrovic, the increased prefrontal activation was found in the ventrolateral and not in the dorsolateral or orbitofrontal part. The BOLD response in this region correlated negatively with activity in ACC. Results from our own laboratory in patients with neuropathic pain also argue for a possible role of the orbitofrontal cortex in the placebo response (Figure 6.1C).

A note on placebo and cerebral responses in depression and Parkinson's disease

Parkinson's disease

de la Fuente-Fernandez and colleagues (2001) used PET to study the involvement of the brain dopamine system in the placebo response in patients with PD. They used [^{11}C]raclopride (RAC) which is an antagonist for the dopamine D2/D3 receptors. By calculating the displacement of the exogenously applied RAC following a pharmacologic or behavioral challenge, one can estimate the amount of endogenously released dopamine. Six PD patients were scanned in a placebo-controlled,

double-blind fashion following the administration of a placebo or an active dopaminergic drug (levodopa). Placebo administration caused a significant decrease in RAC specific binding in the dorsal striatum (caudate and putamen). Interestingly, the magnitude of the decrease in RAC specific binding following a placebo was comparable to that evoked by a therapeutic dose of levodopa. The authors also reported a positive correlation between the degree of dopamine release and the extent of the perceived placebo effect. However, no interaction was found between the effects of placebo and the active drugs: the degree of drug-induced change in RAC binding tended to be lower in patients who responded to placebo. In a following study, the authors also showed a release of dopamine in the ventral striatum (nucleus accumbens) although this was not correlated with the perceived placebo effect (de la Fuente-Fernandez 2002a). The authors concluded that the release of dopamine in the ventral striatum is caused by the expectation of reward – in this case, the anticipation of a therapeutic effect.

A recent study from the laboratory of Benedetti (2004) studied the placebo response in PD at the single cell level. They recorded from 110 single neurons in the subthalamic nucleus (STN) of 11 PD patients during stereotaxic implantation with a deep brain electrode for therapeutic purposes. Activity was recorded before and after the administration of a placebo. It was shown that those patients who showed a manifest clinical placebo response (sense of well-being and improved arm rigidity) also showed a significant reduction in firing frequency of STN neurons compared to pre-placebo. In nonresponders, no change in firing frequency of STN neurons was observed. In addition, the authors also reported a qualitative change in the firing pattern of STN neurons. Whereas the majority of the STN neurons discharged in a bursting type of pattern prior to placebo, the response shifted to a nonbursting pattern in placebo responders. No change in firing pattern was observed in nonresponders.

Depression

Like pain, depression is also strongly susceptible to placebo responses. Recent meta-analyses indicated that placebo accounts for more than 70% of the effectiveness of drugs in studies of depression (Khan et al. 2000; Kirsch and Sapirstein 1997). The primary outcome measure in depression studies is change in mood ratings. Like pain ratings, these subjective measures can be influenced in a variety of ways, e.g. the motivation of the subject and investigator's expectations. However, functional brain measurements can provide an objective physiologic indication of treatment efficacy. A recent report compared brain electrophysiologic activity in subjects treated with antidepressants and placebo. Using quantitative electroencephalography (QEEG),

Leuchter (2002) reported that placebo responders had an increased activity in the prefrontal cortex while those who responded to antidepressants had reduced activity in the same area. In this study, 38% of the patients responded to placebo and 52% to the active medication. This finding indicates that placebo treatment induces changes in brain function that are different from those associated with antidepressants. Mayberg and co-workers (2002) used PET to examine changes in brain glucose consumption (CMRglc) in depressed patients who were treated with antidepressants (fluoxetine) or placebo. After 6 weeks of treatment, patients in both groups showed regional metabolic increases (involving the prefrontal cortex, ACC, posterior insula and posterior cingulate cortex). Fluoxetine was however associated with a number of additional subcortical and limbic changes in CMRglc such as the brainstem, striatum, and hippocampus. The authors argued that the overlapping pattern of changes might be necessary for the therapeutic response and the additional changes observed in the active treatment group might indicate an additional advantage in sustaining a long term response and preventing relapse. Overall, both studies indicate that the placebo effect triggers specific changes in the brain.

Results of brain imaging and single cell studies add important insights into the mechanisms underlying placebo responses. First, they give firm support to the conjecture that placebos alter neural activity in the brain, therefore refuting the objection that placebos are simply the result of a publication bias, as suggested by Hrobjartsson and Götzsche (2001). Second, they provide information about specific brain areas that may mediate the placebo response. When comparing the brain mechanisms involved in placebo analgesia with those involved in other types of placebo (depression, PD), there appear to be striking differences. Although these differences might in part be explained by differences in experimental procedures, this seems to suggest that there are different forms of placebo. This may not be surprising when we consider that there is evidence that not one but multiple mechanisms play a role in placebo such as expectancy, classical conditioning, desire for relief, release of endogenous opioids, etc.

Since placebos are intrinsically inert, these findings also indicate that situational and interpersonal (the interaction between the patient and physician) processes can trigger these specific responses in the brain. This helps to come to a neurobiologic understanding of the patient–doctor relationship, which may open some new therapeutic perspectives (Oh 1994). The therapeutic context and the way the therapist approaches the patient can influence the outcome of, for example, a pathologic pain condition through the modulation of specific neurobiologic systems. If we accept the claim that expectancy of reward plays a pivotal role in placebo analgesia, it must be the job of the therapist to induce positive expectations of rewarding therapeutic outcomes in the patient (Benson and Friedman 1996; Moerman 2002). Obviously, placebos and good bedside manners are not a good panacea, but together comprise a humane aspect of care, which should not be neglected (Benedetti 2002). The factors that generate the placebo effect are clearly also operating in every routine therapeutic intervention, including surgical procedures and pharmacotherapy. Inducing positive expectations will boost the placebo component of the therapy. This will result in a more powerful drug effect at lower doses, thereby reducing the risk of side effects and dependence (Stewart-Williams and Podd 2004).

THE ETHICS OF PLACEBO

There has been a lively debate about the ethical dilemma surrounding the placebo-controlled trial. On the one hand, the adherents of "placebo orthodoxy" argue that methodologic considerations make placebo-controlled trials necessary. On the other hand, the adherents of "active-control orthodoxy" hold that the use of placebo sacrifices medical ethics and the rights and welfare of patients to presumed scientific rigor (Emanuel and Miller 2001).

In October 2000, a revision was made to the Declaration of Helsinki which supports the active-control orthodoxy by reinforcing a clear stance of prohibiting offering placebo instead of proven effective therapy. Recently, the World Medical Association issued a Note of Clarification that allows for a limited use of placebo controls, marking some deviation from the October 2000 revision (Miller and Brody 2002). This note states that placebo-controlled trials may be ethically justifiable despite the availability of proven effective treatments under the following circumstances: (1) when for compelling and scientifically sound methodologic reasons its use is necessary to determine the efficacy or safety of a prophylactic, diagnostic or therapeutic method, and (2) when a prophylactic, diagnostic or therapeutic method is being investigated for a minor condition and the patients who receive placebo will not be subject to any additional risk of serious or irreversible harm.

Given the fact that a number of effective therapies often do exist, the recently revised Declaration of Helsinki raises ethical and methodologic concerns for the conduct of placebo-controlled clinical trials. Opponents of placebo-controlled trials pay little attention to the power of the placebo response given the fact that a large number of patients who are administered placebos show measurable and clinically meaningful improvements (Miller and Brody 2002). The design and conduct of clinical trials could benefit substantially from an exhaustive understanding of the placebo phenomenon, its underlying mechanisms and its interaction with test therapies (Straus and Briggs 2002). Conversely, the design and conduct of clinical trials might lead to a better understanding of the placebo. However, the placebo-controlled trial leaves us with a dilemma: on the one hand, is it unethical to use a placebo control if effective treatments do exist? On the other hand, is a placebo-controlled study the most reliable way to determine the efficacy of an experimental drug (Fleischhacker et al. 2003)?

Alternatives to the placebo-controlled trial should be explored in order to resolve the impasse. One such alternative is the active-control trial in which it can either be shown that the new treatment is superior to the control treatment, or that the new treatment is equivalent or non-inferior in relation to a known effective treatment (Ellenberg and Temple 2000). However, Fleischhacker and colleagues (2003) argued that a comparison between a test drug and placebo is the most powerful method for demonstrating efficacy since replacing placebo with an active control drug can hamper the interpretation of the findings. If the test drug and the standard control group show matching effects in the absence of a placebo group it cannot be determined whether they were both effective or ineffective. Consequently, in active control trials it has to be assumed that the active control drug is effective in order to interpret a result where the test drug showed to be non-inferior. In other words, it must be assumed that if the study did in fact include a placebo group, the placebo would have been inferior to the active control. If this assumption is incorrect, the study has a poor ability to distinguish between treatments: low so-called assay sensitivity (Fleischhacker et al. 2003). If assay sensitivity cannot be assured, active control trials are often uninformative in that they can neither demonstrate the efficacy of a new treatment nor provide a valid comparison to control treatment (Ellenberg and Temple 2000). An interesting example comes from a recent study on the efficacy of the herbal remedy *Hypericum perforatum* (St John's wort) and placebo for treatment of major depression. It was found that St John's wort was not significantly better than placebo (Hypericum Depression Trial Study Group 2002). In the same study, another antidepressant (sertraline) was tested as well. There was no difference in depression scores following placebo and the known effective drug sertraline. One can hence conclude that neither drug was any better than placebo. However, if no placebo condition had been included, it would have been concluded that St John's wort is as effective as the "proven" drug sertraline.

Proponents of the usage of placebos in the clinical practice have used some pragmatic arguments against the active control trial. They assert that a large number of therapies are discarded eventually because they turn out to be ineffective. Despite this, many patients may have benefited from these therapies. In addition, application of a randomized trial gives each patient a 50% chance not to get the new therapy. According to Lasagna, "too often the placebo-treated patients turn out to be the lucky ones in a drug trial, deprived only of a toxic and ineffective chemical." It is further argued that if it is considered unethical to withhold subjects from a known effective treatment, it is equally unethical to deprive these patients of this known effective treatment by testing them with a new investigational drug which may not only be ineffective but even hazardous.

PLACEBOS AND THE ISSUE OF STUDY DESIGN

THE QUESTIONABLE "OBJECTIVITY" OF THE DOUBLE-BLIND DESIGN

Although the randomized double-blind placebo-controlled trial is considered by many as the gold standard, this design is associated with serious methodologic problems. In the traditional double-blind design, neither the investigator nor the subject is aware of the true nature of the intervention. Therefore, in principle, the investigator cannot bias the results by knowing who is receiving active treatment and who a placebo (but see above). The extent to which the double-blind design controls for subject bias is dependent on the instructions that are given by the investigator. Until the obligation of the principle of informed consent became established, it was common to present a placebo as if it were a real drug. In other words, the subject was unaware that they could receive a placebo and expected with 100% certainty to get an active drug. From a methodologic point of view, this is an ideal situation since it mimics best the clinical situation. Since current ethical standards require informed consent, this design is no longer considered as ethically acceptable. In a double-blind design with informed consent, the subject is told beforehand that they are taking part in an experimental investigation and that they have a 50% chance to receive a placebo instead of an active treatment. This changes de facto the subject's expectations with respect to the effect of the administered therapy. From the moment the subject enters the trial, they will use all possible means to try to find out to which of the two conditions they have been allocated – placebo or active treatment? Thereto, they will start focusing attention upon subtle physiologic or psychological cues: do they perceive an increase in heart rate, a dry mouth, dizziness, nausea, has their mood changed...? This self-scrutiny may profoundly affect the result of the trial, not only for the placebo arm but also for the active arm of the trial. Knowing that one may receive a placebo drug may decrease expectation levels and introduce a feeling of uncertainty which may in turn reduce the magnitude of the placebo response. It has been argued that this phenomenon is one of the possible explanations for the low placebo effect in Hrobjartsson and Gotzsche's (2001) study. On the other hand, it might be argued that participation in a double-blind study should heighten the sensitivity and vigilance on the part of both physician and participant, thereby increasing the detection of beneficial or adverse symptoms. Symptoms that normally would go unperceived will be reported as adverse side-effects or as indications of the efficacy of the drug. Empirical support for this position comes from studies showing that the verum effect of a drug was significantly higher in non-placebo-controlled compared to placebo-controlled trials (Eikerman and Diener 2003). Another recent example of potentiating effects of placebo comes from a double-blind sham surgery-controlled trial designed to study the effects of fetal tissue transplants of dopamine neurons in the brain of Parkinson's patients. It was found that 76% of the patients thought they had received the transplant seven days after the procedure (McRae et al. 2004). Therefore, the double-blind procedure fails to provide a manner to test for the pure effects of a therapy, unconfounded by the subject's expectations of receiving a therapy. To complicate matters even more, some of these reactions may differentially affect the effect of active therapy and placebo control (Kaptchuk 2001). Vigilance may increase the effect of the placebo and decrease the effect of the drug or vice versa. Another major concern relating to the double-blind approach is its lack of ecologic validity. Some investigators have described the double-blind procedure as anathema to the human spirit. Randomly subjecting a person to a series of hidden and stringent manipulations with endless observations and measurements is very far removed from daily reality, and may inspire ambivalence, confusion or passivity in the subject.

THE BALANCED PLACEBO DESIGN

The so-called balanced placebo design may overcome some of the flaws associated with the placebo-controlled and the active control trial. As has become clear from the above consideration, there are two experimental factors that can be manipulated independently: the actual therapy (active therapy or placebo) and the instructions given to the subjects. The balanced placebo design uses a 2×2 factorial design in which expectancy and therapy are independently varied. Subjects are informed beforehand that they may be allocated to either an active therapy or a placebo control. In contrast with the classical double-blind procedure in which the subject is left unaware of their treatment allocation, they are informed to which study condition they have been allocated. To do so, a person independent of the

experimenter informs the subject. Although in reality the subject has already been assigned to a particular condition, a procedure that gives the appearance of random assignment is introduced. Half of the subjects are told that they were assigned to the active therapy and the remaining are told that they were assigned to the placebo control (expectancy). In addition, half of the subjects in each group will receive active therapy and the other half placebo (therapy). This means that the balanced placebo design contains four study groups. Subjects in the first group are told they will receive a drug, and they do receive it; subjects in the second group are told they will receive a placebo, but instead they receive an active drug; subjects in the third group are told they will receive an active drug but they receive a placebo; those in the fourth group are told they will receive a placebo and they do in fact get one. Symptom improvement in condition (1) may be due to the combined effect of physiologic and psychological factors. This condition mimics the clinical situation in which subjects know that they are given an active therapy. Whereas improvement in condition (2) must be the result of the pure physiologic effect of the therapy, in condition (3) improvement is the result of pure psychological (expectancy) effects. In the latter condition, the subject is led to believe that they are receiving an active treatment although they receive a placebo. This is different from the traditional double-blind approach with informed consent where the subject is told that they will either receive a placebo or a real treatment. The following pairwise comparisons can be made:

- condition (1) with (3): to which degree do the combined expectancy and physiologic effects exceed the effect of expectancy alone?
- condition (1) with (2): to which degree do the combined expectancy and physiologic effects exceed the physiologic effects?
- condition (2) with (4): assessment of pure physiologic effects
- condition (3) with (4): evaluation of expectancy effects.

This design therefore allows one to assess the pure effects of therapy and expectancy and their interactions. The balanced placebo design is not yet widely used in current research, no doubt because it requires four instead of two experimental groups. Nonetheless, some examples can be found of studies that have used this design. For example, Kirsch and colleagues (1993) compared the effect of double-blind versus deceptive administration of a placebo on alertness and cardiovascular responses. The results showed that placebo had an opposite effect when administered under deceptive compared to double-blind procedures.

The classical double-blind design may not only affect the magnitude of the placebo response but also that of the active therapy. We studied the effect of deep brain stimulation on clinical pain in 7 patients in their daily-life situation and under placebo-controlled laboratory conditions (Marchand et al. 2003). Whereas average pain relief at home was rated as being above 50%, average pain relief during the double-blind laboratory session was less than 10% on the 101-point rating scale. In line with these results, Eikerman and Diener (2000) reported that the efficacy of anti-migraine drugs was significantly higher when measured in non-placebo-controlled compared to placebo-controlled trials. Likewise, the number of adverse effects towards a study-drug was significantly lower in placebo-controlled compared to trials in which the same drug was compared to another active treatment (Rochon et al. 1999).

The balanced placebo design has several advantages: it provides a baseline from which to evaluate drug and placebo effects, and further offers a direct measurement of the effect of active therapy, placebo and their interaction. However, the problem with the balanced placebo design is that it involves some form of deception. Whereas some proposed that, for this reason, the balanced placebo design should only be used in healthy volunteers and not in clinical trials, others have argued that the deception is not more extensive than that occurring in any other placebo design since subjects are informed beforehand about the possibility of receiving a placebo (Marlatt and Rohsenow 1980).

THE SILENT ADMINISTRATION DESIGN

Some of the ethical concerns related to the balanced placebo design can be avoided by using the silent administration design. In this design, a drug is administered without the subject's knowledge and the effects are compared with those occurring when the drug is openly administered. The hidden versus open administration design provides a measurement of the placebo component of a therapy by subtracting the drug effect (hidden administration) from the drug response (open administration). In other words, the design allows the study of the placebo effect without the need to actually include a placebo group (Benedetti et al. 2003a). The two conditions of the silent administration paradigm are similar to conditions (1) and (2) of the balanced placebo design but conditions (3) (told drug/get no drug) and (4) (told no drug/get no drug) of this design are not present. An important difference from the balanced placebo design is that it bypasses the need for deception. The open versus hidden administration design represents an innovative alternative to the classic placebo controlled trial for probing the crucial psychosocial factors involved in any therapy, such as the patient–provider interaction, awareness of treatment and expectancies.

The silent administration approach was pioneered by Ross and co-workers in the early 1960s (Ross et al.

1962). In order to find a way to separate psychological and pharmacologic processes in drug responses, they administered d-amphetamine in either an open (pill) fashion or in disguised form (dissolved in orange juice). The group which received d-amphetamine in disguised form along with neutral instructions regarding its effects did not behave significantly differently from the placebo group (Lyerly et al. 1964). Recently, Amanzio and colleagues (2001) used the silent administration design to study placebo analgesia. Patients received intravenous injections of opioids or nonsteroidal anti-inflammatory drugs for treatment of postoperative pain. In half of the patients, the painkillers were administered openly and with the patients aware of the substance that was injected. In the other half of the patients, the analgesics were administered via a hidden drug-infusion pump and the patient was completely unaware that he or she was receiving a drug. The results showed that hidden injections were far less effective than open injections. In addition, the results of the hidden injections were much less variable than the results of the open administration condition. It was interpreted that the larger amplitude and the larger variability of the response were due to the placebo effect.

SOME MISCONCEPTIONS ABOUT PLACEBO

THE GENUINE PLACEBO RESPONDER

As mentioned at the beginning of this chapter, until recently it was believed that there exists a typical placebo responder, i.e., a person who will respond in a consistent way to a placebo. This is a misconception that can be rejected on the basis of studies that investigated the intra-individual variability of the placebo analgesic response. Lasagna and colleagues (1954) studied the reproducibility of placebo in a group of 69 patients with postoperative pain. Only 14% of the patients were consistent placebo responders; 55% behaved in an inconsistent way; and 31% were consistent nonresponders. Liberman (1964) investigated the effect of placebo on pain under three different situations: during delivery, postpartum pain and experimental pain. There was no correlation between the occurrence of a placebo response in these conditions. Very similar results were obtained in a study by Wolf and colleagues (1957). These investigators tested the intra-individual variability in the placebo response against nausea. The results showed that it was not possible on the basis of between one and six tests to predict whether or not an individual would display a placebo response on subsequent testing. Moreover, even the "pure" reactors, defined on the basis of five previous successive placebo responses, showed no greater incidence of subsequent positive responses than when defined on the basis of one through three previous tests. These results argue against the idea that certain individuals can be characterized as systematic placebo responders. However, a study by Lasagna and colleagues (1954) showed that 95% of individuals responding to a placebo showed pain reduction following the injection of morphine whereas only 54% of the individuals *not* responding to a placebo showed pain reduction following the injection of morphine. This suggests that there might be a shared mechanism common to placebo analgesia and opioid analgesia, a hypothesis which is supported by recent PET imaging findings (see above).

PLACEBO RESPONDERS HAVE A "SPECIAL" PERSONALITY

Closely linked to the above is the mistaken belief that placebo responders have a special personality. As mentioned at the beginning of this chapter, in the early days of the placebo era, it was believed that placebo responders have a special, hysteriform-like personality. Unfortunately, this belief is still widely held. Numerous investigators have tried to link the placebo responder to a certain personality type. However, the results of these studies failed to show a correlation between personality and response to a placebo. Further arguments against this possibility come from the earlier discussed studies that have used drug conditioning procedures or expectancy cues to increase the placebo response rate (Amanzio and Benedetti 1999; Benedetti et al. 2003b). These results show that it is rather the cognitive and situational context that determines the occurrence of a placebo response. When subjects are randomly allocated to a placebo group that will only receive verbal expectancy cues of improvement or to a group that at the same time will be submitted to (pharmacologic) conditioning, the placebo effect is much more pronounced in the latter condition. This potentiation is difficult to reconcile with the personality hypothesis.

A POSITIVE RESPONSE TO A PLACEBO MEANS THAT THE PAIN IS NOT REAL OR IMAGINED

It should by now have become clear that a positive placebo response does not imply that the pain is not real. Although the argument of fictive pain has been often used to explain placebo responses in some spectacular clinical cases, it is difficult to defend with respect to the findings on the placebo effect in experimental pain. In particular, the neuroimaging findings strongly support that placebos selectively affect activity in a network of cortical and subcortical areas, collectively known as the pain matrix (Peyron et al. 2000). This neuroanatomical substrate for placebo has important consequences for the way in which some clinical trials are run. Sometimes trials include a pre-screening phase in

which a placebo is tested. If the patient shows a positive response to placebo, he or she is considered a placebo responder and excluded from further participation because a positive response to a placebo is considered as a proof that the pain has a psychological and not an organic basis. It should be clear from the preceding that this argument is based upon false premises.

PLACEBO IS EQUIVALENT TO NO THERAPY

As mentioned earlier, placebos are inert. However, this does not imply that placebo is equivalent to having no therapy. The placebo effect is not caused by the placebo agent but by the cognitive context that is associated with it. The verbal instruction to the patient, the expectancy of an effect, classical conditioning and the meaning of the situation are processes which produce together the placebo effect.

THIRTY-FIVE PERCENT OF PEOPLE RESPOND TO PLACEBOS

Another common misunderstanding is that with any given therapy, around 35% of the subjects will be placebo responders. The mythical 35% figure seems to have come from a misunderstanding of Beecher's paper. Beecher had calculated that across multiple studies, which were not controlled for natural course of the disease and regression to the mean, about 35% of the subjects show a placebo response. However, a closer inspection of the table in Beecher's paper informs us that there was a high variability in the placebo response across studies. In other words, there is no fixed percentage of the population that will respond to some placebo treatment. Placebo response rates may in fact vary anywhere between 0 and 100%, depending on the meaning and context. In our modern western society that worships high technological procedures, medical interventions involving an impressive amount of high technological complexity (e.g., deep brain stimulation or intracerebral stem cell implants for treatment of movement disorders) produce a higher placebo response rate than do sugar pills (Kaptchuk et al. 2000). A significantly higher placebo response rate occurs when a placebo is delivered intracutaneously compared to when it is delivered *per os* (de Craen et al. 2000). As mentioned earlier, the placebo response rate in a double-blind placebo surgery trial of stem cell transplantation for PD was even 71% in the early period of the trial and then decreased to 67% at 8 months and 33% at 12 months after surgery (McRae et al. 2004). In addition, a significantly higher placebo response rate occurs when patients are given multiple placebo tablets daily compared to when they get only one daily (de Craen et al. 1999). All this can be explained as responses to meaning. Many pills work better than one pill and more advanced technology works better than old-fashioned pills.

THE PLACEBO EFFECT PROVIDES A FIXED EFFECT THAT IS INDEPENDENT OF THE THERAPEUTIC EFFECT OF A PHARMACOLOGIC COMPOUND OR A THERAPY

It is commonly believed that the placebo effect represents a fixed effect independent from the effect of the active therapy (additive placebo model). Additivity is often assumed when comparing an active drug with placebo responses in randomized clinical trials. Since the placebo group receives everything that the active treatment group also receives (e.g., pill or capsule, attention, expectancy for improvement), it is assumed that the *additional* benefit of *adding* an active process can be assessed. However, the interaction between active therapy and expectancy questions the assumption of additivity. For example, increased vigilance as a consequence of participating in double-blind study may increase the drug effect and decrease the placebo response. Furthermore, the magnitude of the placebo response correlates significantly with the magnitude of the effect of the active therapy (Rickels et al. 1970; Moerman 2000).

ANY CLINICAL IMPROVEMENT AFTER THE ADMINISTRATION OF A PLACEBO IS DUE TO A PLACEBO EFFECT

When an individual patient shows improvement following the administration of a placebo, this is not necessarily due to a placebo response. As we have discussed in this chapter, several other factors may be responsible for the improvement, such as regression to the mean, natural course of the disease and additional therapies. For these reasons, it is extremely difficult to reveal placebo responses in individual patients.

CONCLUSION

Over the past decades, considerable progress has been made with respect to our understanding of placebo. Once considered an unpopular topic that was left largely untouched by both basic scientists and clinicians, placebo research has gained momentum. More rigorous methodologic studies have succeeded in more realistically portraying the power of placebo. Thanks to clever experimental set-ups, researchers have pinpointed some of the basic neurophysiologic and psychological mechanisms involved in the placebo response. At the same time, brain imaging techniques begin to unravel the neural circuitry that is at the foundation of the placebo response. Confusion remains about the definition of a placebo and it has been suggested that the term placebo be dropped in favor of the term "meaning response." The time has come to

reconsider the assessment of placebo as an unethical approach to treatment, and to perceive its full potential for improving the well-being of patients.

REFERENCES

Albe-Fessard D, Berkley KJ, Kruger L, et al Diencephalic mechanisms of pain sensation. Brain Res 1985; 356:217–296.

Amanzio M, Benedetti F The neurobiology of placebo analgesia: from endogenous opioids to cholecystokinin. Prog Neurobiol 1997; 52:109–125.

Amanzio M, Benedetti F Neuropharmacological dissection of placebo analgesia: expectation-activated opioid systems vs. conditioning-activated specific subsystems. J Neurosci 1999; 19:484–494.

Amanzio M, Pollo A, Maggi G, et al Response variability to analgesics: a role for non-specific activation of endogenous opioids. Pain 2001; 90:205–215.

An X, Bandler R, Ongur D, et al Prefrontal cortical projections to longitudinal columns in the midbrain periaqueductal gray in macaque monkeys. J Comp Neurol 1998; 40:455–479.

Bantick SJ, Wise RG, Ploghaus A, et al Imaging how attention modulates pain in humans using functional MRI. Brain 2002; 125:310–319.

Batterman RC, Lower WR Placebo responsiveness–influence of previous therapy. Curr Ther Res Clin Exp 1968; 10:136–143.

Battista AF, Wolff BB Levodopa and induced-pain response: a study of patients with Parkinsonian and pain syndromes. Arch Intern Med 1973; 132:70–74.

Becerra L, Breiter HC, Wise R, et al Reward circuitry activation by noxious thermal stimuli. Neuron 2001; 32:927–946.

Beecher HK The powerful placebo. JAMA 1955; 159:1602–1606.

Beecher HK Surgery as placebo. A quantitative study of bias. JAMA 1961; 176:1102–1107.

Benedetti F How the doctor's words affect the patient's brain. Eval Health Prof 2002; 25:369–387.

Benedetti F, Arduino C, Amanzio M Somatotopic activation of opioid systems by target-directed expectations of analgesia. J Neurosci 1999; 19:3639–3648.

Benedetti F, Maggi G, Lopiano L Open versus hidden medical treatments: the patient's knowledge about a therapy affects the therapy outcome. Prev Treat 6: article 1. Available: http://journals.apa.org/prevention/volume6/toc-jun-03.html.

Benedetti F, Pollo A, Lopiano L, et al Conscious expectation and unconscious conditioning in analgesic, motor, and hormonal placebo/nocebo responses. J Neurosci 2003b; 23:4315–4323.

Benedetti F, Colloca L, Torre E, et al Placebo-responsive Parkinson patients show decreased activity in single neurons of subthalamic nucleus. Nat Neurosci 2004; 7:587–588.

Benson H, Friedman R Harnessing the power of the placebo effect and renaming it "remembered wellness." Annu Rev Med 1996; 47:193–199.

Bernard JF, Bester H, Besson JM Involvement of the spino-parabrachio amygdaloid and hypothalamic pathways in the autonomic and affective emotional aspects of pain. Prog Brain Res 1996; 107:243–255.

Blackburn-Munro G, Blackburn-Munro RE Chronic pain, chronic stress and depression: coincidence or consequence? J Neuroendocrinol 2001; 13:1009–1023.

Boileau I, Dagher A, Leyton M, Welfeld K, Booij L, Diksic M, Benkelfat C. Conditioned dopamine release in humans: a positron emission tomography [11C]raclopride study with amphetamine. J Neurosci. 2007; 27:3998–4003.

Bolam JP, Hanley JJ, Booth PA, et al Synaptic organisation of the basal ganglia. J Anat 2000; 196:527–542.

Brewer WF There is no convincing evidence for operant or classical conditioning in adult humans. In: Weimer WB, Palermo DS (eds). Cognition and the Symbolic Processes, Hillsdale : Lawrence Erlbaum Associates NJ, 1974.

Brody H The placebo response. Recent research and implications for family medicine. J Fam Pract 2000; 49:649–654.

Burkey AR, Carstens E, Jasmin L Dopamine reuptake inhibition in the rostral agranular insular cortex produces antinociception. J Neurosci 1999; 19:4169–4179.

Burstein R, Cliffer KD, Giesler GJ Direct somatosensory projections from the spinal cord to the hypothalamus and telencephalon. J Neurosci 1987; 7:4159–4164.

Bushnell MC, Duncan GH Sensory and affective aspects of pain perception: is medial thalamus restricted to emotional issues? Exp Brain Res 1989; 78:415–418.

Bushnell MC, Duncan GH, Dubner R, et al Attentional influences on noxious and innocuous cutaneous heat detection in humans and monkeys. J Neurosci 1985; 5:1103–1110.

Chudler EH, Dong WK The role of the basal ganglia in nociception and pain. Pain 1995; 60:3–38.

Chudler EH, Sugiyama K, Dong WK Nociceptive responses in the neostriatum and globus pallidus of the anesthetized rat. J Neurophysiol 1993; 69:1890–1903.

Chudler EH, Sugiyama K, Dong WK Multisensory convergence and integration in the neostriatum and globus pallidus of the rat. Brain Res 1995; 674:33–45.

Coghill RC, Talbot JD, Evans AC, et al Distributed processing of pain and vibration by the human brain. J Neurosci 1994; 14:4095–4108.

Davis C Regression to the mean or placebo effect? In: Guess HA, Kleinman A, Kusek JW, Engel LW (eds). The Science of the Placebo. Toward an Interdisciplinary Research Agenda. BMJ Books, London, UK. 2002:183–206.

de Craen AJ, Moerman DE, Heisterkamp SH, et al Placebo effect in the treatment of duodenal ulcer. Br J Clin Pharmacol 1999; 48:853–860.

de Craen AJ, Tijssen JG, de Gans J, et al Placebo effect in the acute treatment of migraine: subcutaneous placebos are better than oral placebos. J Neurol 2000; 247:183–188.

de la Fuente-Fernandez R, Stoessl A The placebo effect in Parkinson's disease. Trends Neurosci 2002; 26:302–306.

de la Fuente-Fernandez R, Ruth TJ, Sossi V, et al Expectation and dopamine release: mechanism of the placebo effect in Parkinson's disease. Science 2001; 293:1164–1166.

de la Fuente-Fernandez R, Phillips AG, Zamburlini M, et al Dopamine release in human ventral striatum and expectation of reward. Behav Brain Res 2002a; 136:359–363.

de la Fuente-Fernandez R, Schulzer M, Calne DB, et al The placebo effect in neurological disorders. Lancet Neurol 2002b; 1:85–91.

de Pascalis V, Chiaradia C, Carotenuto E The contribution of suggestibility and expectation to placebo analgesia phenomenon in an experimental setting. Pain 2002; 96:393–402.

Dennis SG, Melzack R Effects of cholinergic and dopaminergic agents on pain and morphine analgesia measured by three pain tests. Exp Neurol 1983; 81:167–176.

Dickey RP, Minton JP Levodopa relief of bone pain from breast cancer. N Engl J Med 1972; 286:843.

Dubner R, Hoffman DS, Hayes RL Neuronal activity in medullary dorsal horn of awake monkeys trained in a thermal discrimination task. Task-related responses and their functional role. J Neurophysiol 1981; 46:444–464.

Duncan GH, Bushnell MC, Bates R, et al Task-related responses of monkey medullary dorsal horn neurons. J Neurophysiol 1987; 57:289–310.

Dworkin RH, Gitlin MJ Clinical aspects of depression in chronic pain patients. Clin J Pain 1991; 7:79–94.

Ebert D, Feistel H, Loew T, et al Dopamine and depression: striatal dopamine D2 receptor SPECT before and after antidepressant therapy. Psychopharmacology 1996; 126:91–94.

Eikerman A, Diener HC Effect of active treatment is lower when using placebo control in clinical trials on acute therapy of migraine. Cephalagia 2003; 23:344–347.

Ellenberg SS, Temple R Placebo-controlled trials and active-control trials in the evaluation of new treatments: 1. Ethical and scientific issues. Ann Intern Med 2000; 133:455–463.

Emanuel EJ, Miller FG The ethics of placebo-controlled trials: a middle ground. N Engl J Med 2001; 345:915–919.

Engel G The need for a new medical model: a challenge for biomedicine. Science 1977; 196:129–136.

Evans FJ Expectancy, therapeutic instructions, and the placebo response. In: White L, Tursky B, Schwartz GE (eds). Placebo: Theory, Research and Mechanisms. Guilford Press, New York, 1985:215–228.

Factor SA, Brown DL, Molho ES Subcutaneous apomorphine injections as a treatment for intractable pain in Parkinson's disease. Mov Disord 2000; 15:167–169.

Fava A, Eden E, Dorerb D, et al The problem of the placebo response in clinical trials for psychiatric disorders: culprits, possible remedies, and a novel study design approach. Psychother Psychosom 2003; 72:115–127.

Faymonville ME, Laureys S, Degueldre C, et al Neural mechanisms of antinociceptive effects of hypnosis. Anesthesiology 2000; 92:1257–1267.

Fleischhacker WW, Czobor P, Hummer M, et al Placebo or active control trials of antipsychotic drugs? Arch Gen Psychiatry 2003; 60:458–464.

Ford B Pain in Parkinson's disease. Clin Neurosci 1998; 5:63–72.

Gear RW, Aley KO, Levine JD Pain-induced analgesia mediated by mesolimbic reward circuits. J Neurosci 1999; 19:7175–7181.

Götzsche PC Is there logic in the placebo? Lancet 1994; 344:25–26.

Gracely RH, McGrath P, Dubner R Validity and sensitivity of ratio scales of sensory and affective verbal pain descriptors: manipulation of affect by diazepam. Pain 1978; 5:19–29.

Gracely RH, Dubner R, Wolskee PJ, et al Placebo and naloxone can alter post-surgical pain by separate mechanisms. Nature 1983; 306:264–265.

Gracely RH, Dubner R, Deeter WR, et al Clinicians' expectations influence placebo analgesia. Lancet 1985; 1 (8419):43.

Grevert P, Albert LH, Goldstein A Partial antagonism of placebo analgesia by naloxone. Pain 1983; 16:129–143.

Grünbaum A Explication and implication of the placebo concept. In: White L, Tursky B, Schwartz GE (eds). Placebo: Theory, Research, and Mechanisms. Guilford Press, New York, 1985.

Hagelberg N, Martikainen IK, Mansikka H, et al Dopamine D2 receptor binding in the human brain is associated with the response to painful stimulation and pain modulatory capacity. Pain 2002; 99:273–279.

Harrington A The Placebo Effect. Harvard University Press, Cambridge, MA, 1997.

Hayes RL, Price DD, Bennett GJ, et al Differential effects of spinal cord lesions on narcotic and non-narcotic suppression of nociceptive reflexes: further evidence for the physiologic multiplicity of pain modulation. Brain Res 1978; 155:91–101.

Helmstetter FJ, Tershner SA, Poore LH, et al Antinociception following opioid stimulation of the basolateral amygdala is expressed through the periaqueductal gray and rostral ventromedial medulla. Brain Res 1998; 779:104–118.

Hergenhahn BR An Introduction to Theories of Learning. Prentice Hall, NJ, 1988.

Hofbauer RK, Rainville P, Duncan GH, et al Cortical representation of the sensory dimension of pain. J Neurophysiol 2001; 86:402–411.

Hrobjartsson A, Götzsche PC Is the placebo powerless? An analysis of clinical trials comparing placebo treatment and no treatment. N Engl J Med 2001; 344:1594–1602.

Hudson PM, Semenenko FM, Lumb BM Inhibitory effects evoked from the rostral ventrolateral medulla are selective for the nociceptive responses of spinal dorsal horn neurons. Neuroscience 2000; 99:541–547.

Hypericum Depression Trial Study Group Effect of Hypericum perforatum (St John's wort) in major depressive disorder: a randomized controlled trial. JAMA 2002; 287:1807–1814.

Kaptchuk TJ Powerful placebo: the dark side of the randomised controlled trial. Lancet 1998; 351:1722–1725.

Kaptchuk TJ, Goldman P, Stone DA, et al Do medical devices have enhanced placebo effects? J Clin Epidemiol 2000; 53:786–792.

Kazdin AE Research Design in Clinical Psychology. Harper & Row, New York, 1980.

Kernbaum S, Hauchecorne J Administration of levodopa for relief of herpes zoster pain. JAMA 1981; 246:132–134.

Khan A, Warner HA, Brown WA Symptom reduction and suicide risk in patients treated with placebo in antidepressant clinical trials: an analysis of the Food and Drug Administration database. Arch Gen Psychiatry 2000; 57:311–317.

Kienle GS, Kiene H The powerful placebo effect: fact or fiction? J Clin Epidemiol 1997; 50:1311–1318.

Kirsch I Specifying nonspecifics: psychological mechanisms of placebo effects. In: Harrington A (ed). The Placebo Effect: An Interdisciplinary Exploration, Harvard University Press, Cambridge, MA, 1997.

Kirsch I, Rosadino MJ Do double-blind studies with informed consent yield externally valid results? An empirical test. Psychopharmacology 1993; 110: 437–442.

Kupers R Is the placebo powerless? N Engl J Med 2001; 345:1278.

Kupers R, Witting N, Jensen TS Brain-imaging studies of experimental and clinical forms of allodynia and hyperalgesia. In: Brune K, Handwerker H (eds). Hyperalgesia: Molecular Mechanisms and Clinical Implications. Progress in Pain Research and Management, vol 30. IASP Press, Seattle, WA, 2004.

Kupers R, Maeyaert J, Boly M, Faymonville M-E, Laureys S, Naloxone-insensitive epidural placebo analgesia in a chronic pain patient, Anesthesiology, 2007 (in press)

Lasagna LL, Mosteller F, Von Felsinger JM, et al A study of the placebo response. Am J Med 1954; 16:770–779.

Laska E, Sunshine A Anticipation of analgesia: a placebo effect. Headache 1973; 13:1–11.

Leuchter AF, Cook IA, Witte EA, et al Changes in brain function of depressed subjects during treatment with placebo. Am J Psychiatry 2002; 159:122–129.

Levine JD, Gordon NC, Fields HL The mechanism of placebo analgesia. Lancet 1978; 2:654–657.

Liberman R An experimental study of the placebo response under three different situations of pain. J Psychiatr Res 1964; 33:233–246.

Lieberman MD, Jarcho JM, Berman S, et al The neural correlates of placebo effects: a disruption account. Neuroimage 2004; 22:447–455.

Liebeskind JC Pain can kill. Pain 1991; 44:3–4.

Lin Y, Morrow TJ, Kiritsy-Roy JA, et al Cocaine: evidence for supraspinal, dopamine-mediated, non-opiate analgesia. Brain Res 1989; 479:306–312.

Lorenz J, Minoshima S, Casey KL Keeping pain out of mind: the role of the dorsolateral prefrontal cortex in pain modulation. Brain 2003; 126:1079–1091.

Lyerly SB, Ross S, Krugman AD, et al Drugs and placebos: the effects of instructions upon performance and mood under amphetamine sulphate and chloral hydrate. J Abn Soc Psych 1964; 68:321–327.

Macedo A, Farre M, Banos JE Placebo effect and placebos: what are we talking about? Some conceptual and historical considerations. Eur J Clin Pharmacol 2003; 59:337–342.

Magni G On the relationship between chronic pain and depression when there is no organic lesion. Pain 1987; 31:1–21.

Magnusson JE, Fisher K The involvement of dopamine in nociception: the role of D(1) and D(2) receptors in the dorsolateral striatum. Brain Res 2000; 855: 260–266.

Marchand S, Kupers RC, Bushnell MC, et al Analgesic and placebo effects of thalamic stimulation. Pain 2003; 105:481–488.

Marlatt GA, Rohsenow DJ Cognitive processes in alcohol use: expectancy and the balanced placebo design. Adv Subst Abuse 1980; 1:159–199.

Mayberg HS, Silva JA, Brannan SK, et al The functional neuroanatomy of the placebo effect. Am J Psychiatry 2002; 159:728–737.

McDonald CJ, Mazzuca SA, McCabe GP How much of the placebo "effect" is really statistical regression? Stat Med 1983; 2:417–427.

McGaraughty S, Chu KL, Bitner RS, et al Capsaicin infused into the PAG affects rat tail flick responses to noxious heat and alters neuronal firing in the RVM. J Neurophysiol 2003; 90:2702–2710.

McRae C, Cherin E, Yamazaki TG, et al Effects of perceived treatment on quality of life and medical outcomes in a double-blind placebo surgery trial. Arch Gen Psychiatry 2004; 61:412–420.

Melzack R, Casey KL Sensory, motivational and central determinants of pain: a new conceptual model. In: Kenshalo DR (ed). The Skin Senses, Springfield, IL, 1968:423–443.

Melzack R, Wall PD Pain mechanisms: a new theory. Science 1965; 150:971–978.

Mersky H, Bogduk N Classification of Chronic Pain. 2nd edn. IASP Task Force on Taxonomy, IASP Press, Seattle, WA, 1994:209–214.

Miley DP, Abrams AA, Atkinson JH, et al Successful treatment of thalamic pain with apomorphine. Am J Psychiatry 1978; 135:1230–1232.

Miller FG Is the placebo powerless? N Engl J Med 2001; 345:1278.

Miller FG, Brody H What makes placebo-controlled trials unethical? Am J Bioeth 2002; 2:3–9.

Moerman DE Cultural variations in the placebo effect: ulcers, anxiety, and blood pressure. Med Anthropol Q 2000; 14:51–72.

Moerman DE The meaning response and the ethics of avoiding placebos. Eval Health Prof 2002; 25: 399–409.

Moerman DE, Jonas WB Deconstructing the placebo effect and finding the meaning response. Ann Intern Med 2002; 136:471–476.

Montgomery GH, Kirsch I Classical conditioning and the placebo effect. Pain 1997; 72:107–113.

Nixon DW Use of L-dopa to relieve pain from bone metastases. N Engl J Med 1975; 292:647.

O'Doherty JP Neural responses during anticipation of a primary taste reward. Neuron 2002; 33:815–826.

Oh V The placebo effect: can we use it better? Br Med J 1994; 309:69–70.

Ongur D, An X, Price JL Prefrontal cortical projections to the hypothalamus in macaque monkeys. J Comp Neurol 1988; 401:480–505.

Pertovaara A, Belczynski CR, Morrow TJ, et al The effect of systemic cocaine on spinal nociceptive reflex activity in the rat. Brain Res 1988; 438:286–290.

Petrovic P, Ingvar M Imaging cognitive modulation of pain processing. Pain 2002; 95:1–5.

Petrovic P, Petersson KM, Ghatan PH, et al Pain-related cerebral activation is altered by a distracting cognitive task. Pain 2000; 85:19–30.

Petrovic P, Kalso E, Petersson KM, et al Placebo and opioid analgesia: imaging a shared neuronal network. Science 2002; 295:1737–1740.

Peyron R, Garcia-Larrea L, Gregoire MC, et al Haemodynamic brain responses to acute pain in humans: sensory and attentional networks. Brain 1998; 122: 1765–1780.

Peyron R, Laurent B, Garcia-Larrea L Functional imaging of brain responses to pain. A review and meta-analysis. Neurophysiol Clin 2000; 30:263–288.

Price DD Psychological and Neural Mechanisms of Pain. Raven Press, New York, 1988.

Price DD Psychological Mechanisms of Pain and Analgesia. IASP Press, Seattle, WA, 1999.

Price DD Psychological and neural mechanisms of the affective dimension of pain. Science 2000; 288:1769–1772.

Price DD, Fields H Where are the causes of placebo analgesia? An experimental behavioral analysis. Pain Forum 1997; 6:44–52.

Price DD, Harkins SW The affective-motivational dimension of pain: a two stage model. APS J 1992; 1:229–239.

Price DD, Milling LS, Kirsch I, et al An analysis of factors that contribute to the magnitude of placebo analgesia in an experimental paradigm. Pain 1999; 84:110–113.

Rainville P, Duncan GH, Price DD, et al Pain affect encoded in human anterior cingulate but not somatosensory cortex. Science 1997; 277:968–971.

Rescorla RA Pavlovian conditioning: it's not what you think it is. Am Psychol 1988; 43:151–160.

Richardson PH Placebo effects in pain management. Pain Rev 1994; 1:15–32.

Rickels K, Hesbacher PT, Weise CC, et al Pills and improvement: a study of placebo response in psychoneurotic outpatients. Psychopharmacologia 1970; 16:318–328.

Riley DE, Lang AE The spectrum of levodopa-related fluctuations in Parkinson's disease. Neurology 1993; 43:1459–1464.

Rochon PA, Binns MA, Litner JA, et al Are randomized control trial outcomes influenced by the inclusion of a placebo group? A systematic review of nonsteroidal antiinflammatory drug trials for arthritis treatment. J Clin Epidemiol 1999; 52:113–122.

Romo R, Schultz W Somatosensory input to dopamine neurones of the monkey midbrain: responses to pain pinch under anaesthesia and to active touch in behavioural context. Prog Brain Res 1989; 80:473–478.

Ross S, Krugman AD, Lyerly SB, et al Drugs and placebos: a model design. Psychol Rep 1962; 10:383–392.

Roth RA Biopsychosocial perspective on the placebo effect: comment on Benedetti et al. Prev Treat 2003; 6:8.

Schultz W Predictive reward signal of dopamine neurons. J Neurophysiol 1998; 80:1–27.

Sesack SR, Pickel VM Dual ultrastructural localization of enkephalin and tyrosine hydroxylase immunoreactivity in the rat ventral tegmental area: multiple substrates for opiate–dopamine interactions. J Neurosci 1992; 12:1335–1350.

Shah PJ, Ogilvie AD, Goodwin GM, et al Clinical and psychometric correlates of dopamine D2 binding in depression. Psychol Med 1997; 27:1247–1256.

Shapiro AK A contribution to the history of the placebo effect. Behav Sci 1960; 5:109–135.

Shapiro AK A historic and heuristic definition of the placebo. Psychiatry 1964; 27:52–58.

Shyu BC, Kiritsy-Roy JA, Morrow TJ, et al Neurophysiological, pharmacological and behavioral evidence for medial thalamic mediation of cocaine-induced dopaminergic analgesia. Brain Res 1992; 572:216–223.

Siegel S Drug anticipatory responses in animals. In: White L, Tursky B, Schwartz GE (eds). Placebo: Theory, Research, and Mechanisms. Guilford Press, New York, 1985:288–305.

Soerensen L, Price DD Endogenous opioid and non-opioid pathways as mediators of placebo analgesia. In: Guess HA, Kleinman A, Kusek JW, Engel LW (eds). The Science of the Placebo. Toward an Interdisciplinary Research Agenda. BMJ Books, London, 2002:183–206.

Soper WY, Melzack R Stimulation-produced analgesia: evidence for somatotopic organization in the midbrain. Brain Res 1982; 18:301–311.

Stewart-Williams S, Podd J The placebo effect. Dissolving the expectancy versus conditioning debate. Psychol Bull 2004; 130:324–340.

Straus SE, Briggs J Conclusions and future directions. In: Guess HA, Kleinman A, Kusek JW, Engel LW (eds). The Science of the Placebo. Toward an Interdisciplinary Research Agenda. BMJ Books, London, 2002.

Suchman AL, Ader R Classic conditioning and placebo effects in crossover studies. Clin Pharmacol Ther 1992; 52:372–377.

Thomas KB Temporarily dependent patient in clinical practice. Br Med J 1974; 1:625–626.

Tracey I, Ploghaus A, Gati JS, et al Imaging attentional modulation of pain in the periaqueductal gray in humans. J Neurosci 2002; 22:48–52.

Turner JA, Deyo RA, Loeser JD, et al The importance of placebo effects in pain treatment and research. JAMA 1994; 271:1609–1614.

Urban MO, Smith DJ Nuclei within the rostral ventromedial medulla mediating morphine antinociception from the periaqueductal gray. Brain Res 1994; 25:9–16.

Valet M, Sprenger T, Boecker H, et al Distraction modulates connectivity of the cingulo-frontal cortex and the midbrain during pain: an fMRI analysis. Pain 2004; 109:399–408.

Vase L, Riley JL, Price DD A comparison of placebo effects in clinical analgesic trials versus studies of placebo analgesia. Pain 2002; 99:443–452.

Voudouris NJ, Peck CL, Coleman G Conditioned placebo responses. J Pers Soc Psychol 1985; 48:47–53.

Voudouris NJ, Peck CL, Coleman G Conditioned response models of placebo phenomena: further support. Pain 1989; 38:109–116.

Voudouris NJ, Peck CL, Coleman G The role of conditioning and verbal expectancy in the placebo response. Pain 1990; 43:121–128.

Wager TD, Rilling JK, Smith EE, et al Placebo-induced changes in FMRI in the anticipation and experience of pain. Science 2004; 303:1162–1167.

Wall PD On the relation of injury to pain. Pain 1979; 6:253–264.

Wall PD The placebo effect: an unpopular topic. Pain 1991; 51:1–3.

Wall PD, Melzack R Textbook of Pain. Lea and Fibiger, Philadelphia, PA, 1999.

Wang H, Wessendorf MW Mu- and delta-opioid receptor mRNAs are expressed in periaqueductal gray neurons projecting to the rostral ventromedial medulla. Neuroscience 2002; 109:619–634.

Watkins LR, Mayer DJ Organization of endogenous opiate and nonopiate pain control systems. Science 1982; 216:1185–1192.

White L, Tursky B, Schwartz G Placebo: Theory, Research and Mechanisms. Guilford Press, New York, 1985.

Wickramasekera I A conditioned response model of the placebo effect: predictions from the model. Biofeedback Self Regul 1980; 5:5–18.

Zubieta JK, Smith YR, Bueller JA, et al Regional mu opioid receptor regulation of sensory and affective dimensions of pain. Science 2001; 293:311–315.

FURTHER READING

Benedetti F The opposite effects of the opiate antagonist naloxone and the cholecystokinin antagonist proglumide on placebo analgesia. Pain 1996; 64:535–543.

Casey KL, Minoshima S, Berger KL, et al Positron emission tomographic analysis of cerebral structures activated specifically by repetitive noxious heat stimuli. J Neurophysiol 1994; 71:802–807.

Craig AD Pain mechanisms: labeled lines versus convergence in central processing. Annu Rev Neurosci 2003; 26:1–30.

Dagher A, Bleicher C, Aston JA, et al Reduced dopamine D1 receptor binding in the ventral striatum of cigarette smokers. Synapse 2001; 42:48–53.

Fields HL, Basbaum AI Central nervous system mechanisms of pain modulation. In: Wall PD, Melzack R (eds). Textbook of Pain. Churchill Livingstone, London, 1999:309–329.

Fields HL, Price DD Towards a neurobiology of placebo analgesia. In: Harrington A (ed). The Placebo Effect. Harvard University Press, Cambridge, MA, 1997:93–116.

Hrobjartsson A The uncontrollable placebo effect. Eur J Clin Pharmacol 1996; 50:345–348.

Iadarola MJ, Berman KF, Zeffiro TA, et al Neural activation during acute capsaicin-evoked pain and allodynia assessed with PET. Brain 1998; 121:931–947.

Ingvar M Pain and functional imaging. Philos Trans R Soc Lond B: Biol Sci 1999; 354:1347–1358.

Kaptchuk TJ Is the placebo powerless? N Engl J Med 2001a; 345:1278.

Kaptchuk TJ The double-blind, randomized, placebo-controlled trial: gold standard or golden calf? J Clin Epidemiol 2001b; 54:541–549.

Kirsch I Hidden administration as ethical alternatives to the balanced placebo design. Prev Treat 2003; 6:5.

Kirsch I, Sapirstein G Listening to Prozac but hearing placebo: a meta-analysis of antidepressant medication. Prev Treat 1998; 1:article 0002a (http://www. journals.apa.org/prevention/volume1/pre0010002a. html).

McDonald CJ Is the placebo powerless? N Engl J Med 2001; 345:1278–1279.

Moerman DE Medicine, Meaning, and the Placebo Effect. Cambridge University Press, London, 2002.

Wall PD Comments after 30 years of the Gate Control Theory. Pain Forum 1996; 5:12–22.

CHAPTER 7

Side effects and numbers-needed-to-harm:

What do we really know about opioid treatment for chronic non-malignant pain?

Elon Eisenberg, MD.

INTRODUCTION

According to recent studies from Europe and the USA, 10–30% of patients with chronic non-malignant pain (CNMP) consume opioids. A review of randomized controlled trials (RCTs) and evidence-based reviews (EBRs) on this topic indicates that assessments of the safety of these drugs are failing to keep pace with data on their efficacy. Data from our analyses of 23 RCTs revealed significant methodological problems that prevented clear conclusions regarding the adverse-event profile of opioids in the treatment of CNMP (Eisenberg et al. 2005 and 2006). This is especially true with respect to assessment of the magnitude (severity) of adverse effects.

The available data do not support the recommended use of long-acting rather than short-acting opioids, as the time course of various side effects and their dose-response relationships are unclear. For the sake of conciseness, we have not in this chapter cited every RCT considered in our earlier systematic reviews, and refer the reader to those reviews for greater detail. Numbers-needed-to-harm (NNH) were calculated and found to be 3.8 for constipation, 5.6 for drowsiness, 5.7 for nausea, 7.4 for dizziness, 9.2 for vomiting, and 8.2 for discontinuation of opioid therapy. The NNH for cognitive impairment could not be calculated. Serious adverse events, such as respiratory depression, abuse or death, as a direct result of opioid therapy were not reported in the 23 RCTs reviewed by us earlier, nor in the subsequent literature that we cite below. Furthermore, data on techniques aimed to control adverse effects, such as opioid rotation, is extremely limited and inconclusive.

EFFICACY VERSUS SAFETY

As we continuously struggle with our inability to reduce chronic pain by more than one-third of its original intensity on average, even with the most advanced and potent available drugs (Loeser 2003), it is clear that the focus of pain research is aimed at improved efficacy. A simple Medline search using the MeSH term *analgesics* yields over 50,000 citations. Given this huge number, the only way of getting valid information on the efficacies of different interventions in specific pain conditions is by isolating the high-quality studies alone and performing a quantitative analysis. Indeed, the number of pain-related EBRs is growing. This chapter reviews the difficulties in conducting an EBR of adverse effects of analgesic interventions, while focusing on the current evidence-based knowledge of the safety of opioids in the treatment of CNMP.

Although the safety of any given treatment is as important as its efficacy, the available evidence on side effects is limited and lags far behind that on efficacy. As McQuay and Moore (1998) note, despite the fact that pain was measured as an outcome in 79% of systematic reviews published between 1966 and 1993, adverse effects were measured in only 14% of them. Recent EBRs do provide general safety information, usually on drug classes, as measured by the numbers of patients reporting an adverse effect or occasionally by NNH. Thus, the number of patients needed to be treated with an anticonvulsant or a tricyclic antidepressant for neuropathic pain in order to get one patient with a minor adverse event (e.g., constipation), also known as "NNH-minor," is approximately three. In other words, roughly one of three patients treated with a drug from these classes will develop a *minor* side effect (Collins et al. 2000). Yet we do not have adequate information regarding the magnitude of any given adverse event – a fact that may compromise our ability to compare the safety of two drugs. For example, in the case of two drugs with an NNH of 3 for dizziness, we do not know if switching a patient from one of these drugs to theother will reduce the *severity* of the dizziness. The same is true for the severity of constipation caused by one opioid versus another and so forth.

METHODOLOGICAL ISSUES RELATED TO QUANTITATIVE ASSESSMENT OF SIDE EFFECTS

Quantitative systematic reviews of pain treatment-related adverse events are often limited by methodological problems and faults of the evaluated trials (see Table 7.1). Perhaps the most relevant limitation of the RCTs is that satisfactory pain relief can rarely be achieved with available drugs. Therefore, the *primary focus* of pain research is still improved efficacy rather than safety.

This notion leads to a second common methodological limitation with respect to the review of adverse events, namely that the *quantification* of their intensities is not yet a standard outcome measure in chronic pain trials. Therefore, in contrast to pain measures that are universally quantitative, adverse events are described only in terms of prevalence or incidence in most studies. A trial comparing one opioid to another may typically show a 15% difference in the prevalence of nausea, for example, without quantitating its severity (such as with a visual analogue or verbal scale). The

Table 7.1 Methodological Limitations Related to RCT-Based Quantitative Assessment of Side Effects

1.	Focus on efficacy rather than safety.
2.	Adverse events are hardly ever used as primary outcome measures.
3.	Avoidance of patients who are at risk for developing AEs.
4.	Only the number of AEs is counted, but not their severity.
5.	No time-related follow-up on the appearance and resolution of AEs.
6.	NNH is different from NNT in that it does not address the magnitude of the AE in any way.
7.	Insufficient quality scores of the RCTs.
8.	Large inter-study methodological differences that preclude quantitative synthesis of data.

equivalent in terms of analgesia would be a 15% difference in the number of patients reporting "pain relief" between the two drugs. Most of us would not be willing to accept this as a valid outcome.

Two steps have been taken to improve quantitation of adverse effects. One is to differentiate "serious" (i.e., events that are life-threatening or require hospitalization) from "non-serious" adverse effects. The other is the introduction of the term NNH, which has become a part of the nomenclature found in EBR. The NNH allows comparisons of the relative safety of different drugs. Taken together, these concepts have led to the introduction of the terms 'NNH minor' and 'NNH major' for mild and serious adverse events, respectively (see, for example, Collins et al. 2000).

Yet, these terms are still based upon notions of prevalence rather than on a true quantitative measure of magnitudes and therefore do not overcome these limitations. The terms numbers-needed-to-treat (NNT) and NNH may seem similar in terms of their preciseness, but a close look shows that they are not. It is true that both terms originate from RCTs. However, NNT refers to the number of patients that need to be treated with a certain drug in order to obtain one patient with a *defined degree* of pain relief (Cook & Sackett 1995), which is usually 50%. In contrast, NNH is the number of patients that need to be treated in order to obtain one patient with an adverse event, regardless of its magnitude. As such, the quantitative assessment of the severity of adverse events is again left untouched.

Lastly, although RCTs are the cornerstones of EBR, they are not regarded as optimal for assessing adverse events because in an attempt to minimize dropouts, they typically exclude patients who are at high risk of developing adverse events.

GUIDELINES FOR THE USE OF OPIOIDS IN CNMP

Along with opioids' well-established use for acute and cancer-related pain, their use for CNMP has expanded dramatically during the past decade. Studies from Europe and the USA estimate that 10–30% of patients with CNMP consume opioids for the management of their pain. A recent study from Denmark showed that 3% of the Danish population use opioids on a regular basis (Eriksen 2003). Not surprisingly, guidelines related to the appropriate use of opioids in CNMP have been issued worldwide (i.e. American Academy of Pain Medicine and the American Pain Society, 2001; Kalso et al., 2003). These guidelines are aimed to close gaps between patients' needs and physicians' prescribing habits, market forces and regulatory requirements, and conceptions and misconceptions regarding opioid usage. Despite the release of these guidelines, two recently published EBRs (Chou et al. 2003; McNicol et al. 2003) reveal that well designed trials with secure evidence on the efficacy and the safety of opioids in chronic use are still missing.

ADVERSE EFFECTS OF OPIOIDS

Common adverse events associated with the use of opioids include nausea, vomiting, constipation, somnolence, dizziness, and cognitive dysfunction. Less common adverse events include myoclonus, pruritus, and possibly paradoxical hyperalgesia. Respiratory depression and addiction are regarded as more serious adverse events. Recent reports indicate that sexual dysfunction may also result from chronic opioid use.

SHORT- VERSUS LONG-ACTING OPIOIDS AND THEIR RELATIONSHIP TO ADVERSE EVENTS

Many of the available guidelines (see Model guidelines 1998) emphasize use of long-acting rather than short-acting opioids for CNMP and some even recommend *not* to use short-acting agents, due to fear of their higher potential for abuse and addiction. Therefore, a key question is whether long-acting opioids produce fewer adverse events than their short-acting counterparts.

In their EBR entitled "Comparative efficacy and safety of long-acting oral opioids for chronic non-cancer pain: a systematic review," Chou et al. (2003) identified 16 RCTs and 8 observational studies that provided appropriate data on the efficacy and safety of these drugs. Only seven of the RCTs cited

provided data specifically relevant to the above question. The quality rating of six of them was poor and the seventh (Jamison et al. 1988) was fair, indicating their relatively low internal validity. Only common adverse events were recorded in these trials, and with the exception of one trial (Jamison et al. 1988) that reported severity on a 10 cm visual analogue scale, all reports were limited to the prevalence of each event. Although no formal safety analysis could be conducted, the authors concluded that overall, there was no pattern favoring either short-acting or long-acting opioids. This EBR could not address the main concern associated with the use of short-acting opioids for CNMP, which is the fear of abuse and addiction. Interestingly, a recent study (Manchikanti et al. 2005) found no significant differences in illicit drug use or opioid misuse between 100 patients given the short-acting opioid hydrocodone and another group who received methadone, a long-acting opioid. Thus, evidence to support advocacy by almost every guideline of long-acting rather than short-acting opioids, remains to be found.

TIME COURSE OF ADVERSE EVENTS

Based on cancer pain studies, opioid-related adverse effects are hypothesized to be time- and dose-related. Such adverse events as nausea and vomiting are usually seen upon initiation of therapy or following dose increments and are expected to resolve over time as a function of tolerance to a stable opioid dosage. Constipation, on the other hand, is unlikely to resolve under similar conditions. In order for us to be able to test this hypothesis in CNMP, we need trials that determine the prevalence of specific adverse effects over time.

Unfortunately, the available RCTs generally do not provide longitudinal adverse events-related information. Only one trial (Kjaersgaard-Andersen et al. 1990) conveyed more accurate information on the prevalence of specific adverse effects over time. This four-week multi-center study evaluated the efficacy and safety of 3 grams of paracetamol (called acetaminophen in North America) plus 180 mg of codeine versus an equal dose of paracetamol alone in the treatment of pain due to osteoarthrosis of the hip. The study was terminated prematurely due to a very high incidence of dropouts (36% during the first week of treatment). Yet, available data show that the total number of reported adverse events dropped from 177 during the first week of treatment to 41 during the fourth week (77% decrease), whereas the number of patients in the study dropped from 83 to 44 (47% decrease). Together, these figures suggest that tolerance to adverse events over time does exist in general. Specifically, the number of events of nausea dropped from 34 to 2, of vomiting from 19 to 1, of dizziness from 26 to 3, and of somnolence from 15 to 5, all showing a greater decrement in symptoms as compared to dropouts. In contrast, events of constipation dropped only from 17 to 9 (47%). This 47% decrease is similar to the dropout rate and indicates, as expected, minimal tolerance to constipation. Another potential adverse effect of opioids is cognitive impairment, whose time course has been the subject of several surveys and at least one controlled trial. This adverse effect will be discussed in greater detail below.

OPIOID DOSAGE AND ADVERSE EVENTS

As mentioned earlier, opioid adverse effects are expected to worsen dose-dependently. Only, two RCTs have compared high versus low doses of the same drug. In one study (Roth et al., 2000) twice-daily doses of 10 or 20 mg of long-acting oxycodone were compared. The results were equivocal: nausea, vomiting, and constipation occured more often with the high dose, somnolence/drowsiness and withdrawal rates were equal, and dizziness occured less frequently with the high dose. In the other study (Rowbotham, 2003), high average daily doses of levorphanol (8.9 mg) were compared to low doses (2.7 mg). The incidences of adverse events in the levorphanol study were not reported, with the exception of higher incidences of dizziness in the high-dose group than in the low-dose group (2 versus 0, respectively) and higher incidences of adverse event-related dropouts (12 versus 3, respectively).

SPECIFIC ADVERSE EFFECTS

COGNITIVE DYSFUNCTION

Cognitive dysfunction is a major concern with the use of opioids. With expectations that some opioid-treated patients will resume daily activities such as working and driving, the safety issue related to possible cognitive impairment bears great significance. Cognitive impairment may result from drowsiness or somnolence, which are common in opioid-treated patients. However, such impairment but may appear without obvious drowsiness or somnolence, and might be even more hazardous under such circumstances. The cognitive evaluation by Rowbotham et al. (2003) of patients who received either high or low dosages of levorphanol over an eight-week period concluded that cognitive impairment was not apparent. Indeed, scores on the Symbol-Digit Modalities Test actually improved in both treatment groups. In contrast, Huse et al. (2001) found impaired cognition in a small group of patients with phantom pain who received an average of 11 mg long-acting morphine per day for four weeks, as compared to the placebo-treated group.

Four other trials provided data on altered cognition, with mixed results. Lloyd (1992) noted altered cognition in 10% of patients receiving long-acting

dihydrocodeine and in 5% of patients taking dextro-propoxyphene plus paracetamol for two weeks. In contrast, Moulin (1996) found a higher incidence of cognitive impairment in patients on a nine-week placebo treatment (15%), as compared to long-acting morphine treatment (9%), but the active placebo used in that study may account for this high figure. In another study with long-acting morphine, Jamison (1998) reported an equal incidence of cognitive impairment in a small group of patients treated by either morphine or placebo over a period of 16 weeks. Raja (2002) found a normal cognitive state in patients who received morphine, methadone or placebo and impaired cognition in those treated with tricyclic antidepressants.

In another prospective study (Sabatowski et al. 2003), a series of computerized tests measured attention, reaction, visual orientation, motor coordination, and vigilance in 21 patients with CNMP who were treated with stable doses of transdermal fentanyl patches for three weeks. In comparison with results of 90 healthy volunteers, none of the performance measures for the fentanyl patients were significantly inferior to those of the controls.

One trial (Tassain et al. 2003) in which the long-term neuropsychological effects of morphine were tested deserves special attention. Of the 28 patients included in the study, 18 received oral sustained morphine (range 40–140 mg/day). The 10 patients who stopped the morphine regimen prematurely because of side effects or insufficient pain relief were followed as a control group. A battery of tests of attention, psychomotor speed and memory was administered, and the effects of morphine on pain, quality of life, mood, subjective memory impairment, and side effects were also investigated. Evaluations were performed at baseline in patients free from opioids and then at 3, 6, and 12 months. No impairment of any neuropsychological variable over time was noted in the morphine-treated patients in comparison with the control group, and a few cognitive parameters even improved. The authors concluded that "12 months treatment with oral morphine does not disrupt cognitive functioning in patients with chronic non-cancer pain and instead results in moderate improvement of some aspects of cognitive functioning, as a consequence of the pain relief and concomitant improvement of well-being and mood." The study can be criticized for its small study population and for the lack of an adequate control group.

Taken together, the above trials indicate that the incidence of cognitive impairment as a result of chronic opioid use does not exceed 10%. At the same time, it should be noted that there is insufficient awareness on the part of investigators in regard to this important adverse event: more than half of the reviewed RCTs do not mention cognitive impairment.

OPIOID-INDUCED PARADOXICAL HYPERALGESIA

A growing number of animal and human studies show that under certain circumstances, opioids can increase pain sensitivity, resulting in hyperalgesia and allodynia. Animal studies have shown reduced thresholds for withdrawal latencies to mechanical and thermal stimuli in response to of various opioids (Mao 2006).

In humans, opioid-induced pain sensitivity has been reported after postoperative infusions of short-acting opioids such as remifentanil, as well as in drug addicts. Guignard et al. (2000) have shown that large doses of intraoperative remifentanil increased postoperative pain and morphine consumption, suggesting that remi-fentanil causes acute opioid tolerance and hyperalgesia. Several researchers suggested as long as 40 years ago that opioid-addicted subjects differ in their sensitivity to pain as compared with normal subjects (Martin and Inglis 1965; Ho and Dole 1979). More recent studies, (Compton et al. 2001; Pud et al. 2006) found shorter withdrawal latencies for cold pressor pain in opioid addicts maintained on methadone and buprenorphine than in opioid-naïve, healthy controls. These results suggest that prolonged opioid use may enhance abnormal pain sensitivity.

In his 2006 review on opioid-induced abnormal pain sensitivity, Mao (2006) stated: "it is difficult to determine whether changes in pain levels occur clinically following opioid administration." In a recent study of this possibility, 142 patients with cancer and chronic non-malignant pain treated with 'regular' dosages of oral opioids were found not to differ in their sensitivity to experimentally evoked mechanical and heat pain versus patients treated with non-opioid drugs (Reznikov et al, 2005). In contrast, a preliminary prospective study in six patients with chronic low back pain showed hyperalgesia to cold (but not heat) following four weeks of morphine treatment (Chu et al. 2006). In conclusion, currently there is no evidence for opioid-induced paradoxical hyperalgesia in patients with CNMP given oral opioids.

SEXUAL DYSFUNCTION

Sexual dysfunction during chronic opioid use has recently gained considerable interest. Although not fully investigated, recent data suggest that chronic exposure to high-dose oral opioid therapy (the equivalent of 200 mg per day of morphine) may cause marked central hypogonadism and sexual dysfunction in males (Rajagopal et al. 2003). The effects of lower doses of opioids, however, are unclear. Although previous studies have indicated that methadone may suppress sexual behavior, these studies were conducted with drug addicts and therefore may be irrelevant to patients suffering from chronic pain. Notably, long-term intra-thecal administration of opioids can cause profound sexual dysfunction and hypogonadism in both males and females with CNMP. Undoubtedly, future opioid trials should add sexual dysfunction to the list of potential adverse events.

SEVERE (MAJOR) ADVERSE EFFECTS

As mentioned earlier, respiratory depression and abuse are key concerns during chronic use of opioids. Yet in the existing RCTs, no mention was made of respiratory depression. It seems, therefore, that respiratory depression is unlikely to occur with commonly-used opioid dosages and that in this respect there is no basis for prescribing a short-acting over a long-acting opioid.

Death or serious injury as a direct result of opioid use was not reported in any of the 23 RCTs cited in this chapter. This is particularly significant in light of the possibility that opioids may reduce alertness and compromise driving ability. The fact that no reports of death or significant injuries have occurred among 1841 opioid users with CNMP is indirect evidence for the relative safety of opioids, at least from this viewpoint. As far as abuse or addiction is concerned, the available RCTs do not address this issue at all. Although not mentioned specifically as an exclusion criterion, it is highly possible that researchers tend to avoid recruiting patients with "abuse or addiction potential" (Dunbar and Katz, 1996). Thus, it is not surprising in the face of such selection bias that abnormal behavior suggesting abuse or addiction has not been reported and that no evidence regarding these risks is currently available. This knowledge gap, along with the growth of prescription drug abuse as a public health issue, including an abuse incidence exceeding conventional street drugs (Katz et al. 2007), highlights the need to further assess the risk of abuse and addiction for obvious medical and legal reasons.

WITHDRAWAL (DROPOUTS) FROM OPIOID TREATMENT DUE TO ADVERSE EVENTS

Of the 23 RCTs reviewed, 17 trials provided information about the number of dropouts due to adverse events. The overall percentage of withdrawals related to adverse events ranges from 4%-40%. In total, 272 of the 1600 patients in whom opioid therapy was initiated (17%) withdrew due to adverse events. For purposes of comparison, placebos were used as a control in 11 of the 23 opioid-related RCTs, of which 8 provided information about dropouts. The results showed that only 20 of the 510 (<4%) placebo-treated patients discontinued treatment due to adverse events. Notably, in those 8 placebo-controlled trials, 112 of the 696 opioid-treated patients (16%) dropped out. Our more recent systematic review of the efficacy and safety of opioids for chronic neuropathic pain of non-malignant origin identified 30 of 206 opioid-treated patients (14.6%) who withdrew due to adverse events during opioid therapy. The NNH for discontinuation of opioid therapy due to adverse effects was calculated to be 11.1 (Eisenberg et al. 2005). This information may seem irrelevant because it refers to different opioids administered in a wide range of dosages for various durations. However, in clinical practice, with opioid rotation and individual titration guiding treatment of CNMP, one can never know which opioid a patient will end up receiving, at what dose, or for how long.

NUMBERS NEEDED TO HARM (NNH)

Even though the term NNH has been in use for a long time, it can barely be found in the opioid-related literature. The calculation of NNH is based on data from RCTs and is conducted in the same way as NNT (Cook and Sackett, 1995). NNH can be calculated for different drugs to allow the comparison of their relative safety or, alternatively, it can be calculated for each adverse event separately to indicate their relative prevalence. A review of the EBRs of opioids used in the treatment of CNMP does not yield helpful information related to either of these alternatives. Therefore, data on the prevalence of the common opioid-related adverse effects was extracted from 12 placebo-controlled trials (see Table 1) and, whenever possible, the NNH for each of the common adverse effects was calculated. The results show that the most common side effect is constipation (NNH = 3.8), followed by drowsiness and nausea with NNHs of 5.6 and 5.7, respectively. The NNHs for dizziness, vomiting, and discontinuation of opioid therapy due to adverse effects are 7.4, 9.2, and 8.2, respectively (see Table 2). Unfortunately, data on cognitive impairment as well as on other adverse effects were insufficient to calculate their NNHs.

MANAGEMENT OF OPIOID-RELATED ADVERSE EVENTS

Adverse effects of opioids often limit the ability to increase the dose as required and can therefore lead to suboptimal pain relief. Various techniques to manageme opioid-related adverse effects have been developed and are extensively utilized in patients with cancer pain. These techniques include reducing opioid dosages, co-administering non-opioid analgesics, rotating opioids, and prescribing drugs to counteract the adverse effects.

CO-ADMINISTERING OPIOIDS AND NON-OPIOID ANALGESICS

Many guidelines on opioids for CNMP emphasize the use of opioids along with other means of pain control to achieve better pain control at lower opioid dosages and to reduce the occurrence of adverse events. However, with the exception of a few studies in which a combination of opioids (usually of the 'weak' variety) and paracetamol were administered, the theory of combining opioids and non-opioids together in the treatment of CNMP has not been tested in clinical trials. Therefore, no safety information is available on the practice of co-administering opioids together with other analgesics, nor is there evidence of the efficacy of the various drugs aimed to counteract adverse effects associated with opioid usage.

OPIOID ROTATION

The technique of opioid rotation, which is frequently used in the treatment of cancer pain and possibly in CNMP as well, refers to the practice of switching from one opioid to another in an attempt to improve analgesia or reduce side effects (Maddocks et al. 1996; McNicol et al. 2003 for review). It is likely that incomplete cross-tolerance between different opioids, different receptor-binding affinities, and possibly a different side-effect profile of opioid metabolites may explain the beneficial effect.

What is the evidence that opioid rotation in CNMP reduces the occurrence of adverse events? This question can be subdivided into two questions: 1) Is there evidence that one long-acting opioid causes fewer adverse effects than another? 2) Do crossover trials in which patients are switched from one opioid to another reveal differences in their side-effect profiles? Unfortunately, only one RCT (Allan et al. 2001) directly compared one opioid (transdermal fentanyl) to another (controlled-release morphine) in a crossover design. This trial found a similar overall incidence of adverse events in both treatment groups. Although significantly fewer events of constipation were caused by fentanyl as compared with morphine (29% versus 48%; p<0.001), the withdrawal rate from the study due to adverse events was higher in the fentanyl-treated group (10% versus 5%). A careful review of this study reveals significant limitations in its design by virtue of recruiting only patients with inadequate responses to morphine, failure to blind patients to the medication they were taking (i.e., the study did not use a double dummy technique), and restricting the treatment course to a relatively short duration (four weeks). Thus, the results of this study indicate that transdermal fentanyl and sustained-release morphine seem to be equally safe in the treatment of CNMP. As this trial is the only attempt made so far to test the opioid rotation hypothesis by conducting a head-to-head comparison of two long-acting opioids, there is insufficient evidence to answer the key question posed above. When choosing to rotate from one opioid to another, clinicians should know that the current rationale for utilizing this strategy in CNMP is based upon extrapolation of data from cancer pain trials (McNicol et al. 2003) or from retrospective CNMP studies (Grilo et al. 2002; Thomsen et al. 1999).

SUMMARY AND CONCLUSIONS

Prescribing opioids for the treatment of CNMP has become a common practice, at least in developed countries. Patients with CNMP who receive opioids are expected to remain active or even to raise their level of activity. The safety of opioid usage is therefore a major concern. Many of the currently available RCTs, which are the cornerstone of evidence-based medicine, suffer from significant methodological weaknesses and were not designed to address safety issues. Evidence regarding the safety of opioid administration for CNMP is therefore far from compelling. At the same time, the available RCT-based data indicate that long-acting opioids are probably as safe as short-acting ones and that there is no clear advantage in using one opioid over another in terms of their side-effect profiles. Serious side effects, such as death, abuse or addiction, and respiratory depression, are rarely reported. Moreover, cognitive impairment is not a common side effect of opioids in CNMP patients. On the other hand, constipation, nausea, drowsiness, dizziness, vomiting, and discontinuation of opioid therapy can be expected to occur frequently, even if their severity and time course have not been thoroughly investigated. Thus, there is an urgent need for large-scale RCTs in which the magnitude and prevalence of side effects associated with opioid usage are the primary outcome measures.

REFERENCES

Allan L, Hays H, Jensen NH, et al. Randomized crossover trial of transdermal fentanyl and sustained-release oral morphine for treating chronic non-cancer pain. *Br Med J* 2001; 322:1154–1158.

American Academy of Pain Medicine and the American Pain Society. State Medical Society of Wisconsin statement on the use of opioids for the treatment of chronic pain. *WMJ* 2001; 100:22,5.

Chou R, Clark E, Helfand M. Comparative efficacy and safety of long-acting oral opioids for chronic non-cancer pain: a systematic review. *J Pain Symptom Manage* 2003; 26:1026–1048.

Chu LF, Clark DJ, Angst MS. Opioid tolerance and hyperalgesia in chronic pain patients after one month of oral morphine therapy: a preliminary prospective study. *J Pain* 2006; 7:43–48.

Collins SL, Moore RA, McQuay HJ, et al. Antidepressants and anticonvulsants for diabetic neuropathy and postherpetic neuralgia: a quantitative systematic review. *J Pain Symptom Manage* 2000; 20:449–458.

Compton P, Charuvastra VC, Ling W. Pain intolerance in opioid-maintained former opiate addicts: effect of long-acting maintenance agent. *Drug Alcohol Depend* 2001; 63:139–146.

Cook RJ, Sackett DL. The number needed to treat: a clinically useful measure of treatment effect. *Br Med J* 1995; 310:452–454.

Dunbar SA, Katz NP. Chronic opioid therapy for nonmalignant pain in patients with a history of substance abuse: report of 20 cases. *J Pain Symptom Manage* 1996; 11:163–171.

Eisenberg E, McNicol ED, Carr DB. Efficacy and safety of opioid agonists in the treatment of neuropathic pain of nonmalignant origin: systematic review and meta-analysis of randomized controlled trials. *JAMA* 2005; 293:3043–3052.

Eisenberg E, McNicol E, Carr DB. Opioids for neuropathic pain. Cochrane Database of Systematic Reviews. Issue 3. Art. No.: CD006146. DOI: 10.1002/14651858. CD006146.

Eriksen J, Jensen MK, Sjogren P, et al. Epidemiology of chronic non-malignant pain in Denmark. *Pain* 2003; 106:221–228.

Grilo RM, Bertin P, Scotto di Fazano C, et al. Opioid rotation in the treatment of joint pain. A review of 67 cases. *Joint Bone Spine* 2002; 69:491–494.

Guignard B, Bossard AE, Coste C, et al. Acute opioid tolerance: intraoperative remifentanil increases postoperative pain and morphine requirement. *Anesthesiology* 2000; 93:409–417.

Ho A, Dole VP. Pain perception in drug-free and in methadone-maintained human ex-addicts. *Proc Soc Exp Biol Med* 1979; 162:392–395.

Huse E, Larbig W, Flor H, et al. The effect of opioids on phantom limb pain and cortical reorganization. *Pain* 2001; 90:47–55.

Jamison RN, Raymond SA, Slawsby EA, et al. Opioid therapy for chronic noncancer back pain. A randomized prospective study. *Spine* 1998; 23:2591–2600.

Kalso E, Allan L, Dellemijn PL, et al. European Federation of Chapters of the International Association for the Study of Pain. Recommendations for using opioids in chronic non-cancer pain. *Eur J Pain* 2003; 7:381–386.

Katz NP, Adams EH, Benneyan JC, et al. Foundations of opioid risk management. *Clin J Pain* 2007; 23:103–118.

Kjaersgaard-Andersen P, Nafei A, Skov O, et al. Codeine plus paracetamol versus paracetamol in longer-term treatment of chronic pain due to osteoarthritis of the hip. A randomised, double-blind, multi-centre study. *Pain* 1990; 43:309–318.

Lloyd RS, Costello F, Eves MJ, et al. The efficacy and tolerability of controlled-release dihydrocodeine tablets and combination dextropropoxyphene/paracetamol tablets in patients with severe osteoarthritis of the hips. *Curr Med Res Opin* 1992; 13:37–48.

Loeser JD. Opiophobia and opiophilia. In: Medrum ML (ed). Opioids and pain relief. A historical perspective, vol. 25. IASP Press, Seattle, WA, 2003: 1–4.

Maddocks I, Somogyi A, Abbott F, et al. Attenuation of morphine-induced delirium in palliative care by substitution with infusion of oxycodone. *J Pain Symptom Manage.* 1996 ;12(3):182–189.

Manchikanti L, Manchukonda R, Pampati V, et al. Evaluation of abuse of prescription and illicit drugs in chronic pain patients receiving short-acting (hydrocodone) or long-acting (methadone) opioids. *Pain Physician* 2005; 8:257–261.

Mao J. Opioid-induced abnormal pain sensitivity: Is it clinically relevant? *Curr Pain Headche Rep* 2006; 10:67–70.

Martin JE, Inglis J. Pain tolerance and narcotic addiction. *Br J Soc Clin Psychol* 1965; 4:224–229.

McNicol E, Horowicz-Mehler N, Fisk RA, et al. Management of opioid side effects in cancer-related and chronic noncancer pain: a systematic review. *J Pain* 2003; 4:231–256.

McQuay H, Moore A. An Evidence-Based Resource for Pain Relief. Oxford University Press, Oxford, 1998: 39–49.

Model guidelines for the use of controlled substances for the treatment of pain: a policy document. Federation of State Medical Boards of the United States, Dallas, TX, 1998.

Moulin DE, Iezzi A, Amireh R, et al. Randomized trial of oral morphine for chronic noncancer pain. *Lancet* 1996; 347:143–147.

Pud D, Cohen D, Lawental E, et al. Opioids and abnormal pain perception: new evidence from a study of chronic opioid addicts and healthy subjects. *Drug & Alcohol Dependence* 2006; 82:218–223.

Raja SN, Haythornthwaite JA, Pappagallo M, et al. Opioids versus antidepressants in postherpetic neuralgia: a randomized, placebo-controlled trial. *Neurology* 2002; 59:1015–1021.

Rajagopal A, Vassilopoulou-Sellin R, Palmer JL, et al. Hypogonadism and sexual dysfunction in male cancer survivors receiving chronic opioid therapy. *J Pain Symptom Manage* 2003; 26:1055–1061.

Reznikov I, Pud D, Reitman L, et al. Oral opioid administration does not produce hyperalgesia in patients with cancer or chronic non-malignant pain. *Br. J Clin Pharmacol* 2005; 60:311–318.

Roth SH, Fleischmann RM, Burch FX, et al. Around-the-clock, controlled-release oxycodone therapy for osteoarthritis-related pain: placebo controlled trial and long-term evaluation. *Arch Intern Med* 2000; 160:853–860.

Rowbotham MC, Twilling L, Davies PS, et al. Oral opioid therapy for chronic peripheral and central neuropathic pain. *N Engl J Med* 2003; 348:1223–1232.

Sabatowski R, Schwalen S, Rettig K, et al. Driving ability under long-term treatment with transdermal fentanyl. *Pain Symptom Manage* 2003; 25:38–47.

Tassain V, Attal N, Fletcher D, et al. Long term effects of oral sustained release morphine on neuropsychological performance in patients with chronic non-cancer pain. *Pain* 2003; 104:389–400.

Thomsen AB, Becker N, Eriksen J. Opioid rotation in chronic non-malignant pain patients. A retrospective study. *Acta Anaesthesiol Scand* 1999; 43:918–923.

Pharmacoeconomics in pain research

Christopher J. Evans • Nathalie Horowicz-Mehler

INTRODUCTION

The general sentiment in North America and Europe is that private and public spending on healthcare is approaching an unsustainable level, and financing and delivery of healthcare is due for substantial changes. The motivation for changing healthcare systems is grounded in improving access to healthcare (e.g., by reducing prescription drug costs for the elderly in the USA or decreasing waiting list times in the UK), which will improve health outcomes. Behind this desire is a network of competing interests that attempts to influence the healthcare system in various ways. Physicians attempt to maximize the health of their patients, often without regard to the cost of care; patients attempt to obtain the care they perceive as best even if there is a lack of empirical evidence to support the use of that care; special interest groups seek to maximize care for their members; and politicians seek to mollify media-inspired campaigns for greater access to medical interventions even when these interventions have no proven value. Decision-makers whether they are patients, healthcare professionals, payers or society in general are becoming increasingly aware of the need to make educated decisions about healthcare spending and how to obtain the best value for the money spent. Pharmacoeconomics is concerned with establishing the relative value of healthcare interventions to healthcare systems and society (Townsend 1987) and provides evidence of the relative risks, benefits and costs of healthcare interventions.

By taking into account various perspectives, pharmacoeconomic research can provide answers for the various decision-makers. From a societal perspective, pharmacoeconomic studies help guide decision-makers away from interventions that show no or poor evidence for a clinical benefit compared to other interventions. Pharmacoeconomic studies can also help allocate resources appropriately within healthcare organizations to allow healthcare to be delivered to subsamples of patients to achieve maximum benefit. From a different perspective, pharmacoeconomic studies, by presenting health outcomes in "understandable" terms, can help health professionals set patient expectations in terms of decreased mortality or morbidity. These studies can also help patients anticipate any indirect cost of treatment that may be accrued in the long term.

Hospital pharmacists or formularies increasingly apply pharmacoeconomic criteria as they deliberate whether to offer new, usually more costly analgesic drugs and devices that achieve results only incrementally superior to existing, less expensive methods. The pharmaceutical industry uses pharmacoeconomic studies to guide decision as to whether the development process for a drug is worth pursuing (Detsky 1993) and make a case for novel agents in front of reimbursement bodies such as the National Institute for Clinical Excellence in the UK. In fact, Australia, New Zealand, the province of Ontario and several other national jurisdictions have mandated pharmacoeconomics assessments as part of the approval or reimbursement process for new drugs. These studies can also help set the price of a new compound as well as guide strategy to launch the drug on the market. Finally from an academic perspective, pharmacoeconomic studies can help model the impact of a disease and identify parameters most influential to the cost or burden of a disease in order to better direct research efforts.

Because acute and chronic pain affects so many people and is costly to treat, various treatment modalities have been subject to pharmacoeconomic evaluations. Overall there has been a trend towards increasing pharmacoeconomic research in pain. From 1996 to 2003 pharmacoeconomic research in this area has increased by two-thirds (Figure 8.1), with most evaluations

conducted in chronic pain. In his review of chronic pain Turk (2002) reports that annual healthcare costs, excluding surgical costs, for chronic pain patients may range from $500 to $35,400, with averages ranging from $12,900 to $18,833 annually.

Pain syndromes affect cost at multiple levels: (1) direct costs managing pain, (2) indirect costs or cost of morbidity such as lost productivity due to disability, and (3) intangible costs such as suffering and grief. In the case of acute pain, postsurgical management drives direct cost while drug use, especially nonsteroidal anti-inflammatory drugs (NSAIDs), drives direct medical costs in chronic pain syndromes. In 2001, there were 40 million surgeries annually in the USA alone (National Center for Health Statistics website). After surgery, 50 to 70% of patients report severe pain and 20 to 40% report experiencing moderate pain. In the USA, 17% of patients seen in primary care report persistent pain, and 2.9 million Americans are treated annually by healthcare professionals specializing in chronic pain (Marketdata Enterprises 1995; Gureje 1998). For these patients, pain is an important motivation for seeking treatment. As a consequence, pain medications are the second most prescribed drugs in both physician offices and emergency rooms. In fact, 30 million patients a day use NSAIDs, making them the most commonly prescribed type of medication in the world. Perhaps as a result, NSAIDs cause the highest

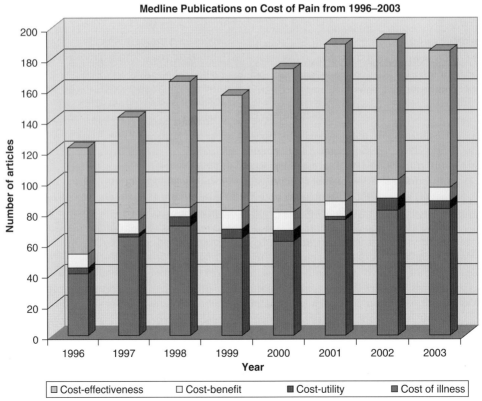

Figure 8.1 Trend in pharmacoeconomic studies in pain.

number of reported serious complications of all medications. Every year, nearly four billion dollars a year are spent treating these complications and about 7600 people actually die from them (Rx magazine).

Often the cost of treating the symptoms of pain is not the largest component of overall costs. The indirect costs, or cost associated with work absences and declines in productivity, also have to be considered. Low back pain and migraine are two areas where the indirect costs are likely to exceed direct medical costs. Frymoyer and Durrett (1997) estimate annual costs of back pain at $33.6 billion for medical care, $11 billion–$43 billion for disability compensation and $4.6 billion for lost productivity. In the UK, Maniadakis and Gray (2000) estimated annual direct medical costs for the treatment of back pain at £1.6 billion with informal care and indirect costs estimated at £10.7 billion annually. A similar relationship is seen in migraine where the indirect costs of treatment are substantial and often overshadow the direct medical costs. Hu (1999) has estimated migraine costs US employers approximately $13 billion a year because of missed work and impaired function. To and Wu (1995) have estimated that in Ontario, Canada, severe migraine headaches may result in $31 million loss in productivity and $2 million in hospitalization costs. In a study looking at the burden of migraine on diagnosed and undiagnosed people with migraine, over 92% of people reported at least some headache-related disability. At the same time, many do not consult physicians for their headaches, and less than half have received a medical diagnosis. However, over 95% of people with migraine reported taking medication for their headaches, mostly over-the-counter medication rather than prescription drugs (Lipton 2001).

Practitioners, the public and politicians are often wary of economics, believing it implies an application of an axe to medical care that seeks to cut costs without regard to the impact on health outcomes. This chapter aims to make pharmacoeconomics techniques more transparent to demonstrate that economic evaluations are concerned with deploying resources to areas where the maximum gain may be obtained. With the premise that evaluations of pain interventions should emphasize "value for money" rather than minimizing the costs of treating pain it is necessary to examine simultaneously safety, efficacy and total treatment costs of any intervention. In this chapter, we outline the most important techniques for evaluating the value of pain interventions. We also consider the main elements of pharmacoeconomic studies and the characteristics of good studies. We conclude by discussing methods for analyzing the results of a pharmacoeconomic study in an appropriate context.

PHARMACOECONOMIC TECHNIQUES

Pharmacoeconomics is a subdiscipline of health economics that concentrates on identifying, measuring and comparing the costs (i.e., resources consumed) and consequences of various interventions. The aim of pharmacoeconomic research is to provide decision-makers, whether they are insurers or clinicians, with information that will enable scarce resources to be distributed efficiently so as to maximize health outcomes. Most pharmacoeconomic studies compare two or more drug interventions in terms of costs and effects. However, their use is not limited to pharmaceuticals, and the techniques of economic evaluations have been employed to examine different strategies, timings, settings and personnel (Drummond et al. 1997). For instance, the use of pain rehabilitation programs can be compared to treatment by general practitioners to determine which is the most "cost-effective." The term "pharmacoeconomics" is slightly misleading as it implies that the discipline is solidly oriented towards economics. In fact, pharmacoeconomics actually pulls from several different areas: epidemiology, clinical

Table 8.1 Types of economic evaluations

Type of study	Identification of consequences	Measurement of consequences	Reporting of cost and effectiveness
Cost-consequence	Single effect	Natural units	No aggregation
Cost-effectiveness	Single effect	Natural units	Incremental cost-effectiveness ratio
Cost-minimization	Assumed equivalent (in practice, for primary outcome)	Natural units (theoretically, none)	Just an examination of cost differences
Cost-utility	Composite effect	QALYs	Incremental cost utility ratio
Cost-benefit	Single effect	Monetary	Benefit to cost ratio

research, medicine, pharmacy and biostatistics. To answer the question of whether a new medication provides good value five types of studies are employed: cost-consequence, cost-minimization, cost-effectiveness, cost-utility and cost-benefit analyses (Eisenberg 1989) (Table 8.1).

COST-CONSEQUENCE ANALYSIS

Cost-consequence analysis (CCA) is the simplest type of pharmacoeconomic study. In a CCA, the impact of the treatment of interest on resource use, costs and health outcomes for an individual or group of pain patients are estimated and reported separately. For example, Pettitt et al. (2000) developed the Arthritis Cost Consequence Evaluation System (ACCES), a pharmacoeconomic model to predict and evaluate the costs and consequences associated with the use of celecoxib in patients with arthritis, compared with other NSAIDs and NSAIDs with gastroprotective agents. The costs included in the model were direct medical costs. Clinical outcomes were the five most common gastrointestinal (GI) consequences of NSAID use: (1) serious GI complications, (2) symptomatic ulcers, (3) anemia with occult bleeding, (4) intolerable diarrhea and (5) GI discomfort a combined endpoint or dyspepsia, abdominal pain and nausea. The sixth clinical outcome considered was loss of efficacy, which often leads to switching of drugs. Since the perspective taken in this model was that of a payer, the model only allowed for direct medical costs to be considered. These costs include the cost of the NSAID itself and any resource utilization that may be associated with side effects or the prevention of side effects resulting from the NSAID (gastroprotective agents, additional physician visits and diagnostic tests resulting from GI discomfort, hospitalizations resulting from serious GI events, etc.).

COST-EFFECTIVENESS AND MINIMIZATION ANALYSIS

The most popular pharmacoeconomic technique in pain research is cost-effectiveness analysis (CEA). There were over 650 cost-effectiveness publications published from 1996 to 2003, nearly ten times greater than that for cost-utility analysis, the second most popular

technique (see Figure 8.1). Cost-effectiveness analysis examines the cost and effectiveness of two or more treatment interventions. The effectiveness of the interventions is measured in natural units (e.g., life years gained or pain free days). In contrast to the CCA, the cost and effect are not only enumerated they are aggregated into a summary measure. The analysis focuses on the incremental cost effectiveness ratio ($C_A - C_B/E_A - E_B$), which will yield a cost per unit of effect gained (e.g., cost per life year gained or cost per pain free day).

For example, Gabriel et al. (1993) conducted a CEA comparing the cost and effect of misoprostol prophylaxis in patients who took NSAIDs to relieve pain from osteoarthritis. The three strategies compared were no prophylaxis, prophylaxis for all who take NSAIDs, and prophylaxis for only the elderly. The results of their study are reported in Table 8.2 and are graphed in Figure 8.2.

The incremental cost-effectiveness ratio for elderly versus no prophylaxis is given as:

$$\frac{\$28,971 - \$25,622}{91.2 - 86} = \frac{\$3349}{5.2} = \$644$$

The incremental cost-effectiveness ratio for all users versus no prophylaxis is given as:

$$\frac{\$32,396 - \$25,622}{95.9 - 86} = \frac{\$6774}{9.9} = \$684$$

The appropriate interpretation of the results of the study is based on the incremental cost-effectiveness ratio. The slopes of the line from the origin to each strategy give the average cost-effectiveness ratio (Figure 8.2). The incremental cost-effectiveness ratio is given by the slope of the line from no prophylaxis to elderly and from no prophylaxis to all users. The interpretation is that it would cost society an additional $644 to prevent one additional GI event if only the elderly were treated. The cost of preventing one GI event by giving misoprostol to all users, compared to no prophylaxis, is $684.

In another example, Frei (2003) developed a Markov model to simulate the resource use and health outcomes of one year of treatment comparing the fentanyl transdermal therapeutic system (fentanyl-TSS) with oral

Table 8.2 Cost-effectiveness of misoprostol for OA patients in NSAIDs

Prophylaxis strategy	Cost*	GI events	GI events averted	Average cost-effectiveness ratio
None	$25,622	14	86	297.9
Elderly	$28,971	8.8	91.2	317.7
All users	$32,396	4.1	95.9	338

*In Canadian dollars.

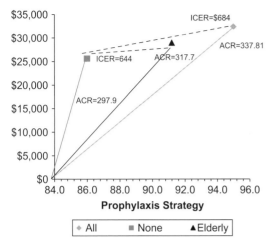

Figure 8.2 Cost-effectiveness of misoprostol for OA patients in NSAIDs.

sustained-release (SR) morphine in outpatients with noncancer pain in Denmark. Effectiveness was assessed in terms of cost per days of good pain control and days on initial treatment. Costs included those of baseline pain management (including breakthrough pain), co-medication costs and control of adverse events. Fentanyl-TSS was more effective than SR-morphine in achieving good pain control (99 versus 64 days, respectively). The incremental cost-effectiveness of fentanyl-TSS versus SR morphine was $10.26 per extra day of good pain control.

Cost-minimization analysis (CMA) is employed when the effectiveness of two or more interventions is assumed to be equivalent. Therefore, in a CMA, the only relevant aspect for decision-makers is the total treatment cost of an intervention. It is relatively rare that two interventions will be completely equivalent (especially if the intervention is a drug), and this type of analysis is used more often with different formulations of the same drug or comparisons to generic versions of the drug.

COST-UTILITY ANALYSIS

Cost-utility analysis (CUA) is a special case of CEA. In a CUA, the effect is measured as a quality adjusted life year (QALY). A QALY is a composite endpoint that incorporates both quality and quantity improvements in life. The "quality" portion of the QALY represents society's or patients' preference for health states. These preferences are represented as utilities. For example, a patient with mild rheumatoid arthritis who exhibits some minor disability, pain and mobility problems may be determined to be at 0.75 of that of perfect health. A patient with chronic low back pain who suffers from an inability to walk more than a block, difficulty driving long distances (which impacts his/her social relationships) and persistent pain may be

determined to have a health state (utility) of 0.50 of perfect health. Assuming these individuals have a life expectancy of 10 years, the QALY derived is 7.5 years (0.75 utilities × 10 years) for the first case and 5 QALYs (0.50 utilities × 10 years) for the second case.

The direct measurement of health state utilities can be relatively easy, as is the case with a simple rating scale, or more cognitively challenging, as with standard gamble or time tradeoff techniques (Torrance 1986). Because direct measurement is fraught with theoretical hurdles and methodologic problems, and is cognitively challenging for survey respondents/patients (Bennett 1996), indirect measurement techniques based on simple surveys have been developed. Three of the most common indirect measures are the EuroQol-5 Dimensions (EQ-5D) (Rabin and de Charro 2001), the Health Utilities Index (HUI) (Furlong 2001) and the Quality of Well-Being Scale (QWB) (Kaplan et al. 1984). In addition, it is possible to derive utilities from quality of life questionnaires as has been demonstrated with utility cross walking from the SF-36 (Brazier et al. 1998). Utility elicitation can be quite involved and readers should refer to other sources for a more in depth discussion (Smith 1993; Bennett and Torrance 1996).

Results from CUAs can be ordered from best to worst on a league table. The league table gives researchers the opportunity to place their findings in a broader context. Examples of general league tables have been reported in the literature in pounds sterling (Williams 1985; Smith 1990) and US dollars (Torrance and Zipursky 1984; Schulman et al. 1991).

One example of a cost-utility study (Evans et al. 1997) compared oral sumatriptan with oral caffeine/ergotamine in the treatment of patients with migraine using a decision tree model. Utilities were assigned to health states using the QWB. From a societal perspective, using sumatriptan resulted in an incremental cost-utility ratio of C$7507 per QALY. From the perspective of the health department, using sumatriptan resulted in an incremental cost-utility ratio of C$29,366 per QALY. Sensitivity analysis showed that the results were robust to relatively large changes in the input variable. The incremental health benefits obtained from using oral sumatriptan rather than oral caffeine/ergotamine were achieved at moderately acceptable incremental costs, if past decisions on the adoption of other health technologies are used as a guide.

COST-BENEFIT ANALYSIS

Cost-benefit analysis (CBA) is unique in that it measures the benefit of a treatment in monetary terms. Benefits are translated into monetary values utilizing one of several possible strategies: human capital approach, revealed preferences, stated preferences or contingent valuation (Drummond et al. 1997). The results are presented as a benefit to cost ratio: as long as the cost of the treatment is lower than the benefit of the treatment, the intervention is deemed worthwhile and should be adopted in medical practice. The advantage of this approach is that it enables a wide range of comparisons to be made. Thus, studies that measure the benefit of the intervention in monetary terms can be compared and ranked in much the same way as in cost-utility studies. For instance, a migraine treatment study that measures the benefit in monetary terms (i.e., by stating the benefit as wages because the migraine patient could work more frequently and more productively) could be compared to a study that examines the effect of seatbelt restraints in automobiles (where the monetary benefit is the dollar value of the additional life years that occur because a certain number of fatalities are avoided).

As a matter of practice it is relatively rare to find true cost-benefit studies. Instead, researchers often conduct "quasi" cost-benefit studies. In a quasi cost-benefit study, the benefit is not measured by the human capital approach, revealed preferences, stated preferences or contingent valuation, but the benefit is determined to be the costs that are avoided by not getting the disorder or disease. There are several variations on this and it is possible to find many examples in the literature where researchers label a cost-benefit study as such when in reality it is a variant on the technique. For example, Loisel and others (2002) conducted a quasi CBA in low back pain that compared an experimental intervention to standard care. The benefit of the treatment was measured as the income replacement cost savings that occurred on the experimental treatment less the additional costs associated with the experimental treatment. Under this situation a positive number (indicating the replacement cost savings associated with the experimental intervention were lower than the cost of the experimental intervention) would suggest that the experimental intervention should be adopted. Over the long-run this proved to be true and the experimental treatment was demonstrated to have monetary benefits that outweighed the monetary cost of the treatment.

PERSPECTIVE AND COSTS

As a matter of pure economic theory it is preferable to utilize opportunity costs (i.e., the value of a resource in its next best alternative use) in economic evaluations. For practical purposes, however, it is difficult to derive this information and proxies for opportunity costs (e.g., charges or average costs) are employed instead.

Direct medical costs include fixed and variable costs associated with the illness and the treatment. Direct medical costs are not limited to only the cost of the intervention, but all costs associated with treatment.

Depending on the type of pain evaluated, these may include: general practitioner (GP) and specialist visits, pharmacologic agents (e.g., NSAIDs, opioids, anticonvulsants, tricyclic antidepressants, NMDA antagonists), anesthesia, physical modalities (e.g., ultrasound, transcutaneous electrical nerve stimulators, diathermy), neuroaugmentation modalities (e.g., spinal column stimulators (SCSs), implantable drug delivery systems (IDDSs)), pain rehabilitation programs (PRPs) (e.g., interdisciplinary pain centers) and alternative medicine (e.g., acupuncture).

Direct nonmedical costs include those costs related to the treatment of the illness or intervention that are nonmedical. Examples in this category include transportation to and from a pain clinic, meals-on-wheels provided to a chronic pain patient with no mobility or babysitting expenses for a pain sufferer so he/she can attend a doctor's appointment. Indirect costs are those costs related to changes in work hours and productivity due to an illness or its treatment. Examples include lost wages because a worker has to quit his or her job due to low back pain or a reduction in productivity while at work due to stomach pain.

The costs used in pharmacoeconomic studies are directly related to the perspective of the study (Figure 8.3). There are several possible perspectives that a pharmacoeconomic study may utilize. The societal perspective is the most comprehensive and is recommended by most researchers as the default perspective (Gold et al. 1996). This perspective includes all relevant viewpoints and costs: direct medical, direct nonmedical and indirect. For example, the economic evaluation reported under the CUA section took the societal perspective.

If the perspective used in a study is that of the insurer only those costs relevant to the insurer are included in the study: direct medical costs. Because insurers do not pay their insured populations for lost wages or babysitting expenses, these costs are excluded when this perspective is employed. In the previous section on cost-consequence analysis the ACCES model developed by Pettitt et al. (2000) included only direct medical costs as the model was developed as a communication tool for formulary committees. If the patient perspective is used, and on the assumption he/she has insurance, the relevant costs include direct nonmedical costs and possibly indirect costs if he/she has no sick leave benefit. A list of possible health outcomes and costs by perspective and type of pain are reported in Table 8.3.

INDIRECT COSTS

As seen in the introduction, indirect costs may account for the majority of overall costs in pain studies, particularly in chronic pain. As such it is worth considering how this data is collected and translated into a

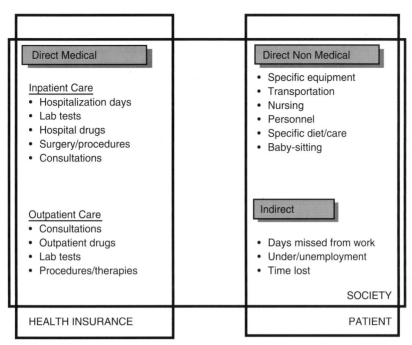

Figure 8.3 Cost and perspective.

Table 8.3 Costs and outcomes by pain type and perspective

	Chronic noncancer pain (e.g., low back pain)	*Acute-recurrent pain (e.g., migraine)*	*Acute pain (e.g., postoperative analgesia) (Goudas and Carr 1996)*
Outcomes	Patient perspective: pain-free days, pain relief as measured by a VAS or VRS, improved physical functioning, improved QoL, QALY Patient and insurer perspective: decreased opioid or NSAID requirement for pain management, treatment satisfaction, treatment compliance	Patient perspective: time to pain relief, duration of pain relief, side effects of analgesia avoided, QALY Patient and insurer perspective: treatment satisfaction, treatment compliance	Patient perspective: pain relief at rest or with activity Payer and employer perspective: hospital length of stay, return to work Patient and insurer perspective: acceptance of and satisfaction with care
Costs	Direct medical: drugs, treatment of side effects (if opioid or NSAID medication), visits to GP, physical therapist, psychotherapist, hospitalization length of stay Indirect: work absences, work productivity, worker's compensation, caregiver time Direct nonmedical: modifications to the house	Direct medical: drugs, visits to general practitioner or specialist Indirect: work absences, work productivity, worker's compensation	Direct medical: drugs (base dose and rescue dose), staff time (physician, ward or home care nurse, pharmacist), patient-controlled analgesia pump and maintenance, disposable supplies. Also cost of potential side effects (nausea, sedation, etc.) and complications (respiratory depression, ileus, etc.). After hospitalization: visits to GP or specialist Indirect: work absences

monetary value (for a fuller discussion on this topic see Evans et al. 2004a). Early cost of illness studies and other economic evaluations dealt only with work absences – an area that is relatively easy to measure. However, researchers have realized that most of the economic loss in chronic pain will come from productivity declines while at work, a concept known as presenteeism, rather than just short absences.

Although archival data on productivity declines is potentially the best source of data for indirect cost estimates it is essentially nonexistent in many occupations (e.g., the productivity of individual office workers does not exist in any accessible database). Given that archival data is difficult to obtain several researchers have developed questionnaires to collect this information directly from patients. None of the questionnaires have been developed specifically for use in a chronic pain population; however, the possibility for adapting the questionnaires to areas of chronic pain is possible. Current productivity questionnaires include the Endicott Work Productivity Scale (EWPS) (Endicott 1997), the Work Productivity and Activity Impairment Questionnaire (Reilly et al. 1993), the Health and Labor Questionnaire (HLQ) (Van Roijen et al. 1996; Hakkaart-van Roijen and Essink-Bot 2000), the Stanford Presenteeism Scale (SPS) (Koopman et al. 2002), the Work Limitations Questionnaire (WLQ) (Lerner et al. 2001), and the Health and Performance Questionnaire (HPQ) (Kessler et al. 2003; see also Chapter 20). One questionnaire has been developed specifically for use in acute recurrent pain (i.e., migraine pain): the Migraine Work and Productivity Loss Questionnaire (MWPLQ) (Lerner et al. 1999; see Chapter 20).

Once information on productivity changes have been measured it is often desirable to translate these estimates into a monetary value. Two approaches are used to attach monetary values to productivity changes: the human capital approach and friction costing. The most frequent method employed is the human capital approach (Berger et al. 2001), which applies an estimate (usually age and sex adjusted) of daily earnings to the time period in which there is a reduction in productivity. In such cases, all changes in employee productivity are monetized. However, this approach has been criticized for providing unreliable estimates of the actual consequences of productivity changes. For instance, an employee who suffers a reduction in productivity at work due to a migraine headache may have his/her work completed by a team member or may make up the work missed on a Saturday. If this is the case, no real economic loss has occurred.

Some authors perceive the friction cost method proposed by Koopmanschap and Rutten (1993, 1996) as a more realistic attempt to derive estimates of productivity changes and work absences. Among other things, this method takes real changes in production into account by incorporating information on the costs of short-term work absences and reduced productivity while at work. Under the friction cost method, there is no monetary value ascribed to an employee who has a temporary illness while at work or a short-term absence. For example, a treatment that increases productivity by reducing migraine symptoms by one day would be given a monetary value under the human capital approach, but would not receive one under the friction costing method.

Gerth et al. (2004) conducted a study to compare rizatriptan to usual care in reducing productivity losses and work absences in migraine sufferers. This study used the MWPLQ to estimate the total work loss resulting from absenteeism and reduced productivity while working with migraine symptoms. The use of rizatriptan was found to lead to a 44% reduction in migraine related work loss compared to usual therapies. The cost of this work loss was estimated by using labor compensation costs held by the US Department of Labor. The study found that if migraine is treated with rizatriptan a representative US company would avoid work loss costs in the region of $800,000 annually.

TIME

In pharmacoeconomic studies, future values must be discounted to their present value to account for the effect of time. This process is used because individuals have a positive time preference for money. For chronic pain studies with durations greater than one year, discounting of both the costs and the effects (if possible) should be conducted according to the following formula:

$$C_{present} = c_0 + \frac{c_1}{(1+r)^1} + \frac{c_2}{(1+r)^2} + \cdots + \frac{c_n}{(1+r)^n}$$

where $C_{present}$ = cost in current dollars, r = discount rate, $c_1 \ldots c_n$ = costs in future years. All costs accrue at the beginning of the year.

Because discounting of health effects is somewhat controversial, and the choice of the discount rate is not always clear (although most analysts in the USA use 5%), researchers usually present results of long-term studies with results undiscounted, both costs and effects discounted and just costs discounted.

Generally, the use of the discount rate is uncomplicated; however, unusual situations arise when the timings of the interventions compared are different. This occurs because alternatives that occur later in time will be favored due to the discount rate alone. Take for example two hypothetical interventions to treat chronic low back pain. Intervention A is a surgical procedure that costs $10,000 and is performed in the first year. Intervention B is a medical treatment that works as well as intervention A, but is given over 5 years at $2,000 per year (for a total of $10,000 – the same as intervention A). However, when the results are discounted, they are:

Intervention A $C_{present} = c_0$
$$C_{present} = \$10,000$$

Intervention B $C_{present} = \$2000 + \dfrac{\$2000}{(1 + 0.05)^1}$

$$+ \frac{\$2000}{(1 + 0.05)^2} + \frac{\$2000}{(1 + 0.05)^3}$$

$$+ \frac{\$2000}{(1 + 0.05)^4}$$

$$C_{present} = \$2000 + \$1905 + \$1814$$
$$+ \$1728 + \$1645 = \$9092$$
$$C_{present} = \$9092$$

In this case, intervention B costs less than A solely due to the discounting. On the assumption that both work equally well and there are no side effects with either treatment, the best financial choice would be to recommend B. However, most physicians and patients would choose A, as the treatment benefit occurs following surgery in the first year, while with treatment B the patient would have to wait for a cure to occur over five years.

VALIDITY OF PHARMACOECONOMIC STUDIES

When assessing the validity of pharmacoeconomic studies two areas are of concern: internal and external validity. Internal validity refers to the accuracy of the results – that is, is the study free of biases? External validity refers to the generalizability of the results. That is, do the results of the study apply to other settings other than where it was conducted? External and internal validity should be thought of as existing on two separate and sometimes competing spectrums. It is possible to have a range of validity, so that you can have a high level of internal validity but a low level of external validity, or even moderate levels of both internal and external validity. However, one situation is never possible: a high level of external validity and a low level of internal validity. It is a necessary precursor to making statements about the generalizability of study results that the results are accurate in the first instance.

The internal validity of a study is influenced by a number of areas. First and foremost is the accuracy of the data which is driven by the study design chosen. It is beyond the scope of this chapter to discuss all possible study designs and their implications for validity; interested readers can refer to Cook and Campbell (1979) and Rothman (1986). In the following paragraphs we cover the main types.

Randomized controlled trials (RCTs) have a high level of internal validity due to the fact that bias is removed from allocation to treatment groups and on

average the study groups will be comparable in all relevant characteristics (assuming formal sample size calculations were performed). The presence of a protocol and strict inclusion and exclusion criteria further improve internal validity so the outcomes of interest can be attributed to the interventions under examination. However, this high level of internal validity often comes at the expense of external validity.

It is common to collect economic information as part of a phase III clinical trial (known as a piggyback study). O'Brien (1996) has identified seven areas where the external validity of a pharmacoeconomic study can be compromised by using data from these trials. First, there is the potential to choose an inappropriate comparison therapy. For a trial to be generalizable it must reflect current medical practice. Placebo controlled trials will not do this under a situation where there is an effective treatment on the market. Second, clinical trials often have gold standard measurement and diagnosis. If this is more invasive, more frequent or utilizes techniques not found in routine practice the trial will not adequately reflect reality. Third, trials may use intermediate rather than final outcomes. For instance, it could be argued that assessment of pain severity is an intermediate outcome and the effect of an intervention on patients' quality of life (pain and physical functioning, emotional well-being, etc.) is a final outcome. Trials that only examine severity on a visual analogue scale fail to capture the many effects pain has on sufferers. Fourth, clinical trials often have inadequate patient follow-up or sample size. It may be necessary to follow chronic pain patients for several years when clinical trials are limited to several months. Fifth, clinical trials often contain protocol driven costs and outcomes. Clinical trials will frequently have more assessments and testing than is done in routine practice and when this information is used in economic evaluations as part of the cost calculations an overestimate of costs will occur (Evans et al. 2003). Sixth, reimbursement of procedures within institutions, specific treatment rules and healthcare system specific delivery mechanisms hamper the generalizability of results within a country, and, more importantly, between countries. Finally, clinical trials have select patient and provider populations. An acute pain trial done in adults may not be generalizable to children and trials conducted in academic centers will not reflect the practice of community hospitals.

Not only are there problems with external validity using data from RCTs in pharmacoeconomic studies, there may also be problems with internal validity. When resource use is collected as part of clinical trials an element of retrospective data collection is introduced through the use of patient self-reports of medical encounters and drug use. Evans and Crawford (1999) reviewed the impact that the use of patient self-reported data has on the validity of estimates in pharmacoeconomic studies and found that the accuracy of recall was affected by the salience of the event, the time elapsed between the episode and the recall of the estimate, the presence of generic recall for healthcare encounters for chronic conditions, the social desirability of the event and several demographic characteristics.

Retrospective study designs, such as administrative claims database studies and decision analytic models, also will have problems with internal validity. The chief limitation of claims databases is that they include only the information that is entered on the claim form. This data may inaccurately reflect the service performed due to up-coding or gaming. Decision analytic models often contain data from a variety of sources and each source must be scrutinized to determine its effect on the level of validity. The presence of data based on expert opinion may lead one to question the accuracy of the results of a decision analytic model; however, the judicious use of experts in pharmacoeconomic studies is generally accepted, even though the validity of this type of data has never been evaluated. When the data used in a pharmacoeconomic study is of questionable internal validity, the robustness of the study findings should be checked with a sensitivity analysis. A sensitivity analysis is a standard method for managing uncertainty. In pharmacoeconomic models the value of one variable (univariate) or several variables (multivariate) is changed over a plausible range and the effect on the results of the model is considered.

The best pharmacoeconomic study design, and most expensive, is a naturalistic or pragmatic trial. A naturalistic study reflects real world treatments by loosening the restriction on patient inclusion and exclusion criteria and by permitting routine medical practice (for instance, by permitting the titration or augmentation of pain medications) not found in clinical trials. The goal of a naturalistic trial is to ensure a high level of both internal and external validity, and if designed correctly these studies provide compelling evidence of cost and effect.

INTERPRETATION

The interpretation of pharmacoeconomic studies can be challenging. Only in the case of cost-benefit and cost-minimization studies is interpretation truly unambiguous. In a CMA the lowest cost choice is chosen as the efficacy of the alternate interventions has been demonstrated to be equivalent. In a CBA as long as the benefit in monetary terms exceeds its costs the intervention is determined to be worthwhile.

In the case of cost-consequence analyses, where the findings are disaggregated the decision-maker must interpret the findings using his own set of values. For instance, in migraine pain, is the additional cost of a new treatment, over a cheaper alternative, "worth it" if the new treatment leads to three fewer missed days at work?

Interpretation of the bulk of pharmacoeconomic studies, cost-effectiveness and cost-utility, are more problematic. When a new intervention costs less than existing treatments and works better it will always be adopted in practice. However, the most common situation in pharmacoeconomic studies is the intervention works better than other interventions, but costs more. Therefore, the question arises: is the additional benefit over the existing therapy worth it given the additional cost? For decades, researchers have grappled with providing adequate decision rules for interpreting results like this.

There are rules of thumbs researchers use for determining whether or not a particular intervention is "cost-effective." The two most frequently referenced are Kaplan and Bush (1982) and Laupacis et al. (1992). The Laupacis estimates (Table 8.4) suggest that interventions that are below a threshold of $20,000 are definitely cost-effective and intervention over $100,000 are likely *not* "cost-effective." Allowing for inflation and differences in exchange rates, most researchers use $50,000 per LYG or QALY gained as the threshold level for cost-effectiveness. Studies with values below this level are definitely considered "cost-effective"; studies between $50,000 and $100,000 are considered good value for money; and studies exceeding $100,000 are believed to be poor value for money. For the most part the use of benchmarks would only apply to chronic pain and migraine studies that used a QALY as an endpoint. Acute pain studies would, by definition, use an endpoint other than life year gained or QALY gained. Endpoints common in acute pain studies, such as time to pain relief, level of pain relief or pain free days, have no published benchmarks.

Recently researchers have questioned the use of these benchmarks as they lack an underlying analytic foundation (Evans et al. 2004b) and other areas need to be examined in order to get an idea of an appropriate benchmark. Hirth et al. (2000) reviewed the literature for the use of thresholds in economic evaluations in order to determine if a consensus could be reached. This review is based on studies that have looked at, among other things, individuals' willingness to pay for gains in life expectancy. The general notion is that if individuals provide the average willingness to pay for a life year then this to some extent represents society's implied cutoff point for the allocation of resources. Values in excess of the estimates from these individuals represent paying "too much" for a life year and represent a poor return on healthcare investment. This review found a tremendous variation in estimates of the cost per QALY. Depending on the method used in the studies estimates ranged from $24,777 to $428,286 per QALY. Excluding the $24,777 estimate as inferior to the others due to the valuation method employed, a median of $265,345 was found. This finding by Hirth and others suggests that the original

Table 8.4 Grades of recommendation for the adoption of appropriate utilization of new technologies

Grade	Recommendation*
A	Compelling evidence for the adoption and appropriate utilization. The new technology is as effective as or more effective than the existing one and is less costly
B	Strong evidence for adoption and appropriate utilization The new technology is more effective than the existing one and costs less than $20,000 per quality adjusted life year (QALY) gained The new technology is less effective than the existing one, but its introduction would save more than $100,000/QALY gained
C	Moderate evidence for adoption and appropriate utilization The new technology is more effective than the existing one and costs $20,000 to $100,000/QALY gained The new technology is less effective than the existing one, but its introduction would save $20,000 to $100,000/QALY gained
D	Weak evidence for adoption and appropriate utilization The new technology is more effective than the existing one and costs more than $100,000/QALY gained The new technology is less effective than the existing one, but its introduction would save less than $20,000/QALY gained
E	Compelling evidence for rejection The new technology is less effective than or as effective as the existing one and is more costly

* Costs in Canadian dollars.
Source: Laupacis A, Feeny D, Detsky A, et al. How attractive does a new technology have to be to warrant adoption and utilization? Tentative guidelines for using clinical and economic evaluations. Canad Med Assoc J 1992; 146(4):473–481.

benchmarks, even when adjusted for inflation, are too low. Their study found that 28 out of 35 estimates of cost per QALY exceeded the $100,000 threshold and 31 of 35 estimates exceeded the $50,000 per QALY threshold. Therefore as a rough rule it appears that absolute lowest boundary for the threshold is $50,000 per QALY and is more likely $100,000 per QALY.

COST ACCEPTABILITY CURVE

As noted in the previous sections there is some confusion as to the correct benchmark to use when

interpreting the results of economic evaluations. Researchers recognize this and it has been suggested that the use of cost-effectiveness acceptability curves improves the interpretation of pharmacoeconomic data. A cost-effectiveness acceptability curve shows the probability a treatment under consideration is "cost-effective" as a function of a particular benchmark (whether it is the maximum or minimum). The advantage of this approach is that it does not make an assumption about the maximum willingness to pay (say $50,000 per life year), but instead allows

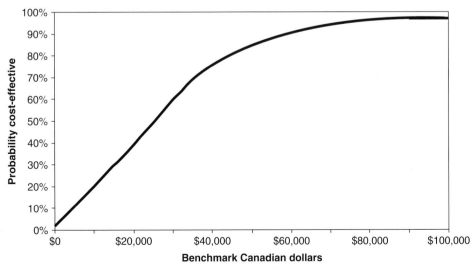

Figure 8.4 Cost acceptability curve.

decision-makers to apply their own maximum and then compare the results of the study to this maximum.

For instance, Figure 8.4 represents a hypothetical cost acceptability curve for a new treatment. If we specify our benchmark to be $50,000 per life year gained the graph shows there is an 80% probability that the therapy is cost-effective. At around $70,000 per life year gained the probability is nearly 100%. In this way we can look at the slope of the cost acceptability curve to determine how likely that a therapy is cost effective: a steep slope implies a better chance of cost-effectiveness than a flat slope.

CONCLUSION

Pharmacoeconomics is a science that examines options. The option under evaluation may be a new pain treatment that costs less and provides the same level of pain relief as existing interventions. Or it may be a pain treatment that costs more than existing medications but leads to better pain relief and physical functioning, or that the pain treatment is most efficacious in one group of patients over another. Other options exist, and the role of pharmacoeconomic research is to determine which option is the best in terms of maximizing overall health outcomes given there is a limited amount of money to spend.

Pharmacoeconomics is not cost containment – in fact it may be quite the reverse. A well-designed pharmacoeconomic study may come to the conclusion that a new and expensive medication is preferable to an older agent if the improvement in outcomes is warranted or if the medication leads to cost offsetting in some other area of direct medical costs (e.g., avoidance of hospitalization or rehabilitation expense). Determining if the new medication provides good value for money is answered by applying the pharmacoeconomic techniques reviewed in the previous section. In a CCA the analysis is easily understood. In general, by making the impact of the treatment of interest as comprehensive and transparent as possible, decision-makers are able to select the information that is most relevant to them and make their own value judgment of whether a therapy is "worth it" (Mauskopf 1998).

In a CMA, there is no need to make a value judgment – the results are unambiguous: since the treatments are proven to be equivalent in outcomes the intervention with the lowest cost is chosen. However, in reality this situation is rare and a more typical result would be that a new intervention costs more and leads to better outcomes. In this case a CEA is more appropriate. The advantage of a CEA is that by aggregating the cost and effect, the economic implications of the therapy become directly entwined with the clinical effect. Thus, statements about the value of the intervention are clearer than in a CCA. Furthermore, not only can researchers compare the interventions in the study under investigation, but they may also compare the results to other cost-effectiveness studies when the same effectiveness endpoint is used.

However, a CEA may not be the most appropriate technique to employ. When an intervention impacts quality of life, as in many chronic pain conditions, a CUA may be more useful. The primary advantage of this type of study is that it is possible to make comparisons across interventions with very different effects. Ultimately, studies that use either QALYs or life years saved as endpoints can be ranked best to worse on a so called league table. Then decision-makers compare findings and consider selecting those interventions with the lowest cost per QALY until the budget for healthcare is exhausted. In this manner, decision-makers will maximize health status given the limited financial resources at their disposal.

Cost-benefit analysis is also a useful technique that avoids some of the interpretation problems associated with CEA and CUA. Since the decision to adopt a medical intervention is only contingent upon the benefit in monetary terms exceeding the costs of the intervention there are no real interpretation issues. However, the main drawback of cost-benefit studies is that the translation of healthcare effects into monetary values is treated with a great deal of skepticism. Therefore, their use in pharmacoeconomics in general and in pain specifically has been limited.

Pharmacoeconomic research plays an important role in understanding overall pain outcomes. Pharmacoeconomics is concerned with demonstrating the relative value of an intervention compared to alternate interventions and seeks to allocate scarce resources to areas that will yield the maximum patient gain. The principles of pharmacoeconomics are relevant to various audiences within the field of pain and the multidimensional nature of pain makes economic evaluations in this area particularly challenging. In this chapter we have set out basic principles of pharmacoeconomics of cost-consequence, cost-minimization, cost-effectiveness, cost-utility and cost-benefit analysis that may be employed in chronic and acute pain interventions. Researchers can use this information as a base to build up a research program or use it as a starting point for further enquiries in the field. The careful design, implementation and reporting of pharmacoeconomic research offers decision-makers, whether they are pain specialists or insurers of pain patients, the ability to consider all relevant patient outcomes and to employ resources to areas that provide the best value for money spent in treating patients with pain.

REFERENCES

Bennett KJ, Torrance GW. Measuring health state preferences and utilities: rating scale, time trade-off, and standard gamble techniques. In: Spilker B (ed). Quality of Life and

Pharmacoeconomics in Clinical Trials, 2nd edn. Lippincott-Raven, Philadelphia, PA, 1996.

Berger M, Murray J, Xu J, et al. Alternative valuations of work loss and productivity. J Occupat Environ Med 2001; 43:18–24.

Brazier J, Usherwood T, Harper R, Thomas K. Deriving a preference-based single index from the UK SF-36 Health Survey. Journal of Clinical Epidemiology 1998; 51 (11):1115–1128.

Cook T, Campbell D. Quasi-Experimentation: Design and Analysis Issues for Field Settings. Houghton Mifflin, Boston, MA, 1979.

Detsky A. Guidelines for economic analysis of pharmaceutical products. Pharmacoeconomics 1993; 3:354–361.

Drummond M, O'Brien B, Stoddart G, Torrance G. Methods for the Economic Evaluation of Health Care Programmes, 2nd edn. Oxford University Press, New York, 1997.

Eisenberg J. Clinical economics: a guide to the economic analysis of clinical practice. JAMA 1989; 262(2): 2879–2886.

Endicott J, Nee J. Endicott Work Productivity Scale (EWPS): a new measure to assess treatment effects. Psychopharmacol Bull 1997; 33:13–16.

Evans C, Crawford B. Patient self reports in pharmacoeconomic studies: their use and impact on study validity. Pharmacoeconomics 1999; 15(3): 241–256.

Evans C, Crawford B, Doyle J. Usefulness of resource utilization estimates from piggyback studies in rheumatoid arthritis. Expert Rev. Pharmacoeconom Outcomes Res 2003; 3(6):685–689.

Evans C, Mertzanis P, Abetz L. Measurement strategies for indirect costs in economic evaluations. Expert Rev Pharmacoeconom Outcomes Res 2004a; 3:703–716.

Evans C, Tavakoli M, Crawford B. Use of quality adjusted life years gained as benchmarks in economic evaluations: a critical appraisal. Health Care Manage Sci 2004b; 7:43–49.

Evans KE, Boan JA, Evans JL, et al. Economic evaluation of oral sumatriptan compared with oral caffeine/ergotamine for migraine. Pharmacoeconomics 1997; 12(5):565–577.

Frei A, Andersen S, Hole P, et al. A one year health economic model comparing transdermal fentanyl with sustained-release morphine in the treatment of chronic noncancer pain. J Pain Palliat Care Pharmacother 2003; 17(2):5–26.

Frymoyer J, Durrett C. The economics of spinal disorders. In: Frymoyer J (ed). The Adult Spine. Lippincott-Raven, Philadelphia, PA, 1997: 143–150.

Furlong W, Feeny D, Torrance GW, et al. The Health Utilities Index system for assessing health-related quality of life in clinical studies. Ann Med 2001; 33:375–384.

Gabriel S, Jaakkimainen RL, Bombardier C. The cost-effectiveness of misoprostol for nonsteroidal anti-inflammatory drug-associated adverse gastrointestinal events. Arthritis Rheumatism 1993; 36:447–459.

Gerth W, Sarma S, Hu XH, et al. Productivity cost benefit to employers of treating migraine with rizatriptan: a specific worksite analysis model. J Occupat Environ Med 2004; 46:48–54.

Gold M, Siegel J, Russell L, et al. Cost-effectiveness in Health and Medicine. Oxford University Press, New York, 1997.

Goudas LC, Carr DB. Postoperative pain control: a survey of promising drugs and pharmacoeconomic criteria for purchasing them. 8th IASP World Congress on Pain: refresher course. Vancouver, Canada, 1996.

Gureje O. Persistent pain and well-being: a World Health Organization study in primary care. JAMA 1998; 280:147–151.

Hakkaart-van Roijen L, Essink-Bot M. Manual Health and Labour Questionnaire. Institute for Medical Technology Assessment, Rotterdam, 2000.

Hirth R, Chernew M, Miller E, et al. Willingness to pay for a quality-adjusted life year: in search of a standard. Med Decision Making 2000; 20:332–342.

Hu XH, Markson L, Lipton R, et al. Burden of migraine in the United States: disability and economic costs. Arch Intern Med 1999; 159:813–818.

Kaplan R, Bush J. Health related quality of life measurement for evaluation research and policy analysis. Health Psychol 1982; 1:61–80.

Kaplan RB, Atkins CJ, Timms R. Validity of a quality of well-being scale as an outcome measure in chronic obstructive pulmonary disease. J Chronic Dis 1984; 37(2):85–95.

Kessler RC, Barber C, Beck A, Berglund P, Cleary PD, McKenas D, Pronk N, Simon G, Stang P, Ustun TU, Wang P. The world Health Organization Health and Work Performance Questionnaire (HPQ). J Occup Environ Med 2003; 45(2):156–174.

Koopman C, Pelletier KR, Murray JF, Berger ML, Turpin RS, Hackleman P, Gibson P, Holmes PM, Bendel T. Stanford Presenteeism scale: health status and employee productivity. J Occup Environ Med 2002; 1(44):14–20.

Koopmanschap M, Rutten F. Indirect costs in economic studies: confronting the confusion. PharmacoEconomics 1993; 4:446–454.

Koopmanschap M, Rutten F. A practical guide for calculating indirect costs of disease. PharmacoEconomics 1996; 10:460–466.

Laupacis A, Feeny D, Detsky A, et al. How attractive does a new technology have to be to warrant adoption and utilization? Tentative guidelines for using clinical and economic evaluations. Canad Med Assoc J 1992; 146:473–481.

Lerner D, Amick B, Malspeis S, et al. The migraine work and productivity loss questionnaire: concepts and design. Quality Life Res 1999; 8:699–710.

Lerner D, Amick B, Rogers W, et al. The work limitations questionnaire. Med Care 2001; 39:72–85.

Lipton RB, Stewart WF, Reed M, et al. Migraine's impact today: burden of illness, patterns of care. Postgrad Med 2001; 109(1):38–45.

Loisel P, Lemaire J, Poitras S, et al. Cost-benefit and cost-effectiveness analysis of a disability prevention model for back pain management: a six year follow up study. Occupat Environ Med 2002; 59(12):807–815.

Maniadakis N, Gray A. The economic burden of back pain in the UK. Pain 2000; 84(1):95–103.

Marketdata Enterprises. Chronic Pain Management Programs: A Market Analysis. Marketdata Enterprises, New York, 1995.

Mauskopf JA, Paul JE, Grant DM, et al. The role of cost-consequence analysis in healthcare decision-making. Pharmacoeconomics 1998; 13(3):277–288.

O'Brien B. Economic evaluation of pharmaceuticals: Frankenstein's monster or vampire of trials. Med Care 1996; 34:DS99–DS108.

Pettitt D, Goldstein JL, McGuire A, et al. Overview of the Arthritis Cost Consequence Evaluation System (ACCES): a pharmacoeconomic model for celecoxib. Rheumatology 2000; 39(suppl 2):33–42.

Rabin R, de Charro F. EQ-5D: a measure of health status from the EuroQol Group. The Finnish Medical Society Duodecim. Ann Med 2001; 33:337–343.

Reilly M, Zbrozek A, Dukes E. The validity and reproducibility of a work productivity and activity impairment instrument. PharmacoEconomics 1993; 4:353–365.

Rothman K. Modern Epidemiology. Little, Brown and Company, Boston, MA, 1986.

Schulman K, Lynn L, Glick H, et al. Cost effectiveness of low-dose Zidovudine therapy of asymptomatic patients with human immunodeficiency virus (HIV) infection. Ann Intern Med 1991; 114:798–802.

Smith GT. The economics of hypertension and stroke. Am Heart J 1990; 119:725–728.

Smith R, Dobson M. Measuring utility values for QALYs: two methodological issues. Health Econ 1993; 2(4):349–355.

To T, Wu K Health care utilization and disability of migraine: the Ontario health survey. Canad J Public Health 1995; Revue Canadienne de Sante Publique. 86(3):195–199.

Torrance GW. Measurement of health state utilities for economic appraisal: a review. J Health Econ 1986; 5:1–30.

Torrance G, Zipursky A. Cost-effectiveness of antepartum prevention of Rh immunization. Clinics Perinatol 1984; 11(2):267–281.

Townsend RJ. Postmarketing drug research and development. Drug Intell Clin Pharm 1987; 21(1 Pt 2): 134–136.

Turk D. Clinical effectiveness and cost-effectiveness of treatments for patients with chronic pain. Clin J Pain 2002; 18:355–365.

Van Roijen L, Essink-Bot M, Koopmanschap M, et al. Labor and health status in economic evaluation of health care: the health and labor questionnaire. Int J Technol Assess Health Care 1996; 12:405–415.

Williams A. Economics of coronary artery bypass grafting. Br Med J 1985; 291:326–329.

FURTHER READING

Koch H. The Management of Chronic Pain in Office Based Ambulatory Care: National Ambulatory Medical Care Survey (Advanced Data from Vital and Health Statistics, No. 123; DHHS Publication No. PHS 86-1250). US Public Health Service, Hyattsville, MD, 1986.

National Center for Health Statistics Fast stats. Available at http://www.cdc.gov/nchs/fastats (accessed June 21, 2004).

Rx magazine. Available at http://rx.magazine.tripod.com/sh_20000410.htm (accessed June 21, 2004).

Clinical analgesic drug trials: targets, research strategies and individualizing outcome measures

James Witter • Raymond A. Dionne

INTRODUCTION

Despite better understanding of pain over the past two decades, few truly novel molecular entities designed to address a fundamentally new pathophysiologic mechanism underlying pain have entered the analgesic clinic to date. The same compounds that are the mainstays of analgesic medicines in use today, the opioids and aspirin-like drugs, have been in use to relieve pain for centuries. Virtually all "new" analgesic drugs approved since 1980 are derivatives of opioids or aspirin-like drugs, reformulations of existing drugs and combinations, or are older drugs being given by different routes of administration (Table 9.1). This disturbing trend seems to reflect new drug development in general (Figure 9.1); no unique "targeted" analgesic is in use today that differs in substantial ways from those drugs available for years that were developed by the trial-and-error methodology of yesterday. Why such an apparent gap in the translation of new knowledge and technologies into different, and maybe better, treatment of one of the oldest problems known to humans? Why no apparent attempts to better control pain in this Decade of Pain Control and Relief? This chapter suggests new strategies for the clinical evaluation of investigational drugs and presents a rationale for evidence-based outcome measures that focus on the responses of the individual patient.

WHY HAVE SCIENTIFIC ADVANCES FAILED TO TRANSLATE INTO IMPROVED PAIN RELIEF?

A recent workshop on analgesic drug development (Dionne and Witter 2003) identified several strategic barriers (Table 9.2) to enhancing the process of drug discovery and development that may be responsible for the paucity of new analgesics introduced into clinical practice. Most striking is the dichotomy between the development of highly specific candidate molecules with selective actions for a molecular nociceptive mechanism in vitro and the practice of pain medicine where multiple drugs acting through diverse, presumably additive, mechanisms is the norm. The notion that there is a class of drug, a universal analgesic, that can intrinsically reduce all pain is obsolete and has to be abandoned (Scholz and Woolf 2002).

The dichotomy between preclinical research and pain medicine is historic as most pain research in the past 150 years studied transient pain that does

Table 9.1 Analgesic gap in research versus new analgesics

Year	Number of publications per year	Cumulative number of approvals
1980	895	0
1981	1051	1
1982	1240	5
1983	1222	5
1984	1378	9
1985	1423	10
1986	1614	11
1987	1543	14
1988	1486	15
1989	1498	17
1990	1498	20
1991	5341	24
1992	5835	27
1993	5968	30
1994	6629	31
1995	7473	33
1996	8439	38
1997	9332	39
1998	9883	42
1999	10720	43
2000	10880	46
2001	11494	48

Publications from Pubmed search using terms for that year. Approvals from PDR and FDA website.

not result in tissue damage and may have little relevance to clinical medicine as a model of disease (Dionne and Witter 2003). The mechanistic complexity of tissue injury, inflammation, signal transduction, gene expression and ascending and descending pain pathways results in multiple molecular and cellular events that operate alone and in combination with the peripheral and central nervous system to produce different forms of pain (Figure 9.2). Even if these simplistic schematics adequately explained the neurophysiology of pain transduction and transmission, the molecular events occurring at each level are driven by gene expression that changes over time and plastic changes in the nervous system. Although the development of animal models has increased our understanding of chronic pain, there is still not a good link

between animal models and many chronic pain conditions in humans. In addition, the seemingly infinite polymorphisms in the human genome make it unlikely that selectively blocking one or two receptors would likely interfere with the cascade of mediators, multiple pathways and redundancy in pain signaling.

Analgesic drug development is highly dependent on the use of animal models to screen putative analgesics, characterize the pharmacokinetics of candidate molecules to describe dosing intervals, and to better understand the mechanisms that contribute to the pain experience. Ideally, preclinical animal models are surrogates for the human condition (Dionne and Witter 2003). Animal models can be combined with information generated by anatomy and histochemistry to investigate the contribution of a receptor or channel on the animal's behavior. This composite information allows us to predict the mechanism of novel drugs in pain states, but they do not necessarily predict the response of a human to a particular drug.

Why do preclinical predictions based on animal models fail? Woolf suggests that pain is not a unitary experience and that it is unrealistic to expect that a single "magic bullet" is going to operate on all of the different mechanisms that contribute to different kinds of pain (Dionne and Witter 2003). Understanding of analgesic mechanisms provides an opportunity to move forward to new ways of assessing analgesics in both animal models and clinical conditions based on understanding of the mechanisms involved rather than the empirical way that has driven analgesic development in the past. The symptoms that comprise the pain experience are the result of specific and identifiable changes in the nervous system; analgesics act because they interfere with the mechanisms that produce the pain, not through some unique intrinsic pain relieving action. The way to move forward in analgesic drug development is to measure multiple signs and symptoms in patients, not just global measures, to look at the natural history, to validate mechanistic hypotheses, and to gain insight into the mechanisms that operate in the individual patient (Dionne and Witter 2003).

Classic analgesic combinations such as an opioid and an aspirin-like drug are based on a strategy of blocking more than one pathway to result in additive analgesia, usually with fewer side effects than increasing the dose of the opioid. These approaches have been the mainstay of analgesic therapy for generations. The search for single agents with greater efficacy or reduced side effect liability was reinforced by the introduction of the nonsteroidal anti-inflammatory drugs (NSAIDs) which demonstrated efficacy comparable to or greater than opioid combinations but with fewer side effects for single doses in clinical models of acute pain, e.g. the surgical removal of impacted third molars. While meta-analysis indicates that the oral surgery model is predictive of analgesic activity in other postoperative

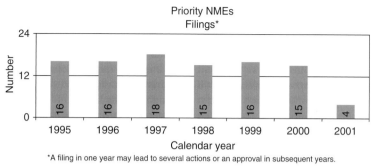

Figure 9.1 Number of priority new molecular entities (NMEs): 1995–2001 (CDER Report to the Nation: 2001; http://www.fda.gov/cder/reports/rtn/2001/rtn2001.htm).

pain settings (Barden et al. 2004), it is unlikely that findings from single dose studies for acute inflammatory pain can be extrapolated to multiple doses, or other clinical conditions where different pain mechanisms predominate such as neuropathic pain states. Individuals with moderate low back pain, for example, might be responsive to a single agent, but patients with more severe disease might be better studied and managed by maintaining baseline drugs and evaluating supplementary drugs. Cancer pain management is an example of multimodal therapy with multiple drugs. Evaluation of a single drug alone may result in the apparent failure of potentially useful drugs.

Another methodologic impediment to analgesic drug development is the temporal differentiation between acute and chronic pain, e.g., 3–6 months, that is often used as a criterion for study entry. Divergent physiologic processes may occur early in the development of pain chronicity. Studies based on a 3- to 6-month criterion might miss critical points for evaluating an intervention aimed at preventing the development of chronic pain and subsequent irreversible changes. Clinical differences between acute and chronic pain suggesting that they are distinctive pain states is not true; acute pain refers to pain at certain times after an initiating event that may be transient, and chronic pain refers to the persistence of pain mechanisms in that patient (Dionne and Witter 2003). The most widely used clinical model for studying analgesic drug efficacy, i.e., the oral surgery model, involves acute

Table 9.2 Barriers to analgesic drug development

While drug development focuses on single agents, chronic pain management is usually combination chemotherapy; regulatory practices need to consider evaluation of new analgesics as concurrent supplementary medications
Current research methods and clinical trials for chronic pain are done with a relatively narrow subset of patients not representative of the heterogeneity of the patient population, e.g., osteoarthritis, low back pain
Temporal differentiation of acute and chronic pain, i.e., greater than 3–6 months, as inclusion criteria may miss interventions that act on plasticity in the nervous system that occur early in the development of a disorder
No consensus pain measurement exists that is useful across different diseases and patients, limiting comparisons across studies and generalizations based on pooling studies
The FDA Guidance for analgesics needs to be revised including for chronic pain indications, the common use of combination drug therapy needs to be addressed, and individual response variability and post-marketing safety issues that are best monitored in large-scale trials need to be considered
Animal models of chronic pain are useful for studying mechanisms of pain and analgesia but do not predict the response of humans to a particular drug
Novel therapies should be designed to treat the mechanisms that contribute to the pain experience, as exemplified by the development of the coxibs based on knowledge of the expression of COX-2 following tissue injury
Translating scientific advances into improved pain relief will require a cooperative effort among the pharmaceutical industry, the regulatory agencies, funding agencies, the biomedical research community, professional societies, and clinicians to improve clinical trials methodology, outcome measures, and better study of the epidemiology of pain

Reproduced with permission from Dionne RA and Witter J. Clin J Pain 2003; 19:139–147.

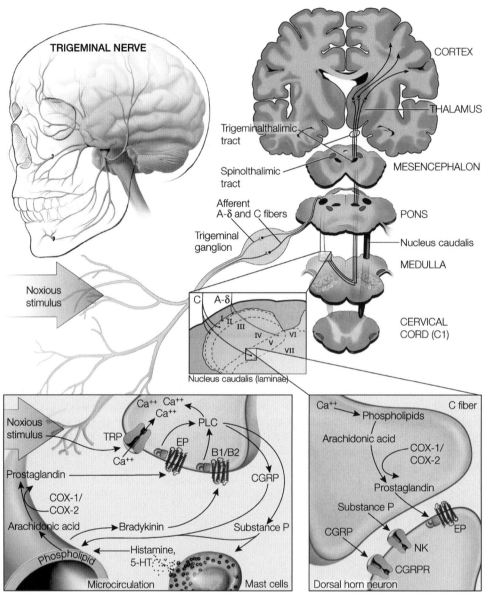

Figure 9.2 Multiple targets and pathways in periphery, dorsal horn and higher CNS that mitigate against specific single agents, including gene expression and polymorphisms; hence, specificity will never work – see list in Scholz and Woolf (2002).

inflammation of 2–3 days' duration. Other clinical models are needed to study the transition from acute injury to chronic pain in order to develop evidence-based criteria for characterizing events related to the development of chronic pain and evaluate pre-emptive interventions that might prevent this transition.

NOVEL TARGETS FOR ANALGESIC DRUGS

An example of the need to consider novel targets for analgesic drugs is the role of glial cells in nociception

and glia-driven clinical pain syndromes. The failure of presently available analgesics to control hyperalgesia and allodynia might lie in glia, as this cell type was not considered when presently available drugs were developed (Watkins and Maier 2003). Emerging evidence demonstrates that astrocytes, microglia and the release of proinflammatory cytokines in the spinal cord are active participants in the creation and maintenance of pain facilitation induced by inflammation and damage to peripheral tissues, peripheral nerves, spinal nerves and the spinal cord (Watkins and Maier 2003). Glial activation following injury results in an enhanced ability to function beyond the basal state, including increased production of proinflammatory substances. Spinal cord glial cells are powerful modulators of pain, producing hyperalgesia and allodynia by releasing substances that act on neurons in pain pathways. Most evidence supports a role for glia-derived proinflammatory cytokines, including tumor necrosis factor (TNF), interleukin (IL)-1, and IL-6 (Watkins and Maier 2003). Both astrocytes and microglia can release proinflammatory cytokines upon activation and both glia and neurons express receptors for them (Watkins et al. 1999).

Perispinal injection of antagonists of proinflammatory cytokines prevents and/or reverses allodynia and hyperalgesia in virtually every animal model tested (Watkins and Maier 2003). Another approach to block the effects of proinflammatory cytokines released from activated glia is to interfere with intra-cellular signaling cascades, most prominently being p38 MAP kinase. Compounds that inhibit p38 MAP kinase inhibit allodynia and hyperalgesia induced by peripheral nerve injury, peripheral tissue inflammation, peripheral nerve injury, spinal nerve injury, spinal cord inflammation and perispinal substance P and NMDA administration in animal models (Watkins and Maier 2003). Recent demonstration of analgesic efficacy for an orally administered MAP kinase inhibitor (SCIO-469) in comparison to an NSAID (Tong 2004) suggests that extrapolation to chronic inflammatory conditions may result in novel analgesics by targeting nontraditional analgesic targets.

MULTIPLE ACTIONS AT MULTIPLE SITES GENERALLY RESULT IN GREATER ANALGESIA

The importance of multiple mechanisms of action for analgesic efficacy is illustrated by inhibitors of cyclooxygenase (COX) in animal models of nociception. While selective COX-2 inhibitors have demonstrated analgesic efficacy comparable to dual COX-1/COX-2 inhibitors in clinical models (Morrison et al. 1999; Dionne and Berthold 2001), recent animal studies suggest that COX-1 in the spinal cord plays an important role in postoperative pain (Zhu et al. 2003). Using the Brennan rat paw incision model (Brennan et al. 1996), both the COX-1 preferring inhibitor ketorolac and the COX-1 selective inhibitor SC-560 were antinociceptive at intervals up to 5 days postincision. Ketorolac is generally considered to be nonselective but is actually several-fold more selective for COX-1 (Warner et al. 1999). The COX-2 selective inhibitor NS-398, in comparison, was inactive in this model (Zhu et al. 2003). COX-1 immunoreactivity in the spinal cord increased ipsilaterally on day 1, peaked on day 2, and declined thereafter in cells with a morphology suggestive of glia. These results argue that COX-1 enzyme is also important in spinal mechanisms of postoperative pain and suggest that drugs targeted at this site, in addition to

peripheral and central COX-2, would be more efficacious for pain than drugs selective for COX-2 only. Demonstration of safety for intrathecal ketorolac in humans (Eisenach et al. 2002) will soon permit assessment of the central effects of NSAIDs, possibly paving the way for central administration of drugs acting on both COX-1 and COX-2.

The importance of central mechanisms of COX-mediated pain has also been demonstrated for the S(+) isomer of ketoprofen. Oral administration of S(+) ketoprofen demonstrates analgesic activity in an animal model of nociception that is significantly attenuated by intrathecal administration of tropisetron, a high affinity $5\text{-}HT_1/5\text{-}HT_2/5\text{-}HT_7$ receptor antagonist (Diaz-Reval et al. 2004). The ability of S(+) ketoprofen to activate serotonergic mechanisms, possibly involving 5-HT release, appears to contribute to its antinociceptive effect. Another COX-related analgesic mechanism, other than suppression of peripheral prostanoid production, involves investigational drugs having dual COX and 5-lipoxygenase (5-LOX) inhibitory effects. Compounds capable of inhibiting COX-1, COX-2 and 5-LOX are showing promise as anti-inflammatory and analgesic agents (De Gaetano et al. 2003). These examples of multiple actions and sites of analgesic activity for the NSAID class, traditionally thought to produce analgesia largely by inhibiting the peripheral effects of COX, are consistent with greater analgesic efficacy for drugs acting at multiple targets for analgesia.

REINVENTING ANALGESIC DRUGS WITH MULTIPLE BUT SELECTIVE ACTIONS

The evolution of analgesic drug development has paralleled other areas of pharmacology. The identification and isolation of the active ingredient of naturally occurring compounds, e.g., opium and willow-bark, was followed by structural modifications to develop semisynthetic and synthetic analogs, e.g. heroin and aspirin, followed by structure–activity-directed screening to identify drugs with greater specificity for the therapeutic effect without retaining the full spectrum of adverse effects. The futility of this latter approach is exemplified by several decades of efforts to identify an optimal opiate drug (Eddy 1973) that resulted in thousands of molecules that differed in potency, pharmacokinetic properties, and routes of administration. It was belatedly recognized, however, that this series of opioid compounds retained the ability to produce similar analgesia and side effects, dependence liability and the development of tolerance, when evaluated at equi-analgesic doses; problems that continue to plague opioid agonists to this day. Recognition of the role of COX in pain and inflammation (Vane et al. 1971) led to the development of NSAIDs with greater analgesic and anti-inflammatory efficacy but these agents retained much of the toxic potential of the aspirin-like drugs. Estimates of greater than 10,000 deaths annually (Wolfe et al. 1999) were attributed to NSAIDs before recognition of these problems and the introduction of selective COX-2 inhibitors resulted in changes in clinical practice that appear to have increased gastrointestinal safety. Increasing selectivity for the COX-2 isoform appears to have increased gastrointestinal safety (Bombardier et al. 2000; Silverstein et al. 2000) but may be at the expense of cardiovascular safety (Topol 2004).

The COX-2 experience and the development of other increasingly specific drugs for traditional analgesic targets or novel ones, e.g., NK-1 antagonists, have not resulted in any therapeutic benefits. The multiplicity of receptors, cells, molecular-genetic events initiated by tissue injury and transmitted to the CNS by multiple pathways logically suggests targeting these multiple events to determine which series or combinations of targets yield effective analgesia for specific diseases and diverse patients.

Classic analgesic combinations arose out of the necessity to provide greater analgesia without the dose-related adverse effects associated with increasing the dose of opioids and the ceiling of analgesic activity attributed to aspirin-like drugs. While generally recognized as an effective strategy for combinations of aspirin or acetaminophen plus an orally effective opioid such as codeine or oxycodone, the therapeutic limitations of fixed doses and adverse effects limit their clinical utility for many applications. As described above, the multitude of analgesic mechanisms and pathways also limit the utility of drugs combinations aimed primarily at opiate receptors and peripheral COX activity.

An alternative is to selectively target multiple analgesic mechanisms with a single drug or combination of drugs with selective actions beyond traditional analgesic mechanisms. This approach can be extended to preemptive strategies to inhibit pain and inflammatory pathways rather than attempt to attenuate them after the inflammatory cascade, for example, has contributed to the development of sensitization. The preoperative administration of NSAIDs has been demonstrated in dozens of acute pain clinical trials (for a review, see Dionne and Berthold 2001) to delay the onset of pain as the local anesthesia dissipates. This strategy also can decrease pain intensity over the initial 4–12 hours postsurgery. Similarly, use of a local anesthetic intraoperatively (to patients undergoing surgery with general anesthesia) or administered prior to the onset of postoperative nociceptive barrage will decrease pain at 24–48 hours. While these strategies involving approved drugs fall under the realm of "off-label" therapeutics, they illustrate the potential for novel pharmacologic strategies to be administered preemptively to interfere with nociceptive and inflammatory processes prior to their onset.

SELECTIVE ACTIONS AT MULTIPLE TARGETS VERSUS NONSELECTIVE MECHANISMS OF ACTION: LESSONS FROM ANTIDEPRESSANTS

The novel antidepressant duloxetine provides an example of a molecule with multiple selective actions with advantage for both increased efficacy and decreased adverse effects. Antidepressants currently in use modulate monoamine neurotransmission, take 6–8 weeks to exert their effects and are only efficacious in 60–70% of patients. The first generation of antidepressants, e.g., iproniazid and imipramine, affected many systems and had multiple mechanisms of actions. This results in a wide spectrum of drug activity, resulting in multiple clinical effects but a wide range of adverse effects. The limitations of the adverse effect profile led to the development of analogs of these drugs to minimize such undesirable effects, analogous to early efforts to develop opioids that retained analgesic activity but minimized their adverse effects.

A second wave of antidepressants focused on the development of selective reuptake inhibitors with increasing tolerability and safety (Wong and Licino 2004) compared to tricyclic antidepressants. This strategy of developing antidepressant drugs with more specific mechanisms of action is at odds with the heterogeneous nature of major depressive disorders and appears to have reduced clinical activity (Wong and Licino 2004). The next phase in antidepressant drug therapy is the development of molecules that have selective mechanisms but act at multiple sites, i.e., serotonin and norepinephrine, resulting in greater effects than selective reuptake inhibitors for just one of these sites. Recognition of genetic variation in patients' responses to antidepressants, combined with the technological advances made possible by the human genome project, has helped accelerate pharmacogenomic studies to develop even more novel, individualized and more efficacious treatments (Wong and Licino 2004). Recognition that multiple peripheral and central receptors and pathways exist for pain and that increasing selectivity leads to decreased analgesic activity provides a rationale for similar approaches in the development of analgesic drugs. Combining several selective but additive actions in one molecule or combination of molecules to develop optimal therapeutic ratios has improved clinical benefit with adverse effect profile appropriate for the disease and patient population of interest. Design of clinical studies capable of detecting small increments in efficacy, e.g., 20–25%, and additive effects of the same order would be a prerequisite to demonstrate the analgesic activity of each ingredient and additive effects when in combination. Effect size of this magnitude might vary between individuals of varying genetic background and previous pain experiences, making the development of scales capable of detecting effects that are meaningful for an individual patient (i.e., responder analysis), even if the overall mean effect for the group is modest, an important new goal in analgesics (Dionne et al. 2005).

OPTIMIZING ANALGESIA BY DEVELOPING INDIVIDUALIZED THERAPY

The need to select the correct drug and dose for the individual patient has been sought by clinicians for a long time (Reidenberg 2003). Individualization of drug therapy traditionally involves both drug selection and dose titration, customarily as a clinical decision for the individual patient. This strategy is evolving to apply to populations in making the decision to start a drug discovery program or whether to market a drug (Reidenberg 2003). Factors contributing to individualization of drug therapy at the population level include pharmacokinetics and pharmacogenetics, increasing understanding of the molecular biology contributing to disease processes and drug effects, and drug epidemiology. As research continues to subdivide diseases into smaller groups of more homogeneous patients, drug discovery is identifying compounds with activity for these narrowly defined diseases (Reidenberg 2003). Pharmacovigilance and drug monitoring also promise to identify variations in responses to drugs that help to permit better matching the individual patient with the correct drug and dose. Analgesic drug development, conversely, has been largely based on the mean responses of groups of patients with the same clinical condition given the same drug and dose, making identification of individual variation in efficacy or toxicity difficult to detect.

In a classic clinical trial design, the mean responses of a group of subjects administered an investigational analgesic is usually compared to the mean responses of other groups of subjects administered placebo and to a standard analgesic drug or therapeutic regimen. The efficacy of the medication is compared statistically by comparing the mean responses of the placebo and experimental treatment groups. In pivotal analgesic trials, a failure to demonstrate a "significant" difference between treatment groups often forms the basis for considering the drug not worthy of further development. Similarly, mean efficacy for an investigational compound comparable to the standard treatment but with a higher incidence of adverse effects forms the basis for considering the investigational compound to not have a therapeutic advantage and, hence, not worthy of further development. Little consideration is given to the efficacy or safety of the investigational treatment in individual subjects or subgroups of the patient sample tested, some of whom may have a very good response to the treatment or demonstrate greater toxicity that taints the responses of the group as a whole.

The responses of the individual subjects in a clinical trial should be considered in the development and assessment of analgesic drugs where the individual genetic composition, past experiences, gender, ethnicity, expectations, disease processes and inflammation-induced gene expression varies widely across subjects. It is unlikely that an analgesic drug would be uniformly effective under such heterogeneous conditions. Assessment of the individual patients' responses relative to generally accepted criteria for pain relief in comparison to the proportion of individuals who respond in appropriate control groups may reveal subgroups for whom the treatment is particularly effective or results in unusual toxicity. Outcomes from this responder analysis approach might include identification of drugs with therapeutic value for chronic pain resistant to normal therapies, development of drug classes with particular promise for pain in a particular condition, but not necessarily all type of pain, and identification of molecular-genetic markers for predicting analgesic drug actions in individual patients.

INDIVIDUAL VARIATION IN RESPONSES TO PAIN

Recent brain imaging studies provide evidence that subjective ratings of pain magnitude are closely related to objectively measured neural activity in a number of cortical regions recognized to be important in pain processing (Coghill et al. 2003). Inter-individual differences in these subjective reports of pain magnitude were closely related to the objectively measured degree of activation in these brain regions, providing evidence that differences in pain report across patients reflect differences in the actual pain experience (Coghill et al. 2003). In another recent study, preoperative ratings of experimental pain were significantly correlated with postoperative pain ratings following elective caesarian section, suggesting that individual pain sensitivity is consistent across indices of experimental and clinical pain following surgical injury (Granot et al. 2003). While this study lacked controls to assess inter-individual differences in the use of pain scales such as the visual analog scale, these results suggest the possibility that simple preoperative tests can predict individual differences in the pain experience after surgery (Coghill and Eisenach 2003).

Evidence is also emerging from functional brain imaging studies that neural circuitry underlying expectation influences pain perception and that variability across individuals may be related to differences in the degree of uncertainty associated with expectation (Ploghaus et al. 2003). Experimental manipulation of subjects presented with either painfully hot as well as innocuous warm stimulation and color cues revealed that expectation of the painful heat activated sites that could be distinguished from those activated by the painful heat (Ploghaus 2003). Uncertainty about the impending nature of an impending event produces anxiety, resulting in anxiety-induced hyperalgesia that is associated with activation of the hippocampus, anterior cingulated cortex and insula. Ploghaus and colleagues point out that while functional neuroimaging has provided an understanding of which brain areas are activated by acute painful stimulation, research on the neural pathways underlying pain modulation by cognitive, emotional, pharmaceutical and other factors has only just begun. The influence of cognitive factors such as expectation clearly varies across subjects based on past experiences and is more likely to confound measurements across subjects rather than assessment of individual responses, at least over the duration of an analgesic study where these cognitive factors are not likely to change.

While the development of plasticity in the nervous system in response to pain is becoming generally accepted, identification of its manifestation in humans is still problematic. Examination of patients with fibromyalgia, which is considered to be an exaggerated hyperexcitability of the nociceptive system, reveals lower pain thresholds and greatly reduced tolerance to cold pain (Desmeules et al. 2003). While the development of quantitative sensory testing methods holds promise as a method to identify patients with central hyperalgesia and other manifestations of sensitization, it is not possible at present to stratify subjects in clinical trials on the basis of possible central sensitization. Averaging in the mean responses of subjects in a clinical trial, some of whom may have altered pain responses due to central sensitization, might fail to discriminate patients who may benefit from a centrally acting analgesic, such as drugs acting at NMDA receptors. Use of individual responses might identify a subgroup benefiting from an intervention that is active against the unique pain mechanism, but not particularly useful for other types of pain, acute inflammatory pain for example.

Age differences in postoperative pain and analgesic responses have been documented (Gagliese and Katz 2003) but may be scale dependent. Older men had significantly lower pain scores following radical prostatectomy than younger men on the McGill Pain Questionnaire but did not demonstrate any differences on a simple VAS scale. Measurement of the change in pain from day one to day two following surgery was detected similarly by both scales, indicating they are both sensitive, but the level of pain appeared to be better captured by verbal descriptor scales of pain qualities than non-verbal measures of pain intensity. Age differences that might explain this difference include varying cognitive abilities or linguistic skills across age groups or age-related changes in the neurobiology of pain mechanisms. Use of mean responses across a group of subjects might not detect a meaningful change in pain intensity in response to an analgesic drug if subjects varied sufficiently in age to make the standard VAS less sensitive to responses in elderly subjects than in younger subjects.

WIDE INDIVIDUAL VARIATION IN RESPONSE TO ANALGESICS

Inter-individual differences in analgesic response to morphine are well recognized; a recent report (Aubrun et al. 2003) demonstrated a nonlinear relationship between morphine dose and the initial VAS score. The range in the mean dose required to relieve pain (13.2 mg) in 3045 patients was 1–48 mg, representing a range of 0.02–0.83 mg/kg (Riou, personal communication). The approximate 40-fold range in response to a single agent given in a controlled fashion to permit quantification of individual difference in opioid requirements following surgery demonstrates the wide inter-individual variation in analgesic responsiveness that is inherent in any patient sample. While it is assumed that randomization minimizes this difference across subjects, administration of a fixed dose of morphine to patients on the sensitive end of the population would be much greater than the dose needed to produce adequate analgesia and would likely result in CNS depression. Conversely, administration of the mean dose for this large sample, 13.2 mg, to morphine insensitive patients would result in inadequate analgesia and the need for continued titration to achieve adequate pain relief. Evaluation of an investigational analgesic with potency similar to morphine at a fixed dose will likely produce similar results: inadequate analgesia in some patients, clinically useful analgesia in others and excessive adverse effects in others. The assessment of the overall efficacy and safety of an investigational drug using a mean effect in a sample responding similar to those in the report by Aubrun and colleagues (2003) might fail to detect efficacy or predict an undesirable side effect profile, thereby masking the response of individual patients experiencing adequate analgesia with an acceptable side effect profile.

The potential importance of individual variability to drug responsiveness is illustrated by the drug trastuzumab (Herceptin) used in the treatment of breast cancer. The response rate in the general patient population is a very modest 6%, but it is nearly 100% effective in a subgroup of 15–20% of patients who express the HER-2 receptor. Given the otherwise poor prognosis for women with metastatic breast cancer, the ability to target a highly effective treatment to those with a biomarker for responsiveness makes the mean results of the group meaningless in comparison to the individual responses of those in the subgroup. This phenomenon should be considered in the development and assessment of analgesic drugs where the individual genetic composition, past experiences, gender, ethnicity, expectations, disease processes and inflammation-induced gene expression varies widely across subjects.

MEASUREMENT OF INDIVIDUAL ANALGESIC RESPONSES

Sample size estimates for trials comparing means are calculated from standard formulae requiring definition of Type I and Type I error rates, standard deviation (SD), and the delta to be observed in the means of the treatment groups of interest. For clinical outcomes that engender a single endpoint such as a blood pressure measure, this approach has many advantages. However, for clinical outcomes that require consideration of more than one endpoint, a composite approach is better able to encompass and accommodate these important variables. These composite endpoints can then be grouped into an index that is then capable of defining, at the individual level, whether any particular patient did or did not achieve the endpoints in this composite index during the study with the drug of interest. New clinical trials can then be powered based upon calculations that take into account the proportion of patients that "responded" to the outcomes measures in the index. This approach has the advantage of grouping clinically important outcomes into a metric that defines the individual as an individual, not the individual's contribution to a "group" outcome. Therefore, decisions may be made on the basis of looking directly at the response of the individual as part of the group rather than having to infer that person's response to the variable of interest as part of a large group mean or average response. In the latter situation, there is no way to understand whether two or more clinical outcomes of interest occurred in the same person, whereas in the responder approach this has been prospectively designed into the interpretation of data and so there is no doubt. Therefore, for a clinical outcome in which the response of the individual is key to proper interpretation of results, the responder approach offers the flexibility, both clinically and statistically, to best capture the patient's experience with the drug. Results similar to these can only be addressed with a means approach after substantial statistical efforts such a multivariate analysis with their problems with imputation artifacts and bias.

PHARMACOGENETIC APPROACHES TO IDENTIFY INDIVIDUAL DIFFERENCES IN ANALGESIC RESPONSES

The principle behind pharmacogenomics is the belief that the responses of a patient to a drug regimen (the phenotype) can be related to some facet of their genetic composition (the genotype). If demonstrated in a sufficient number of individuals, it might be possible to derive a causal relationship between genetics and therapeutic responses. The example of Herceptin, described above, demonstrates the potential for pharmacogenomic success but, to date, few other success stories have emerged (Willis and Lesney 2003). Another promise of pharmacogenomics is the ability to identify potential adverse reactions that occur in a subset of individuals who react poorly to a treatment, sometimes related to metabolites of the parent drug. Given that most drugs are withdrawn from the market due to patient safety considerations, it may be more cost effective to identify individuals likely to experience toxicity due to a drug class, a particular drug or a drug dose. With an estimated 10 million single nucleotide polymorphisms in the human genome, the challenges may be related more to the ability to identify the relationship between single nucleotide polymorphisms or their haplotypes to individual variations in pain responsiveness and analgesia.

The possible role of genetic factors in pain sensitivity was assessed in sibling pairs using experimental pain stimuli in comparison to polymorphisms for the mu and delta opioid receptor subtypes (Kim et al. 2003). Moderate, but significant, intraclass correlation coefficients were demonstrated from sibling pairs for pain sensitivity similar to the degree of correlation seen for inherited traits such as body mass and longevity. Gender differences in experimental pain perception were also evident, suggesting the need to analyze males and females separately for genetic influences on pain sensitivity. A functional polymorphism in a delta opioid receptor gene resulted in differences in pain sensitivity that was dependent both on gender and the characteristics of the applied stimuli. These data, although preliminary and in need of replication in larger samples, suggest that pain is familial and that individual responses to pain is heritable, being influenced by polymorphisms in genes for molecules involved in pain perception. Other studies suggest a role for COMT polymorphisms on pain perception in humans (Zubieta et al. 2003) but this effect may vary by stimulus (Kim et al. 2004).

Sensory input in humans is filtered through an individual's genetic composition, prior learning, current physiologic status, idiosyncratic appraisals, expectations, current mood states and sociocultural environment (Turk 2003). These influences manifest as variability in pain sensitivity, perception, and tolerance. The relative contribution and interactions of these many factors to inter-individual variations in pain is currently unknown. Considering the complexity of pain mechanisms, the impact of psychological factors and the hundreds to thousands of molecules involved, wide inter-individual differences and a broad range of responses to painful experimental (Figure 9.3, upper panel) and clinical stimuli (Figure 9.3, lower panel) are not surprising (Kim et al. 2004).

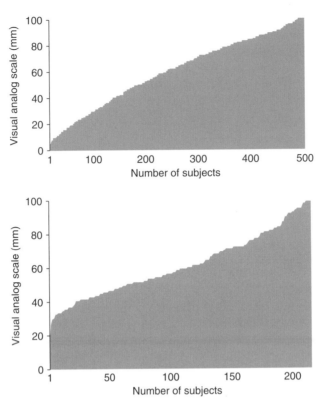

Figure 9.3 Broad range of responses to painful experimental stimuli (upper panel) and clinical stimuli (lower panel).

Target molecules for genetic variation include specialized pain transducing receptors expressed in primary afferent neurons, such as the heat/capsaicin sensing vanilloid receptor ionophore 1 (VR1), which is a heat-gated ion channel that has been proposed to mediate responses of small-diameter sensory neurons to moderate thermal stimuli (Caterina et al. 1997). Pain modulatory molecules expressed both centrally and peripherally, i.e., the opioid receptor genes, may also impact on individual pain sensitivity. Target molecules also include genes generally expressed that may have an influence on neurotransmitter metabolism, i.e. catechol O-methyltransferase (COMT) (Mannisto and Kaakkola 1999). An initial step for identifying genetic polymorphisms that may be associated with pain perception in humans is evaluating the effects of candidate genes, such as the VR1, the opiate delta receptor (OPRD1) and the COMT loci, on variation in experimental pain responses and their interactions with gender, ethnicity, and psychological factors on pain sensitivity in humans.

Recent observations suggest that gender, ethnicity and psychological state interact with genetic polymorphisms of molecules with important roles in sensory pain transduction. Gender was confirmed as an important factor in the response to both hot and cold experimental pain stimuli but was influenced by psychological factors characterized as harm avoidance, novelty seeking and persistence (Kim et al. 2004). Polymorphisms in genes that modulate nociceptive transduction (TRPV1) and opioid analgesia (OPRD1) also predict alterations in pain sensitivity. These results support complex interactions between pain sensitivity and genetic variation, gender, ethnicity and psychological factors. Moderate heritability estimates combined with these findings that TRPV1 and OPRD1 are linked to responses to painful stimuli support a genetic contribution to pain sensitivity in humans. Considering the genetic factors inherent in gender, ethnicity and psychological temperament, it is likely that genotypes functionally most important to pain have yet to be determined and may provide a basis for individualizing analgesic drug treatment.

HOW CAN WE TRANSLATE SCIENTIFIC ADVANCES INTO IMPROVED PAIN RELIEF?

Translating scientific advances into improved pain relief may be enhanced by developing a framework for change in the analgesic drug development process. A necessary first step is to improve clinical trials methodology in this area by developing consensus outcome measures for pain relief that are subjected to validation in clinical trials to provide an evidence-based approach to evaluating candidate analgesics. Useful drugs might have an anti-hyperalgesic effect, for example, that would be missed if only evaluating their activity of spontaneous pain. Such measures need to be sensitive to detect subtle therapeutic effects but robust enough to withstand the increased variability associated with multisite trials.

Individual responses (i.e., responder analyses) need to be considered in developing outcome measures for analgesic trials. Treatments that are effective for subgroups of patients within the population need to be detectable with prospectively designated outcome measures and may permit development of drugs with greater efficacy or safety for some patients, but not necessarily be detectable in large groups traditionally used in clinical trials. Individual responder measures might also help to identify genetic factors associated with the development and progression of chronic pain or responsiveness to the drug being evaluated.

It is likely that the potential of genomics and proteomics will permit a better description of the molecular-genetic basis of acute and chronic inflammation. These new tools and thinking will also probably lead to a deeper understanding of the plasticity in the nervous system that is thought to be an important component of chronic pain that no longer depends on obvious peripheral injury. It is likely that this new knowledge will lead to new drugs entering the drug development pipeline of the future. Existing clinical trial settings may only be capable of detecting drugs with a mechanism of action similar to already approved drugs that have been used to validate the clinical model, while screening out chemical entities with novel mechanisms of action. This circular process may lead to a failure to detect drugs acting through non-opioid or non-NSAID mechanisms as the investigational analgesic might not advance beyond the initial proof-of-concept studies. Given the high cost of analgesic drug development, new clinical models should be validated for the detection of non-traditional mechanisms of action – possibly including genotypically defined subgroups – that optimizes the chances for detecting useful drugs that might otherwise fail in a pivotal study.

The proceedings of the NIH-FDA workshops (Dionne and Witter 2003), the IMMPACT initiative and other workshops (Dionne et al. 2005) all support the need to enhance the scientific basis for analgesic drug development. The large unmet need for management of pain and suffering associated with chronic diseases such as cancer in vulnerable populations and at the end of life drives the search for new analgesics with greater efficacy and less morbidity than currently available drugs. Concern that emerging scientific opportunities are not translating into improved therapy for pain should motivate the development of improved, evidence-based strategies for target identification, development of drugs with additive selective actions, improved methods and the eventual development of interventions that interfere with the transition from acute pain and inflammation to chronic pain. Chronic pain that is treated from an understanding of its mechanistic and clinical perspectives, takes into consideration the wide inter-individual variation in pain and the response to analgesics, and is evaluated in models sensitive to these differences might be pain that is ultimately cured.

CONCLUSION

Despite better understanding of pain over the past two decades, few truly novel molecular entities designed to address a fundamentally new pathophysiologic mechanism underlying pain have entered the analgesic clinic to date. Understanding of analgesic mechanisms provides an opportunity to move forward to new ways of assessing analgesics in both animal models and clinical conditions based on understanding of the mechanisms involved rather than the empirical way that has driven analgesic development in the past. The way to move forward in analgesic drug development is to measure multiple signs and symptoms in patients, not just global measures, to look at the natural history, to validate mechanistic hypotheses, and to gain insight into the mechanisms that operate in the individual patient.

REFERENCES

Aubrun F, Langeron O, Quesnel C, et al. Relationship between measurement of pain using visual analog score and morphine requirements during postoperative intravenous morphine titration. Anesthesiology 2003; 98:1415–1421.

Barden J, Edwards JE, McQuay HJ, et al. Pain and analgesic response after third molar extraction and other postsurgical pain. Pain 2004; 107:86–90.

Bombardier C, Laine L, Reicin A, et al. Comparison of upper gastrointestinal toxicity of rofecoxib and naproxen in patients with rheumatoid arthritis. VIGOR Study Group. N Engl J Med 2000; 343:1520–1528.

Brennan TJ, Vandermeulen EP, Gebhart GF. Characterization of a rat model of incisional pain. Pain 1996; 64:493–501.

Caterina M, Schumacher M, Tominaga M, et al. The capsaicin receptor: heat activated ion channel in the pain pathway. Nature 1997; 389(23):816–24.

Coghill RC, Eisenach J. Individual differences in pain sensitivity: implications for treatment decisions. Anesthesiology 2003; 98:1312–1314.

Coghill RC, McHaffie JG, Yen YF. Neural correlates of interindividual differences in the subjective experience of pain. Proc Natl Acad Sci USA 2003; 100:8538–8542.

De Gaetano G, Donati MB, Cerletti C. Prevention of thrombosis and vascular inflammation: benefits and limitations of selective or combined COX-1, COX-2, and

5-LOX inhibitors. Trends Pharmacol Sci 2003; 24:245–252.

Desmeules JA, Decraschi C, Rapiti E, et al. Neurophysiologic evidence for central sensitization in patients with fibromyalgia. Arthritis Rheumatism 2003; 48:1420–1429.

Diaz-Reval MI, Ventura-Martinez R, Deciga-Campos M, et al. Evidence for a central mechanism of action of S-(+)-ketoprofen. Eur J Pharmacol 2004; 483(2–3):241–248.

Dionne RA, Berthold CB. Therapeutic uses of non-steroidal anti-inflammatory drugs in dentistry. Crit Rev Oral Biol Med 2001; 12:315–330.

Dionne RA, Witter J. NIH-FDA analgesic drug development workshop: translating scientific advances into improved pain relief. Clin J Pain 2003; 19:139–147.

Dionne RA, Bartoshuk L, Mogil J, et al. Individual responder analyses for pain: does one pain scale fit all? Trends Pharmacol Sci 2005; 26:125–130.

Eddy NB, May EL. The search for a better analgesic. Science 1973; 181:407–414.

Eisenach JC, Curry R, Hood DD, et al. Phase I safety assessment of intrathecal ketorolac. Pain 2002; 99:599–604.

Gagliese L, Katz J. Age differences in postoperative pain are scale dependent: a comparison of measures of pain intensity and quality in younger and older surgical patients. Pain 2003; 103:11–20.

Granot M, Lowenstein L, Yarnitsky D, et al. Postcesarean section pain prediction by preoperative experimental pain assessment. Anesthesiology 2003; 98:1422–1426.

Kim HS, Neubert JK, Iadarola MJ, et al. Genetic influence on pain sensitivity: evidence of heritability associated single nucleotide polymorphisms in opioid receptor genes. In: Proceedings of the World Congress on Pain. IASP Press, Seattle, WA, 2003: 513–520.

Kim H, Neubert JK, Dionne RA, et al. Genetic influence on variability in human acute experimental pain sensitivity associated with gender, ethnicity and psychological temperament. Pain 2004; 389(109):488–496.

Mannisto P, Kaakkola S. Catechol-O-methyltransferase (COMT) biochemistry, molecular biology, pharmacology, and clinical efficacy of the new selective COMT inhibitors. Pharmacol Rev 1999; 51(4):593–628.

Morrison BW, Daniels SE, Kotey P, et al. Rofecoxib, a specific cyclooxygenase-2 inhibitor, in primary dysmenorrhea: a randomized controlled trial. Obstet Gynecol 1999; 94:504–508.

Ploghaus A, Becerra L, Borras C, et al. Neural circuitry underlying pain modulation: expectation, hypnosis, placebo. Trends Cognitive Sci 2003; 7:197–200.

Reidenberg MM. Evolving ways that drug therapy is individualized. Clin Pharmacol Therap 2003; 74:197–202.

Scholz J, Woolf CJ. Can we conquer pain? Nature Neurosci 2002; suppl 5:1062–1067.

Silverstein FE, Faich G, Goldstein JL, et al. Gastrointestinal toxicity with celecoxib vs. nonsteroidal anti-inflammatory drugs for osteoarthritis and rheumatoid arthritis: the CLASS study. A randomized controlled trial. Celecoxib Long-Term Arthritis Safety Study. JAMA 2000; 284:1247–1255.

Tong SE, Daniels SE, Montano T, et al. SCIO-469, a novel P38A MAPK inhibitor, provides efficacy in acute post-surgical dental pain [abstract]. Clin Pharmacol Therap 2004; 75:P3.

Topol EJ. Failing the public health, Merck and the FDA. N Engl J Med 2004; 351:1707–1709.

Turk DC, Dworkin RH, Allen RR, et al. Core outcome measures for chronic pain clinical trials: IMMPACT recommendations. Pain 2003; 106:337–345.

Vane JR. Inhibition of prostaglandin synthesis as a mechanism of action for aspirin-like drugs. Nat New Biol 1971; 231:232–235.

Warner TD, Giuliano F, Vojnovic I, et al. Nonsteroid drug selectivities for cyclo-oxygenase-1 rather than cyclo-oxygenase-2 are associated with human gastrointestinal toxicity: a full in vitro analysis. Proc Natl Acad Sci USA 1999; 96:7563–7568.

Watkins LR, Maier SF. Glia: a novel drug discovery target for clinical pain. Nature Rev Drug Discov 2003; 2:973–985.

Watkins LR, Hansen MK, Nguyen KT, et al. Dynamic regulation of pro-inflammatory cytokine, interleukin-1β: molecular biology for non-molecular biologists. Life Sci 1999; 65:449–481.

Willis RC, Lesney MS. Pharmacogenomics: looking toward the payoff. Mod Drug Discov 2003; July:30–34.

Wolfe MM, Lichenstein DR, Singh G. Gastrointestinal toxicity of non-steroidal anti-inflammatory drugs. N Engl J Med 1999; 340:1888–1899.

Wong ML, Licino J. From monoamines to genomic targets: a paradigm shift for drug discovery in depression. Nature Rev Drug Discov 2004; 3:136–151.

Zhu XY, Conklin D, Eisenach JC. Cyclooxygenase-1 in the spinal cord plays an important role in postoperative pain. Pain 2003; 104:15–23.

Zubieta JK, Heitzeg MM, Smith YR, et al. COMT val15met genotype affects mu-opioid neurotransmitter responses to a pain stressor. Science 2003; 299(5610):1240–1243.

CHAPTER 10

Systematic reviews and meta-analyses of intervention studies

Athina Tatsioni • Joseph Lau

INTRODUCTION

The randomized controlled trial is generally considered the reference standard for the evaluation of therapeutic interventions, but uncertainties may arise when small clinical trials produce statistically nonsignificant results, and controversies may occur when trials report discrepant findings. Pain management is an area that crosses boundaries between specialties, often requiring the participation of health professionals from different disciplines. The study of analgesics still poses problems more than 50 years after Beecher first described the methods of measuring pain and pain relief (Denton and Beecher 1949; Houde et al. 1965). Problems can be diverse and various, starting with the many possible comparisons of drugs, doses, routes of administration and pain conditions that make comparisons difficult. The task for monitoring therapeutic developments and arriving at a coherent understanding of the appropriate use of interventions in this field, as in almost any field in medicine, becomes more complicated due to the overwhelming number of clinical studies that are published annually. Some 10,000 randomized controlled trials were identified for pain interventions in a study by Jadad et al. in 1996, of which over 4000 were in pharmacologic interventions in acute pain (Jadad et al. 1996). These numbers assuredly have greatly increased since then. In addition to the complexity of comparisons, a large number of randomized trials may be irrelevant to current medical practice, be overtly biased or be unusable for many other reasons.

The systematic review has been developed as a solution to assess comprehensively a large number of articles, to identify relevant studies and to summarize available evidence on specific clinical questions. It applies rigorous and transparent methods to minimize bias. Clear and precise research questions are formulated and then, a comprehensive literature search is conducted often using multiple databases. Selection of articles is based on carefully defined criteria, and selected articles are critically appraised for their methodologic quality and applicability to the target population. When appropriate, data which address a common outcome can be combined in a meta-analysis (Greenland and Robins 1994; Chalmers and Altman 1995; Lau et al. 1997).

Systematic reviews and meta-analyses are also useful to identify information gaps and limitations of existing literature. In 1986, the World Health Organization (WHO) released guidelines for cancer pain relief, which included the "three step using analgesic ladder" (WHO 1986). Their aim was to improve the management of cancer pain worldwide by using a limited number of inexpensive and well-known analgesics following a set of simple principles (WHO 1986; Cleeland 1990; Jacox et al. 1994). More than 10 years after the release of the first ladder draft of the guidelines, a systematic review showed that no controlled studies had yet been conducted to assess the proportion of patients in whom the use of the "ladder" results in adequate analgesia (Jadad and Browman 1995).

Since the early 1980s, systematic reviews and meta-analyses have increasingly been published in the medical literature. Applying the search term "meta-analysis" in MEDLINE in 2004 yielded more than 5000 articles. In a systematic review of pain treatments including 80 meta-analyses for analgesic interventions, two-thirds of the meta-analyses identified were published since 1990 (Jadad et al. 1996). Through 2000 there have been over 80 separate meta-analyses published for chronic pain (Fishbain et al. 2000).

Current initiatives, such as the Cochrane Collaboration, aim to produce and disseminate systematic reviews of randomized trials on healthcare interventions and to update them regularly with data from new randomized trials (Bero and Rennie 1995). Over 1800 completed systematic reviews and over 1300 protocols are included in the 4th quarter issue (2003) of the Cochrane Library. It has been estimated that at least 10,000 Cochrane reviews will be needed to cover most topics in healthcare interventions (Mallet and Clarke 2003). Another approach, taken by the US Agency for

Healthcare Research and Quality (AHRQ), is to produce comprehensive evidence reports and technology assessments on multiple and broad questions covering prevalence, diagnosis, and treatments. These reports and technology assessments are based on systematic reviews of the literature and include experimental and observational studies, as well as analyses of databases.

The purpose of this chapter is to provide users of systematic reviews and meta-analyses with an understanding of methods and limitations, with special emphasis on randomized controlled trials of pain interventions.

BASIC STEPS OF CONDUCTING A SYSTEMATIC REVIEW (TABLE 10.1)

FORMULATING THE RESEARCH QUESTION AND ESTABLISHING A PROTOCOL

Arguably the most important step in conducting a systematic review is formulating answerable research questions. Well-defined questions help to define the boundaries of the review protocol, the literature search strategy, the inclusion criteria and the analytic methods, as well as in the interpretation of the results.

The questions to be answered should be clearly defined. The PICO approach (i.e., patient, intervention, comparator and outcome) to specify parameters to be addressed is an increasingly common method to formulate research questions. For example, in the AHRQ evidence report on Cancer Pain Treatment, the basic question of "How to treat cancer pain?" is not one that

Table 10.1 Steps for conducting systematic reviews and meta-analyses

Steps	Tasks
Develop protocol	Formulate an answerable question Define and present robust research plan
Conduct literature search	Collect data from several different sources
Select studies Assess study quality	Assess features of studies that are important for the proper interpretation of the evidence
Extract data	Extract data, compare and resolve all discrepancies
Estimate treatment effect	Assess magnitude of the treatment effect using the appropriate effect measure
Choose statistical model*	Summarize the data using an appropriate statistical model (fixed effects model or random effects model)
Report results	Make a summary presentation of results by forest plots, scatter plots, box plots
Perform sensitivity analysis*	Assess heterogeneity using meta-regression analysis, subgroup analysis
Interpret results	Assess for publication bias

*Steps for meta-analysis.

is directly answerable (Goudas et al. 2001). This question was reformulated into six major questions and 20 more specific and directly answerable subquestions. After defining the target population and setting, interventions and comparators, the outcomes are then specified. The following research question could serve as an example: "What is the efficacy (e.g., pain intensity, the need for rescue medications) of NSAIDs compared to opioids in the management of patients with metastatic bone pain?" Only by formulating a series of well-focused and answerable research questions would we be able to attempt to answer the broader question. For the evaluation of most interventions, the PICO approach assumes that the type of studies to be analyzed is the randomized controlled trial. One might broaden this approach by including experimental as well as observational studies.

It is crucial that the reviewers develop a robust protocol, a detailed analytical plan, and a careful presentation plan equal to that of any good-quality clinical trial. Issues of multiple comparisons, specification of endpoints and data analysis also pertain to systematic reviews and meta-analyses. Exploratory analyses suggested by the data need not be prohibited and may even lead to hypotheses more interesting than the primary endpoint, but such analyses should be identified as exploratory. However, published data seldom allow one to construct such detailed subgroup analysis. The search strategy, data sources, and inclusion and exclusion criteria for the studies considered should be delineated. The modes of data extraction and validation should be specified. Analysis plans should be specified before the study begins, and the presentation of the results should follow a specified format.

PERFORMING THE LITERATURE SEARCH

Comprehensive searches of the literature should be conducted in systematic reviews to minimize bias in the selection of relevant articles (Helmer et al. 2001). Articles may need to be identified and collected from different sources. Because it is readily available and free, the literature search generally starts with the MEDLINE database. Through the efforts of volunteers worldwide performing manual searches of journals to identify controlled trials and retagging previously incorrectly indexed controlled trials, the Cochrane Library's Controlled Trials Registry is becoming an increasingly valuable source for searches. Depending on the topic and the availability of resources, additional electronic databases such as EMBASE (the electronic equivalent of Excerpta Medica) should also be searched.

Recent investigators have suggested the presence of a "Tower of Babel bias" in the publication of randomized trials (Egger et al. 1996). Egger at al. found that authors selectively publish positive studies in English language journals but negative studies in their native language journals. Thus, limiting the search to English-language evidence may distort results of a systematic review. However, a reverse language bias may also occur. Vickers et al. found that studies from certain countries consistently report mostly positive results (Vickers et al. 1998). Thus, including every study from these countries may also lead to biased conclusions. In many medical disciplines, the non-English literature of randomized trials has never been large, is shrinking even further, or may be of generally dubious quality. Before routinely committing to a specific approach, it would be useful to understand the contribution of different languages to the literature of the potential field.

Bibliographic databases are likely to become more inclusive and even larger in the future. However, electronic search strategies currently fail to identify all pertinent studies. Depending on the specific topic as well as the search strategy (sensitive strategies will identify a high proportion of relevant literature but at the cost of manually screening through many irrelevant articles), MEDLINE searches may identify 30–90% of relevant randomized controlled trials (Dickersin et al. 1994), although our experience suggests that the problem may not be that serious. In meta-analyses of analgesic interventions, MEDLINE identified 86% of the reports indexed by the US National Library of Medicine (Jadad et al. 1996). Reasons for missed retrieval include indexing errors and incorrect terms in the search strategy. Subject-specific databases, such as BIOSIS, CINAHL, and PsychLit, should be searched when appropriate.

Other methods for identifying information include manually searching through relevant journals, screening reference lists and trial registries, and personally contacting pharmaceutical and medical device companies, as well as colleagues and researchers who may be aware of other published or unpublished studies. Surveys of authors of previous studies, content experts, and colleagues who may know additional studies may yield low response rates (Hetherington et al. 1989). Other initiatives involve a proposal that would require the prospective registration of trial protocols in various medical fields, a concept proposed as the only means of ensuring access to complete information (Simes 1986; Stern and Simes 1997).

SELECTING STUDIES AND PERFORMING QUALITY ASSESSMENT ON THE ORIGINAL STUDIES

Studies identified through the literature search should be evaluated according to a pre-specified protocol using parameters defined in the PICO approach discussed earlier. Failure to adhere to a well-defined protocol may produce misleading results, especially if the exclusion of a relevant study or the inclusion of an inappropriate study leads to alteration of statistical significance of the meta-analysis. Some valid reasons for excluding a study from an analysis are the lack of reported data for an outcome, or extreme differences in patient or disease characteristics. Another reason is poor quality of study design. The studies included in a meta-analysis must have high degree of internal validity to produce reliable results, and issues related to the study quality should be incorporated into the meta-analysis.

Assessing the quality of a study can sometimes be difficult because quality can be inferred only from published information and often these data are poorly reported or unavailable. The quality of randomized trials has been assessed with scales that attempt to score various components of the study design, analysis, and reporting. One of the earliest scales assessed more than 30 different elements (Chalmers et al. 1981). Other scales, such as the one by Jadad (1993), focus on three study design and reporting issues including the adequacy of random assignment, blinding and patient withdrawals. A comprehensive review of the various quality scales was published by Moher et al. (1995). It concluded that among all the 25 quality scales that were examined in the review article, only one had evolved with standard scale development techniques. A recent empirical study called into question the validity of the use of any quality scales (Juni et al. 1999). This study examined 26 quality scales that calculated a score based on the evaluation of 3 to 35 quality-related items in one meta-analysis of 17 randomized controlled trials. It found that different quality scales could result in different conclusions; hence quality scales are inconsistent among themselves. The use of specific factors related to study quality has also been proposed. Although the use of specific quality measures may be appropriate in specific well-defined areas in which there is pertinent evidence, findings of associations with treatment effect cannot be generalized to all clinical areas or meta-analyses (Balk et al. 2002). Thus, it may be better to examine the impact of individual quality factors such as the adequacy of random assignment or masking on the summary estimate (Ioannidis and Lau 1998).

PERFORMING QUANTITATIVE SYNTHESIS OF DATA

Meta-analyses are often performed when there is sufficient amount of appropriate data to provide a more precise estimate of treatment effect. The most common type of meta-analysis involves a weighted average of the outcomes of the individual studies using one of the several statistical methods. Before undertaking a meta-analysis on a study question, appropriateness of combining studies should be assessed. Provided that more than one study addressed the study question, homogeneity should be identified among the studies. In the AHRQ report for Management of Cancer Pain (Goudas

et al. 2001), the possibility of performing a meta-analysis was evaluated by examining the following conditions that contributed to homogeneity among included studies:

- Whether the study evaluated pain as an outcome and which assessment instrument was used (i.e., VAS, Likert scale)
- Whether pain assessment data were provided and in what format (e.g., mean and standard deviation of VAS measures, graphical, descriptive)
- The study design, including its time course
- The study population (e.g., type of cancer, demographic characteristics, length of assessment period).

Meta-analysis can sometimes be performed on several studies evaluating different drugs belonging to the same class (i.e., different NSAIDs) to determine the class effect. However, when there are too few studies (two or three), such meta-analysis can be misleading. For example, two studies of different NSAIDs do not necessarily constitute a class effect because there are many different types of NSAIDs, and therefore a meta-analysis should not be performed. In addition, each of the studies used in the meta-analysis must have appropriately defined outcome measures and the necessary numerical data (outcome estimates and standard error or confidence intervals).

MEASURES OF TREATMENT EFFECT

Unless pain is assessed systematically using a validated scale across studies, it is difficult to judge the benefits, or lack thereof, of any analgesic regimen, let alone to compare one regimen with another (Jadad 1993; Max 1996; McQuay and Moore 1998). The 0–10 cm visual or verbal analog scales for both pain intensity and relief are validated and easily administered. Their use is common but by no means universal in clinical trials of pain relief. Categorical pain intensity and pain relief scales have also been used. Trials may report their results on 0–4 or 0–5 categorical scales. Some authors have suggested transforming a continuous scale to a categorical one, or vice versa. However, the validity of combining results of a categorical scale with those of a continuous scale has not been resolved.

Previous reports (Moore et al. 1996, 1997) have examined the hypothesis that, for pharmacologic interventions in acute pain, a relationship exists between the descriptive mean value for summed categorical pain relief (TOTPAR) and a dichotomous description of the same data set, and that knowing the relationship enables the conversion of descriptive mean values for pain relief into dichotomous data (relief of at least 50% pain) that can be used with confidence in meta-analysis. Similar results were shown when exploring whether mean data for categorical pain intensity scales and VAS for both pain intensity and relief could also be converted to the same dichotomous outcome, relief of at least 50% pain (Moore et al. 1997).

The number-needed-to-treat (NNT) has been proposed as an easy to interpret metric to communicate treatment effects for clinicians and patients. The number-needed-to-harm (NNH) has also been suggested as a metric to interpret harmful effects of treatments. NNT is calculated as the inverse of risk difference and requires dichotomous data; it involves defining a clinical endpoint, and comparing the rate of that event in a treatment group with the rate in a comparator group (Cook and Sackett 1995). Proponents argue for its usefulness in the comparisons of harms and benefits from treatment (Laupacis 1988; Sackett et al. 1989). Criticisms against its use has centered on its statistical properties and its name, which encourages individuals to think of it as precise and without probabilistic content (Hutton 2000). Additionally, patients can often misinterpret the meaning of NNT and it is suggested it should not be used alone to communicate risk to patients (Sheridan et al. 2003). On the other hand, patients are best able to interpret the benefits of treatment when presented as absolute risk reduction or in a relative risk reduction format with a given baseline risk disease (Sheridan et al. 2003).

In randomized controlled trials, "effect size" is generally referred to as the difference between outcomes in treatment arms of the study, not pretreatment versus post-treatment comparisons in the experimental group. Different approaches have been used to measure the outcome according to the setting in which it is appropriate.

When the outcomes reported by available large studies, which will be combined, are heterogeneous and not amenable to categorizing the effect size on the same scale, or when pain intensity has not been reported using a VAS, a qualitative score may be assigned for the effect size. The group of heterogeneous outcomes in pain treatment literature may include drug consumption, pain relief or quality of life related indices. In order to maintain consistency and directionality of the effect, pain management experts may characterize such outcomes as large, modest, as small beneficial effect or no beneficial effect (Goudas et al. 2001).

The issue that arises then is whether a single question about the overall effectiveness of an intervention could be asked of a patient which would be both simple to administer and provide relevant information about effectiveness. Collins et al. (2001) sought to answer this question in acute pain. They investigated the potential of using this simple global estimation as a measure of treatment efficacy by comparing it with at least 50% max-TOTPAR, a validated outcome of percentage of the maximum possible pain relief. This paper supports the view that a single global question about the overall effectiveness of an acute pain intervention can provide estimates of analgesic efficacy equivalent to those obtained by multiple questioning about pain relief (Collins et al. 2001).

The magnitude of the treatment effect may be expressed and summarized by different measures. For continuous outcomes, correlation coefficients or the mean difference in event rate between treatment and control groups and the standardized mean difference can be used when the scales used to measure the treatment effect differ among trials. The standardized mean difference (or "effect size") is the ratio of the difference between the mean in the treatment group and the mean in the control group divided by the standard deviation in the control group. The use of means to describe asymmetrically distributed data has been shown to yield erroneous conclusions (McQuay et al. 1996). Information for many thousands of published papers becomes invalid for use in meta-analysis because analgesic trials conventionally have reported data as means. Transformation of continuous metric to categorical (TOTPAR) or dichotomous (50% TOTPAR) metric may deal more successfully with this problem.

For binary data, measures of the treatment effect include the risk difference (and its inverse, the NNT), the risk ratio, and the odds ratio (McQuay and Moore 1997). The risk difference is the difference in the event rates of the treatment and control groups, whereas the odds ratio and risk ratio provide relative measures of the treatment effect. Ideally, all measures should be considered because they provide complementary information (Sinclair and Bracken 1994).

In practice, risk and odds ratios tend to be more consistent across studies than risk differences. In some cases, either the odds or the risk ratio may seem more appropriate, but in most circumstances, one ratio functions as well as the other for summarizing the data (Deeks et al. 1997). The practical advantages of the odds ratio include the ability to take any positive value and its direct correspondence to logistic regression when binary data are considered. The advantage of the risk ratio is that it does not inflate the magnitude of the treatment effect, as the odds ratio does when it is used as a proxy for risk ratio, especially when the event rates are high.

CHOOSING A STATISTICAL MODEL

To summarize the data, each study is given a weight that depends on the precision of its results. The weight is generally estimated as the inverse of the variance of the estimated treatment effect in each study. This variance of the estimated treatment effect has two components: the variance of the individual study (the within-study variance) and the variance between different studies (the between-study variance). The simplest approach to thinking about combining different results is to assume that all studies have approximated the same fixed truth and that differences among the observed treatment effects are only the results of random error. In this case, the between-study variance is assumed to be zero, and the calculations are performed with what are called "fixed-effects models." Fixed-effects models are exemplified by the Mantel–Haenszel method (Mantel and Haenszel 1959) and the Peto method (Fleiss 1993) in the case of dichotomous data.

On the other hand, if the "truth" itself is not fixed but is believed to vary within a range of values, then each study can be seen as addressing a different true treatment effect, and these treatment effects derive from a distribution of truths with a variance equal to the between-study variance. In this case, calculations are performed with random effects models, which add the between-study variance to the within-study variance of each study. The most commonly used random effects model is that proposed by DerSimonian and Laird (1986). More sophisticated, fully Bayesian approaches may also be used to calculate the between-study variance (Smith et al. 1995). Fixed- and random-effects methods have also been developed for continuous outcomes (Hedges and Olkin 1985).

Ideally, both fixed- and random-effects calculations should be performed and their results compared. When the results are significantly heterogeneous, the fixed-effects models are counterintuitive and should be avoided. Usually, fixed- and random-effects estimates are similar, but exceptions can occur (Borzak and Ridker 1995). In terms of precision, random effects are almost invariably associated with larger confidence intervals when heterogeneity is present because between-trial uncertainty is introduced. Compared to the DerSimonian and Laird estimates, fully Bayesian methods may result in even wider confidence intervals.

Generally, Mantel–Haenszel estimates work well even with small numbers (Emerson 1994), whereas random effects estimates are unstable. The Peto fixed-effects model may be associated with large bias when the data are unbalanced (Greenland and Salvan 1990). With the increasing popularity of meta-analysis, several easy-to-use software programs to combine data have become available (Egger et al. 1998). However, the informed researcher should be aware of the preceding caveats and should understand which formulas the software uses.

A common problem of using meta-analysis to combine studies with continuous data is that the outcomes (e.g., pain score and standard error) may be reported as the pre- and post-treatment group means for the treatment and control group; however, correlated standard errors might not be reported. In such cases, assumptions need to be made to estimate the correlated standard error in order to perform a meta-analysis (Ballantyne et al. 1998).

TOTPAR is calculated as the area under the curve of pain relief/intensity (categorical scale) against time,

and the percentage of the maximum possible for this summary measure is then calculated (% maxTOTPAR) (Cooper 1991). Finally, if NNT is used it is calculated according to the method of Cook and Sackett (1995).

Figure 10.1 shows the typical summary presentation of the results of a meta-analysis. Each study is shown with its point estimate and confidence intervals (CI; typically the 95% CI). The summary estimate and its 95% CI are also presented.

PUBLICATION BIAS

Even comprehensive searches of the literature (including gray literature) and the use of other less formal methods, such as personal communication, may not produce an unbiased sample of studies when conducting a meta-analysis. Research with statistically significant results is potentially more likely to be submitted, published or published more rapidly than work with null or non-significant results (Easterbrook et al. 1991; Ioannidis 1998). A meta-analysis of only the identified published studies may lead to an overoptimistic conclusion. This problem is known as publication bias (Begg and Berlin 1989).

Funnel plot has been proposed as a method to assess the potential for publication bias. Small studies have greater variation in their estimation of the treatment effect and will be found to have more scattering around the mean effect, compared to the larger studies. In a funnel plot, the weight of each study, the sample size or the inverse of the variance, is plotted against the size of its treatment effect in a meta-analysis. This plot should be shaped like an inverted funnel if there is no publication bias while asymmetric funnel plots may suggest publication bias. Nevertheless, there needs

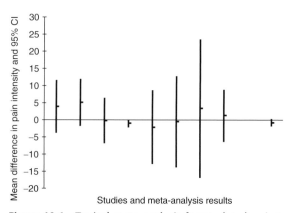

Figure 10.1 Typical meta-analysis forest plot showing the estimates and the 95% confidence intervals of 8 studies and the overall meta-analysis result (rightmost plot). Data are from a meta-analysis comparing controlled-released morphine versus oral aqueous morphine. (Goudas L, Carr DB, Bloch R, et al. Management of Cancer Pain, AHRQ Publication No. 02-E002. Agency for Health Care Research and Quality, Rockville, MD, 2001.)

to be a range of studies with varying sizes for a funnel plot to be useful. It should also be stressed that a skewed funnel plot may be caused by factors other than publication bias, such as the study quality, the different intensity of intervention, differences in underlying risk, choice of effect measure and chance (Tang and Liu 2000; Thornton and Lee 2000). Finally, funnel plot interpretation is subjective and is only an informal method.

Formal statistical tests have also been described to assess publication bias, such as the rank correlation test by Begg and Mazumdar (1994), the linear regression test suggested by Egger (1997) as well as the "trim and fill" method (Duval and Tweedie 2000). Besides these methods, which are based on funnel plot, other statistical methods handling publication bias include the Rosenthal's file drawer method, the estimation of the number of the unpublished studies and the selection modeling method. Although selection modeling seems to be a promising method, further research is needed on this field.

Methods for detecting or correlating for publication bias are based on certain assumptions that may not be true in all circumstances. These methods may introduce bias themselves if the assumptions are not valid. For the time being, it would be difficult to offer practical advice on which test to use as they appear to come to contrasting conclusions a large proportion of time (Sutton et al. 2000).

PERFORMING THE SENSITIVITY ANALYSIS

A common criticism of meta-analysis is that the analyst is combining apples and oranges. There is a widespread misconception that the goal of meta-analysis is to force heterogeneous results from individual studies into a single estimate. Although obtaining a single treatment effect may be appropriate in many circumstances, a more interesting application of meta-analysis is to explore heterogeneity among different trials and to understand possible reasons for these differences. The test most commonly used for heterogeneity is based on the chi-square distribution but tends to be insensitive, so a high p-value is generally recommended to be significant at $P < 0.10$ (Lau et al. 1997). However, the failure to detect heterogeneity among different trial results does not mean that it does not exist. Significant heterogeneity suggests that the studies perhaps should not be combined to yield a single overall estimate. The analyst should try to identify reasons for heterogeneity among the studies.

Meta-regression analysis. Meta-regression analysis uses the individual study as the unit of observation in assessing the relationship between the magnitude of the treatment effect and different predictors (Smith et al. 1993; Thompson 1993; Berlin and Antman 1994). Predictors may be study-specific (e.g., the dose or route of

administration of a drug) or ecologic variables in which a mean or median value is taken as characteristic of the study group of patients (e.g., mean age or percentage of men).

In addition to these potentially subjective covariates, others are always available in clinical trials, regardless of the topic, and may thus be used as standard probes in the assessment and interpretation of among-study heterogeneity. These other covariates include the sample size, the variance of the results and the rate of events in the control group.

Meta-regression analyses of the treatment effect on sample size or variance may be useful in assessing the potential for publication bias, in particular the lack of publication of small studies with negative results (Egger et al. 1997).

The control rate reflects the risk of the study cohort and should therefore be interpreted cautiously because it does not predict for individual patients. Patients enrolled even in trials with fairly strict enrollment criteria may still be widely heterogeneous (Ioannidis and Lau 1997). Generally, the minority of high-risk patients tends to contribute the majority of the events of interest. Thus, a meta-regression analysis suggesting that benefit is seen only when the event rate of the entire control group is above, say, 7% may simply be reflecting the fact that a high-risk portion of the control group experienced an event rate of, say, 30% or higher and that these patients were those who benefited from the treatment.

META-ANALYSIS OF INDIVIDUAL PATIENT DATA (MIPD)

Most meta-analyses conducted to date used summary data from individual studies or subgroups thereof. Meta-analyses using individual patient data (MIPD) from all the pertinent studies are not new, but only a relatively small number have been conducted. The MIPD approach provides several clear advantages, such as closer involvement of the participating investigators and trialists; the ability to verify and update the data collected within the included studies; the possibility of more detailed time-to-event analyses; the ability to generate individual-based predictive models; and the chance to assess the effect of various predictors at the individual patient level to avoid potential ecologic fallacies of using summary data (Stewart and Clarke 1995). The disadvantages of this approach include the potential for retrieval bias when trials whose data are not retrievable are excluded; the potentially lower quality of updated data that have been accumulated after the end of the main follow-up period of a randomized trial (such as extensive crossovers or incomplete information on many patients); and the time and effort required to obtain data from a multitude of investigators and trialists groups. The first two reasons could theoretically make MIPD even less reliable than meta-analyses of published group data in some circumstances. Such studies should be encouraged, however, and may become the way of the future, especially with prospective meta-analyses. Early reports have suggested that the estimates obtained by MIPD may occasionally differ from the estimates of conventional meta-analyses of the literature on the same topic (Stewart and Parmar 1993; Jeng et al. 1995), but the extent and frequency of the discrepancies need to be evaluated in a larger number of examples.

QUALITY OF META-ANALYSES

A large number of meta-analyses are published each year and their overall quality is becoming a concern (Moher and Olkin 1995; Bailar 1997). Results in a review on assessing quality of meta-analyses on chronic pain treatment showed that half of the procedures examined were not adequately implemented (Fishbain 2000). These procedures included publication bias, data extraction, assessment of quality of included studies and homogeneity of included studies (Fishbain 2000). In a previous study (Jadad and McQuay 1996), meta-analyses of analgesic interventions showed that there were methodologic deficiencies that may limit the validity of their conclusions. Problems were described in reporting the method used to assess the validity of the combined studies, in the description of design features of the primary studies and to a lesser extent in the description of the clinical setting, the outcome variables, the statistical methods for combining data or the conclusion of the analysis (Jadad and McQuay 1996). Moreover, several examples have been identified showing conflicting results between separate meta-analyses evaluating the same intervention (Jadad and McQuay 1996).

In an effort to address standards for improving the quality of reporting of meta-analyses of clinical randomized controlled trials, the Quality of Reporting of Meta-analyses (QUOROM) conference was held in October 1996 (Moher et al. 1999). The QUOROM group consisted of clinical epidemiologists, clinicians, statisticians, editors and researchers. In conference, the group was asked to identify items they thought should be included in a checklist of standards. Whenever possible, checklist items were guided by research evidence suggesting that failure to adhere to the item proposed could lead to biased results. The conference resulted in the QUOROM statement, which consists of a checklist and a flow diagram (Moher et al. 1999). The checklist described a way that might be appropriate to present the abstract, introduction, methods, results and discussion sections of a report of a meta-analysis. It is organized into 21 headings and subheadings and encourages authors to provide readers with information regarding search strategies, selection criteria, validity assessment, data abstraction, study characteristics, quantitative data synthesis and trial flow (Moher et al. 1999). The flow diagram provides information about the progress of randomized trials throughout the review process regarding the numbers of RCTs identified, included and excluded and the reasons for exclusion of trials (Moher et al. 1999).

READING AND INTERPRETING A META-ANALYSIS

Systematic reviews and meta-analyses, like any clinical study, must be read carefully and their strengths and limitations recognized. The same rules for conducting a meta-analysis should be applied to its interpretation. The published article should provide the protocol and data from individual studies in sufficient detail to allow the reader to verify the results. Several authors have described the sources of bias and error during the design, conduct and analysis of meta-analyses (Goldman 1979; Fleiss and Gross 1991; Thompson and Pocock 1991; Felson 1992) and at least one instrument has been developed according to conventional methodologic standards to assess the methodologic rigor or scientific quality of review articles (Oxman and Guyatt 1991). Authors have pointed out that meta-analyses of pain literature should be scrutinized closely (Fishbain 1996; Max 1996; Goodkin et al. 1998; McQuay and Moore 1998).

The basic questions that the clinician and investigator should ask are as follows:

- Was the meta-analysis performed according to a defined protocol?
- Were the questions well formulated and would the answers to them be clinically useful?
- Was a thorough literature search implemented and the search strategy reported adequately?
- Were explanations provided for exclusion of studies?
- Were the studies used in the meta-analysis assessed for their internal validity?
- Were the treatments well described and similar to what I would plan to use?
- Were the patients included in the meta-analysis similar to my patients?
- Were the clinical outcomes well defined and useful?
- Were the characteristics of the individual studies listed with sufficient detail to allow an assessment of the appropriateness of their inclusion?
- Were the outcome data provided for the treatment and control groups?
- Was the definition of the treatment effect meaningful?
- Were the confidence intervals, rather than p values, given for the statistically combined results?
- Did the meta-analysis provide an estimate of the baseline risk?
- Were limitations of the meta-analysis discussed?

Considering the overwhelming number of clinical studies on pain interventions that is continuously increasing, it is very important to combine the data that are available to form valid recommendations for clinical practice. Systematic reviews and meta-analyses have proved to play a major role for this in several fields such as pain treatment. Nevertheless, even these procedures are still evolving and may present with certain limitations.

CONCLUSION

Systematic reviews and meta-analyses have been developed as a solution to comprehensively assess a large number of articles, to identify relevant studies and to summarize available evidence on specific clinical questions. Pain management is an area with great complexity, regarding the number of published trials and the diversity of comparisons. Consequently, systematic reviews and meta-analyses could play a major role in evaluating pain interventions. The methods that are applied in systematic reviews and meta-analyses should be rigorous and transparent, their main purpose being to minimize bias.

REFERENCES

Bailar JC 3rd. The promise and problems of meta-analysis. N Engl J Med 1997; 337:559–561.

Balk E, Bonis P, Moskowitz H, et al. Correlation of quality measures with estimates of treatment effect in meta-analysis of randomized controlled trials. JAMA 2002; 287:2973–2982.

Ballantyne JC, Carr DB, deFerranti SD, et al. The comparative effects of postoperative analgesic therapies on pulmonary outcome: cumulative meta-analysis of randomized controlled trials. Anesth Analg 1998; 86:598–612.

Begg CB, Berlin JA. Publication bias and dissemination of clinical research. J Natl Cancer Inst 1989; 81:107–115.

Begg CB, Mazumdar M. Operating characteristics of a rank correlation test for publication bias. Biometrics 1994; 50:1088–1101.

Berlin JA, Antman EM. Advantages and limitations of meta-analytic regressions of clinical trials data. Online J Curr Clin Trials 1994, Doc No 134.

Bero L, Rennie D. The Cochrane Collaboration: preparing, maintaining, and disseminating systematic reviews on the effects of health care. JAMA 1995; 274:1935–1938.

Borzak S, Ridker PM. Discordance between meta-analyses and large-scale randomized, controlled trials. Ann Intern Med 1995; 123:873–877.

Chalmers I, Altman DG. Systematic Reviews. BMJ Publishing, London, 1995.

Chalmers TC, Smith H Jr, Blackburn B, et al. A method for assessing the quality of a randomized control trial. Controlled Clin Trials 1981; 2:231–249.

Cleeland CS. Demonstration projects for cancer pain relief. In: Foley KM, Bonica JJ, Ventafridda V, Callaway MV

(eds). Advances in Pain Research and Therapy. Raven Press, New York, 1990.

Collins SL, Edwards J, Moore RA, et al. Seeking a simple measure of analgesia for mega-trials: is a single global assessment good enough? Pain 2001; 91(1–2):189–194.

Cook RJ, Sackett DL. The number needed to treat: a clinically useful measure of treatment effect. Br Med J 1995; 310:452–454.

Cooper SA. Single-dose analgesic studies: the upside and downside of assay sensitivity. In: Max MB, Portenoy RK, Laska EM (eds). The Design of Analgesic Clinical Trials: Advances in Pain Research and Therapy. Raven Press, New York, 1991.

Deeks JJ, Altman DG, Dooley G, et al. Choosing an appropriate dichotomous effect measure for meta-analysis: empirical evidence of the appropriateness of the odds ratio and relative risk. Controlled Clin Trials 1997; 18:84S–85S.

Denton JE, Beecher HK. New analgesics. JAMA 1949; 141:1051–1057.

DerSimonian R, Laird N. Meta-analysis in clinical trials. Controlled Clin Trials 1986; 7:177–188.

Dickersin K, Scherer R, Lefebvre C. Identifying studies for systematic reviews. Br Med J 1994; 309:1286–1291.

Duval S, Tweedie R. Trim and fill: a simple funnel plot based method of testing and adjusting for publication bias in meta-analysis. Biometrics 2000; 56(2):455–463.

Easterbrook P, Berlin JA, Gopalan R, et al. Publication bias in clinical research. Lancet 1991; 337:867–872.

Egger M, Zellweger T, Antes G. Randomised trials in German language journals. Lancet 1996; 347:1047–1048.

Egger M, Smith GD, Schneider M, et al. Bias in meta-analysis detected by a single, graphical test. Br Med J 1997; 315:629–634.

Egger M, Sterne JAC, Smith GD. Meta-analysis software [BMJ website]. BMJ 1998;316:221–225 (17 January). Available at: http://bmj.com.archieve/7126/7126ed9.htm.

Emerson JD. Combining estimates of the odds ratio: the state of the art. Stat Meth Med Res 1994; 3:157–178.

Felson D. Bias in meta-analysis. J Clin Epidemiol 1992; 45:885–892.

Fishbain DA. Meta-analysis results: application to pain forum format. Pain Forum 1996; 5:279–280.

Fishbain D, Cutler R, Rosomoff H, et al. What is the quality of the implemented meta-analytic procedures in chronic pain treatment meta-analysis? Clin J Pain 2000; 16(1):73–85.

Fleiss JL. The statistical basis of meta-analysis. Stat Meth Med Res 1993; 2:121–145.

Fleiss JL, Gross AG. Meta-analysis in epidemiology, with special reference to studies of the association between exposure to environmental tobacco smoke and lung cancer: a critique. J Clin Epidemiol 1991; 44:127–139.

Goldman L, Feinstein AR. Anticoagulants and myocardial infarction: the problems of pooling, drowning and floating. Ann Intern Med 1979; 90:92–94.

Goodkin K, Feaster DJ, Baldewicz T. Meta-analysis: a time for closer scrutiny in applications to pain research? Pain Forum 1998; 7:100–103.

Goudas L, Carr DB, Bloch R, et al. Management of Cancer Pain. Evidence Report/Technology No. 35 (prepared by the New England Medical Center Evidence-based Practice Center under Contract No 290-97-0019). AHRQ

Publication No. 02-E002. Agency for Health Care Research and Quality, Rockville, MD, 2001.

Greenland S, Robins J. Invited commentary: ecologic studies: biases, misconceptions, and counterexamples. Am J Epidemiol 1994; 139:747–760.

Greenland S, Salvan A. Bias in the one step method for pooling study results. Stat Med 1990; 9:247–252.

Hedges LV, Olkin I. Statistical methods for meta-analysis. Academic Press, Orlando, FL, 1985.

Helmer D, Savoie I, Green C, et al. Evidence-based practice: extending the search to find material for the systematic review. Bull Med Libr Assoc 2001; 89(4):346–352.

Hetherington J, Dickersin K, Chalmers I, et al. Retrospective and prospective identification of unpublished controlled trials: lessons from a survey of obstetricians and pediatricians. Pediatrics 1989; 84:374–380.

Houde RW, Wallenstein SL, Beaver WT. Clinical measurement of pain. In: De Stevens G (ed). Analgesics. Academic Press, New York/London, 1965.

Hutton JL. Number needed to treat: properties and problems. J R Stat Soc A 2000; 163:403–419.

Ioannidis JP. Effect of the statistical significance of results on the time to completion and publication of randomized efficacy trials. JAMA 1998; 279(4):281–286.

Ioannidis JP, Lau J. The impact of high risk patients on the results of clinical trials. J Clin Epidemiol 1997; 50:1089–1098.

Ioannidis JP, Lau J. Can quality of clinical trials and meta-analyses be quantified? [commentary]. Lancet 1998; 352:590–591.

Jacox A, Carr DB, Payne R. New clinical practice guidelines for the management of pain in patients with cancer. N Engl J Med 1994; 330:651–655.

Jadad AR. Meta-analysis of randomised clinical trials in pain relief [thesis]. Oxford University, 1993.

Jadad AR, Browman GP. The WHO analgesic ladder for cancer pain management: stepping up the quality of its evaluation. JAMA 1995; 274(23):1870–1873.

Jadad AR, McQuay HJ. Meta-analysis to evaluate analgesic interventions: a systematic qualitative review of their methodology. J Clin Epidemiol 1996; 49(2):235–243.

Jadad AR, Caroll D, Moore A, et al. Developing a database of published reports of randomized clinical trials in pain research. Pain 1996; 66:239–246.

Jeng GT, Scott JR, Burmeister LF. A comparison of meta-analytic results using literature vs. individual patient data. Paternal cell immunization for recurrent miscarriage. JAMA 1995; 274:830–836.

Juni P, Witschi A, Bloch R, et al. The hazards of scoring the quality of clinical trials for meta-analysis. JAMA 1999; 282(11):1054–1060.

Lau J, Ioannidis JPA, Schmid CH. Quantitative synthesis in systematic reviews. Ann Intern Med 1997; 27:820–826.

Laupacis A, Sackett D, Roberts R. An assessment of clinically useful measures of the consequences of treatment. N Engl J Med 1988; 318:1728–1733.

Mallett S, Clarke M. How many Cochrane reviews are needed to cover existing evidence on the effect of health care interventions? ACP J Club 2003; July/August: A11–A12.

Mantel N, Haenszel W. Statistical aspects of the analysis of data from retrospective studies of disease. J Natl Cancer Inst 1959; 22:719–748.

Max B. Collecting better data about drug treatments for chronic pain. In: Cohen B, Campbell B (eds). Pain Treatment Centers at the Crossroads: A Practical and Conceptual Reappraisal. IASP Press, Seattle, 1996.

McQuay HJ, Moore RA. Using numerical results from systematic reviews in clinical practice. Ann Intern Med 1997; 126:712–720.

McQuay H, Moore A. An Evidence-Based Resource for Pain Relief. Oxford University Press, Oxford, 1998.

McQuay H, Carroll D, Moore A. Variation in the placebo effect in randomized controlled trials of analgesics: all is as blind as it seems. Pain 1996; 64:331–335.

Moher D, Olkin I. Meta-analysis of randomized controlled trials: a concern for standards. JAMA 1995; 274:1962–1964.

Moher D, Jadad AR, Nichol G, et al. Assessing the quality of randomized controlled trials: an annotated bibliography of scales and checklists. Controlled Clin Trials 1995; 16:62–73.

Moher D, Cook D, Eastwood S, et al. for the QUOROM Group. Improving the quality of reports of meta-analyses of randomised controlled trials: the QUOROM statement. Quality of Reporting of Meta-analyses. Lancet 1999; 354:1896–1900.

Moore A, McQuay H, Gavaghan D. Deriving dichotomous outcome measures from continuous data in randomized controlled trials of analgesics. Pain 1996; 66:229–237.

Moore A, McQuay H, Gavaghan D. Deriving dichotomous outcome measures from continuous data in randomized controlled trials of analgesics: verification with independent data. Pain 1997; 69:127–130.

Oxman AD, Guyatt GH. Validation of an index of the quality of review articles. J Clin Epidemiol 1991; 44:1271–1278.

Sackett D. Inference and decision at bedside. J Clin Epidemiol 1989; 42:309–316.

Sheridan SL, Pignone MP, Lewis CL. A randomized comparison of patients' understanding of number needed to treat and other common risk reduction formats. J Gen Intern Med 2003; 18:884–892.

Sinclair JC, Bracken MB. Clinically useful measures of effect in binary analyses of randomized trials. J Clin Epidemiol 1994; 47:712–720.

Simes RJ. Publication bias: the case for an international registry of clinical trials. J Clin Oncol 1986 Oct; 4(10): 1529–1541.

Smith GD, Song F, Sheldon RA. Cholesterol lowering and mortality: the importance of considering initial level of risk. Br Med J 1993; 306:1367–1373.

Smith TC, Spiegelhalter DJ, Thomas A. Bayesian approaches to random effects meta-analysis: a comparative study. Stat Med 1995; 14:2685–2699.

Stern JM, Simes RJ. Publication bias: evidence of delayed publication in a cohort study of clinical research projects. BMJ 1997 Sep 13; 315(7109):640–645.

Stewart LA, Clarke MJ. Practical methodology of meta-analyses (overviews) using updated individual patient data. Cochrane Working Group. Stat Med 1995; 14:2057–2079.

Stewart LA, Parmar MKB. Meta-analysis of the literature or of individual patient data: is there a difference? Lancet 1995; 341:418–422.

Sutton AJ, Duval SJ, Tweedie RL, et al. Empirical assessment of effect of publication bias on meta-analyses. Br Med J 2000; 10(320(7249)):1574–1577.

Tang JL, Liu JLY. Misleading funnel plot for detection of bias in meta-analysis. J Clin Epidemiol 2000; 53:477–484.

Thompson SG. Controversies in meta-analysis: the case of the trials of serum cholesterol reduction. Stat Meth Med Res 1993; 2:173–192.

Thompson SG, Pocock SJ. Can meta-analysis be trusted? Lancet 1991; 338:1127–1130.

Thornton A, Lee P. Publication bias in meta-analysis: its causes and consequences. J Clin Epidemiol 2000; 53:207–216.

Vickers A, Goyal N, Harland R, et al. Do certain countries produce only positive results? A systematic review of controlled trials. Controlled Clin Trials 1998; 19:159–166.

World Health Organization. Cancer Pain Relief. World Health Organization, Geneva, 1986.

CHAPTER 11

Applying the ICF and ICF Core Sets for chronic widespread pain

Alarcos Cieza • Gerold Stucki

INTRODUCTION

There are a large number of health conditions that present chronic generalized pain or chronic widespread pain (CWP). Although there is not a universally accepted definition of CWP, there is increasing agreement that CWP represents pain involving several regions of the body. This conceptualization has been applied both in the diagnosis of fibromyalgia (Wolfe et al. 1990) as well as in epidemiologic studies (Macfarlane et al. 1996).

All conditions associated with CWP carry a high level of burden. Problems in functioning, psychological distress, fatigue, poor sleep quality and difficulties in activities of daily living (ADL) have consistently been reported as related to CWP in the literature (Yunus et al. 1981; Prescott et al. 1993; Wolfe et al. 1995; Aaron et al. 2002; Leveille et al. 2001). However, no systematic framework that covers the spectrum of symptoms and limitations in functioning of patients with CWP has been established so far.

Therefore, it would be valuable for clinical practice, research, and teaching to define the spectrum of symptoms and limitations in functioning of patients with CWP.

The approval of the new International Classification of Functioning, Disability and Health (ICF) (World Health Organization 2001) enables us to define the typical spectrum of problems in functioning of patients with CWP under consideration of influential environmental factors and using a globally agreed-upon language of functioning and health.

The objective of this chapter is to outline how the ICF can serve as a new global language of functioning and health and hence become a new approach for our understanding of the impact of CWP. The specific aims are to (1) introduce the ICF and the ICF Core Sets for CWP, (2) demonstrate how the ICF can be used to compare the content of health status measures, (3) demonstrate how the ICF and the ICF Core Sets can be used in clinical practice and (4) point to future applications of the ICF and ICF Core Sets for CWP.

THE INTERNATIONAL CLASSIFICATION OF FUNCTIONING DISABILITY AND HEALTH

The ICF is the World Health Organization's (WHO) framework for measuring health and disability at both individual and population levels. While the

International Classification of Diseases (ICD-10) classifies diseases as causes of death, ICF classifies health.

The ICF, as a classification, provides the means to map the different constructs and domains to describe the process of functioning and disability (WHO 2001; Stucki et al. 2002a). Accordingly, the ICF contains lists of so-called ICF categories organized in three different components: (1) *Body Functions and Structures*, (2) *Activities and Participation* and (3) *Environmental Factors*. Body Functions (b), Body Structures (s) and Activities and Participation (d) belong to the part *Functioning and Disability*. Environmental factors belong to the part *Contextual Factors*. *Personal Factors*, which constitute the fourth component of the classification and belong to the part *Contextual Factors* as well, have not yet been classified. The ICF categories represent the units of the ICF classification. Within the hierarchical code system of the ICF classification, the ICF categories are designated by the letters b, s, d, and e, followed by a numeric code starting with the chapter number (one digit), followed by the second level (two digits) and the third and fourth levels (one digit each). Thus, within each chapter, there are individual two-, three- or four-level categories.

The understanding of the interactions between the components of the ICF is shown in Figure 11.1.

A health condition is an umbrella term for disease, disorder, injury or trauma and may also include other circumstances, such as aging, stress, congenital anomaly or genetic predisposition. It may also include information about pathogeneses and/or etiology. There are (possible) interactions with all components of functioning: *body functions* and *structures*, *activity and participation*.

Body functions are defined as the physiologic functions of body systems, including psychological functions. *Body structures* are the anatomical parts of the body, such as organs, limbs and their components. Abnormalities of function, as well as abnormalities of structure, are referred to as *impairments*, which are defined as a significant deviation or loss (e.g., deformity) of structures (e.g., joints) and/or functions (e.g., reduced range of motion (ROM), muscle weakness, pain, fatigue).

Activity is the execution of a task or action by an individual and represents the individual perspective of functioning. *Participation* refers to the involvement of an individual in a life situation and represents the societal perspective of functioning. Difficulties at the activity level are referred to as *activity limitation* (e.g., limitations in mobility, such as walking and climbing steps). Problems an individual may experience in his/her involvement in life situations are denoted as *participation restriction* (e.g., restrictions in community life, recreation and leisure, but may be in walking, too, if walking is an aspect of participation in terms of life situation).

The contextual factors represent the complete background of an individual's life and living situation. Within the contextual factors, the *environmental factors* constitute the physical, social and attitudinal environment in which people live and conduct their lives. These factors are external to individuals and can have a positive or negative influence, i.e., they can represent a *facilitator* or a *barrier* for the individual. *Personal factors* are the particular background of an individual's life and living situation and comprise features that are not part of a health condition, i.e., gender, age, race, fitness, lifestyle, habits and social background. Risk factors could thus be described in both personal factors (e.g., lifestyle, genetic kit) and environmental factors (e.g., architectural barriers, living and work conditions). Risk factors are not only associated with the onset, but interact with the disabling process at each stage.

Within this context, *functioning* is an umbrella term for body functions, body structures, activities and participation. Functioning denotes the positive aspects of the interaction between an individual (with a health condition) and the contextual factors of this individual.

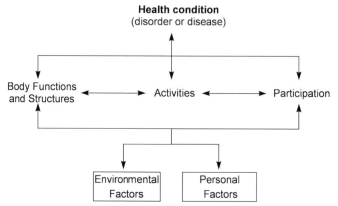

Figure 11.1 The current framework of functioning and disability: the WHO International Classification of Functioning, Disability and Health (ICF).

Disability is an umbrella term for impairments at the body level, activity limitations, and participation restrictions. Disability denotes the negative aspects of the interaction between an individual (with a health condition) and the contextual factors of this individual.

ICF CORE SETS FOR CWP

All member states of the WHO are now called upon to implement the ICF into a number of sectors that include, besides health, education, insurance, labor, health and disability policy and health statistics. To implement the ICF into medicine and other fields, practical tools need to be developed. Considering the length of the classification with more than 1400 categories, the main challenge is feasibility. To address this challenge, so-called ICF Core Sets have been jointly developed by the ICF Research Branch of the German WHO Collaborating Center for the Family of International Classifications (DIMDI) in Munich and the Classification, Assessment and Surveys (CAS) team at the WHO in cooperation with a number of international societies, including the European League Against Rheumatism (EULAR), the Bone and Joint Decade and the European Union health monitor project (Stucki et al. 2002a).

In a first project, ICF Core Sets have been developed for 12 burdensome chronic conditions, including the musculoskeletal health conditions chronic widespread pain, low back pain, osteoarthritis, osteoporosis, and rheumatoid arthritis (Cieza et al. 2004a,b,c; Dreinhöfer et al. 2004; Stucki et al. 2004). In this project, the development of ICF Core Sets is in line with the current concept in outcomes and quality-of-life research of condition-specific measures (Guyatt et al. 1993), i.e., it is based on the assumption that different conditions are associated with typical problems in functioning and represents an attempt to link the use of the ICF with the International Classification of Diseases (ICD-10). Therefore, the ICF Core Sets represent a link between specific conditions or diseases and relevant ICF categories. Since the requirements to describe functioning in association with a condition are different for a comprehensive multidisciplinary assessment and a clinical study, a Comprehensive ICF Core Set as well as a Brief ICF Core Set is needed (Cieza et al. 2004d).

The **Comprehensive ICF Core Set** for a specific condition is a list of ICF categories that includes as few categories as possible to be practical, but as many as necessary to be sufficiently comprehensive to describe the prototypical spectrum of problems in functioning and health in a comprehensive, multidisciplinary assessment. The Comprehensive ICF Core Sets are intended for the diagnosis or so-called assessment of functioning in multi-professional settings, e.g., rehabilitation, and may be used in the teaching and training of students and young specialists when taking the patient's history and when performing a physical examination.

Instead, the **Brief ICF Core Set** for a specific condition includes a list of ICF categories with as few categories as possible to be practical, but as many as necessary to be sufficiently comprehensive to describe the prototypical spectrum of limitations of functioning and health in clinical studies. The **Brief ICF Core Set** may also serve as a short checklist to assess functioning in daily busy clinical practice.

While a Comprehensive ICF Core Set should include all typical problems in functioning of patients with a condition, the Brief ICF Core Set aims to include only the most important ICF categories across cultures and countries to be practical in any situation or setting.

Tables 11.1 and 11.2 show the ICF categories of the components *body functions* and *activities and participation* of the *Comprehensive ICF Core Set for CWP*. The ICF categories in bold type represent the categories selected for the *Brief ICF Core Set* in the corresponding components. Overall, the Comprehensive ICF Core Set for CWP includes 66 ICF categories, which reflect the complex functional problems encountered in patients with CWP and also the crucial influence of patients' surroundings and life situations on their functioning and health.

Consistent with the main *body functions* affected in CWP, *neuromusculoskeletal- and movement-related functions* and *mental functions* are broadly covered in the Comprehensive ICF Core Set (Croft et al. 1993; Aaron et al. 2002; Clauw and Crofford 2003; Giesecke et al. 2003).

Further *body functions* related to sensory functions, like *exercise tolerance functions*, and *sexual functions*, are also included. The body function *sensation of pain* could either be missing in the Comprehensive ICF Core Set for CWP.

The body function *content of thought*, which includes somatization, was also included in the Comprehensive ICF Core Set. The process of somatization has been widely discussed in the literature as a relevant factor in relation to CWP and FM (MacBeth et al. 2001; Winfield 2001; Staud 2002).

The concept generally found in the literature in relation to mental functions affected in CWP is psychological distress, usually understood as depressive mood, anxiety, and somatoform disorders (MacBeth et al. 2002). It has been shown that CWP has been associated with high levels of psychological distress both in clinical samples and in the general population (Croft et al. 1993; Croft et al. 1994; Fishbain et al. 1997; White et al. 2002). Moreover, research suggests that 40–50% of patients with chronic pain suffer from depression (Romano and Turner 1985) and that anxiety and anger are highly prevalent (Fernandez and Turk 1995).

Cognitive deficits have been reported in multiple-site musculoskeletal pain (Kewman et al. 1991) and

Table 11.1 International Classification of Functioning, Disability and Health (ICF): categories of the component "body functions" included in the Comprehensive ICF Core Set for CWP. Brief ICF core set in bold.

ICF code	ICF category title
b122	Global psychosocial functions
b126	Temperament and personality functions
b130	**Energy and drive functions**
b134	**Sleep functions**
b140	Attention functions
b147	**Psychomotor functions**
b152	**Emotional functions**
b1602	**Content of thought**
b164	Higher-level cognitive functions
b180	Experience of self and time functions
b260	Proprioceptive function
b265	Touch function
b270	Sensory functions related to temperature and other stimuli
b280	**Sensation of pain**
b430	Hematological system functions
b455	**Exercise tolerance functions**
b640	Sexual functions
b710	Mobility of joint functions
b730	**Muscle power functions**
b735	Muscle tone functions
b740	Muscle endurance functions
b760	**Control of voluntary movement functions**
b780	Sensations related to muscles and movement functions

CWP: chronic widespread pain.

in patients with fibromyalgia (Glass and Park 2001). Concretely, deficits in performance in complex cognitive tasks (Cote and Moldofsky 1997), reduced psychomotor speed (Sletvold et al. 1995) and memory problems have been reported in patients with fibromyalgia. Psychomotor functions, attention functions and higher-level cognitive functions were included in the Comprehensive ICF Core Set to address these problems.

Limitations and *restrictions* in *activity and participation* may, indeed, be most relevant to patients with CWP.

This is reflected not only by the fact that 27 categories of this component, as compared to the 23 *body functions* considered relevant, have been included, but also by the fact that eight of nine ICF chapters of this component are represented in the Comprehensive ICF Core Set. Besides the life areas, such as *mobility*, *self-care* and *domestic life*, which have been reported in the literature

Table 11.2 International Classification of Functioning, Disability and Health (ICF): categories of the component "activities and participation" included in the Comprehensive ICF Core Set for CWP. Brief ICF core set in bold.

ICF code	ICF category title
d160	Focusing attention
d175	**Solving problems**
d220	Undertaking multiple tasks
d230	**Carrying out daily routine**
d240	**Handling stress and other psychological demands**
d410	Changing basic body position
d415	Maintaining a body position
d430	**Lifting and carrying objects**
d450	**Walking**
d455	Moving around
d470	Using transportation
d475	Driving
d510	Washing oneself
d540	Dressing
d570	Looking after one's health
d620	Acquisition of goods and services
d640	**Doing housework**
d650	Caring for household objects
d660	Assisting others
d720	Complex interpersonal interactions
d760	**Family relationships**
d770	**Intimate relationships**
d845	Acquiring, keeping and terminating a job
d850	**Remunerative employment**
d855	Non-remunerative employment
d910	Community life
d920	**Recreation and leisure**

CWP: chronic widespread pain.

as areas affected by CWP (Leveille et al. 2001; MacBeth et al. 2002; White et al. 2002), other issues related to *solving problems, carrying out daily routine, handling stress and other psychological demands, interpersonal interactions and relationships, work and employment,* and *recreation and leisure,* which are frequently reported in the literature in association with other health conditions or under the umbrella term health-related quality of life (HRQoL) (Petrak et al. 2003) or functional status (Aaron et al. 2002), were considered relevant and selected by the group of experts.

The relevance of environmental factors regarding the functioning of patients with CWP is reflected by the fact that 15 categories representing 20% of the categories of the Comprehensive ICF Core Set belong to the component *environmental factors.*

It is important to note that the ICF Core Sets for CWP are preliminary versions. Current users must be aware of the procedures and limitations which are described in the introduction paper on ICF Core Set development for patients with chronic conditions (Cieza et al. 2004d) and in the paper on CWP (Cieza et al. 2004a). The preliminary ICF Core Sets for CWP will need to be tested extensively in field studies. The testing needs to be performed throughout the world in different countries, cultures and settings, in the hands of different professionals, for subsets of patients with varying personal and disease characteristics. Despite the fact that the patient perspective has been addressed in the empiric data collection of the preliminary studies, the ICF Core Sets will also require a close examination and possibly even modification by patient focus groups throughout the world. Focus-groups techniques are currently being developed in a cooperation of the ICF Research Branch with the German Patient Organizations. After the testing which will be coordinated by the ICF Research Branch in Munich under the auspices of the CAS Team at the WHO and in close collaboration with a number of international organizations, the ICF Core Sets will finally be approved and recommended for general use by an international panel based on the review of the evidence from the testing.

LINKING HEALTH STATUS MEASURES TO THE ICF

Many studies compare the psychometric properties of health status measures, but content comparisons are scarcely represented in the literature. This is probably due to the varying use of concepts, scales and items in the different health status measures. The ICF as a universal framework of functioning and health enables the content comparison of health status measures. The results of such comparison provide information on which contents are covered by which measure. Thus, the use of the ICF as a reference tool for comparison can provide clinicians and researchers with new insights when selecting health status measures for clinical studies (Cieza et al. 2004a).

The first question when selecting health status measures is to decide on what should be measured based on the study endpoints, the population to be studied and the intervention. The ensuing question regarding how to measure or which measure to use may be answered based on the content comparison of the possible candidate measures.

There exist many different health status measures that can be selected when planning a study for patients with pain. Both generic measures, which allow comparing effects across conditions, populations and interventions, as well as condition- or symptom-specific measures for chronic pain, which may cover pain and aspects of functioning and health more associated with a condition, can be considered.

Four instruments frequently used in studies with patients with chronic pain are: the Brief Pain Inventory (BPI) (Daut et al. 1983; Cleeland and Ryan 1994; Chapter 22), the Pain Disability Index (PDI) (Tait et al. 1987; Chapter 17), the West Haven–Yale Multidimensional Pain Inventory (WHYMPI) (Kerns et al. 1985; Kerns and Rosenberg 1995; Chapter 17) and the Short Form 36 (SF-36) (Ware and Sherbourne 1992; Chapter 1). These four health status measures have all been linked to the ICF separately by two trained health professionals on the basis of ten linking rules which enable health status measures to be linked to the ICF in a specific and precise manner (Cieza et al. 2002a, b; 2005).

The most important of these linking rules are numbers two and three, which state, respectively, that each item of an outcome measure should be linked to the most precise ICF category and that if one item encompasses different concepts, the information in each concept should be linked.

Consensus between health professionals is used to decide which ICF category should be linked to each item/concept of the two questionnaires. To resolve disagreements between the two health professionals concerning the selected categories, a third person trained in the linking rules is consulted.

After linking each health status measure to the ICF, the latter is used as a cardinal reference to compare the contents of the health status measures. The results of this content comparison are presented in Table 11.3.

The digits contained in the columns with the headings BPI, PDI, WHYMPI and SF-36 represent the frequency with which the ICF categories are addressed in the corresponding health status measures. Generally, the ICF categories were linked to just one item/concept of a questionnaire, as it is indicated by a "1" in the tables. A higher number indicates that either the measure contains a determined concept more than once or that the ICF did not differentiate in greater detail, and, therefore, several items or concepts of items from a specific measure had to be linked to the same ICF

Table 11.3 Frequencies showing how often listed ICF categories are addressed in the BPI, the PDI, the WHYMPI and the SF-36

ICF category	BPI	PDI	WHYMPI	SF-36
b1300 Energy level				4
b28134 Sleep functions	1	1		
b28147 Psychomotor functions				
b28152 Emotional functions	1		4	7
b1528 Emotional functions, other specified	1			1
b28280 Sensation of pain	12	7	12	2
b28019 Pain in body part, unspecified	1			
b28289 Sensation of pain, other specified and unspecified	3			
b28440 Respiration functions		1		
d230 Carrying out daily routine	1		1	2
d4102 Kneeling				1
d4105 Bending				1
d4154 Maintaining a standing position	1			
d430 Lifting and carrying objects				1
d4300 Lifting	1			
d4309 Lifting and carrying, unspecified				1
d4459 Hand and arm use, unspecified				1
d450 Walking	2			
d4500 Walking short distances				1
d4501 Walking long distances				2
d4551 Climbing				2
d4559 Moving around, unspecified				1
d475 Driving		1		
d5 SELF-CARE		1		
d510 Washing oneself		1		
d5101 Washing whole body				1
d540 Dressing		1		1
d550 Eating		1		
d6 DOMESTIC LIFE		1		
d640 Doing housework	1		1	
d6409 Doing housework, unspecified				1
d649 Household tasks, other specified and unspecified				1
d7 INTERPERSONAL INTERACTIONS AND RELATIONSHIPS	1			
d750 Informal social relationships			1	
d760 Family relationships			1	
d7701 Spousal relationships			1	

d7702 Sexual relationships		1		
d850 Remunerative employment	1	1	2	1
d855 Non-remunerative employment		1		
d859 Work and employment, other specified and unspecified				2
d920 Recreation and leisure	1	1	2	
d9205 Socializing		1	1	2
d9209 Recreation and leisure, unspecified				2
e110 Products or substances for personal consumption	1			
e1101 Drugs	4			
e1151 Assistive products and technology for personal use in daily living	1			
e5800	1			

category. For example, for the SF-36, the ICF category b152 Emotional functions was chosen to link a number of different feelings: "feeling depressed or anxious," "emotional problems," "very nervous," "I felt so down in the dumps nothing could cheer me up," "I felt calm and peaceful," "I felt downhearted and blue" and "Have you been a happy person?" If there were different categories for different feelings, the named items would have been linked to different categories.

As can be seen in Table 11.3, it is possible to study the differences as well as the commonalities of health status measures regarding their representation of body functions, activities, participations and environmental factors.

In relation to the linking of health status measures to the ICF, one could also take advantage of the ICF Core Sets described above. Adding the Comprehensive or Brief ICF Core Set for CWP to the comparison, it would be possible to examine whether and to what extent the compared measures cover the prototypical spectrum of problems encountered in patients with CWP as defined by the ICF Core Sets. Without being in competition with other health status measures, the ICF Core Sets can be the basis for the definition of what should be measured. The content comparison of health status measures based on the ICF can then facilitate the definition of how to measure or which measure to use.

USING THE ICF AND ICF CORE SETS IN CLINICAL PRACTICE

The ICF framework is increasingly being applied in clinical practice to structure patient problems, particularly in multidisciplinary care and for rehabilitation purposes (Stucki et al. 2002b; Stucki and Sangha 2003; Stucki and Sigl 2003). Physicians and health professionals can use the ICF framework and the ICF Core Sets to identify and document patients' complaints when taking a patient's history and to identify and document clinical findings of a clinical examination. The ICF Core Sets may be particularly useful for trainees, but may also be of value in the hands of experienced clinicians, since physicians may underestimate patients' functional problems.

The use of an ICF sheet (Steiner et al. 2002) based on the ICF framework, either on paper or in an electronic form, facilitates understanding of the relationship between selected target problems and impaired body functions and structures and psychosocial and environmental factors which exacerbate or help to minimize them (Figure 11.2). The use of an ICF sheet and the ICF Core Sets can be used to improve the internal reporting and documentation and to structure multidisciplinary care (McBeth et al. 2001).

FURTHER DEVELOPMENTS AND USE OF THE ICF AND ICF CORE SETS FOR CWP

For the first time in the history of medicine, there now exists a universally agreed-upon conceptual framework and classification for functioning, disability and health. The already ongoing adoption of the ICF by clinicians and health professionals, researchers, health authorities, healthcare providers and insurers is likely to trigger a number of important developments. Language influences the way people think and, consequently, act.

Since the ICF now includes contextual factors, which interact with the components *body functions* and *structures, activity and participation*, it is likely that people who work with the ICF will probably increasingly consider these factors and interactions. Also, the now neutral terms *body functions* and *structures, activity and participation* as compared to the prior "negative" terms impairment, disability and handicap may stimulate a more positive view and bring a more resource-oriented perspective into medicine.

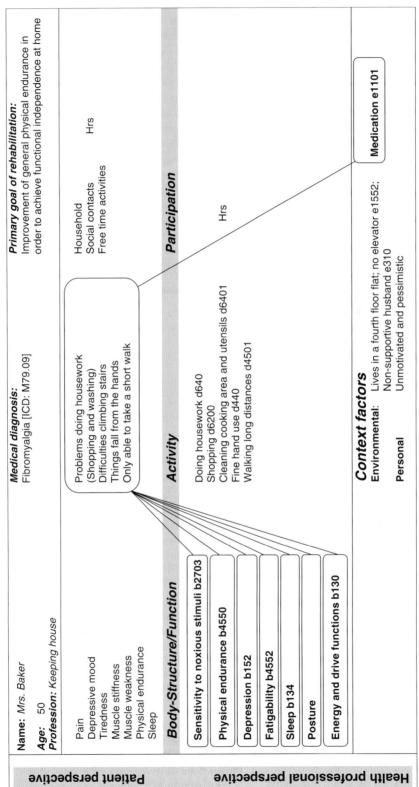

Figure 11.2 How the ICF components can be used to structure patient problems (listed in the upper section "patient perspective") as well as findings, and observations by the rehabilitation team (listed in the lower section "health professional perspective"). Lines between the selected target problems from the patient perspective (circled in the upper section) and impaired body functions and structures as well as the given personal and environmental factors (circled in the lower section) denote their hypothesized relationship. Note that the wording denotes patients' words or special medical terms and not text from ICF categories.

The ICF as a common language for functioning will likely change multi-professional communication, which is highly important in chronic and complex conditions. As illustrated in Figure 11.2, the ICF will become the basis for multi-professional patient assessment, goal setting, intervention management and evaluation. The ICF may also improve communication between patients and health professionals. It will be easier for patients with CWP to understand their functioning and health, rehabilitation goals, and an intervention plan based on a language they can understand. Similarly, the ICF will become an important part for the education of all professionals involved in the care of patients with CWP.

The ICF may provide new ways for outcomes research. Currently we are faced with "competing" instruments in many areas. The linking of items to the ICF (Cieza et al. 2002b) provides the unique opportunity to compare health-status instruments and to standardize items and instruments. The components of the ICF are the basis for research into their interactions and will lead to a better understanding of functioning, disability and health (Stucki 2003). Most importantly, the components are a practical framework for designing longitudinal prognostic studies on the negative and positive factors related to functioning and health in persons with a specific health condition or within a specific context.

Finally, the ICF will be used by health agencies, healthcare providers and insurances in many ways. It will, for example, be used for expert opinion or as a framework to develop expert systems, case-management, health reporting and health statistics, quality assurance and bench marching, healthcare planning and case management. The ICF may also be used for the development of prospective payment systems. In all these situations a mass of information must be handled and analyzed. Redundant data collection must be avoided, and decisions need to be made based on relevant data only. The ICF provides a framework for data collection and a terminology for comparing data on all aspects encompassing functioning.

The research community or regulatory agencies may use the ICF and ICF Core Sets to define what should be measured when reporting a clinical study or when defining the minimal requirements to be met for approval. It would thus be valuable to define first what categories should be covered when referring to functioning and health on patients with CWP and only then deciding how to measure these categories.

CONCLUSION

The new ICF by the WHO provides both a framework and a classification to comprehensively represent the experience of patients with CWP. It is a universal language understood by health professionals, researchers,

policy makers, patients and patient organizations alike. The ICF is a promising new framework and classification to assess the impact of CWP. The ICF can also be used as a reference tool for comparison of health status measures. This kind of comparison can provide clinicians and researchers with new insights when selecting health status measures for clinical studies. Moreover, the ICF framework, e.g., in the form of an ICF sheet differentiating the patient and the professional perspective, can be used in clinical practice to structure patient problems. The ICF and practical tools, such as the ICF Core Sets for CWP, are useful for clinical practice, outcome and rehabilitation research, education, health statistics and regulation.

REFERENCES

Aaron LA, Arguelles LM, Ashton S, et al. Health and functional status of twins with chronic regional and widespread pain. J Rheumatol 2002; 29:2426–2434.

Cieza A, Brockow T, Ewert T, et al. Linking health-status measurements to the International Classification of Functioning, Disability and Health. J Rehabil Med 2002a; 34:1–6.

Cieza A, Brockow T, Ewert T, et al. Linking health-status measurements to the International Classification of Functioning, Disability and Health. J Rehabil Med 2002b; 34:205–210.

Cieza A, Stucki G, Weigl M, et al. ICF Core Sets for chronic widespread pain. J Rehabil Med 2004a; 44 (suppl):63–68.

Cieza A, Stucki G, Weigl M, et al. ICF Core Sets for low back pain. J Rehabil Med 2004b; 44(suppl):69–74.

Cieza A, Schwarzkopf SR, Sigl T, et al. ICF Core Sets for osteoporosis. J Rehabil Med 2004c; 44(suppl):81–86.

Cieza A, Ewert T, Üstün TB, et al. ICF Core Set development for patients with chronic conditions. J Rehabil Med 2004d; 44(suppl):9–11.

Cieza A, Geyh S, Chatterji S, Kostanjsek N, Ustun TB, Stucki G. ICF linkage rules: an update based on lessons learned. J Rehabil Med 2005; 37:212–218.

Clauw DJ, Crofford LJ. Chronic widespread pain and fibromyalgia: what we know, and what we need to know. Best Pract Res Clin Rheumatol 2003; 17:685–701.

Cleeland CS, Ryan KM. Pain assessment: global use of the Brief Pain Inventory [review]. Ann Acad Med Singapore 1994; 23:129–138.

Cote KA, Moldofsky H. Sleep, daytime symptoms, and cognitive performance in patients with fibromyalgia. J Rheumatol 1997; 24:2014–2023.

Croft P, Rigby AS, Boswell R, et al. The prevalence of chronic widespread pain in the general population. J Rheumatol 1993; 20:710–713.

Croft P, Schollum J, Silman A. Population study of tender point counts and pain as evidence of fibromyalgia. Br Med J 1994; 309(6956):696–699.

Daut RL, Cleeland CS, Flanery RC. Development of the Wisconsin Brief Pain Questionnaire to assess pain in cancer and other diseases. Pain 1983; 17:197–210.

Dreinhöfer K, Stucki G, Ewert T, et al. ICF Core Sets for osteoarthritis. J Rehabil Med 2004; 44(suppl): 75–80.

Fernandez E, Turk DC. The scope and significance of anger in the experience of chronic pain. Pain 1995; 61:165–175.

Fishbain DA, Cutler R, Rosomoff HL, et al. Chronic pain-associated depression: antecedent or consequence of chronic pain? A review. Clin J Pain 1997; 13:116–137.

Giesecke T, Williams DA, Harris RE, et al. Subgrouping of fibromyalgia patients on the basis of pressure-pain thresholds and psychological factors. Arthritis Rheum 2003; 48:2916–2922.

Glass JM, Park DC. Cognitive dysfunction in fibromyalgia. Curr Rheumatol Rep 2001; 3:123–127.

Guyatt GH, Feeny DH, Patrick DL. Measuring health-related quality of life. Ann Intern Med 1993; 15:622–629.

Kerns RD, Rosenberg R. Pain-relevant responses from significant others: development of a significant-other version of the WHYMPI scales. Pain 1995; 61:245–249.

Kerns RD, Turk DC, Rudy TE. The West Haven–Yale Multidimensional Pain Inventory (WHYMPI). Pain 1985; 23:345–356.

Kewman DG, Vaishampayan N, Zald D, et al. Cognitive impairment in musculoskeletal pain patients. Int J Psychiatry Med 1991; 21:253–262.

Leveille SG, Ling S, Hochberg MC, et al. Widespread musculoskeletal pain and the progression of disability in older disabled women. Ann Intern Med 2001; 135:1038–1046.

MacBeth J, Macfarlane GJ, Benjamin S, et al. Features of somatization predict the onset of chronic widespread pain: results of a large population-based study. Arthritis Rheum 2001; 44:940–946.

MacBeth J, Macfarlane GJ, Silman AJ. Does chronic pain predict future psychological distress? Pain 2002; 96:239–245.

Macfarlane GJ, Croft PR, Schollum J, et al. Widespread pain: is an improvement classification possible? J Rheumatol 1996; 23:1628–1632.

Petrak F, Hardt J, Kappis B, et al. Determinants of health-related quality of life in patients with persistent somatoform pain disorder. Eur J Pain 2003; 7:463–471.

Prescott E, Jacobsen S, Kjoller M, et al. Fibromyalgia in the adult Danish population: II. A study of clinical features. Scand J Rheumatol 1993; 22:238–242.

Romano JM, Turner JA. Chronic pain and depression: does the evidence support a relationship? Psychol Bull 1985; 97:18–34.

Sletvold H, Stiles TC, Landro NI. Information processing in primary fibromyalgia, major depression and healthy controls. J Rheumatol 1995; 22:137–142.

Staud R. Somatization does not fit all fibromyalgia patients: comment on the article by Winfield. Arthritis Rheum 2002; 46:564–565.

Steiner WA, Ryser L, Huber E, et al. Use of the ICF model as a clinical problem-solving tool in physical therapy and rehabilitation medicine. Phys Ther 2002; 82:1098–1107.

Stucki G. Understanding disability. Ann Rheum Dis 2003; 62:289–290.

Stucki G, Sangha O. Principles of rehabilitation. In: Hochberg, Silman, Smolen, Weinblatt, Weisman (eds). Rheumatology, 3rd edition, vol 1. Mosby of Elsevier, 2003:517–530.

Stucki G, Sigl T. Assessment of the impact of disease on the individual. Best Pract Res Clin Rheumatol 2003; 17:451–473.

Stucki G, Cieza A, Ewert T, et al. Application on the International Classification of Functioning, Disability and Health (ICF) in clinical practice. Disabil Rehabil 2002a; 24:281–282.

Stucki G, Ewert T, Cieza A. Value and application of the ICF in rehabilitation medicine. Disabil Rehabil 2002b; 24:932–938.

Stucki G, Cieza A, Geyh S, et al. ICF Core Sets for rheumatoid arthritis. J Rehabil Med 2004; 44(suppl):87–93.

Tait RC, Pollard CA, Margolis RB, et al. The pain disability index: psychometric and validity data. Arch Phys Med Rehabil 1987; 68:438–441.

Ware JE, Sherbourne CD. The MOS 36-item short-form health survey (SF-36). A. Conceptual framework and item selection. Med Care 1992; 30:473–483.

White KP, Nielson WR, Harth M, et al. Chronic widespread musculoskeletal pain with or without fibromyalgia: psychological distress in a representative community adult sample. J Rheumatol 2002; 29:588–594.

Winfield JB. Does pain in fibromyalgia reflect somatization? Arthritis Rheum 2001; 44:751–753.

Wolfe F, Ross K, Anderson J, et al. The prevalence and characteristics of fibromyalgia in the general population. Arthritis Rheum 1995; 38:19–28.

Wolfe F, Smythe HA, Yunus MB, et al. The American College of Rheumatology 1990 Criteria for the Classification of Fibromyalgia. Report of the Multicenter Criteria Committee. Arthritis Rheum 1990; 33:160–172.

World Health Organization. International Classification of Functioning, Disability and Health: ICF. WHO, Geneva, 2001.

Yunus MB, Masi AT, Calabro JJ, et al. Primary fibromyalgia (fibrositis): clinical study of 50 patients with matched normal controls. Semin Arthritis Rheum 1981; 11:151–171.

12 Assessment of acute pain and condition-specific health-related quality of life

Scott A. Strassels • Daniel B. Carr

INTRODUCTION

In many countries, concern about rising healthcare costs has resulted in intense attention devoted to understanding the outcomes of medical care. These data provide objective information that help guide decision- and policy-makers, clinicians, and patients about the results of using medical interventions or the decision to forego use of an intervention. In 2004, in the USA, for example, national health expenditures were estimated to be $1.9 trillion, a 7.9% increase over spending in 2003, with a growth rate in this segment of the US economy more than twice that of the gross domestic product (Levit et al. 2004). Yet, while these estimates by themselves provide important information about the economics of healthcare, the picture they paint is far from complete. It is also important to understand these data within a context that allows healthcare providers, decision-makers, payers, and consumers to make well-informed decisions about how to make use of healthcare resources. Such an environment exists when healthcare costs are considered with measures of clinical and patient-reported outcomes. Since medical practice, clinical research, and, increasingly, reimbursement decisions rely heavily on assessment of evidence of clinical, economic, and patient-centered reports of benefit, use of these measures is becoming increasingly necessary, regardless of where treatment takes place (Schyve 1995).

Healthcare outcomes are the results of using (or foregoing the use of) healthcare resources. These outcomes are generally described in terms of clinical events, economic costs, and patient-reported measures, such as health-related quality of life (HRQL; also called health status), a multidimensional concept used to summarize an individual's health from their own perspective, or in combining different types of outcomes in a summary measure. For example, a cost-effectiveness ratio presents an estimate of cost per some measure of a clinical event or, in a cost-utility analysis, the cost per quality-adjusted event is reported, which takes into account patients' preferences for that event (Drummond et al. 1997). While clinical data are readily available from physical examination and diagnostic tests, information about the effect of healthcare interventions from the patient's perspective is important because it provides additional insight into how an individual is directly affected by a medical condition or treatment.

Within the context of pain, assessment and management are widely acknowledged to be important dimensions of patient care and a standard by which the quality of medical care may be assessed (Carr et al. 1992; American Pain Society Quality of Care Committee 1995; Joint Commission on Accreditation of Healthcare Organizations 2001). Furthermore, the assessment of pain in adults and children has been well described, and most clinicians consider pain intensity and analgesia the primary outcomes of pain treatment (Chapman and Loeser 1989; Keefe et al. 1996; Song and Carr 1999; Turk and Melzack 2001). Yet, while pain intensity is important, just as nociception is the keystone of pain-related suffering, it reflects only one dimension of the pain experience (Chapman and Gavrin 1999). This gap in understanding the consequences of pain is important because suboptimally treated acute pain is common, and acute pain is a risk factor for the development of chronic pain (Perkins and Kehlet 2000). Furthermore, although pain is commonly a dimension of HRQL instruments, the effects of acute pain on HRQL are incompletely described and understood.

Therefore, the purpose of this chapter is to describe the measurement of condition-specific HRQL among persons with acute pain. While HRQL instruments are broadly classified as being generic or disease-specific, generic HRQL instruments provide insight about health-related domains that are not age, treatment, or disease specific, while disease-specific instruments allow measurement of aspects of HRQL that may be unique to a group of affected individuals and focus on how dimensions of that condition affect HRQL. For example, the SF-36 contains questions about the amount of bodily pain experienced during the previous four weeks, and how much that pain affected the person's ability to perform their normal work (Ware et al. 1993). In contrast, questions about pain in a condition-specific instrument would be expected to focus on how the person's HRQL is affected by pain related to that condition. Thus, we wanted to know if disease- or condition-specific HRQL instruments have been used to assess acute pain, which conditions have been studied in this way, and whether using specific HRQL instruments contributed to understanding acute pain beyond that gained by use of generic HRQL questionnaires.

METHODS

In order to identify the pertinent literature, we searched the Cochrane Library (2004, number 1), Embase Drugs and Pharmacology (1991–2004, 3rd quarter), and PubMed. PubMed is an online service of the National Library of Medicine, and includes more than 14 million citations for biomedical articles from Medline and

other life sciences journals dating from the 1950s (PubMed 2007). We used these search terms: health-related quality of life, pain, quality of life, questionnaire, and survey. The purpose of this study was to evaluate the effects of acute pain on disease-specific health-related quality of life, using postoperative pain within three months of surgery as the model. In addition, we specifically excluded studies that report the effects of chronic or cancer-related pain on HRQL, the effects of pain on generic HRQL, and studies in which the questionnaire used was specific to pain, but which did not include other dimensions of HRQL. We also excluded articles not published in English and we searched the bibliographies of selected articles to identify other papers of interest.

RESULTS

ARTHRITIS

The Western Ontario and McMaster Universities Osteoarthritis Index (WOMAC) includes 24 questions pertaining to pain (5 items), stiffness (2 items), and physical function (17 items; WOMAC Osteoarthritis Index 2004; Bellamy et al. 1988). It was developed in 1982 and has been shown to be valid, reliable, and sensitive. It is widely used in trials of interventions to treat osteoarthritis of the hip and knee, and has been tested with some success to assess outcomes in other rheumatologic conditions (Wolfe and Kong 1999). It is also available in 65 languages as well as formats including Likert-type or visual analog scales (see also Chapter 16).

In a report of a study comparing the use of the WOMAC and the SF-36, 86 persons who underwent total hip replacement and 108 individuals who had total knee replacement surgery for osteoarthritis completed these instruments preoperatively and every three months for a year (Bachmeier et al. 2001). While preoperative pain in this population is expected to be significant, individuals who undergo this procedure are likely to have mainly acute pain following their surgery.

As measured by the WOMAC, these investigators found that pain decreased, physical functioning improved, and stiffness in the operative joint decreased over the first three months after surgery, relative to preoperative scores in each surgical group. While we anticipate that postoperative functioning will increase dramatically, and that pain will diminish over time, these data are also useful to provide additional insights into the effect of pain after surgery. In this study, for example, not only do the WOMAC scores indicate pain intensity, they also can be used to correlate pain with functioning and joint functioning.

Another instrument that may be suitable for use to assess the outcomes of acute pain in terms of condition-specific HRQL is the Treatment Outcomes in Pain Survey, or TOPS (Rogers et al. 2000a,b; Chapter 17).

The TOPS was designed to assess the condition-specific HRQL of persons being treated in outpatient multidisciplinary clinics for chronic noncancer pain. Although targeted at persons with chronic pain, we have used questions from the TOPS to enhance measurement of acute postoperative pain outcomes during the first month following total joint replacement or radical prostatectomy surgery (Strassels et al. 1999, 2004). In addition, a version of the TOPS is being developed for use in persons with cancer-related pain (Orkin et al. 2003).

NEPHRECTOMY

The Postoperative Recovery Scale (PRS) is a validated scale that builds off the Acute (1-week) SF-36 by including a series of visual analog scales to more fully describe the effect of postoperative pain on HRQL (Pace et al. 2003). There are three versions of the PRS: preoperative, postoperative inpatient, and postoperative outpatient. In contrast to the scoring algorithm used for the SF-36, the PRS score is obtained by summing the scores for each item. Higher scores indicate better HRQL.

In a report of persons who underwent open ($n = 33$) or laparoscopic ($n = 38$) nephrectomy, study participants completed the PRS preoperatively twice, on each day of their hospital stay, and then 2, 4, and 8 weeks, and 3, 6, and 12 months, after being discharged from the hospital (Pace et al. 2003). These authors observed that, while preoperative scores were similar between groups, HRQL was slightly higher among the open nephrectomy patients prior to discharge, although differences were not statistically significant. After hospital discharge, HRQL was statistically significantly higher among persons in the laparoscopic surgery group starting at two weeks after leaving the hospital and continuing through the end of the study. In addition, postdischarge differences between surgical groups gradually increased through three months after discharge, after which, the mean PRS scores began to converge. While it is difficult to directly interpret the clinical significance of PRS scores because they are an unweighted sum of responses and do not reflect scale-specific functioning as in the SF-36, it is worth noting that the differences observed persisted through the year after surgery, and that the median time for persons to reach 75% of their preoperative PRS score was 33 days in the laparoscopic surgery group and 90 days among persons in the open procedure group. When considered with the time spent in the hospital after surgery and days needed before returning to work, these data support the argument that HRQL differences reflect meaningful information.

POSTOPERATIVE ANALGESIA AND SURGICAL COMPLICATIONS

The relation between postoperative analgesia and major complications has also been examined. In a meta-analysis of large studies identified from Medline and the Cochrane Library databases, investigators sought to assess the evidence that analgesia reduces the morbidity or mortality by at least 50% (Liu and Wu 2007). These authors concluded that the evidence included in this analysis allowed neither confirmation nor denial of an effect of analgesia on morbidity or mortality, despite the evidence that epidural analgesia has proven benefits. These results were attributed to the low incidence of major complications, although, as the authors of the accompanying editorial pointed out, the restrictive inclusion criteria may have contributed to the relatively counterintuitive findings (White and Kehlet 2007).

IMPINGEMENT SYNDROME

A group of 28 persons who underwent decompression surgery to treat impingement syndrome of the shoulder were evaluated with the University of California, Los Angeles (UCLA) shoulder rating scale and the Constant-Murley (CM) shoulder scoring system (O'Connor et al. 1999). Each of these scales includes subjective assessment of pain and functioning, and objective measurements of range of motion and strength. Scores on these domains are summed to provide an instrument score. Study participants were evaluated before surgery and six weeks, three months, and six months postoperatively. The authors sought to compare the disease-specific measures to the SF-36 and the visual analog scale to measure pain intensity. In general, scores from all the instruments used improved over time, and, in terms of a standardized response mean and effect size, the UCLA scale was judged to be the most sensitive of these scales at three months after surgery. As with other instruments scored by summing across multiple domains, an important limitation of these scales is that insight about how an individual domain affects the overall scale is lost.

ORAL SURGERY

Another model of assessing patient outcomes and HRQL is third molar surgery (Shugars et al. 1996). This model is useful to study acute pain because most persons who have this surgery are relatively young and otherwise healthy. A 14-item instrument that includes domains of oral function, general function, pain, and other symptoms was used for these studies. The "other symptoms" category includes swelling, bruising, bleeding, nausea, bad taste or breath, food impaction, and lip numbness. Twenty persons who underwent outpatient third molar surgery completed a diary that included the HRQL instrument each evening for 14 days, starting on the first postoperative day. These investigators found that, as expected, median pain levels on a 0–10 scale (10 = most intense pain imaginable) were highest on the first and second postoperative days and declined fairly rapidly after that over the study period.

In a similar study of 630 persons who had all four third molars removed and used the same HRQL instrument, the investigators also assessed pain with a seven-point Likert-type scale, anchored by no pain at one end and worst pain imaginable at the other end (White et al. 2003). In this study, scores of five or more were interpreted as representing substantial interference with functioning. These authors found that about a third of patients had pain at their first postoperative clinic visit, and that 9% of people reported pain at any postoperative visit. More than half of patients reported having severe pain during the previous 24 hours on the first postoperative day, although 20% of persons had severe pain on average during that time. A week after surgery, 15% of persons reported having had severe pain during the previous 24 hours and 5% had severe pain on average.

CONCLUSION

Outcomes research studies the results of medical care (Foundation for Health Services Research 1994). It involves "the rigorous determination of what works in medical care and what does not" and states that "outcomes research, by informing the content of policy positions, payment rules, and practice guidelines, presumably both solves the problems of quality and cost that beset healthcare and does so by scientific rather than political means" (Tanenbaum 1993). This evidence-based approach to healthcare, exemplified by the Cochrane Collaboration, has been accompanied by a shift toward identification of patient-centered health outcomes (Gerteis et al. 1993; Straus et al. 2005; Alderson et al. 2003).

Pain is a highly individual experience, and, as a result, understanding of the effects of a person's pain experience depends on much more than unidimensional measurements of pain intensity, or by measurements obtained by subtracting threshold from tolerance (Chapman et al. 1985; Turk and Okifuji 1999). While generic HRQL instruments (the SF-36, in particular) are much more commonly used than condition-specific questionnaires, some investigators have used the latter type of survey to assess acute pain and its effects in persons with certain conditions, and a few of these reports have been discussed in this report. There are presently relatively few examples of the use of condition-specific HRQL instruments to assess acute pain, in part because it is difficult to separate acute pain from chronic in the setting of common diseases, such as arthritis, and because most attention to date has focused on long-term outcomes. In addition, minimal clinically significant differences in instrument scores are not always known. Nonetheless, the existing reports we found indicate that the information from condition-specific instruments represents a valuable addition to data available from generic questionnaires.

REFERENCES

American Pain Society Quality of Care Committee. Quality improvement guidelines for the treatment of acute pain and cancer. JAMA 1995; 274:1874–1880.

Bachmeier CJM, March LM, Cross MJ, et al. for the Arthritis Cost and Outcome Project Group. A comparison of outcomes in osteoarthritis patients undergoing total hip and knee replacement surgery. Osteoarthritis Cartilage 2001; 9:137–146.

Bellamy N, Buchanan WW, Goldsmith CH, et al. Validation study of WOMAC: a health status instrument for measuring clinically important patient relevant outcomes to antirheumatic drug therapy in patients with osteoarthritis of the hip or knee. J Rheumatol 1988; 15:1833–1840.

Carr DB, Jacox AK, Chapman CR, et al. Acute Pain Management: Operative or Medical Procedures and Trauma. Clinical Practice Guideline No. 1. AHCPR Pub. No. 92–0032. Agency for Health Care Policy and Research, Public Health Service, US Department of Health and Human Services, Rockville, MD, 1992.

Chapman CR, Gavrin J. Pain: suffering: the contributions of persistent pain. Lancet 1999; 353:2233–2237.

Chapman CR, Loeser JD (eds). Issues in Pain Management, Advances in Pain Research and Therapy, vol 12. Raven Press, New York, 1989.

Chapman CR, Casey KL, Dubner R, et al. Pain measurement: an overview. Pain 1985; 22:1–31.

Drummond MF, O'Brien B, Stoddart GL, et al. Methods for the Economic Evaluation of Health Care Programs, 2nd edn. Oxford University Press, New York, 1997.

Foundation for Health Services Research. Health Outcomes Research: A Primer. Association for Health Services Research website, 1994. Available at: http://www.academyhealth.org/publications/glossary.pdf (accessed August 6, 2004).

Gerteis M, Edgman-Levitan S, Daley J, et al. (eds). Through the Patient's Eyes: Understanding and Promoting Patient-Centered Care. Jossey-Bass, San Francisco, 1993.

Higgins JPT, Green S (eds). Cochrane Reviewers' Handbook 4.2.6 [updated September 2006]. In: The Cochrane Library, Issue 4. John Wiley, Chichester, UK, 2006.

Joint Commission on Accreditation of Healthcare Organizations. Pain Assessment and Management Standards: Hospitals. Joint Commission on Accreditation of Healthcare Organizations (JCAHO), 2001. Available at: http://www.jcrinc.com/subscribers/perspectives.asp?durki=3243 (accessed May 12, 2004).

Keefe FJ, Holzberg AD, Beaupré PM. Contributions of pain behavior assessment and pain assessment to the developments of pain clinics. In: Cohen MJM, Campbell JN (eds). Pain Treatment Centers at a Crossroads: A Practical and Conceptual Reappraisal, Progress in Pain Research and Management, vol 7. IASP Press, Seattle, WA, 1996:79–100.

Levit K, Smith C, Cowan C, et al and the Health Accounts Team. Health spending rebound continues in 2002. Health Affairs 2004; 23:147–159.

Liu SS, Wu CL. Effect of postoperative analgesia on major postoperative complications: a systematic update of the evidence. Anesthesia & Analgesia 2007;104:689–702.

O'Connor DA, Chipchase LS, Tomlinson J, et al. Arthroscopic decompression: responsiveness of disease-specific and health-related quality of life outcome measures. Arthroscopy. J Arthroscopic Relat Surg 1999; 15:836–840.

Orkin FK, Polomano RC, Burton AW, et al. Comparison of pain outcomes and HRQOL using the Treatment Outcomes in Pain Survey (TOPS) in cancer-related pain. 6th Annual European Congress for the International Society of Pharmacoeconomics and Outcomes Research, Barcelona, Spain, November 9–11, 2003.

Pace KT, Dyer SJ, Stewart RJ, et al. Health-related quality of life after laparoscopic and open nephrectomy. Surg Endoscopy 2003; 17:143–152.

Perkins FM, Kehlet H. Chronic pain as an outcome of surgery: a review of predictive factors. Anesthesiology 2000; 93:1123–1133.

PubMed. Home page. 2007. Available at: http://www. ncbi.nlm.nih.gov/entrez/query.fcgi (accessed May 12, 2007).

Rogers WH, Wittink H, Wagner A, et al. Assessing individual outcomes during outpatient multidisciplinary chronic pain treatment by means of an augmented SF-36. Pain Med 2000a; 1:44–54.

Rogers WH, Wittink HM, Ashburn MA, et al. Using the "TOPS," an outcomes instrument for multidisciplinary outpatient pain treatment. Pain Med 2000b; 1:55–67.

Schyve PM. Outcomes as performance measures [Appendix A]. In: Schoenbaum SC, Sundwall DN, Bergman D, et al. (eds). Using Clinical Practice Guidelines to Evaluate Quality of Care: Agency for Health Care Policy and Research, Rockville, MD, 1995:27–34.

Shugars DA, Benson K, White RP, et al. Developing a measure of patient perceptions of short-term outcomes of third molar surgery. J Oral Maxillofac Surg 1996; 54:1402–1408.

Song SO, Carr DB. Pain and memory. Pain Clin Updates 1999; 7(1):1–4.

Strassels SA, Carr DB, Cynn DJ, et al. SF-36 versus SF-12 scores in persons at home one month after surgery [abstract]. 9th World Congress on Pain, 1999, Abstract 325:599.

Strassels SA, McNicol E, Wagner AK, et al. Persistent postoperative pain, health-related quality of life, and functioning one month after hospital discharge. Acute Pain 2004; 6:95–104.

Straus SE, Richardson WS, Glasziov P, et al. Evidence-based Medicine: How to Practice and Teach EBM. New York; Churchill Livingstone, 2005.

Tanenbaum SJ. What physicians know. N Engl J Med 1993; 329:1268–1271.

Turk DC, Melzack R (eds). Handbook of Pain Assessment, 2nd edn. Guilford Press, New York, 2001.

Turk DC, Okifuji A. Assessment of patients' reporting of pain: an integrated perspective. Lancet 1999; 353:1784–1788.

Ware JE Jr., Snow KK, Kosinski M, et al. SF-36 Health Survey Manual and Interpretation Guide. The Health Institute, Boston, MA, 1993.

White RP, Shugars DA, Shafer DM, et al. Recovery after third molar surgery: clinical and health-related quality of life outcomes. J Oral Maxillofac Surg 2003; 61:535–544.

White PF, Kehlet H. Postoperative pain management and patient outcome: Time to return to work! Anesthesia & Analgesia 2007;104:487–489.

Wolfe F, Kong SX. Rasch analysis of the Western Ontario MacMaster questionnaire (WOMAC) in 2205 patients with osteoarthritis, rheumatoid arthritis, and fibromyalgia. Ann Rheum Dis 1999; 58:563–568.

WOMAC Osteoarthritis Index. Online. 2004. Available at: http://www.womac.org/womac/index.htm (accessed May 12, 2004).

CHAPTER 13

Pediatrics and pain outcomes

Suellen M. Walker

INTRODUCTION

Recent advances in pediatric pain management have been reliant on multiple factors including: knowledge of the developmental neurobiology of pain processing and developmental pharmacokinetics of analgesic agents; improved age-appropriate tools for pain assessment; and increased awareness of the impact of pain management on short and long-term outcomes. However, as there is limited information available from randomized controlled trials many pediatric treatments are still empirically based (Fitzgerald and Howard 2003; Howard 2003b). The ethics of placebo-controlled trials continue to be debated (Miller and Brody 2002; Michels and Rothman 2003), and in children active controls rather than placebo are usually employed. Both parental consent and child assent need to be gained (Erb et al. 2002) and difficulties with recruitment often lead to small sample sizes or the need to include a wide age range which encompasses significant developmental changes. The relative lack of specific pediatric drug testing and labeling studies has been recognized by the US Food and Drug Administration (FDA) and Congress in the USA (Department of Health and Human Services 2001), and marketing incentives have been provided to manufacturers who conduct trials in children for a range of indications including pain management. Although this has increased the number of pediatric drug trials and resulted in labeling changes for some drugs (e.g., over-the-counter ibuprofen is now recommended for children down to 6 months of age), there has been little impact on drugs with low sales or those lacking patent protection, and few studies have been conducted in neonates.

Guidelines for pediatric pain management are based on current best levels of evidence, but despite increases in the quality and quantity of data in recent years, pediatric evidence lags behind that available for adult management. In the Second Edition of a national guideline for acute pain management (ANZCA 2005) the proportion of pediatric citations based on level I and II evidence has increased to 50%, compared with only 8% of pediatric but 67% of adult recommendations in the First Edition (Walker et al. 2006). Specific acute pain guidelines for neonates and infants are being updated (Anand et al. 2005b; Berde et al. 2005; RACP 2005), but evidence is not available for all clinical settings (Walker 2005), and suggestions for improved study design have been outlined with the aim of stimulating further research (Anand et al. 2005a). In older children, meta-analyses of analgesic interventions are becoming available, but conclusions are often limited by methodological deficiencies in the primary studies (Hollis et al 2000; Steward et al, 2003; Ansermino et al, 2003; Moiniche et al, 2003) (Hamunen and Kontinen 2005).

One factor delaying the development of evidence-based pediatric practice has been the lack of validated and standardized outcome measures. The evaluation of different outcome measures in pain management requires consideration of the context in which it is measured, the validity of surrogate outcomes, to whom the outcome is relevant, and differentiation of statistically and clinically significant changes. As neonates, preverbal and cognitively impaired children cannot provide self-report of pain, there is an increased reliance on surrogate outcomes and parental assessment in pediatric practice. Multiple pain measurement tools have been developed for neonates and infants but none has emerged as clearly superior (Franck et al. 2000; Howard 2003a). Evidence for analgesic efficacy of individual treatments is available for acute procedural and postoperative pain, but there is insufficient data to allow comparison of the effect size of different agents, or to determine the most appropriate intervention or combination of treatments in different settings. Agreement is needed on a minimal set of well-validated measures of acute pain intensity (Ohlsson et al. 2000; Hicks et al. 2001) to allow comparison and combination of data from different studies. Importantly, two recent systematic reviews have analysed the psychometric properties of self-report and behavioural tools for acute pain assessment in children and adolescents with the aim of recommending outcome measures for clinical trials (Stinson et al. 2006; von Baeyer and Spagrud 2007). As awareness of the prevalence of chronic pain in children and adolescents has increased, specific pediatric outcome tools for assessing pain intensity as well as more global aspects such as quality of life, disability and psychological function are becoming available. This chapter aims to describe outcomes currently being assessed and utilized in the management of pediatric acute and chronic pain. Many of these measures are still being validated rather than being used to assess treatment efficacy, but represent important tools for future trials.

OUTCOMES IN ACUTE PAIN MANAGEMENT

PAIN INTENSITY

Pain measurement scales

The ability to measure pain is an important component of overall pain assessment. This allows evaluation of the intensity of pain and the response to treatment in individual patients, and also provides an essential outcome measure for determining the efficacy of different interventions in controlled trials. Verbal self-report is considered the gold standard of pain measurement in adults, but as children's understanding of pain and their ability to describe it changes with age, measurement tools must be appropriate to the different stages of development. A large number of scales have been developed for neonates and infants, encompassing a number of surrogate measures (e.g., physical signs such as increased heart rate) or behavioral responses (e.g., facial characteristics and cry). Choice of the most appropriate tool depends on the age of the infant, the stimulus (e.g., procedural or postoperative pain), and the purpose of the measurement (e.g., clinical care or research). In older children, age-appropriate scales for self-report need to consider the child's ability to differentiate levels of intensity and separate the emotional from the physical components of pain.

Behavioral measures

Noxious stimuli produce a series of behavioral responses in neonates and infants that can be used as surrogate measures of pain (McGrath 1998; Gaffney et al. 2003). Differential responses to noxious and non-noxious stimuli can be recognized in premature neonates, and these behaviors become more robust and recognizable with increasing postconceptional age (PCA) (Johnston et al. 1996). Behavioral changes included in pain coding systems include: cry, changes in facial activity, movement of torso and limbs, consolability, and sleep state. Cry can be described in terms of its presence or absence, duration, and amplitude or pitch. Changes in facial activity have been reported to be less variable and more consistent in infants. The actions most often descriptive of pain following procedural interventions in preterm to 3 month neonates are brow bulge (bulging, creasing, and vertical furrows above and between brows); eye squeeze (eyes closed with squeezing or bulging of eyelids); nasolabial furrow (deepening of furrow from nostril wings down to and beyond lip corners); open lips; and a taut tongue (Grunau and Craig 1987; Craig 1998). In infants and young children, behavioral items which predict analgesic demand in the postoperative period are crying, facial expression, posture of the trunk, posture of the legs, and motor restlessness (Buttner and Finke 2000).

The reliability and validity of behavioural measures is best established for short sharp pain associated with procedural interventions, but measures for assessing postoperative pain have also been validated. The behaviour of infants having a large number of procedures may become habituated or sensitised depending on the temporal proximity of repeated procedures, motor development and previous handling (Holsti et al.

2006; Holsti and Grunau 2007). Overlap with manifestations of other states of distress (e.g. hunger and fatigue) can further reduce the specificity of the response, and specific measures for pain-related distress or anxiety are available (von Baeyer and Spagrud 2007). Therefore, the developmental age of the child and the context in which the score is being obtained need to be considered. In infants and children, FLACC and CHEOPS (see Table 13.1B) have been recommended as tools for acute procedural and postoperative pain, the COMFORT scale for children in intensive care, and the Parents Postoperative Pain Measure (PPPM) for postoperative pain managed by parents at home (von Baeyer and Spagrud 2007).

Physiologic measures

Changes in physiologic parameters which have been associated with procedural interventions in infants and assumed to indicate the presence of pain include: increases in heart rate, respiratory rate, blood pressure, intracranial pressure, cerebral blood flow and palmar sweating; and decreases in oxygen saturation, transcutaneous carbon dioxide tension, and vagal tone (Sweet and McGrath 1998). These changes are reduced by analgesia and therefore are useful surrogate outcome measures of pain, but as such are only a substitute for a clinically meaningful endpoint.

Physiologic parameters such as heart rate are influenced by many clinical conditions, and not all variability can be specifically attributed to pain. Changes in response to brief procedural pain have been determined, but effects of ongoing or repeated pain are unclear. Physiologic parameters alone cannot determine the presence or absence of pain, and do not always parallel behavioral responses. Some changes require complex recording equipment and analysis (e.g., heart rate variability) and therefore are only suited to research studies. Although changes in physiologic parameters may indicate the presence of acute procedural pain, the ability to differentiate levels of pain intensity is limited. A weak correlation ($r = 0.25$) has been found between clinician ratings of painfulness and the degree of change in heart rate during different procedures. Although an overall increased magnitude of physiologic response occurred with increasingly invasive procedures, there was considerable overlap (i.e., an increase of 20–30 beats per minute in heart rate could occur in response to all severity of procedures) (Porter et al. 1999b).

Changes in hormonal and metabolic hormones (e.g., catecholamines, cortisol, insulin, glucose, beta-endorphin) occur as part of the "stress response" to surgery and have been used as surrogate outcome measures (Anand and Hickey 1987). Although analgesics have been shown to modify this response, and there is an important association with reduced morbidity (Anand et al. 1987; Anand and Hickey 1992), these changes cannot be directly correlated with pain intensity or relief. As results are not immediately available, such measures are suited to research rather than acute clinical management. Longer term changes in cortisol levels have been noted during, and for several months after, neonatal intensive care (Grunau et al. 2005; Grunau et al. 2007).

Using near-infrared spectroscopy, functional activation of the somatosensory cortex has been demonstrated following blood sampling in premature neonates (Bartocci et al. 2006; Slater et al. 2006). The potential for measures of cortical activation to be modified by analgesia and provide a quantifiable surrogate outcome in research studies is being investigated.

Composite measures

Many scales have been developed which incorporate both physiological and behavioural parameters to determine an overall pain score. Some examples are included in Table 13.1 but a wider range of measures, their strengths and limitations, and issues of testing reliability and validity are discussed more fully in recent reviews (Johnston et al. 2003; Franck et al. 2000) (Stinson et al. 2006; von Baeyer and Spagrud 2007). As there is no "gold standard" for pain measurement in neonates and infants, the validity of one scale is often assessed against another scale (Blauer and Gerstmann, 1998), and as yet no single scale has been universally adopted.

The ability of composite measures to differentiate levels of pain intensity with different procedural interventions requires further evaluation. The response to endotracheal suctioning (as assessed by the Premature Infant Pain Profile, PIPP) was reduced in neonates during infusions of morphine or midazolam but not placebo. Therefore, the sensitivity of this measure in differentiating a sedative effect from an analgesic effect was questioned (Anand et al. 1999). In a subsequent larger study, no difference in response to endotracheal suctioning (as assessed by PIPP, NIPS and observer VAS) was found in neonates receiving routine morphine (10mcg/kg/hr) infusions or placebo. However, the correlation between the different measures was relatively low, and the use of rescue morphine in both groups did not correlate with the recorded pain scores. Therefore, limited sensitivity of these measures for relatively mild to moderate pain may have influenced the results (Simons et al. 2003). Similarly, morphine has been reported to be less effective in early life, but pain scores (DAN scale) ranged from 0 to the maximum of 10 following heel stick in both morphine and placebo groups (Carbajal et al. 2005). Further research is needed to improve the sensitivity, specificity, and generalizability of pain-assessment tools, and contextual factors need to be more fully incorporated (Franck et al. 2000), to increase the utility and reliability of these scales as outcome measures.

Table 13.1 Examples of acute pain intensity measurement tools
Table 13.1A Neonates

Scale	Indicators	Score	Validity	Reliability	Utility	Reference
Premature Infant Pain Profile (PIPP)	Gestational age Behavioral state Heart rate Oxygen saturation Brow bulge Eye squeeze Nasolabial furrow	Each scored on 4-point scale (0, 1, 2, 3); 6 or less = minimal pain, >12 = moderate to severe pain	Content and construct validity	Inter-rater reliability; intra-rater reliability; internal consistency	Procedural pain preterm and term neonates; postoperative pain in term neonates	Stevens et al. (1996)
Neonatal Infant Pain Scale (NIPS)	Facial expression Cry Breathing patterns Arms Legs State of arousal	Each scored on 2- (0, 1) or 3-point (0, 1, 2) scale; total score: 0–7	Content, construct and concurrent validity $r = 0.53$–0.84	Inter-rater reliability; internal consistency	Preterm and term neonates; procedural pain	Lawrence et al. (1993)
Neonatal Facial Coding Scale (NFCS)	Brow bulge Deep nasolabial fold Eyes squeezed shut Open mouth Taut tongue	Presence or absence of action during discrete time intervals scored	Content and construct validity; convergent validity $r = 0.89$	Inter-rater and intra-rater reliability > 0.85	Preterm to 3 months; procedural pain	Grunau and Craig (1987)
Crying, Requires oxygen, Increased vital signs, Expression, Sleeplessness (CRIES)	Cries Oxygen saturation Heart rate/BP Expression Sleeplessness	Each scored on 3-point scale (0, 1, 2); total score: 0–10	Content, construct, discriminant and concurrent validity $r = 0.49$–0.73	Inter-rater reliability	32–60 weeks Postoperative pain	Krechel and Bildner (1995)
Modified Behavioral Pain Scale	Facial Cry Movements	Total score 0–10	Construct and concurrent validity $r = 0.68$–0.74	Inter-rater and test/retest reliability	2–4 months Immunization pain	Taddio et al. (1995)

Table 13.1B Composite scales for infants and children

Scale	Indicators	Score	Validity	Reliability	Utility	Reference
Children's Hospital of Eastern Ontario Pain Scale (CHEOPS)	Cry Facial expression Verbal expression Torso position Touch Leg position	Each scored as 0, 1, 2 or 3; total 4–13	Content, criterion and construct validity	Inter-rater reliability; internal consistency	1–7 years Postoperative pain Procedural pain	McGrath et al. (1985)
FLACC	Face Legs Activity Cry Consolability	Each scored on 3-point scale (0, 1, 2); total 0–10	Content, criterion and construct validity	Inter-rater reliability; test/retest reliability	Young children Postoperative pain	Merkel et al. (1997)
Objective Pain Scale (OPS)	Blood pressure Crying Movement Agitation Verbal expression/body language	Each scored 0, 1 or 2; total 0–10	Content, criterion and construct validity	Inter-rater reliability	8 months to 13 years Postoperative pain	Norden et al. (1991)
COMFORT scale	Alertness Calmness/agitation Respiratory response Physical movement Muscle tone Facial expression MAP HR	Score 8–40	Content and criterion validity	Inter-rater reliability	Newborn to adolescent Distress in PICU; postoperative pain 0- to 3-year-olds	Ambuel et al. (1992) Van Dijk et al. (2000)

Table 13.1C Self-report tools for children

Scale	Components	Properties	Anchors	Validity	Utility	Reference
Poker Chip	4 chips = pieces of "hurt"	Concrete ordinal	± White "no pain" chip; 1 chip = "a little hurt"; 4 chips = "most hurt you could ever have"	Adequate convergent validity; correlates with overt behaviors in injection pain	4–8 years	Hester (1979)
Faces Pain Scale	7 graded drawings of faces	Ordinal	No pain/hurt (neutral face, not smiling) to most pain/hurt possible (open mouth, closed eyes, furrowed brow, no tears)	Inter-rater reliability; test/retest reliability; sensitivity to stimulus intensity; good construct validity	6–8 years	Bieri et al. (1990)
Faces Pain Scale – Revised	6 faces	More closely conforms to linear interval scale			5–12 years	Hicks et al. (2001)
Oucher	6 color photographs of young children + 100 point corresponding vertical scale	Ordinal Ratio/interval in older children as numerical scale also	No hurt to biggest hurt you can have	Reliable, adequate content validity	3–12 years Different ethnic versions available	Beyer and Wells (1989)
Colored Analogue Scale	Modification of 10 cm horizontal VAS; scored 0–10 in 0.25 increments	Ratio/interval properties in children > 7–8 years	Gradations in color (white to dark red) and area (progressively wider tetragon); labels "no pain" to "most pain"	Reliable and valid	5 years and above	McGrath et al. (1996)

Tables adapted from Franck et al. (2000); Howard (2003a); Finley and McGrath (1998); Gaffney et al. (2003); Stevens et al. (2000).

MAP = mean arterial pressure; HR = heart rate.

Content validity = adequacy of sampling of content area (e.g., does behavioral scale incorporate all necessary behaviors?).

Criterion validity = correlation with "gold standard"; more approximate measure as no "gold standard" for infant pain measurement.

Construct validity = measures particular construct related to pain such as intensity; supported by ongoing studies; convergent validity (correlation between constructs that have theoretical relation, e.g., increased HR and pain); discriminant validity (test correlation against unrelated construct, e.g., musical talent and pain) (Johnston 1998; Stevens et al. 2000).

Self-report

The reliability and validity of self-report pain intensity measures have recently been reviewed (Stinson et al. 2006). No single scale is applicable across all age ranges. Self-report of pain is usually possible by 4 years of age but will depend on the cognitive and emotional maturity of the child and requires adequate explanation of an age- appropriate tool. Young children can differentiate "more", "less" or "the same" and therefore use tools such as the Poker Chip (now called Pieces of Hurt Tool) scale to choose how many "pieces of hurt" represent their pain. Scores in preschool children may be needed to be supplemented with a behavioural measure to improve reliability in clinical trials (Stinson et al. 2006). Children aged 4–5 years can use a faces pain scale, but have limited capacity to appraise current pain and match it to previous experience, and they are more likely to choose the extremes of the scale (Hicks et al. 2001). As a result, the numbers ascribed to different faces may not represent an interval scale with equidistant points, and non-parametric statistics are more appropriate for analysis. In scales anchored with smiling or tearful faces, pain may be confused with other emotional states such as happiness/sadness or anxiety. In clinical practice, standardised use of the same tool throughout an institution may be more important than which tool is chosen. In research trials, the Faces Pain Scale-Revised has been recommended for acute procedure-related, postoperative and disease-related pain for children aged 4 to 12 years (Stinson et al. 2006).

Between 7 and 10 years children develop skills with measurement, classification and seriation (i.e., putting things in ascending or descending order). Visual analogue scales are now appropriate and can be analyzed as interval scales with parametric statistics. A variety of scales have been used, consisting of a vertical or horizontal line with verbal, facial or numerical anchors. In younger children more concrete simple anchor words such as no hurt/biggest hurt are more appropriate than no pain/worst pain possible. The upper end of the scale is less static than in adults as it will change with the individual child's ability to objectify, label and remember previous pain experiences (Gaffney et al. 2003). It is not until 10–12 years of age that children can clearly discriminate the sensory intensity and the affective emotional components of pain and report them independently (McGrath et al. 1996). Verbally competent children aged 12 years and above can understand and use the McGill Pain Questionnaire (Gaffney et al. 2003).

Standardized instruction is vital for each scale, but it cannot be assumed that different scales are understood in the same way, especially if the anchor points are named in different ways. Good correlation between some self-report scales has been reported, but this depends on the age of the child and the clinical context. For example, correlation between a behavioral scale (FLACC) and a faces scale was shown for children aged 5–7 years but not for younger children (Willis et al. 2003). Correlation between the Faces Pain Scale-Revised (FPS-R) and a visual analogue scale has been reported for brief pain in children between 5 and 12 years, although further validation in children with disease-related pain is required. Many scales have a different range of options, and a compromise must be made between the ability of younger children to differentiate between a large number of choices, and the potential for greater differentiation of intensity with increased choices. In the FPS-R, the number of faces was reduced from 7 to 6 with the aim of developing a common metric (i.e., all scales producing scores of 0–5 or 0–10). This would allow a more universal language for reporting scores, but the ability of each measure to conform to a theoretical linear metric needs to be tested (Hicks et al. 2001).

Children with cognitive impairment

Assessment of pain is difficult in children with cognitive impairment and communication problems, and can contribute to inadequate provision of analgesia. Neonates at risk for neurologic impairment required more procedural interventions in intensive care, but received less analgesia (Stevens et al. 2003). A retrospective chart review of children who had undergone spine fusion surgery found that pain was assessed less frequently in cognitively impaired children and they received less analgesia (Malviya et al. 2001). Behaviours reported by caregivers to be associated with potentially painful stimuli and which discriminate these from distressful or calm events, have been compiled in the Pediatric Pain Profile (Hunt et al. 2004) and the Non-Communicating Children's Pain Checklist (NCCPC) (Breau et al. 2001). Validity of a revised scale (NCCPC-R) has now been assessed in a larger number of patients aged 3–18 years (Breau et al. 2002b) and a postoperative version has also been developed (NCCPC-PV) (Breau et al. 2002a). In the assessment of postoperative pain in children with cognitive impairment, scores on the FLACC scale correlate with parental pain report and are reduced after analgesia (Voepel-Lewis et al. 2002).

Methodologic difficulties with use of pain intensity as outcome measure

Lack of a standardized measure

The lack of a universally accepted measure of pain in children makes direct comparison and combination of data from controlled trials difficult. This is in part insurmountable as different measures will always be required for different age groups, but could be improved with more standardized use of assessment tools in clinical trials (Stinson et al. 2006; von Baeyer and Spagrud 2007). Meta-analyses and systematic reviews of post-tonsillectomy pain have highlighted these methodological problems: the effect of dexamethasone on pain could not be analyzed "due to missing data and varied outcome measurement tools" (Steward et al. 2003); the efficacy of perioperative local anaesthetic could not be confirmed as "some studies included inappropriate, possibly post-hoc outcome measures such as 'global pain scores' which may have resulted in bias" (Hollis et al. 2000); and limited conclusions on the clinical efficacy of systemic analgesics could be drawn due to the variable methodology and limited sensitivity of many trials (Hamunen and Kontinen 2005).

In adult studies, dichotomous data can be derived from visual analogue scores, i.e., the proportion of patients achieving 50% of maximum TOTPAR (total pain relief = area under curve of pain relief against designated time period, e.g., 4 or 6 hours) (Moore et al. 1997). This allows calculation of the number needed to treat (NNT; i.e., number treated to achieve 50% relief in one patient) in a meta-analysis and construction of a league table of the efficacy of different drugs (Kalso et al. 2001). Similar quantitative analyses cannot be conducted with currently available pediatric data. As an alternative, when analyzing data relating to the use of nonsteroidal anti-inflammatory drugs (NSAIDs) following tonsillectomy, Moiniche et al. (2003) qualitatively evaluated if NSAIDs provided inferior, superior or equal analgesia to opioids in individual trials, and concluded that overall NSAIDs were equianalgesic to opioids.

Age range

As recruitment is difficult in pediatric clinical studies, children from a wide range of ages may be included in the sample. If an analgesic agent is being investigated, the same dose is usually given based on the weight of the child (e.g., mg/kg). However, developmental changes in pharmacokinetics and pharmacodynamics (particularly in neonates and infants) may mean that the dose cannot be assumed to be equianalgesic at all ages. Many studies include children aged from 1 to 15 years, and this necessitates using different scales encompassing both categorical and interval data. As the sensitivity and characteristics of scales differ, a 20% reduction in pain score may not represent the same change in intensity on multiple scales, and this has implications for statistical analysis.

Effect size: clinically versus statistically significant change

Statistically significant changes that are relevant to the researcher are often reported in clinical trials, but may not correlate with a clinically significant change for individual patients. A reduction in pain intensity by 30–35% has been rated as clinically meaningful by adult patients with postoperative pain (Jensen et al. 2002) or acute pain in the emergency department (Lee et al. 2003). Children capable of self-report can give an indication of the intensity of pain that is clinically significant, as they rated a score of 3 or greater on the Faces Pain Scale (0–6) as the level they felt warranted pharmacologic intervention (Gauthier et al. 1998). However, the degree of change following an analgesic that is deemed clinically relevant is more difficult to determine in pediatric studies. As preverbal children cannot report the degree of change, assumptions must necessarily be made from changes in surrogate behavioral and physiologic parameters, but will be influenced by the sensitivity of the measure. Use of topical local anesthetic rather than placebo for circumcision reduced the increase in heart rate by 12–27 beats per minute (Taddio et al. 2000), and although this is likely to represent a decrease in pain intensity it cannot be determined if this is a clinically significant or acceptable reduction in pain intensity. Evaluation of the efficacy of analgesic interventions cannot be based on "statistically significant" changes in single parameters.

Parent and child report

The relationship between observer ratings of pain and the child's self-report are influenced by many factors including: the type of pain (e.g., brief needle versus postoperative pain); the clinical context; expectations of pain and availability of relief; cultural and temperamental influences; the child's coping strategies; and who is observing the pain (e.g., parent or nurse). Many analgesic studies are performed in children undergoing day case surgery, and therefore there is an increased reliance on parental assessment and management of pain following discharge. Parental ratings of pain often show poor levels of agreement with children's self-report, and both underestimation (Chambers et al. 1998) and overestimation of children's pain has been reported (Chambers et al. 1999). Correlation between different observers may be more difficult in children with cognitive impairment. No concordance was found between parental assessment of pain and the observed behavioral response in children with autism, whereas much better correlation was found for a control group of children (Nader et al. 2004).

Improved education of parents and use of a more structured form of assessment may improve correlation with the child's report. The Postoperative Pain Measure for Parents (PPMP) is a 15-item behavioral checklist based on nonverbal pain cues for children aged 7–12 years (Chambers et al. 1996). Good correlation between PPMP scores and child-rated pain ($r = 0.61$) has been reported. The score is reduced by analgesia, is specific for pain not anxiety, and can discriminate between low pain and moderate/high pain surgery

(Finley et al. 2003). The reliability and validity of this scale has more recently been demonstrated in younger children aged 2 to 6 years (Chambers et al. 2003).

Comparison group in controlled trials

It is very rare in current pediatric trials for the control group to receive only a placebo and no active treatment. Studies tend to compare two active treatments, or the effect of addition of an active drug or placebo to an analgesic regime. With this design, it is often difficult to distinguish a difference in pain scores between the two groups (Williams et al. 2002; Ansermino et al. 2003). This may reflect a true lack of difference between the two groups, or the difference may be masked by the use of supplemental analgesia. Alternatively, this may represent a type II error if the outcome measure lacks sensitivity or the sample size is too small.

Degree of surgical stimulus

Children with different types of surgery may be included in studies to increase the sample size, but must be equally distributed between treatment groups. Although both herniotomy and orchidopexy may be considered as lower abdominal day case surgery, different intensities of postoperative pain and analgesic requirement have been demonstrated (Ho and Keneally 2000). If the surgery is relatively mild, changes in treatment groups may be difficult to detect. Following myringotomy, no difference was found between patients receiving paracetamol alone and those receiving a combination of paracetamol, codeine and promethazine (Painstop®) as pain scores were low in both groups and there was minimal additional postoperative analgesic required (Ragg and Davidson 1997).

ANALGESIC CONSUMPTION

Total dose

A reduction in analgesic consumption when an active rather than placebo drug is added to an analgesic regime is often used as a measure of analgesic efficacy. The amount of supplemental analgesia required in the two groups can be used for statistical analysis, but the clinical significance of any change will depend upon demonstration of improved efficacy with the combination or a reduction in side effects resulting from the lower dose of supplemental analgesia. NSAIDs have been shown to reduce opioid requirements in several postoperative models, but this is of increased significance if there is an associated reduction in opioid-related side effects without introduction of new side effects (e.g., NSAID-related bleeding) (Forrest et al. 1997). Following spinal fusion, ketorolac had a beneficial effect as pain scores were lower than a group who received placebo. A reduction in PCA opioid requirement was also demonstrated, but was of limited impact as an outcome as there was no associated reduction in side effects (Munro et al. 2002).

The total dose of analgesia received will also be dependent on the trigger for administration, which may be controlled by the child (e.g., PCA), his/her nurse, or his/her parent. As in adults, the dose of opioid delivered via PCA can be used in older children but factors other than pain may influence the dose administered (e.g., individual variability in opioid requirements, education and understanding of device, presence of side effects) (Peters et al. 1999). In neonatal and infant studies, administration of additional analgesia will be dependent on the nurse or clinician assessment. Often poor correlation is found between reported pain scores and supplemental analgesia (Simons et al. 2003), suggesting that other factors may influence analgesic administration. Neonates at risk of neurologic impairment were given less analgesia despite undergoing a higher number of painful procedures, and a perceived increased risk of side effects or difficulty with assessment may have contributed (Stevens et al. 2003). Fifty-one percent of children aged 6 to 16 years were found to be undermedicated for postoperative pain as they reported pain scores above a level that they felt warranted analgesic intervention (Gauthier et al. 1998). Following day case surgery, parents giving analgesia on a "prn" basis tend to administer insufficient analgesia, even when they judge their child to be experiencing clinically significant pain (Finley et al. 1996). Therefore, it cannot be assumed that all children are receiving sufficient analgesia to titrate them to the same pain score or the same level of comfort, and this may limit the applicability of analgesic consumption as an outcome measure.

Time to first analgesic

The time to first analgesia can be used to compare two treatment groups. In individual studies this may be represented as the time period before supplemental analgesia or as Kaplan-Meier survival curves: e.g. cumulative proportion of children requiring extra analgesia over time. A higher number of children receiving 1.5 mg codeine required analgesia 2 and 4 hours following tonsillectomy, compared with a group receiving 0.15 mg morphine. As these doses are relatively equianalgesic, differences may reflect genetic polymorphism in codeine metabolism (Williams et al, 2002). Such studies require the return of pain prior to analgesia, and therefore the trigger for administration will influence the results. In a meta-analysis examining addition of clonidine to caudal local anaesthetic, studies used different criteria from a range of scales (eg. VAS >4/10 or 6/10; CHEOPS >6 or >9).The difference in duration between treatment groups was combined rather than the raw data, revealing a statistically significant increase in time to analgesia (144.7 minutes) (Ansermino et al. 2003). The authors questioned if this represented a clinically important improvement, but the final result may have been influenced by the sensitivity of the data.

GLOBAL SATISFACTION

Global ratings of satisfaction allow patients to evaluate the unpleasantness or inconvenience of the intervention, the personal meaningfulness of any improvement in their pain and function, and the unpleasantness and meaning of any adverse events. This can be difficult in younger children as they have limited language to describe their pain, and limited experiences with which to compare their current pain. Results need to be considered in the context of the family, particularly as parents are the primary decision makers about current and future care. Outcomes relevant to the researcher or parent may not always be relevant to the child. Fasting leads to dissatisfaction in children and therefore earlier resumption of diet and a reduction in vomiting (e.g., with use of steroids and tonsillectomy) (Steward et al. 2003) may contribute greatly to overall satisfaction and be more relevant to the child than a small but statistically significant reduction in pain score.

Satisfaction may be difficult to predict and influenced by expectations. A comparison of epidural versus intravenous morphine following dorsal rhizotomy reported lower pain scores and less muscle spasm in the epidural group. However, parents from both groups believed the postoperative pain was less than anticipated, perceived relief as adequate, and were very satisfied (Malviya et al. 1999).

Standardized questionnaires may improve the evaluation of satisfaction, and have been utilized in adults to assess changes in quality of care, such as the impact of an acute pain service on outcomes (Miaskowski et al. 1999). Versions of the Total Quality Pain Management (TQPM) instrument have been tested in parents and children (8–12 years). It comprises a visual analogue scale to assess current and previous pain intensity, and a questionnaire with five domains: communication about pain after surgery; therapeutic effects and side effects of the pain medications; duration of pain and perceived intent of doctors and nurses to relieve pain; ratings of pain experienced and pain expected; and satisfaction with pain management. Parents and children tended to agree in responses about communication, response to analgesics and pain duration, but children tended to be less satisfied and were less likely than their parents to say that "everything is fine" (Foster and Varni 2002). Further research is required to investigate the importance of discrepancies between child and parent report, and to establish the validity of these instruments in different settings and different age groups.

MORBIDITY AND MORTALITY

Side effects

Clinical analgesic trials usually focus on and are powered for efficacy. The incidence of side effects may be low in small trials, and can be difficult to accurately determine from meta-analysis if studies vary in the manner of reporting (e.g., vomiting may be reported as absent/present, with no indication of frequency or severity) or the method of reporting (e.g., a diary is often more sensitive than spontaneous reporting or direct questioning). Information on rare and serious adverse events may only be found in large epidemiologic studies (Kalso et al. 2002).

Many pediatric studies fail to show a difference in the incidence of side effects, either because there is no difference or because the difference is too small to be detected in a small sample. Statistically significant differences in opioid dose (e.g., reduction in opioid dose by adding NSAIDs, or increases in morphine dose when PCA is compared with continuous infusion) may not be associated with significant differences in the incidence of nausea and vomiting (Peters et al. 1999; Munro et al. 2002). As the baseline incidence of vomiting is relatively high following tonsillectomy, changes due to treatment can be easier to detect in these patients. The probability of vomiting was related to morphine dose by logistic regression, and doses above 0.1 mg/kg were associated with a greater than 50% incidence of vomiting (Anderson et al. 2000). A systematic review found no difference in analgesia between NSAIDs and opioids following tonsillectomy, but the risk of emesis was significantly reduced when NSAIDs were utilized (Moiniche et al. 2003).

Respiratory outcomes

The role of postoperative pain management in improving cardiac and respiratory outcomes, hastening resumption of gastrointestinal function, and reducing thromboembolic complications has been an important area of investigation in adults; with the main focus being comparisons between regional and systemic analgesic techniques (Rathmeel et al. 2003). However, as ischemic heart disease and chronic obstructive pulmonary disease are rare in children, these outcomes are less relevant to pediatric studies.

The impact of different analgesic regimes on perioperative pulmonary complications has been evaluated by meta-analysis in adults (Ballantyne et al. 1998). In pediatric studies, retrospective case series (McNeely et al. 1997; Hodgson et al. 2000) report improvements in respiratory function and reduced need for mechanical ventilation with regional analgesia techniques, but these were nonrandomized and uncontrolled studies. In a blinded randomized controlled trial, children receiving intravenous morphine had lower respiratory rates and oxygen saturation than children managed with epidural analgesia, but the degree of difference was of limited clinical significance (Wolf and Hughes 1993).

The incidence of postoperative apnea is an important respiratory outcome in neonates. Following inguinal herniorrhaphy performed under general anesthesia, a strong inverse relationship was found between postoperative apnea and gestational age; and the operative use of opioids was one of eleven risk factors associated with apnea (Cote et al. 1995). A meta-analysis of spinal versus general anesthesia for inguinal herniorrhaphy in premature infants reported a reduction in postoperative apnea in the spinal group, but only when infants having preoperative sedation were excluded. A reduction in use of postoperative ventilation was noted in the spinal group but this was of borderline statistical significance, and as the analysis included only 108 patients, the authors noted a need for further large randomized controlled trials with adequate blinding, follow-up and intention to treat analysis (Craven et al. 2003).

Surgical outcomes

Analgesic regimes may affect surgical outcomes, and the impact of non-steroidal anti-inflammatory drugs (NSAIDs) on post-tonsillectomy bleeding has been evaluated in meta-analyses. However, these analyses have included different trials, defined the primary outcome in different ways, and used different methodology. This has led to different results and recommendations which include: (i) bleeding is increased by aspirin but not ibuprofen and diclofenac (7 trials) (Krishna et al. 2003); (ii) risk of bleeding and reoperation is increased (number needed to harm, NNH = 29) and NSAIDs should not be used (7 trials) (Marret at al. 2003); (iii) risk of reoperation (NNH 60) but not bleeding is increased and NSAIDs should be used cautiously (25 trials) (Moiniche et al. 2003); and (iv) NSAIDs do not increase the risk of bleeding or reoperation but further studies are required (13 pediatric trials) (Cardwell et al. 2005). These reports emphasise the difficulty in making definitive conclusions when different outcome measures are used in individual trials, particularly when evaluating relatively rare complications in small trials, and different methodologies are used in meta-analyses.

Stress response

In early studies, improved perioperative analgesia in neonates undergoing cardiac surgery was associated with a reduction in the stress response (assessed by changes in plasma catecholamines, cortisol, and steroid hormones) and reduction in postoperative morbidity and mortality (Anand et al. 1987; Anand and Hickey 1992). However, the stress response is a surrogate outcome that does not directly reflect pain, and an association rather than a direct causal link exists between increased analgesia and reduced morbidity.

An inverse relationship has been shown between opioid dose and extent of rise in glucose, cortisol and catecholamines (Duncan et al. 2000), but the threshold for a clinically significant change is not clear. Perioperative increases in adrenaline, glucose and ACTH were greater in children receiving systemic morphine compared with epidural bupivacaine following abdominal surgery, but "acceptable analgesia" was achieved in both groups (Wolf et al. 1993). Further research is required to establish the degree of change in stress response which affects clinically significant outcomes.

Neurologic outcome and mortality

It has been postulated that analgesia may decrease the fluctuations in cerebral blood volume and intracranial pressure caused by neonatal reactions to painful procedures, thereby improving neurological outcome (Simons et al, 2003). Several studies in ventilated preterm neonates have compared the effect of routine morphine versus placebo infusions on neonatal death, severe intraventricular haemorrhage (IVH, grade III or IV), or periventicular leukomalacia. The incidence of poor neurologic outcome was reduced by morphine (10–30 mcg/kg/hr) when compared with midazolam or placebo infusion (4% vs 32% vs 24% respectively; n=67), but no difference was found in neurobehavioural outcomes at 36 weeks PCA (Anand et al, 1999). A reduction in IVH from 40% in the placebo group to 23% in a routine morphine group was subsequently reported (n=150). Both groups could receive open-label morphine if judged to be in pain or distress, and this was administered to 27% in the morphine group and 40% in the placebo group (Simons et al. 2003). A much larger trial (n=898) found no improvement in neurological outcome with routine morphine infusions, and initially reported that neonates given open-label morphine were more likely to develop severe IVH (Anand et al. 2004). However, a subsequent analysis found that IVH and death were associated with pre-exisiting hypotension, and morphine was not a contributing factor (Hall et al. 2005). It is possible that neonates with early neurological impairment exhibited signs of irritability that were misinterpreted as pain. These studies demonstrate how not only the sensitivity, but also the specificity, of pain measures can impact on reported outcomes in this patient group.

MEASUREMENT OF HYPERALGESIA

In adults, there is a correlation between reported pain intensity and the threshold and intensity of the flexion reflex. Opioid analgesia reduces both pain intensity and the strength of the reflex withdrawal (Willer 1985). The mechanical sensory threshold for hindlimb withdrawal can be determined in infants by applying progressively increasing mechanical stimuli (von Frey hairs) to the foot or lower leg. In premature infants, the threshold is low and increases with postnatal age, and the latency and amplitude of the reflex response correlates with the intensity of the mechanical stimulus (Fitzgerald et al. 1988; Andrews and Fitzgerald 1999). Tissue injury and inflammation result in a reduction in the mechanical threshold, which can be reversed by topical local anesthesia (Fitzgerald et al. 1989; Jain and Rutter 2000). Although not evaluating "pain," measurement of reflex thresholds and hyperalgesia may provide a surrogate quantifiable outcome for evaluating the extent of tissue injury and the response to analgesic interventions in neonates and infants.

Tactile stimulation of the abdomen triggers a reflex contraction of abdominal muscles producing ipsilateral flattening of the abdominal wall. This abdominal skin reflex has been used as a quantitative measure of skin wound sensitivity following unilateral abdominal surgery. The mechanical threshold was decreased on the side of surgery (by up to 78%) compared with the contralateral side, and increased following administration of analgesia. Although this initial study was not controlled adequately to evaluate the efficacy of different analgesic agents, this methodology provides a potential outcome measure for future studies (Andrews and Fitzgerald 2002).

LONG-TERM EFFECTS OF NEONATAL PAIN

Significant reorganization of synaptic connections occurs in the postnatal period. Activity within sensory pathways is required for normal development, but abnormal or excessive activity related to pain and injury during the neonatal period may alter normal development and produce persistent changes (Fitzgerald and Walker 2003). In laboratory studies, the degree of long-term change varies with the type and severity of injury (Walker et al. 2003). These findings are of considerable importance as pain and injury in neonates may have effects on nociceptive processing that differ in mechanism and duration from that experienced by older children and adults. The evidence for long-term consequences following early pain is outlined in review articles (Goldschneider and Anand 2003; Fitzgeraldand Walker 2003; Grunau et al. 2006; Grunau and Tu 2007).

Behavioral responses

Neonates requiring intensive care management undergo a large number of potentially painful interventions (Porter et al. 1999b; Stevens et al. 2003). Longitudinal studies suggest that early pain may have long-term effects upon pain-related behavior and the perception of pain, which vary with the age at follow-up. At 18 months of age extremely low birth weight (ELBW) ex-premature neonates were judged by their parents to be less sensitive to pain; higher somatization was noted at 4.5 years; at 8–10 years images of medically related pain were rated higher than psychosocial pain, and the duration of intensive care stay correlated with higher pain affect (Grunau 2000; Goldschneider and Anand 2003). However, it is difficult to isolate the effects of pain and its management from the effects of concurrent illness during the neonatal period, or from

social and environmental factors that will influence subsequent neurobehavioral development. A meta-analysis of case-control studies of children born preterm (<37 weeks gestation) and evaluated after 5 years reported reduced cognitive test scores and alterations in behavior including an increased incidence of attention-deficit/hyperactivity disorder (ADHD) (Bhutta et al. 2002). At 8 years of age, ELBW or very preterm (weight <1000 g or gestational age <28 weeks) neonates scored significantly below normal birth weight (>2500 g) controls on full scale IQ, verbal comprehension, perceptual organization, and processing speed. Increased behavioral problems, including attentional difficulties, internalizing behavior problems, immature adaptive skills and increased somatic complaints, were also reported by parents and teachers of the ex-premature group (Anderson et al. 2003). Many of these factors may effect self-report and the behavioral response to pain.

Alterations in behavioral responses to subsequent stimuli have been noted days and months following interventions in term neonates. Infants who underwent repeated heel lances in the first 24–36 hours of life had higher median scores for grimacing and crying (compared to normal controls) during a subsequent venepuncture in the hand (Taddio et al. 2002). Males who were circumcised without analgesia during the neonatal period displayed an increased response (measured as percentage facial action, percentage cry duration and visual analogue pain scores by blinded observers) to routine vaccination at 4–6 months of age (Taddio et al. 1995, 1997). Long-term changes may be modified by analgesia at the time of neonatal surgery (Taddio et al. 1997; Peters et al. 2003), but current outcome measures lack the sensitivity and trial sizes are too small to confirm the degree of change. Further studies are required.

Hyperalgesia

Hyperalgesia has been demonstrated in the area of injury following repeated heel pricks in neonates (Fitzgerald et al. 1989). Laboratory studies have shown persistent reductions in sensory thresholds in the region of neonatal skin wounds (Reynolds and Fitzgerald 1995), but this has not been extensively evaluated in clinical studies. Using the abdominal skin reflex, a reduction in mechanical sensory threshold was found on the ipsilateral abdomen in infants with prenatally diagnosed unilateral hydronephrosis, suggesting the presence of referred visceral hyperalgesia. In these infants the reflex did not show the normal developmental change (i.e., increase in threshold and reduction in radiation of the reflex with increasing age) during the first year of life, and the threshold was still lower than in control infants 3 months following corrective surgery (Andrews et al. 2002). This may provide an objective outcome measure for the evaluation of long-term effects of early injury.

Quantitative sensory testing (QST) allows evaluation of the response to a number of sensory modalities (eg. thermal and mechanical thresholds) in children aged 5 years and above (Meier et al, 2001). Longterm changes in sensory function have been demonstrated 9–14 years following intensive care (Hermann et al. 2006) and surgery (Schmelzle-Lubiecki et al. 2007) in the neonatal period. QST has also been used to quantify thermal and mechanical allodynia in children with different chronic pain states, such as Complex Regional Pain Syndrome (Sethna et al. 2007) and migraine (Zohsel et al. 2006). It is not yet clear if these measures will have a role as outcome measures in clinical trials of interventions for pediatric chronic pain.

COST

In adult practice, the impact of perioperative care and pain management on hospital stay and cost has become an important outcome measure, but has not been systematically evaluated in the pediatric setting. Children managed with epidural analgesia following surgery for idiopathic scoliosis were discharged from hospital 0.5 days earlier than a group receiving PCA opioids (Van Boerum et al. 2000). Although representing a statistically significant change, factors such as the time of discharge and ability to use the bed for the remainder of the day will influence if this translates into a cost saving outcome. Retrospective studies comparing the use of epidural analgesia and systemic opioid analgesia in children following fundoplication report reduced hospital stay (8 versus 13 days) (Wilson et al. 2001) and a 20% reduction in hospital charges (McNeely et al. 1997) in the epidural group. Neonates receiving epidural analgesia following congenital diaphragmatic hernia repair had a reduced requirement for postoperative ventilation, but as children with a worse prognosis were excluded from this group (Hodgson et al. 2000) a reduction in morbidity and cost cannot be solely attributed to the analgesic regime. These findings need confirmation in prospective randomized trials.

As a large proportion of pediatric surgery is now performed on a day stay basis, inadequate analgesia or side effects of treatment that require hospital admission will significantly increase cost. The probability of admission for vomiting after tonsillectomy has been related to morphine dose by logistic regression, and the rate of admission is 10% with a dose of 0.1 mg/kg or above (Anderson et al. 2000). The incidence of vomiting is reduced with the use of NSAIDs but this may be associated with an increased risk of postoperative bleeding, and therefore the relative benefits need to be assessed. In a recent meta-analysis evaluating the NNH associated with NSAID use and tonsillectomy, the question was raised: "is avoiding PONV in 11 patients worth the potential risk and expense of bringing 2 patients back to the operating room for bleeding?" (Moiniche et al. 2003).

Indirect costs to the parent and family also need to be considered. In a recent study evaluating a measure of patient and parent satisfaction with acute postoperative care, children expected to miss an average of 10 days of school and parents required an average of 7.4 days away from work to care for their child (Foster and Varni 2002).

OUTCOMES IN PEDIATRIC CHRONIC PAIN MANAGEMENT

INTRODUCTION

Children may experience chronic pain in association with medical illnesses such as juvenile arthritis and sickle cell disease, or in association with cancer and/or its treatment. In addition, many chronic recurrent pain syndromes (e.g., headache, recurrent abdominal pain) are relatively common and can occur in up to 25% of children (Perquin et al. 2000a; Berde et al. 2003; Schanberg et al. 2003). Neuropathic pain is also increasingly recognized in children and may be related to traumatic or surgical injury (e.g., phantom limb pain), complex regional pain syndromes (CRPS), or tumor involvement. Chronic pain requires recognition and appropriate management in childhood, as it can have significant social and emotional consequences for the child and family; physical and psychological sequelae; and disability that may impact on overall health and school attendance (American Pain Society Position Statement). As in acute pain management, appropriate age-specific outcome measures are required to determine the overall impact of chronic pain on physical and social function, assess the efficacy of different treatments, and develop evidence-based practice. At this stage, many pharmacologic treatments are extrapolated from adult studies (e.g., use of tricyclic antidepressants for neuropathic pain) and there are relatively few controlled trials determining the safety and efficacy of treatment in pediatric patients (Hamalainen et al. 1997a,b). Developmental issues of pain experience also require clarification as the pattern of pain experience, level of reporting, types of coping strategies, and social interactions vary significantly throughout childhood and adolescence (Hunfeld et al. 2002).

The outcome most extensively reported in the pediatric chronic pain literature is pain severity derived from reports of intensity and frequency. Functional and psychological consequences have been relatively neglected (Palermo 2000), and there is a need for controlled trials including other domains of pain experience such as mood, function, disability, school attendance, quality of life, impact on family, healthcare use and medication use. Many scales are now being developed (see Table 13.2), but have been utilized

Table 13.2 Examples of scales for different domains of pain experience in children and adolescents
Table 13.2A Mental health scales

Scale	Age range	Items	Domains	Subscales	Score	Reference
Children's Depression Inventory	7–17 years: reading level 1st grade	27-item self-report symptom-oriented scale	Negative mood, interpersonal problems, ineffectiveness, anhedonia, negative self-esteem		Each item has 3 choices, select one that best describes last 2 weeks: 0 = no symptoms, 1 = mild, 2 = definite symptoms	Kovacs (1992)
Revised Children's Manifest Anxiety Scale (RCMAS)	6–19 years: reading level grades 3–4; recommend reading out to grades 1 and 2	37-item self-report	28 anxiety items 9 lie (social desirability) items	Anxiety subscales: physiologic factor, worry/oversensitivity factor, concentration anxiety factor	Yes or no	Reynolds and Richmond (1978)

Table 13.2B Coping scales

Scale	Items	Domains	Subscales	Score	Reference
Pain Response Inventory for Children		(i) Active coping; (ii) passive coping; (iii) accommodative coping	Each has subscales		Walker et al. (1997)
Waldron/Varni Pediatric Pain Coping Inventory	41 items		Cognitive self-instruction; seek social support; strive to rest and be alone; cognitive refocusing; problem solving/self-efficacy	Rate how often coping strategies used on 3-point scale	Varni et al. (1996)
Coping Strategies Questionnaire (CSQ-C)	44-item measure	(i) Cognitive strategies; (ii) behavioral strategy	(i) Diverting attention, reinterpreting pain sensations, ignoring pain sensations, calming self-statements, praying or hoping, catastrophizing; (ii) increasing behavioral activity level	How often use strategy to cope with pain using 7-point scale: 0 = never, 6 = always	Schanberg et al. (1997)
Pain Coping Questionnaire		(i) Approach; (ii) problem-focused avoidance; (iii) emotion-focused avoidance	(i) Information seeking, problem solving, seeking social support, positive self-statements; (ii) positive self-statements, behavioral distraction, cognitive distraction; (iii) externalizing, internalizing/catastrophizing	Grade how often use each strategy: 1 = never, 5 = very often	Reid et al. (1998)
Pain Catastrophizing Scale for Children (PCS-C)	13 items		Rumination; magnification; helplessness	5-point response scale: 0 = not at all, 4 = extremely	Crombez et al. (2003)

*see also BAPQ Table 13.2C

Table 13.2C Quality of life

Scale	Items	Domains	Subscales	Score	Reference
Quality of Life Headache in Youth (QLH-Y)		Psychological functioning; physical functioning; social functioning; functional status	(i) Stress, harmony and vitality, fatigue, depression, cheerful mood, optimism; (ii) somatic symptoms; (iii) at home, at school, interaction with peers, interaction with siblings; (iv) impact on activities of daily life and leisure	Assess impact on daily life 2 VAS scales: satisfaction with life and health	Langeveld et al. (1996)
QOL Questionnaire for Adolescents with Chronic Pain (QLA-CP)		Psychological functioning; functional status; physical status; social functioning; satisfaction with life in general; satisfaction with health			Merlijn et al. (2002)
Pediatric Quality of Life Inventory (PedsQL)	Arthritis module: 22 items	Pain and hurt, daily activities, treatment, worry, communication			Varni et al. (2002)
Impact on Family Scale	24 items	Economic burden; familial/social impact; personal strain; mastery			Hunfeld et al. (2001)
Bath Adolescent Pain Questionnaire (BAPQ)	61 items	Social functioning; physical functioning; depression; general anxiety; pain specific anxiety; family functioning; development			Eccleston et al. (2005)

Table 13.2D General health and disability

Scale	Items	Domains	Score	Reference
Childhood Health Assessment Questionnaire (CHAQ)	30-item questionnaire	Dressing and personal care, rising, eating, walking, hygiene, reach, grip, activities	Assess performance over last week	Singh et al. (1994)
Children Somatization Inventory (CSI)	35-item questionnaire	Self-reported somatic complaints	5-point Likert scales (1 = no problems, 5 = many problems)	Walker and Greene (1989)
Functional Disability Inventory (FDI)	15-item questionnaire	School, home, recreation, social interactions	Difficulty in activities: 5-point scale, 0–4	Walker and Greene (1991)

predominantly in cross-sectional studies rather than in controlled longitudinal studies evaluating the efficacy of different treatment strategies.

INCIDENCE

The reported incidence of chronic pain in children varies in different studies due to use of different research designs (e.g., investigation of specific conditions such as headache rather than more global sources), different measurement instruments (retrospective questionnaire versus prospective diary), and variable inclusion criteria or definitions. Recent prevalence data for some conditions include: arthritis, 3 to 460 per 100,000; sickle cell disease, 28 to 120 per 100,000; limb pain, 4.2 to 33.6%; recurrent abdominal pain, 6 to 15%; migraine, 4 to 27%; and non-migraine headache, 6.3 to 29% (McGrath 1999; Hamalainen and Masek 2003). Although accounting for 40% of referrals to a pediatric chronic pain clinic, the overall incidence of neuropathic pain in children and adolescents is unknown (Berde et al. 2003).

There is no clear consensus regarding the definition of chronic pain in children, but Dutch epidemiologic studies found that 25% of children reported "pain existing recurrently or continuously for more than 3 months" (Perquin et al. 2000). Questionnaires were completed by the parent (for children aged 0–7 years; $n = 1946$) or the child (8–18 years; $n = 3477$). As this was a community-based study, chronic recurrent pains such as limb pain, headache and abdominal pain were the most common conditions, and in subsequent publications the authors refer to these conditions as "chronic benign pain" or "chronic pain and no documented physiologic etiology" (Perquin et al. 2001; Merlijn et al. 2003; Perquin et al. 2003). Fifty percent of chronic pain sufferers had pain in multiple sites, and in one-third this pain was frequent and intense (at least once per week and 50 mm on a 0–100 mm visual analogue scale). The prevalence of chronic pain increased with age, with a peak in girls aged 12–14 years. Gender differences have also been noted in the intensity of pain (higher intensity in girls) and site of pain (increased headache and abdominal pain in girls, increased back and limb pain in boys) (Perquin et al. 2000a; Merlijn et al. 2003).

PAIN-SPECIFIC MEASURES

Pain intensity

Age-specific measures of pain intensity are applicable to both acute and chronic pain. Many chronic pain assessment tools include a visual analogue scale for older children (Varni et al. 1987; Abu-Saad et al. 1990). In addition to pain intensity, the frequency and duration of chronic pain episodes need to be evaluated. This can be achieved with a retrospective questionnaire or prospective diary, but the former will be influenced by recall errors (van den Brink et al. 2001). In children aged 9–16 years with recurrent headaches, reports from a retrospective questionnaire and a prospective diary completed 3 months later were compared. Both headache intensity and duration were overestimated on the questionnaire compared to the diary (assuming no major changes in the disease process). The size of the recall error was predicted by age, depression, and headache severity (van den Brink et al. 2001). Older children overestimated intensity on the questionnaire more than younger children, and more severe headaches were associated with less overestimation.

Calculation of change in pain severity

For the purposes of assessment in individuals and for comparison amongst different groups, a measure that captures the overall pain experience in a given time period is often calculated. For example, intensity ratings over a week may be summated to give the "Pain Index" (Eccleston et al. 2002). The percentage change from baseline can be calculated for individual patients to determine the degree of change with time, or to determine if a specific treatment provides an analgesic effect in a controlled trial. Although often chosen as the primary outcome, the degree of change in pain intensity that is statistically significant may not always correlate with a change that individual patients perceive as clinically significant. Although this issue has been discussed in relation to adult studies (Turk 2001; McQuay et al. 2003), it has not been evaluated in pediatric trials. In adults, the number of patients achieving a 50% reduction in pain is often used as the outcome measure, and has also been used in a meta-analysis of psychological therapies for headache in children aged 7–18 years (Eccleston et al. 2002). The odds-ratio for a 50% pain reduction was 9.62 and the number needed to treat was 2.32, indicating that psychological treatments were effective in reducing headache pain. At this stage, there are insufficient controlled trials and meta-analyses conducted from pediatric trials to compare the efficacy of different treatments.

PSYCHOLOGICAL FUNCTION (MOOD AND COPING)

Interaction of biologic processes, psychological factors and social/environmental factors will influence the overall experience of chronic pain in children. Questionnaires provide information rapidly and can be utilized for research but must be validated in pediatric age groups, rather than being simply adapted from adult measures. The multiple domains of pain experience that can affect perceived pain intensity and quality of life are best assessed by age-appropriate measures developed specifically for patients with pain. Child mental health measures of depression and anxiety (see Table 13.2A) may be utilized to assess mood, but in children with chronic pain and associated somatic complaints, total scores may be disproportionately high. Disease-specific (e.g., rheumatoid arthritis or headache) rather than generic scales may not be generalizable to all pain conditions, and measures need to be sensitive to changes with time due to fluctuations in disease activity. Although many instruments have been used to assess the impact of chronic pain in adolescents, relatively few have been specifically evaluated in this population (Eccleston et al. 2006). The Bath Adolescent Pain Questionnaire (BAPQ) has been validated in adolescents with chronic pain and assesses multiple domains including physical disability, mood, social and family functioning, and school attendance (Eccleston et al. 2005).

Outcome measures

A number of outcome scales have been utilized in cross-sectional studies to investigate their validity in community samples, their ability to distinguish differences between pain and nonpain cohorts, or their sensitivity to changes in disease activity. If shown to be valid, reliable and reproducible, these scales may be utilized as outcome measures in future controlled trials that critically assess or compare different treatments. A further challenge will be to determine which measure is most appropriate for different ages, different treatments, and different outcomes. In 18 trials of psychological therapies for the management of pediatric chronic pain, 47 distinct measurement instruments were used with each study including between 1 and 6 measures. The primary outcome was often unclear, and incomplete reporting and use of unreliable measurement instruments limited the ability to combine data in a meta-analysis (Eccleston et al. 2002).

Developmental changes

Normal developmental changes that influence behavior, language skills, memory, and cognitive function have marked effects on pain reporting at different ages. Therefore, tools need to be age-appropriate. Most questionnaires are only applicable to the reading level and comprehension of children aged over 7–8 years. In younger children and developmentally delayed or cognitively impaired children, many measures are dependent on parental report. Psychological parameters also change with time, and children have less stable coping patterns with changes towards maladaptive patterns during adolescence (Gil et al. 1997). The effect of age-related changes in coping style on chronic pain requires further evaluation in longitudinal studies (Schanberg et al. 1997).

Parent versus child reports

Discrepancies have been noted between parent and child reports of the intensity of pain experienced by the child and his/her behavioral and cognitive responses to chronic pain. Children rate worst pain higher than parents, but also report better health-related quality of life. Many coping strategies cannot be adequately assessed by parents, and children report higher levels of positive self-statements, lower levels of internalizing/catastrophizing, and use more cognitive self-instruction than reported by their parents. Parents report higher use of observable behavioral responses (strive to rest and be alone, and seek social support) (Reid et al. 1998; Sawyer et al. 2004).

Disease activity

Fluctuations in disease activity can produce variability in the frequency and severity of pain. A positive correlation between physician rating of disease activity and reported pain intensity has been found using the Varni Pediatric Pain Questionnaire (Varni et al. 1987). However, many studies have shown that only a proportion (28–33%) of pain variance is uniquely explained by disease severity. Scores on the Pain Control and Rational Thinking factor of the Coping Strategies Questionnaire for Children (CSQ-C) accounted for an additional 21–22% of variability in pain rating (Schanberg et al. 1997). The effects of coping style were evident even after controlling for age, disease duration, and disease severity, thus emphasizing the importance of including psychological factors in overall assessment.

Coping style

Many psychological factors, such as coping style, have been used in regression models to examine predictors of present pain intensity. However, correlations between psychological factors and pain conditions must not be confused with causal effects. When compared with a control group, adolescents with chronic pain are more likely to use emotion-focused avoidance coping strategies (Merlijn et al, 2003). In this case, emotions are freely expressed, and strategies reflect a lack of effort to regulate feelings when in pain. The related subscales of externalizing and internalizing/catastrophizing are incorporated in several questionnaires (see Table 2.2). Higher scores on this measure are associated with more emotional distress, less coping effectiveness, and higher levels of pain (Reid et al, 1998). Gender has also been shown to influence coping style in adolescents with chronic pain; females used more social support and internalizing/catastrophizing; whereas males used more behavioural distraction (Keogh and Eccleston 2006). Children with more severe headache have been shown to require more social support, use behavioural and cognitive distraction techniques less often, and are less likely to seek information (Bandell-Hoekstra et al, 2002). As well as being associated with increased pain intensity, a relationship has been shown between catastrophizing and pain related disability (Crombez et al, 2003).

PHYSICAL FUNCTION AND DISABILITY

Disability

The degree of disability and functional impairment associated with chronic pain is an important outcome in pediatric patients. Different "measures" have been reported and include: (1) simple descriptive terms (e.g., bedridden or confined to wheelchair, nonambulatory without crutches; Sherry et al. 1999); (2) generic measures of standardized physical activities (e.g., time to walk 10 meters, number of sit to stand movements within 1 minute; Eccleston et al. 2003); and (3) disease-specific measures (e.g., number of joints involved in JRA). More detailed questionnaires encompass several domains of function in different settings (e.g., Functional Disability Inventory, FDI) or combine aspects of function and general health (e.g., Childhood Health Assessment Questionnaire, CHAQ) (see Table 13.2D). As many chronic pain syndromes have a variable course with fluctuating symptoms (e.g., headache) or a tendency to relapse (e.g., CRPS), trials of different treatments need to be controlled and have detailed outcome measures to ensure that changes in function with time can be ascribed to treatment rather than the natural history of the underlying condition. In adolescents with chronic pain, pain intensity was a significant predictor of functional disability, and depression but not anxiety was also associated with worse function (Gauntlett-Gilbert and Eccleston 2007).

School attendance

School attendance is an important functional outcome in children, although it will also be influenced by parental attitudes and needs. In 18 trials of psychological therapies for chronic pain management, only 4 reported school attendance as an outcome measure (Eccleston et al. 2002). A mean of 4.1 days of school absenteeism per month has been reported in children with chronic benign pain (Perquin et al. 2001). In a group of 57 adolescents with chronic pain for a mean duration of 4.02 years, only 14 were in full time education. Three months following a program of interdisciplinary cognitive behavior therapy, school attendance had improved from a mean of 3.28 to 5.69 sessions per week (Eccleston et al. 2003).

QUALITY OF LIFE

Quality of life is a global outcome measure that encompasses a broad range of physical and psychological characteristics relating to function and satisfaction. Questionnaires with multiple items in different domains (e.g., psychological function, physical status, functional status, social functioning, and satisfaction with health) have been developed to provide an overall measure of quality of life (see Table 13.2C). The negative influence of chronic pain on quality of life has been confirmed in a number of pediatric studies (Hunfield et al. 2001; Bandell-Hoekstra et al. 2002; Frare et al. 2002; Merlijn et al. 2003). Adolescents with the highest headache severity reported the lowest quality of life and the most problems with regard to physical functioning, impact on daily and leisure activities, physical symptoms other than headache, and social functioning at home (Bandell-Hoekstra et al. 2002). Pain, quality of life, and the individual's ability to cope all interact within a set of personal and situational variables (Frare et al. 2002). A bi-directional relationship has been suggested, in which headache influences quality of life, quality of life influences headache, and coping strategies act upon both (Bandell-Hoekstra et al. 2002).

INTERACTION WITH FAMILY

Outcomes in pediatric care must incorporate interactions within the family, and include both the influence of the family on the child (e.g., reinforcement and modeling) and the effect of the child on the family (e.g., personal and financial impact of caring for the child). In infants and young children parents have essential roles in assessing and reporting the child's pain, presenting him/her for medical care, and compliance with subsequent treatment. In older children, discrepancies between parental and child report can occur on measures of pain intensity, coping style, and quality of life. The parent version of the Bath Adolescent Pain Questionnaire (BAPQ-P) provides more structured evaluation of parental report (Eccleston et al. 2007).

When compared to a matched group without pain, adolescents with chronic pain had more "significant others" with pain (Merlijn et al. 2003), and it has been suggested that this may lead to modeling of pain behavior. Rewarding behavior by parents and peers (i.e, gifts, increased time spent pampering or spoiling, excusing from regular chores) may reinforce pain behaviors, and has been assessed by the Illness Behavior Encouragement Scale. However, both increased (Walker et al. 1993) and decreased (Merlijn et al. 2003) parental encouragement of pain behavior has been reported in different chronic pain groups. The family's ability to organize daily activities in a meaningful way for all family members has been found to be predictive for successful coping and improved quality of life (Frare et al. 2002). Parental variables have also been shown to alter during treatment of their child in an interdisciplinary pain management program, and these may have a mediating effect on their child's subsequent outcome (Eccleston et al. 2003).

HEALTHCARE UTILIZATION AND COST

With an increasing realization of the prevalence of chronic pain in children and adolescents comes an increased awareness of the potential cost associated with healthcare utilization, medication use, long term disability and loss of income for parents while caring for the child. (Sleed et al. 2005).

In a retrospective questionnaire of children reporting chronic or recurrent pain for over 3 months, 57% had consulted a physician, 39% had used medication, and 30% had used both (Perquin et al. 2000b). In a subsequent prospective study, 31% had consulted a general practitioner, 14% a specialist, 11% a physiotherapist, and 2.8% a psychologist (Perquin et al. 2001). In comparisons of chronic pain and control groups, no difference was found in general practitioner visits (average 2.6 contacts per year) (van Ekeelen et al. 2002), but another study from the same group reported a 6.4% hospital admission rate for children with chronic pain compared to 4% for the total pediatric pain population (Perquin et al. 2001).

Medication use is a useful outcome measure in adult studies, both in terms of cost and reliance on a passive coping strategy, but it has not been extensively investigated in children. Only 6 of 18 trials assessing psychological therapies for chronic recurrent pain reported medication use as an outcome (Eccleston et al. 2002). In a prospective diary, 53% of children with chronic recurrent pain used medication, but in the majority of cases this was paracetamol (28%) or NSAIDs (11%) and the mean number of medications used was 1.3 (Perquin et al. 2001). As a result, the direct cost of medication is likely to be relatively low in pediatric patients when compared with adults. However, self-administration of over-the-counter medications is relatively common in adolescents (58–96% depending on type of pain), who begin to self-administer between the ages of 11 and 12, often without first checking with an adult (Chambers et al. 1997).

Chronic pain in childhood may predispose to pain and disability in adulthood, and it has been proposed that early intervention may facilitate learning of adaptive rather than maladaptive coping strategies (Schanberg et al. 1997). This hypothesis has not been investigated in controlled longitudinal studies. The likelihood of ongoing symptoms varies with the underlying condition, and current data is influenced by the study inclusion criteria and design. In children with chronic benign pain, 48% still experienced chronic pain at one-year follow-up, and 30% at two years (Perquin et al. 2003). Reported rates of residual symptoms for CRPS Type 1 vary widely from 8 to 54%, and relapse rates also vary (Wilder et al. 1992; Sherry et al. 1998). Associations have been found between recurrent abdominal pain and increased anxiety and medication use in adulthood (Campo et al. 2001). Higher levels of functional disability, school or work absence, and clinic visits have also been reported at 5-year follow-up of children with recurrent abdominal pain (Walker et al. 1995, 1998).

Families of children who consult medical practitioners for chronic benign pain report a higher financial burden due to pain (Perquin et al. 2001). The indirect costs of parental time and loss of income due to chronic pain within the family require further evaluation.

CONCLUSION

Significant advances have been made in the understanding and management of acute and chronic pain in children. Further development of evidence-based practice will be enhanced by the use of validated and standardized outcome measures that are appropriate for children at different stages of development and in different clinical settings. Outcome measures that evaluate global aspects of pain experience (e.g., sensory changes, behavioral responses, psychological measures, and functional outcomes) need to be developed and validated to assess long-term consequences from pain and injury in the neonatal period, and evaluate the degree to which chronic pain during childhood extends into adulthood.

REFERENCES

Abu-Saad HH, Kroonen E, Halfens R. On the development of a multidimensional Dutch pain assessment tool for children. Pain 1990; 43:249–256.

Ambuel B, Hamlett KW, Marx CM, et al. Assessing distress in pediatric intensive care environments: the COMFORT scale. J Pediatr Psychol 1992; 17:95–109.

Anand KJ, Aranda JV, Berde CB, et al. Analgesia and anesthesia for neonates: study design and ethical issues. Clin Ther 2005a; 27(6):814–843.

Anand KJ, Hall RW, Desai N, et al. Effects of morphine analgesia in ventilated preterm neonates: primary outcomes from the NEOPAIN randomised trial. Lancet 2004; 363(9422):1673–1682.

Anand KJ, Hickey PR. Pain and its effects in the human neonate and fetus. N Engl J Med 1987; 317:1321–1329.

Anand KJ, Hickey PR. Halothane-morphine compared with high-dose sufentanil for anesthesia and postoperative analgesia in neonatal cardiac surgery. N Engl J Med 1992; 326:1–9.

Anand KJ, Johnston CC, Oberlander TF, et al. Analgesia and local anesthesia during invasive procedures in the neonate. Clin Ther 2005b; 27(6): 844–876.

Anand KJ, Sippell WG, Aynsley-Green A. Randomised trial of fentanyl anaesthesia in preterm babies undergoing surgery: effects on the stress response. Lancet 1987; 1(8524):62–66.

Anand KJ, Barton BA, McIntosh N, et al. Analgesia and sedation in preterm neonates who require ventilatory support: results from the NOPAIN trial. Neonatal Outcome and Prolonged Analgesia in Neonates. Arch Pediatr Adolesc Med 1999; 153:331–338.

Anderson BJ, Ralph CJ, Stewart AW, et al. The dose-effect relationship for morphine and vomiting after day-stay tonsillectomy in children. Anaesth Intensive Care 2000; 28:155–160.

Anderson P, Doyle LW. Victorian Infant Collaborative Study Group. Neurobehavioral outcomes of school-age children born extremely low birth weight or very preterm in the 1990s. JAMA 2003; 289:3264–3272.

Andrews KA, Fitzgerald M. The cutaneous flexion reflex in human neonates: a quantitative study of threshold and stimulus/response characteristics, following single and repeated stimuli. Dev Med Child Neurol 1999; 41:696–703.

Andrews K, Fitzgerald M. Wound sensitivity as a measure of analgesic effects following surgery in human neonates and infants. Pain 2002; 100:35–46.

Andrews KA, Desai D, Dhillon HK, et al. Abdominal sensitivity in the first year of life: comparison of infants with and without prenatally diagnosed unilateral hydronephrosis. Pain 2002; 99:281–288.

Ansermino M, Basu R, Vandebeek C, et al. Nonopioid additives to local anaesthetics for caudal blockade in children: a systematic review. Paediatr Anaesth 2003; 13:561–573.

Australian and New Zealand College of Anaesthetists and Faculty of Pain Medicine. Acute pain management: Scientific Evidence (2nd edition). Melbourne: Australian and New Zealand College of Anaesthetists, 2005. www.anzca.edu.au/publications/acutepain.htm.

Ballantyne JC, Carr DB, deFerranti S, et al. The comparative effects of postoperative analgesic therapies on cumulative meta-analyses of randomized controlled trials. Anesth Analg 1998; 86:598–612.

Bandell-Hoekstra IE, Abu-Saad HH, Passchier J, et al. Coping and Quality of Life in relation to headache in Dutch schoolchildren. Eur J Pain 2002; 6:315–321.

Bartocci M, Bergqvist LL, Lagercrantz H, et al. Pain activates cortical areas in the preterm newborn brain. Pain 2006; 122(1–2):109–117.

Berde CB, Jaksic T, Lynn AM, et al. Anesthesia and analgesia during and after surgery in neonates. Clin Ther 2005; 27 (6):900–921.

Berde CB, Lebel AA, Olsson G. Neuropathic pain in children. In: Schechter NL, Berde CB, Yaster M (eds). Pain in Infants, Children, and Adolescents, 2nd edn. Lippincott Williams and Wilkins: Philadelphia, PA 2003:58–70.

Beyer JE, Wells N. The assessment of pain in children. Pediatr Clin North Am 1989; 36:837–854.

Bhutta AT, Cleves MA, Casey PH, et al. Cognitive and behavioral outcomes of school-aged children who were born preterm: a meta-analysis. JAMA 2002; 288:728–737.

Bieri D, Reeve RA, Champion GD, et al. The Faces Pain Scale for the self-assessment of the severity of pain experienced by children: development, initial validation, and preliminary investigation for ratio scale properties. Pain 1990; 41:139–150.

Blauer T, Gerstmann D. A simultaneous comparison of three neonatal pain scales during common NICU procedures. Clin J Pain 1998; 14:39–47.

Breau LM, Camfield C, McGrath PJ, et al. Measuring pain accurately in children with cognitive impairments: refinement of a caregiver scale. J Pediatr 2001; 138:721–727.

Breau LM, Finley GA, McGrath PJ, et al. Validation of the Non-communicating Children's Pain Checklist-Postoperative Version. Anesthesiology 2002a; 96:528–535.

Breau LM, McGrath PJ, Camfield CS, et al. Psychometric properties of the non-communicating children's pain checklist-revised. Pain 2002b; 99:349–357.

Buttner W, Finke W. Analysis of behavioural and physiological parameters for the assessment of postoperative analgesic demand in newborns, infants and young children: a comprehensive report on seven consecutive studies. Paediatr Anaesth 2000; 10:303–318.

Campo JV, Di Lorenzo C, Chiappetta L, et al. Adult outcomes of pediatric recurrent abdominal pain: do they just grow out of it? Pediatrics 2001; 108:E1.

Carbajal R, Lenclen R, Jugie M, et al. Morphine does not provide adequate analgesia for acute procedural pain among preterm neonates. Pediatrics 2005; 115 (6):1494–1500.

Cardwell M, Siviter G, Smith A. Non-steroidal anti-inflammatory drugs and perioperative bleeding in paediatric tonsillectomy. Cochrane Database Syst Rev 2005:(2):CD003591.

Chambers CT, Reid GJ, McGrath PJ, et al. Development and preliminary validation of a postoperative pain measure for parents. Pain 1996; 68:307–313.

Chambers CT, Reid GJ, McGrath PJ, et al. Self-administration of over-the-counter medication for pain among adolescents. Arch Pediatr Adolesc Med 1997; 151:449–455.

Chambers CT, Reid GJ, Craig KD, et al. Agreement between child and parent reports of pain. Clin J Pain 1998; 14:336–342.

Chambers CT, Giesbrecht K, Craig KD, et al. A comparison of faces scales for the measurement of pediatric pain: children's and parents' ratings. Pain 1999; 83:25–35.

Chambers CT, Finley GA, McGrath PJ, et al. The parents' postoperative pain measure: replication and extension to 2–6-year-old children. Pain 2003; 105:437–443.

Cote CJ, Zaslavsky A, Downes JJ, et al. Postoperative apnea in former preterm infants after inguinal herniorrhaphy. A combined analysis. Anesthesiology 1995; 82:809–822.

Craig KD. The facial display of pain. In: Finley GA, McGrath PJ (eds). Measurement of Pain in Infants and Children. Progress in Pain Research and Management, vol 10 IASP Press: Seattle, WA 1998:103–122.

Craven PD, Badawi N, Henderson-Smart DJ, et al. Regional (spinal, epidural, caudal) versus general anaesthesia in preterm infants undergoing inguinal herniorrhaphy in early infancy. Cochrane Database Syst Rev 2003; 3CD003669.

Crombez G, Bijttebier P, Eccleston C, et al. The child version of the pain catastrophizing scale (PCS-C): a preliminary validation. Pain 2003; 104:639–646.

Department of Health and Human Services, US Food and Drug Administration The Pediatric Exclusivity Provision.

Status Report to Congress, January 2001 (http://www.fda.gov/cder/pediatric/index.htm).

Duncan HP, Cloote A, Weir PM, et al. Reducing stress responses in the pre-bypass phase of open heart surgery in infants and young children: a comparison of different fentanyl doses. Br J Anaesth 2000; 84:556–564.

Eccleston C, Jordan A, McCracken LM, et al. The Bath Adolescent Pain Questionnaire (BAPQ): development and preliminary psychometric evaluation of an instrument to assess the impact of chronic pain on adolescents. Pain 2005; 118(1–2): 263–270.

Eccleston C, Jordan AL, Crombez G. The impact of chronic pain on adolescents: a review of previously used measures. J Pediatr Psychol 2006; 31(7):684–697.

Eccleston C, McCracken LM, Jordan A, et al. Development and preliminary psychometric evaluation of the parent report version of the Bath Adolescent Pain Questionnaire (BAPQ-P): A multidimensional parent report instrument to assess the impact of chronic pain on adolescents. Pain 2007 (EPub Jan 22).

Eccleston C, Morley S, Williams A, et al. Systematic review of randomised controlled trials of psychological therapy for chronic pain in children and adolescents, with a subset meta-analysis of pain relief. Pain 2002; 99:157–165.

Eccleston C, Malleson PN, Clinch J, et al. Chronic pain in adolescents: evaluation of a programme of interdisciplinary cognitive behaviour therapy. Arch Dis Child 2003; 88:881–885.

Erb TO, Schulman SR, Sugarman J. Permission and assent for clinical research in pediatric anesthesia. Anesth Analg 2002; 94:1155–1160.

Finley GA, McGrath PJ, Forward SP, et al. Parents' management of children's pain following "minor" surgery. Pain 1996; 64:83–87.

Finley GA, Chambers CT, McGrath PJ, et al. Construct validity of the parents' postoperative pain measure. Clin J Pain 2003; 19:329–334.

Fitzgerald M, Walker S. The role of activity in developing pain pathways. In: Dostrovsky JO, Carr DB, Koltzenburg M (eds). Proceedings of the 10th World Congress on Pain. Progress in Pain Research and Management, vol 24IASP Press: Seattle, WA 2003:185–196.

Fitzgerald M, Shaw A, MacIntosh N. Postnatal development of the cutaneous flexor reflex: comparative study of preterm infants and newborn rat pups. Dev Med Child Neurol 1988; 30:520–526.

Fitzgerald M, Millard C, McIntosh N. Cutaneous hypersensitivity following peripheral tissue damage in newborn infants and its reversal with topical anaesthesia. Pain 1989; 39:31–36.

Forrest JB, Heitlinger EL, Revell S. Ketorolac for postoperative pain management in children. Drug Saf 1997; 16:309–329.

Foster RL, Varni JW. Measuring the quality of children's postoperative pain management: initial validation of the child/parent Total Quality Pain Management (TQPM) instruments. J Pain Sympt Manage 2002; 23:201–210.

Franck LS, Greenberg CS, Stevens B. Pain assessment in infants and children. Pediatr Clin North Am 2000; 47:487–512.

Frare M, Axia G, Battistella PA. Quality of life, coping strategies, and family routines in children with headache. Headache 2002; 42:953–962.

Gaffney A, McGrath PJ, Dick B. Measuring pain in children: developmental and instrument issues. In: Schechter NL, Berde CB, Yaster M (eds). Pain in Infants, Children, and Adolescents, 2nd edn. Lippincott Williams and Wilkins: Philadelphia, PA 2003:128–141.

Gauntlett-Gilbert J, Eccleston C. Disability in adolescents with chronic pain: Patterns and predictors across different domains of functioning. Pain 2007 (EPub Jan 22).

Gauthier JC, Finley GA, McGrath PJ. Children's self-report of postoperative pain intensity and treatment threshold: determining the adequacy of medication. Clin J Pain 1998; 14:116–120.

Gil KM, Wilson JJ, Edens JL. The stability of pain coping strategies in young children, adolescents, and adults with sickle cell disease over an 18-month period. Clin J Pain 1997; 13:110–115.

Goldschneider KR, Anand KJS. Long-term consequences of pain in neonates. In: Schechter NL, Berde CB, Yaster M (eds). Pain in Infants, Children, and Adolescents, 2nd edn. Lippincott Williams and Wilkins: Philadelphia, PA 2003:58–70.

Grunau RV, Craig KD. Pain expression in neonates: facial action and cry. Pain 1987; 28:395–410.

Grunau R, Tu M. Long-term consequences of pain in human neonates. In: KJ Anand, BJ Stevens, P McGrath (eds). Pain in Neonates and Infants. Third Edition. Elsevier: Edinburgh. 2007:45–55.

Grunau RE, Haley DW, Whitfield MF, et al. Altered basal cortisol levels at 3, 6, 8 and 18 months in infants born at extremely low gestational age. J Pediatr 2007; 150 (2):151–156.

Grunau RE, Holsti L, Haley DW, et al. Neonatal procedural pain exposure predicts lower cortisol and behavioral reactivity in preterm infants in the NICU. Pain 2005; 113 (3):293–300.

Grunau RE, Holsti L, Peters JW. Long-term consequences of pain in human neonates. Semin Fetal Neonatal Med 2006; 11(4):268–275.

Hall RW, Kronsberg SS, Barton BA, et al. Morphine, hypotension, and adverse outcomes among preterm neonates: who's to blame? Secondary results from the NEOPAIN trial. Pediatrics 2005; 115 (5):1351–1359.

Hamalainen M, Masek BJ. Diagnosis, classification, and medical management of headache in children and adolescents. In: Schechter NL, Berde CB, Yaster M (eds). Pain in Infants, Children, and Adolescents, 2nd edn. Lippincott Williams and Wilkins: Philadelphia, PA 2003:58–70.

Hamalainen ML, Hoppu K, Santavuori P. Sumatriptan for migraine attacks in children: a randomized placebo-controlled study. Do children with migraine respond to oral sumatriptan differently from adults? Neurology 1997a; 48:1100–1103.

Hamalainen ML, Hoppu K, Valkeila E, et al. Ibuprofen or acetaminophen for the acute treatment of migraine in children: a double-blind, randomized, placebo-controlled, crossover study. Neurology 1997b; 48:103–107.

Hamunen K, Kontinen V. Systematic review on analgesics given for pain following tonsillectomy in children. Pain 2005; 117(1–2):40–50.

Hermann C, Hohmeister J, Demirakca S, et al. Long-term alteration of pain sensitivity in school-aged children with early pain experiences. Pain 2006; 125 (3):278–285.

Hester NK. The preoperational child's reaction to immunization. Nurs Res 1979; 28:250–255.

Hicks CL, von Baeyer CL, Spafford PA, et al. The Faces Pain Scale-Revised: toward a common metric in pediatric pain measurement. Pain 2001; 93:173–183.

Ho D, Keneally JP. Analgesia following paediatric day-surgical orchidopexy and herniotomy. Paediatr Anaesth 2000; 10:627–631.

Hodgson RE, Bosenberg AT, Hadley LG. Congenital diaphragmatic hernia repair: impact of delayed surgery and epidural analgesia. S Afr J Surg 2000; 38:31–34.

Hollis LJ, Burton MJ, Millar JM. Perioperative local anaesthesia for reducing pain following tonsillectomy. Cochrane Database Syst Rev 2000; 2:CD001874.

Holsti L, Grunau RE. Initial validation of the Behavioral Indicators of Infant Pain (BIIP). Pain 2007.

Holsti L, Grunau RE, Whifield MF, et al. Behavioral responses to pain are heightened after clustered care in preterm infants born between 30 and 32 weeks gestational age. Clin J Pain 2006; 22(9):757–764.

Howard RF. Acute pain management in children. In: Rowbotham DJ, Macintyre PE (eds). Clinical Pain Management. Acute Pain. Arnold: London 2003a:437–462.

Howard RF. Current status of pain management in children. JAMA 2003b; 290:2464–2469.

Hunfeld JA, Perquin CW, Duivenvoorden HJ, et al. Chronic pain and its impact on quality of life in adolescents and their families. J Pediatr Psychol 2001; 26:145–153.

Hunfeld JA, Perquin CW, Bertina W, et al. Stability of pain parameters and pain-related quality of life in adolescents with persistent pain: a three-year follow-up. Clin J Pain 2002; 18:99–106.

Hunt A, Goldman A, Seers K, et al. Clinical validation of the paediatric pain profile. Dev Med Child Neurol 2004; 46 (1):9–18.

Jain A, Rutter N. Local anaesthetic effect of topical amethocaine gel in neonates: randomised controlled trial. Arch Dis Child Fetal Neonatal Ed 2000; 82:F42–F45.

Jensen MP, Chen C, Brugger AM. Postsurgical pain outcome assessment. Pain 2002; 99:101–109.

Johnston CC, Stevens B, Yang F, et al. Developmental changes in response to heelstick in preterm infants: a prospective cohort study. Dev Med Child Neurol 1996; 38:438–445.

Johnston CC, Stevens BJ, Boyer K, et al. Development of psychologic responses to pain and assessment of pain in infants and toddlers. In: Schechter NL, Berde CB, Yaster M (eds). Pain in Infants, Children, and Adolescents, 2nd edn. Lippincott Williams and Wilkins: Philadelphia, PA 2003:85–104.

Kalso E, Edwards J, McQuay HJ, et al. Five easy pieces on evidence-based medicine (3). Eur J Pain 2001; 5:227–230.

Kalso E, Edwards J, McQuay HJ, et al. Five easy pieces on evidence-based medicine (5). Eur J Pain 2002; 6:409–412.

Keogh E, Eccleston C. Sex differences in adolescent chronic pain and pain-related coping. Pain 2006; 123(3): 275–284.

Krechel SW, Bildner J. CRIES: a new neonatal postoperative pain measurement score. Initial testing of validity and reliability. Paediatr Anaesth 1995; 5:53–61.

Krishna S, Hughes LF, Lin SY. Postoperative hemorrhage with nonsteroidal anti-inflammatory drug use after tonsillectomy: a meta-analysis. Arch Otolaryngol Head Neck Surg 2003; 129:1086–1089.

Langeveld JH, Koot HM, Loonen MC, et al. A quality of life instrument for adolescents with chronic headache. Cephalalgia 1996; 16:183–196.

Lawrence J, Alcock D, McGrath P, et al. The development of a tool to assess neonatal pain. Neonatal Netw 1993; 12:59–66.

Lee JS, Hobden E, Stiell IG, et al. Clinically important change in the visual analog scale after adequate pain control. Acad Emerg Med 2003; 10:1128–1130.

Malviya S, Pandit UA, Merkel S, et al. A comparison of continuous epidural infusion and intermittent intravenous bolus doses of morphine in children undergoing selective dorsal rhizotomy. Reg Anesth Pain Med 1999; 24:438–443.

Malviya S, Voepel-Lewis T, Tait AR, et al. Pain management in children with and without cognitive impairment following spine fusion surgery. Paediatr Anaesth 2001; 11:453–458.

Marret E, Flahault A, Samama CM, et al. Effects of postoperative, nonsteroidal, antiinflammatory drugs on bleeding risk after tonsillectomy: meta-analysis of randomized, controlled trials. Anesthesiology 2003; 98:1497–1502.

McGrath P. Chronic pain in children. In: Crombie IK, Linton SJ, LeResche L, Von Korff MM (eds). Epidemiology of Pain. IASP Press: Seattle, WA 1999:81–102.

McGrath PA, Seifert CE, Speechley KN, et al. A new analogue scale for assessing children's pain: an initial validation study. Pain 1996; 64:435–443.

McGrath PJ. Behavioural measures of pain. In: Finley GA, McGrath PJ (eds). Measurement of Pain in Infants and Children. Progress in Pain Research and Management, vol 10IASP Press: Seattle, WA 1998:83–102.

McGrath PJ, Johnson G, Goodman JT. CHEOPS: a behavioural scale for rating postoperative pain in children. In: Fields HL, Dubner R, Cervero F (eds). Advances in Pain Research and Therapy, vol 9Raven Press: New York 1985:395–402.

McNeely JK, Farber NE, Rusy LM, et al. Epidural analgesia improves outcome following pediatric fundoplication. A retrospective analysis. Reg Anesth 1997; 22:16–23.

McQuay HJ, Barden J, Moore RA. Clinically important changes: what's important and whose change is it anyway? J Pain Sympt Manage 2003; 25:395–396.

Meier PM, Berde CB, DiCanzio J, et al. Quantitative assessment of cutaneous thermal and vibration sensation and thermal pain detection thresholds in healthy children and adolescents. Muscle Nerve 2001; 24:1339–1345.

Merkel SI, Voepel-Lewis T, Shayevitz JR, et al. The FLACC: a behavioral scale for scoring postoperative pain in young children. Pediatr Nurs 1997; 23:293–297.

Merlijn VP, Hunfeld JA, van der Wouden JC, et al. Shortening a quality of life questionnaire for adolescents with chronic pain and its psychometric qualities. Psychol Rep 2002; 90:753–759.

Merlijn VP, Hunfeld JA, van der Wouden JC, et al. Psychosocial factors associated with chronic pain in adolescents. Pain 2003; 101:33–43.

Miaskowski C, Crews J, Ready LB, et al. Anesthesia-based pain services improve the quality of postoperative pain management. Pain 1999; 80:23–29.

Michels KB, Rothman KJ. Update on unethical use of placebos in randomised trials. Bioethics 2003; 17:188–204.

Miller FG, Brody H. What makes placebo-controlled trials unethical? Am J Bioeth 2002; 2:3–9.

Moiniche S, Romsing J, Dahl JB, et al. Nonsteroidal antiinflammatory drugs and the risk of operative site bleeding after tonsillectomy: a quantitative systematic review. Anesth Analg 2003; 96:68–77.

Moore A, McQuay H, Gavaghan D. Deriving dichotomous outcome measures from continuous data in randomized controlled trials of analgesics: verification from independent data. Pain 1997; 69:127–130.

Munro HM, Walton SR, Malviya S, et al. Low-dose ketorolac improves analgesia and reduces morphine requirements following posterior spinal fusion in adolescents. Can J Anaesth 2002; 49:461–466.

Nader R, Oberlander TF, Chambers CT, et al. Expression of pain in children with autism. Clin J Pain 2004; 20:88–97.

Norden J, Hannallah R, Getson P. Concurrent validation of an objective pain scale for infants and children. Anesthesiology 1991; 75:A934.

Ohlsson A, Taddio A, Jadad AR, et al. Evidence-based decision making, systematic reviews and the Cochrane collaboration: implications for neonatal analgesia. In: Anand KJS, Stevens BJ, McGrath PJ (eds). Pain in Neonates, 2nd revised and enlarged edn. Pain Research and Clinical Management, vol 10Elsevier: Amsterdam 2000:251–268.

Palermo TM. Impact of recurrent and chronic pain on child and family daily functioning: a critical review of the literature. J Dev Behav Pediatr 2000; 21:58–69.

Perquin CW, Hazebroek-Kampschreur AA, Hunfeld JA, et al. Pain in children and adolescents: a common experience. Pain 2000a; 87:51–58.

Perquin CW, Hazebroek-Kampschreur AA, Hunfeld JA, et al. Chronic pain among children and adolescents: physician consultation and medication use. Clin J Pain 2000b; 16:229–235.

Perquin CW, Hunfeld JA, Hazebroek-Kampschreur AA, et al. Insights in the use of health care services in chronic benign pain in childhood and adolescence. Pain 2001; 94:205–213.

Perquin CW, Hunfeld JA, Hazebroek-Kampschreur AA, et al. The natural course of chronic benign pain in childhood and adolescence: a two-year population-based follow-up study. Eur J Pain 2003; 7:551–559.

Peters JW, Bandell-Hoekstra IE, Huijer Abu-Saad H, et al. Patient controlled analgesia in children and adolescents: a randomized controlled trial. Paediatr Anaesth 1999; 9:235–241.

Peters JW, Koot HM, de Boer JB, et al. Major surgery within the first 3 months of life and subsequent biobehavioral pain responses to immunization at later age: a case comparison study. Pediatrics 2003; 111:129–135.

Porter FL, Wolf CM, Miller JP. Procedural pain in newborn infants: the influence of intensity and development. Pediatrics 1999b; 104:e13.

Ragg P, Davidson A. Comparison of the efficacy of paracetamol versus paracetamol, codeine and promethazine (Painstop) for premedication and analgesia for myringotomy in children. Anaesth Intensive Care 1997; 25:29–32.

Reid GJ, Gilbert CA, McGrath PJ. The Pain Coping Questionnaire: preliminary validation. Pain 1998; 76:83–96.

Reynolds CR, Richmond BO. What I think and feel: a revised measure of children's manifest anxiety. J Abnorm Child Psychol 1978; 6:271–280.

Reynolds ML, Fitzgerald M. Long-term sensory hyperinnervation following neonatal skin wounds. J Comp Neurol 1995; 358:487–498.

Royal Australasian College of Physicians, Division of Paediatric and Child Health.. Guideline Statement: Management of Procedure-related Pain in Neonates. www.racp.edu.au/index.cfm?objectid=A4254F55-2A57-5487-DFE129631BCB4C59.

Sawyer MG, Whitham JN, Roberton DM, et al. The relationship between health-related quality of life, pain and coping strategies in juvenile idiopathic arthritis. Rheumatology 2004; 43:325–330.

Schanberg LE, Lefebvre JC, Keefe FJ, et al. Pain coping and the pain experience in children with juvenile chronic arthritis. Pain 1997; 73:181–189.

Schanberg LE, Anthony KK, Gil KM, et al. Daily pain and symptoms in children with polyarticular arthritis. Arthritis Rheum 2003; 48:1390–1397.

Schmelzle-Lubiecki BM, Campbell KA, Howard RH, et al. Long-term consequences of early infant injury and trauma upon somatosensory processing. Eur J Pain 2007(EPub Feb 21).

Sethna NF, Meier PM, Zurakowski D, Berde CB: Cutaneous sensory abnormalities in children and adolescents with complex regional pain syndromes. Pain 2007 (EPub Feb 26).

Sherry DD, Wallace CA, Kelley C, et al. Short- and long-term outcomes of children with complex regional pain syndrome type I treated with exercise therapy. Clin J Pain 1999; 15:218–223.

Simons SH, van Dijk M, van Lingen RA, et al. Routine morphine infusion in preterm newborns who received ventilatory support: a randomized controlled trial. JAMA 2003; 290:2419–2427.

Singh G, Athreya BH, Fries JF, et al. Measurement of health status in children with juvenile rheumatoid arthritis. Arthritis Rheum 1994; 37:1761–1769.

Slater R, Cantarella A, Gallella S, et al. Cortical pain responses in human infants. J Neurosci 2006; 26(14):3662–3666.

Sleed M, Eccleston C, Beecham J, et al. The economic impact of chronic pain in adolescence: methodological considerations and a preliminary costs-of-illness study. Pain 2005;119(1–3):183–190.

Stevens B, Johnston C, Petryshen P, et al. Premature Infant Pain Profile: development and initial validation. Clin J Pain 1996; 12:13–22.

Stinson JN, Kavanagh T, Yamada J, et al. Systematic review of the psychometric properties, interpretability and feasibility of self-report pain intensity measures for use in clinical trials in children and adolescents. Pain 2006;125 (1–2):143–157.

Steward DL, Welge JA, Myer CM. Steroids for improving recovery following tonsillectomy in children. Cochrane Database Syst Rev 2003; 1:CD003997.

Sweet SA, McGrath PJ. Physiological measures of pain. In: Finley GA, McGrath PJ (eds). Measurement of Pain in Infants and Children. Progress in Pain Research and Management, vol 10IASP Press: Seattle, WA 1998:59–82.

Taddio A, Goldbach M, Ipp M, et al. Effect of neonatal circumcision on pain responses during vaccination in boys. Lancet 1995; 345:291–292.

Taddio A, Katz J, Ilersich AL, et al. Effect of neonatal circumcision on pain response during subsequent routine vaccination. Lancet 1997; 349:599–603.

Taddio A, Ohlsson K, Ohlsson A. Lidocaine-prilocaine cream for analgesia during circumcision in newborn boys. Cochrane Database Syst Rev 2000; 2:CD000496.

Taddio A, Shah V, Gilbert-MacLeod C, et al. Conditioning and hyperalgesia in newborns exposed to repeated heel lances. JAMA 2002; 288:857–861.

Van Boerum DH, Smith JT, Curtin MJ. A comparison of the effects of patient-controlled analgesia with intravenous opioids versus epidural analgesia on recovery after surgery for idiopathic scoliosis. Spine 2000; 25:2355–2357.

van den Brink M, Bandell-Hoekstra EN, Abu-Saad HH. The occurrence of recall bias in pediatric headache: a comparison of questionnaire and diary data. Headache 2001; 41:11–20.

van Dijk M, de Boer JB, Koot HM, et al. The reliability and validity of the COMFORT scale as a postoperative pain instrument in 0 to 3-year-old infants. Pain 2000; 84:367–377.

Varni JW, Thompson KL, Hanson V. The Varni/Thompson Pediatric Pain Questionnaire: I. Chronic musculoskeletal pain in juvenile rheumatoid arthritis. Pain 1987; 28:27–38.

Varni JW, Waldron SA, Gragg RA, et al. Development of the Waldron/Varni pediatric pain coping inventory. Pain 1996; 67:141–150.

Varni JW, Seid M, Knight T, et al. The PedsQLTM in pediatric rheumatology: reliability, validity and responsiveness of the Pediatric Quality of Life Inventory™ Generic Core Scale and Rheumatology Module. Arthritis Rheum 2002; 46:714–725 (see: http://www.pedsql.org/).

Voepel-Lewis T, Merkel S, Tait AR, et al. The reliability and validity of the Face, Legs, Activity, Cry, Consolability observational tool as a measure of pain in children with cognitive impairment. Anesth Analg 2002; 95:1224–1229.

von Baeyer CL, Spagrud LJ. Systematic review of observational (behavioral) measures of pain for children and adolescents aged 3 to 18 years. Pain 2007;127(1–2):140–150.

Walker SM. Management of procedural pain in NICUs remains problematic. Paediatr Anaesth 2005;15(11):909–912.

Walker SM, Macintyre PE, Visser E, et al. Acute pain management: current best evidence provides guide for improved practice. Pain Med 2006;7(1):3–5.

Walker LS, Greene JW. Children with recurrent abdominal pain and their parents: more somatic complaints, anxiety, and depression than other patient families? J Pediatr Psychol 1989; 14:231–243.

Walker LS, Greene JW. The functional disability inventory: measuring a neglected dimension of child health status. J Pediatr Psychol 1991; 16:39–58.

Walker LS, Garber J, Greene JW. Psychosocial correlates of recurrent childhood pain: a comparison of pediatric patients with recurrent abdominal pain, organic illness, and psychiatric disorders. J Abnorm Psychol 1993; 102:248–258.

Walker LS, Garber J, Van Slyke DA, et al. Long-term health outcomes in patients with recurrent abdominal pain. J Pediatr Psychol 1995; 20:233–245.

Walker LS, Smith CA, Garber J, et al. Development and validation of the Pain Response Inventory for Children. Psychol Assess 1997; 9:392–405.

Walker LS, Guite JW, Duke M, et al. Recurrent abdominal pain: a potential precursor of irritable bowel syndrome in adolescents and young adults. J Pediatr 1998; 132:1010–1015.

Walker SM, Meredith-Middleton J, Cooke-Yarborough C, et al. Neonatal inflammation and primary afferent terminal plasticity in the rat dorsal horn. Pain 2003; 105:185–195.

Wilder RT, Berde CB, Wolohan M, et al. Reflex sympathetic dystrophy in children. Clinical characteristics and follow-up of seventy patients. J Bone Joint Surg Am 1992; 74:910–919.

Willer JC. Studies on pain. Effects of morphine on a spinal nociceptive flexion reflex and related pain sensation in man. Brain Res 1985; 331:105–114.

Williams DG, Patel A, Howard RF. Pharmacogenetics of codeine metabolism in an urban population of children and its implications for analgesic reliability. Br J Anaesth 2002; 89:839–845.

Willis MH, Merkel SI, Voepel-Lewis T, et al. FLACC Behavioral Pain Assessment Scale: a comparison with the child's self-report. Pediatr Nurs 2003; 29:195–198.

Wilson GA, Brown JL, Crabbe DG, et al. Is epidural analgesia associated with an improved outcome following open Nissen fundoplication? Paediatr Anaesth 2001; 11:65–70.

Wolf AR, Hughes D. Pain relief for infants undergoing abdominal surgery: comparison of infusions of i.v. morphine and extradural bupivacaine. Br J Anaesth 1993; 70:10–16.

Wolf AR, Eyres RL, Laussen PC, et al. Effect of extradural analgesia on stress responses to abdominal surgery in infants. Br J Anaesth 1993; 70:654–660.

Zohsel K, Hohmeister J, Oelkers-Ax R, et al. Quantitative sensory testing in children with migraine: preliminary evidence for enhanced sensitivity to painful stimuli especially in girls. Pain 2006;123(1–2):10–18.

CHAPTER 14

Headache

Douglas C. McCrory • Alvin E. Lake III • Joel R. Saper

INTRODUCTION

Headache disorders are very common in the population. Headache attacks are episodes of head pain that occur intermittently with varying severity. Between attacks, most headache sufferers are asymptomatic. However, about 1.5% of the general population experience daily headache, and some experience continuous, unremitting pain (Scher et al. 1998). Different headache disorders have remarkably different patterns. This chapter will focus on the major primary headache disorders of migraine, tension-type headache and cluster headache; the International Classification of Headache Disorders includes a comprehensive list of secondary causes of headache and less common primary headache disorders (Classification Subcommittee of the International Headache Society 2004). The headache field has developed tools for use in clinical trials to measure the benefits of therapeutic interventions. Measurement of their impact is complicated by the variety of symptoms and time courses of different common headache disorders. The tools used to assess the impact of therapy aimed at relief of acute attacks differ markedly from those used to assess the impact of preventive or long-term treatments. This chapter describes specific outcome measurement approaches used in clinical trials of common primary headache disorders to assess the benefits of treatment. The main primary headache disorders of migraine, tension-type headache and cluster headache have salient differences in the duration of attacks, severity of attacks, associated symptoms and disability. These differences require that measurement approaches must be tailored to specific headache diagnoses. Facial pain and other less common primary and secondary headache disorders differ greatly in their clinical presentation, treatment and measurement, and are beyond the scope of this chapter.

PRIMARY HEADACHE DISORDERS

MIGRAINE

Migraine manifests in attacks lasting a few hours to 3 days, with a median frequency of one per month. Current 1-year migraine prevalence in adults is about 12% in the Americas and Europe, with higher rates among women (15–18%) than men (6%) (Lipton et al. 2001; Rasmussen 2001). Approximately 27.9 million US adults suffer with migraine (Lipton et al. 2001). Prevalence appears to be higher in whites than in blacks, and for both women and men, prevalence is highest in middle adulthood (30–49 years of age), and, in the USA, among those with lower socioeconomic status (Stewart et al. 1992). However, population-based studies outside the USA have not shown an association between migraine and socioeconomic status, educational level, or occupation (Rasmussen 1992; O'Brien et al. 1994).

In an American survey, 80% of people with migraine reported some degree of disability because of it and, globally, migraine is 19th in the list of all causes of years lived with disability (World Health Organization 2001). Because migraine affects people particularly during their productive years, its economic impact is high. In addition to suffering directly from its symptoms, people with migraine consistently score poorly on scales of general physical and mental ill-health. The level of disability is directly related to the frequency and severity of headaches. In one epidemiologic population-based migraine study, the 20% of participants with the most frequent and severe headaches accounted for 77% of the lost workdays due to migraine (von Korff et al. 1998).

The discrete attacks that characterize migraine are primarily marked by head pain, which is typically severe enough to cause disability. The International Headache Society (IHS) diagnostic criteria for migraine require the presence of at least two of four pain symptoms (unilateral headache, pulsatile pain, moderate–severe in intensity, aggravated by normal activity) and one of two related symptoms that contribute to disability experienced by migraineurs (nausea or emesis, or both light and sound sensitivity) (Classification Subcommittee of IHS 2004). Other symptoms of migraine, such as premonitory symptoms or aura, provide some discrimination of different diagnostic subtypes but, for most patients, have little impact on health or disability. Only in certain infrequent varieties – e.g., hemiplegic or basilar-type migraine – may aura be significantly disabling.

While an attack frequency of once per month is typical, there is a great deal of variability, especially between individuals. A relatively small proportion of migraine sufferers have very frequent attacks. The recently revised new appendix criteria of the IHS define *chronic migraine* as migraine headaches occurring ≥ 8 days/month for ≥ 3 months, in a patient who is experiencing headache (either tension-type or migraine) ≥ 15 days/month for at least 3, in the absence of overly frequent reliance on analgesic or abortive medication. *Medication overuse headache* is defined as headache occurring ≥ 15 days/month that has developed or markedly worsened during at least 3 months of overuse of abortives or analgesics: the use of either (1) ergotamines, triptans, opioids, or combination analgesics on a regular basis for ≥ 10 days/month; or (2) simple analgesics or a any combination of the ergotamines, triptans, opioids or combination analgesics for ≥ 15 days/month,

in the absence of overuse of any one class alone months (Headache Classification Committee: Olesen et al. 2006).

TENSION-TYPE HEADACHE

Tension-type headache (TTH) is the most common headache disorder. Most is episodic, with occasional attacks of bilateral pressure-type pain lasting from 1 to 3 hours. Tension-type headaches are typically less severe than migraine attacks; the head pain is not as intense, migrainous symptoms are absent, and they are associated with less disability for usual activities. However, despite their milder nature, TTHs are more common and frequent than migraine.

In its chronic and much more disabling subtype, chronic tension-type headache (CTTH) is present on more days than not (>15 days per month for at least 6 months). Estimates of the prevalence of this group of conditions in Europe and USA are as high as 1 in 25 of the entire adult population, with about 1.5% experiencing headache every day (Scher et al. 1998). Such frequent headache often occurs in patients who also experience migraine, and is associated with long-term morbidity and disability. Patients with persistent and severe chronic daily headache (often a combination of CTTH and migraine or chronic migraine) are the most likely to seek treatment at specialized headache centers (Saper et al. 1999) and have a poorer quality of life than those with episodic migraine (Monzon and Lainez 1998).

CLUSTER HEADACHE

Cluster headache has a lower prevalence (lifetime about 0.07%), and at any given time most people with the disorder are not in a cluster period. It is unique among the primary headache disorders in affecting more men than women (about 6:1). Typically occurring in bouts of a few weeks each year with periods of full remission between, it is characterized by frequent (daily or more often), short-lasting (15–120 minutes) but excruciating unilateral localized frontal or periorbital pain accompanied by marked but similarly localized autonomic symptoms. Headaches often occur during sleep. In its rarer chronic subtype there are no periods of remission. In contrast to migraineurs who may function to a greater or lesser extent during attacks, cluster headache sufferers are typically totally nonfunctional during the headache, with a return to functioning after the headache subsides.

APPROACHES TO ASSESSMENT: ACUTE VERSUS PREVENTIVE

The headache field has incorporated two views of headache: as episodic attacks on the one hand, and as a chronic health disorder on the other. This dichotomy

Table 14.1 Outcome assessment for treatment of acute headache attacks

Headache disorder	Outcome domain	Data collected	Outcome measures
Migraine	Head pain	Headache intensity Recurrence Use of rescue Rx Headache relief	Headache response Pain-free response Sustained pain-free response
	Nausea/vomiting	Presence, severity	
	HRQoL/disability	Various instruments; e.g., MQoLQ	Unclear
	Other associated symptoms	Presence, severity	
Tension-type headache	Head pain	Headache intensity Headache relief	Same as migraine
Cluster	Head pain	Headache intensity Relapse	Aborted attack Time to meaningful relief Time to complete relief Headache intensity
	Associated autonomic symptoms	Presence, severity	

Table 14.2 Outcome assessment for treatment of chronic headache or prevention of acute headache attacks

Headache disorder	Outcome domain	Data collected	Outcome measures
Migraine	Head pain	Migraine attack frequency (headache diary)	Number of attacks per 28 days Number of days with headache Response rate
	Disease-specific HRQoL/disability	Various instruments; e.g., MIDAS, HIT, HIT-6, MSQoL, MSQ	Unclear; e.g., significant differences on subscale scores
	Generic HRQoL	Various instruments; e.g., MOS-SF-36; SF-20; SF-12; SF-8	Unclear; e.g., significant differences on subscale scores
Chronic migraine or chronic TTH	Head pain	Attack frequency Attack severity Attack duration	Responder rate Headache index
Episodic tension-type headache	Head pain	Headache attack frequency	Number of attacks per 28 days Number of days with headache Response rate
Cluster	Head pain	Attack frequency	Number of attacks per 7 days Responder rate

is preserved in the design of clinical trials of headache treatments. In order to assess the benefit of symptomatic treatment of individual headache attacks outcome measures used in acute headache treatment trials must capture the variety of manifestations which include head pain, but also nausea, vomiting, phonophobia, photophobia, and temporary disability (Table 14.1).

In order to assess the long-term benefits associated with treatment, outcome measures must capture the effects of short-term attacks that accrue over time, as well as effects of persistent symptoms associated with the various chronic headache syndromes, including chronic migraine and chronic tension-type headache (Table 14.2).

In the following section, the types of instruments and questions often used to elicit data from patients in clinical trials of headache treatment are reviewed, followed by discussion of the outcome measures derived from these basic data. The IHS has developed consensus recommendations for the design of clinical trials in migraine (Tfelt-Hansen et al. 2000). Revised in 2000, these guidelines discuss the measurement approaches and preferred outcome measures for randomized control trials.

Because migraine has been the focus of the vast majority of clinical research and methodologic development in the field of headache, by necessity most of this chapter will focus on migraine. Methods for measuring outcomes in tension-type headache, cluster headache and other headache disorders have generally been borrowed or adapted from those used for migraine. Consequently, most of the important concepts are presented in the discussion on migraine; the shorter sections on TTH and cluster headache describe briefly how measures have been adapted to the particulars of these disorders.

MEASURING HEADACHE SYMPTOMS AND EFFECTS IN ACUTE MIGRAINE

Headache pain

Headache pain assessment

Head pain is the primary symptom of headache disorders and is almost always the principal focus of outcome assessment in headache trials. One or both of two approaches are commonly used. Headache intensity may be rated at baseline and following treatment. Alternatively, a patient may be asked directly to judge the improvement in headache pain following treatment, termed *headache relief*. Headache intensity and headache relief are commonly assessed using categorical scales or continuous visual analogue scales (VAS). Categorical scales used to measure headache intensity usually consist of four categories (none, mild, moderate, and severe) (Keele 1948), while those used to measure headache relief commonly include five categories (none, slight, moderate, good, and complete). These fundamental pain assessments in the form of categorical and/or continuous data collected from patients are used to calculate a variety of outcome measures used in clinical trials.

Outcome measures

Headache response or relief Headache response at 2 hours has been the most common primary efficacy endpoint in recent migraine trials, particularly clinical trials of triptan drugs. It is defined as the percentage of patients with a decrease in headache intensity from severe or moderate at baseline to mild or no pain within 2 hours after treatment (Tfelt-Hansen et al. 2000). There is empirical evidence that a change in headache intensity from moderate to mild is not perceived by patients as equivalent to a change from severe to mild: patient-rated satisfaction with these outcomes were 35% versus 77%, respectively, in one study (Massiou et al. 1997).

Pain-free response Although headache response has been widely used, it has been criticized for being less

clinically relevant than pain-free response, which is currently recommended as the primary endpoint for clinical trials of acute migraine (Tfelt-Hansen et al. 2000). Pain-free response uses the same data collected from a patient regarding headache intensity on a 4-point ordinal scale (none, mild, moderate, severe), but is defined as the percentage of patients with a decrease in headache intensity from severe or moderate at baseline to no pain within a specified time (usually 2 hours for migraine trials).

The implications of using headache relief versus pain-free response as the primary outcome measure is illustrated by a study comparing oral sumatriptan with a combination of aspirin and lysine acetylsalicylate (LAS) and metoclopramide (aspirin 900 mg/LAS 1620 mg + metoclopramide 10 mg) (Oral Sumatriptan and Aspirin-plus-Metoclopramide Comparative Study Group 1992). The study concluded that there was no significant difference between the two treatments in providing headache relief: 56% (74/133) of patients taking sumatriptan reported relief at 2 hours, compared with 45% (62/138) of patients taking aspirin + metoclopramide ($p = 0.078$). However, the same trial found that sumatriptan was significantly more effective at providing pain-free response at 2 hours: 26% (35/133) of patients taking sumatriptan reported pain-free response at 2 hours, compared with 14% (19/138) of patients taking aspirin + metoclopramide ($p = 0.016$). Although equivalent on one efficacy parameter (headache relief), a significant difference in a more clinically relevant secondary outcome (pain-free response) may have been underemphasized. The improved pain-free response must be weighed against the higher cost and significantly higher rate of adverse events associated with sumatriptan.

The standard 4-point scale for measuring headache pain intensity has been adapted to different purposes. One trial examined the question of whether sumatriptan, taken during the aura phase while the headache is still grade 0 or 1, prevents or delays the development of a grade 2–3 headache (Bates et al. 1994).

Pain assessments at later time points are often measured, but because patients who do not have pain relief at 2 hours are usually allowed to repeat treatment or use rescue medication (prohibited before the primary outcome assessment), the proportion of patients experiencing headache relief at later time points is often confounded by retreatment or use of rescue medication. Nevertheless, the headache response at later time points is important to patients; several approaches have been used to capture these data.

Headache recurrence Recurrence of headache after initially successful treatment has been identified as a possible clinical problem with sumatriptan. The trials that report such data use widely varying definitions of headache recurrence, so comparing results across trials has been difficult. Furthermore, headache recurrence is conditional on headache relief during the first 2 hours. That is, only patients who have relief of their headache from baseline can have a recurrence. Thus, in randomized controlled trials, if there is a large discrepancy in initial rate of headache relief between active and control treatments, then the numbers of subjects who could have a recurrence might be quite different.

Sustained pain-free response A more stringent outcome measure, sustained pain-free response, measures the proportion of patients who achieve a pain-free response at 2 hours, and maintain pain-free status until 24 hours after baseline (i.e., have no recurrence of headache). This outcome was proposed as a simpler measure that is clinically important to patients and avoids the conditional nature of headache recurrence by itself. It is not confounded by rescue medication which is typically prohibited during the first 2 hours; use of rescue medication after 2 hours for a recurrent headache would represent a failure to maintain pain-free status. In essence it is a composite measure that incorporates initial response, no use of rescue medication and absence of recurrence.

Other pain-related outcome measures Other pain-related measures include: (1) time to "meaningful" pain relief (usually defined subjectively); and (2) time to "onset of action" (defined as first noticeable pain relief). Studies of the effect of treatment of acute attacks often allow patients/subjects to treat multiple separate attacks and gather data on the results of such treatment. Such data allow investigators to estimate the consistency of response across attacks within individuals (Tfelt-Hansen et al. 2000).

Functional disability and quality of life

The approaches used to measure functional disability within headache attacks have not been standardized. Common approaches in the literature are to use simple verbal scales of 3, 4 or 5 categories. The IHS guidelines recommend the following 4-point categorical scale:

0: No disability: able to function normally.
1: Performance of daily activities mildly impaired: can still do everything but with difficulties.
2: Performance of daily activities moderately impaired: unable to do some things.
3: Performance of daily activities severely impaired: cannot do all or most things, bed rest may be necessary.

Recently, an instrument was developed and validated to assess disease-specific quality of life and/or disability over a short term period. The 24-hour Migraine Quality of Life Questionnaire (MQoLQ) assesses migraine-related quality of life during a 24-hour period after taking medication for an acute attack (Hartmaier et al. 1995). The instrument consists of 15 questions, comprising five domains: (i) work functioning, (ii) social

functioning, (iii) energy/vitality, (iv) migraine symptoms, and (v) feelings/concerns. For each domain, three questions answered on a 7-point scale (1 indicating maximum impairment and 7 indicating no impairment) are used to calculate a domain score by summing the response to the three corresponding questions (domain score range is from 3 to 21). Although this instrument has been shown to be sufficiently responsive to assess the impact of migraine and migraine therapy on health-related quality of life during an acute migraine attack, it has not seen widespread use (Santanello et al. 1997).

The IHS concludes that short-term functional disability is an appropriate secondary efficacy measure for clinical trials, but that currently available instruments are not well suited for use in acute treatment trials (Tfelt-Hansen et al. 2000). The clinical significance of changes in HRQoL measures over the short term is uncertain. Several other instruments are designed to assess disability or HRQoL over longer periods of time; these instruments are discussed later in the chapter.

Associated symptoms

Effects on associated symptoms such as nausea, vomiting, photophobia, and phonophobia are usually measured using simple assessments of presence or absence of these symptoms at defined time points, or categorical scales measuring their severity. Except in rare studies of the effect of antinauseant drugs as adjunct treatments for acute migraine, nausea and vomiting is considered as a secondary outcome.

Medication-related outcomes

Medication use is often considered as a behaviorally based surrogate outcome for headache pain. The rate and timing of use of rescue medication can imply lack of efficacy of the initial treatment. Since limiting the use of rescue medication is a stated goal of migraine treatments according to some guidelines (Silberstein 2000), this is also a clinically relevant outcome.

Global evaluation of study medication is often assessed using a simple verbal scale (very poor, poor, no opinion, good, very good). It has the advantage that each patient assimilates the efficacy of the medication as well as the tolerability in making these ratings.

MEASURING ACUTE HEADACHE SYMPTOMS AND EFFECTS IN TENSION-TYPE HEADACHE

Headache pain intensity is more difficult to measure in tension-type headache because the spectrum of pain is less severe than that associated with migraine. Thus the 4-point categorical verbal rating scale commonly used in migraine may be too insensitive. The IHS recommends using a visual analogue scale (VAS) (e.g., 100 mm line from "none" to "very severe") instead of or in addition to the categorical scale (Schoenen 1995).

Another strategy for improving the sensitivity of the pain assessment is to ask patients to rate not only the severity of the headache, but also the degree of relief of headache at a time point after therapy. This may be done on a categoric scale (0 = no relief; 1 = a little relief; 2 = some relief; 3 = much relief; 4 = complete relief). Sometimes, the headache relief scale allows for increasing pain (e.g., −1 = worsening) (Langemark and Olesen 1987).

Recommended outcome measures related to head pain assessment are pain-free response defined as the percentage of patients pain-free at 2 hours after treatment (Steiner et al. 2004). Other secondary endpoints include headache intensity difference (the arithmetic change in headache intensity score) at 2 hours and at other time points after treatment. This can be calculated based on a verbal rating scale (with categories scored numerically as an interval scale) or with continuous ratings from a 100 mm VAS.

When continuous pain ratings are used over multiple time points, it is possible to construct a time–response curve and calculate measures such as the SPID (sum of pain intensity differences, PID), of PAR (pain relief) and TOTPAR (sum of PARs) used in other pain syndromes. These measures have sometimes been renamed to reflect headache as the type of pain as HID (headache intensity difference), SHID (sum of HIDs at every time interval), HER (headache relief) and TOTHER (sum of HERs at every time interval) (Pfaffenrath and Isler 1993).

One drawback to the summed time–response parameter is that the clinical interpretation is less clear. The 2-hour pain-free response rate may be interpreted as the probability of obtaining a clinically significant response. Other measures such as time to meaningful relief also have a clear clinical interpretation. The IHS argues that the ease of clinical interpretation is an important consideration in selecting efficacy parameters that needs to be considered, along with statistical properties and data collection issues (Schoenen 1995). Finally, as with migraine, additional outcomes may focus on functional disability, rate and timing of use of rescue medication, and global evaluation of study medication.

MEASURING ACUTE HEADACHE SYMPTOMS AND EFFECTS IN CLUSTER HEADACHE

To evaluate efficacy and comparative effectiveness and tolerability in aborting or suppressing the acute attack requires some modifications to the approaches used with migraine and tension-type headache. Headache intensity measurements are made on a 5-point (rather than 4-point) verbal rating scale (0 = no pain; 1, 2, 3,

4 = mild, moderate, severe, excruciating pain) to accommodate the greater severity of cluster headache pain. Multiple fixed time points are generally recommended (5, 10 and 15 minutes after treatment and every 15 minutes thereafter for up to 3 hours); however, the agitation that accompanies acute cluster headache attacks may make such frequent assessments impractical (Steiner et al. 2004).

The IHS guideline for controlled trials of drugs in cluster headache recommends as the primary endpoint the *"aborted attack"* rate, defined as the percentage of patients in whom the attack is effectively stopped (headache intensity reduced to mild or no pain) within a prescribed time interval (which may be as short as 10 minutes) (Lipton et al. 1995). Because cluster headaches are typically short lasting but intense, longer assessment intervals of 1–2 hours are not clinically relevant. The increased emphasis on timing or speed of relief suggests also a methodology that directly measures time to a defined level of pain relief as might be obtained with a stop watch: time to meaningful relief or time to "complete" relief (mild or no pain).

Other secondary endpoints recommended for use in cluster headache trials that differ from those used in migraine include: (1) rate of relapse, defined as the return of headache of moderate or greater intensity within 1 hour in patients reporting an aborted attack; and (2) effect on associated autonomic symptoms.

ASSESSING BENEFITS OF PREVENTIVE OR LONG-TERM TREATMENT

Assessing changes in the pattern of headache attacks over time is a challenge that requires different approaches. Preventive treatments usually aim to reduce the frequency of recurrent headaches rather than abort or relieve individual acute episodes. Data on individual episodes or attacks may be important to record and consider, but such information should be integrated over the long time duration (of weeks to months) during which preventive treatments are expected to have their effect. The same outcome domains are important to consider – headache pain, other symptoms of migraine (nausea, vomiting, photophobia, phonophobia), and other outcomes (medication use, functional status (disability), and quality of life) – but the time course is entirely different.

One key distinction is whether data about headache attacks is obtained from the patient at or near the time of symptoms or by asking patients to recall their headache experience over a protracted period of time; most preventive drug studies are conducted over a treatment period of 8 to 12 weeks, with an assessment period lasting at least 4 weeks. Data based on contemporaneous and timed (usually daily) recording of headache symptoms are preferred to those based on global or retrospective assessments.

MEASURING CHRONIC SYMPTOMS OR EFFECT IN MIGRAINE

Headache pain or attacks

Assessment

Headache diaries are often used in clinical trials, and less often in clinical practice, to record headache symptoms on a daily basis. At a minimum, headache diaries should indicate the occurrence of a headache; other information about the attack (severity, duration, associated symptoms) may assist with evaluating the burden, and other information about antecedent events is sometimes used clinically to identify triggers, or potential causes of headache attacks.

Although not preferred, global or retrospective assessments are common in clinical trials, particularly in those designed prior to the publication of IHS guidelines (Tfelt-Hansen et al. 2000). There is empirical evidence that headache diaries are more accurate and less biased than global or retrospective assessments (Penzien et al. 1994).

Outcome measures

Migraine frequency (number of attacks) To confirm effectiveness and evaluate comparative efficacy and tolerability in migraine prevention, appropriate primary endpoints include (1) frequency of attacks per specified unit time (usually 4 weeks) measured during treatment after a specified period (usually 8 weeks) and (2) response rate: percentage of patients with a reduction in frequency of 50% or more after a specified treatment period. In determining migraine frequency, the number of attacks is recorded regardless of duration; however, since migraine attacks may by definition last up to 72 hours, rules are needed to distinguish an attack of long duration from two attacks and between attacks and relapses. A migraine attack that is interrupted by sleep or that temporarily remits spontaneously and then recurs within 48 hours after its onset should be recorded as one attack and not two (Tfelt-Hansen et al. 2000). An attack treated successfully with medication but with relapse within 48 hours counts as one attack.

Headache days or migraine days An alternative outcome of "migraine days" (defined as any day on which symptoms of migraine are present) per 4 weeks is often used to assess the burden of chronic headache. For migraine days, the rules for counting attacks do not apply. While migraine days may be a more appropriate measure for long-duration migraines, as in so-called transformed or chronic migraine, it has drawbacks in assessing the burden of short duration headaches that might occur more than once per day. This is more of a problem with cluster or tension-type headache.

Response rate Data on headache frequency can also be used to calculate the *response rate*, which is defined as the percentage of subjects with a 50% or greater reduction in attack frequency during treatment compared to baseline assessment. The choice of 50% as the threshold is arbitrary. The IHS guidelines suggest that a clinical rationale might suggest a different threshold; indeed thresholds of 25, 30, 40 and 50% have appeared in the literature, but 50% is the most commonly used threshold and is generally acknowledged to be clinically relevant (Tfelt-Hansen et al. 2000). It may be insufficiently sensitive to clinically meaningful treatment effects, however, and so is a poor choice for a primary outcome measure.

Headache index Headache indices are composite outcomes that use a mathematical formula to combine headache frequency, intensity and/or duration into a single outcome measure. Indices may be difficult to meaningfully compare between patients, and may have a wider range and variance than frequency measures. They have been criticized because there is no consistent definition of headache index and weights applied to the components are arbitrary and their effects may be increased by multiplication. Studies have shown that headache frequency is significantly correlated with both headache intensity and duration (Penzien et al. 1994), which suggests that measuring headache frequency alone may be sufficient in some cases.

While making a strong case and preference for frequency of attacks (followed by headache days) as the primary outcome measure for episodic (not necessarily chronic) migraine, the IHS guidelines also acknowledge that a headache index may more accurately reflect the patient's overall level of suffering (Tfelt-Hansen et al. 2000). For patients with chronic daily headache (chronic migraine, CTTH, or a mixture of both), some researchers have argued that significant reductions in the headache index (most commonly 50%) may be the more appropriate outcome measure (Lake and Saper 2002).

For example, a double-blind, placebo-controlled randomized outcome study of tizanidine for chronic daily headache found significant reduction on the primary variable of headache index (frequency × severity × duration) for active treatment over placebo (54% versus 19%, $p < 0.015$) but not for total headache days (30% versus 22%). In this case, the headache index reduction appeared to be primarily due to a reduction in the number of severe headache days (55% versus 21%, $p < 0.035$), with more modest but significant reductions in peak and average headache intensity and duration (Saper et al. 2002b).

The appropriateness of a frequency measure as the primary endpoint may depend on the frequency of headache. For example, a post hoc analysis of patients with true daily headaches versus those with at least one headache-free day per month, who had received tizanidine for chronic daily headache (predominantly migraine), found a mean reduction of 42% in headache days for those who had at least one headache-free day at baseline (mean of 19.6 days, versus 11.3 days during third month on drug), but only 10% in those with daily headaches at baseline (28 days, versus 25 days). In contrast, reductions in the headache index for these two groups were more substantial (67.2% versus 35.5%, $P < 0.002$) (Lake and Saper 2003). There are few studies that have focused on patients with true daily headaches who are not in analgesic rebound. This subgroup may have particular difficulty in achieving headache-free days.

Headache indices have been used extensively in past trials, including studies of behavioral treatment where the interventions are designed to both prevent headaches and help reduce the intensity and duration of pain when an attack occurs. Interpreting older literature requires familiarity with them.

Drug consumption and medication overuse headache (analgesic rebound) Drug consumption for symptomatic or acute treatment totaled over an evaluation period may be used as a secondary outcome measure. It is critical in studies of preventive treatment that cases of medication overuse headache (e.g., consumption of certain analgesic and abortive medications that may exceed 2 days/week) be distinguished from episodic or chronic daily headaches without medication overuse. Most studies of preventive treatment make the overuse of medication an exclusionary condition. When the over-consumption of analgesic or abortive medication is believed to play a significant role in the frequency, severity, and intractability of headache, reductions in drug use may be part of the therapeutic intervention and, thus, its use as an outcome measure is problematic (Bigal et al. 2004). However, in long-term follow-up, maintaining appropriate limits on the frequency of using drugs with the potential for rebound may be a critical outcome measure associated with preventing relapse (Grazzi et al. 2002; Katsarava et al. 2003).

Disease-specific quality of life and disability

Health-related quality of life (HRQoL) measures provide information beyond that captured by clinical measures. It includes patient-reported physical, mental/emotional, and social aspects of health. Because HRQoL assesses the impact of a medical condition on functional health and well-being, as reported by the individual with the condition, it is useful in understanding the wide variability of individual responses to similar disease conditions.

HRQoL instruments can be either condition-specific or generic; both types of measures have been applied to headache conditions. Though these measures of function assess the same underlying concepts, condition-specific measures are generally more sensitive and more responsive to condition-specific changes, while generic measures make it possible to compare disease burden and outcomes across diseases and treatments.

Generic HRQoL instruments

A number of recent studies have used the Medical Outcomes Study Short Form (SF)-36, SF-20, SF-12, and SF-

8 Health Surveys to assess impact of migraine on functional health and well-being (Solomon 1995, 1997; Dahlof et al. 1997; Cohen et al. 1999; Turner-Bowker et al. 2003). The SF-20, SF-12, and SF-8 are shorter alternative forms that include a subset of the original SF-36 items. Data on the SF-20 and SF-36 demonstrated that chronic headache disorders were associated with significant limitations in all eight health domains of patient well-being and functioning (Solomon 1997). Furthermore, the SF-20 outcomes profiles for each of the common benign headache disorders (migraine, tension-type headache, mixed headache, and cluster headache) appear to be unique for the specific headache diagnosis. However, while these generic HRQoL measures provide a practical and efficient method of describing the burden of migraine in population studies, they are not sufficiently responsive to changes associated with treatment to be useful as outcome measures for clinical trials of preventive drugs or other long-term treatment approaches.

Disease-specific HRQoL instruments

Several standardized questionnaires have been developed specifically for headache or migraine, including the Henry Ford Hospital Headache Disability Inventory (HDI), Migraine Specific Quality of Life (MSQoL) questionnaire, Migraine Disability Assessment (MIDAS), Headache Impact Test (HIT; see http://www.headachetest.com/), and the Migraine Specific Quality of Life questionnaire (MSQ). Like the generic quality-of-life measures, these measures have proven to be very useful in quantifying the burden of migraine in population studies (Stewart et al. 1999); however, unlike the generic measures, disease-specific measures display greater responsiveness and can be used to evaluate the effectiveness of headache treatment (Solomon et al. 1995; Adelman et al. 1996; Cohen et al. 1996; Jhingran et al. 1996; Dahlof et al. 1997; Lofland et al. 1999).

The HDI is an empirically derived 25-item headache disability inventory which has demonstrated strong internal consistency/reliability, construct validity (Jacobson et al. 1994), and test–retest reliability (Jacobson et al. 1995). However, it has not shown very good responsiveness to changes associated with treatment (Jacobson et al. 1995) and has not been extensively used.

The MSQoL questionnaire is a 20-item instrument that assesses the long-term quality-of-life effects of migraine (Wagner et al. 1996). The MSQoL meets established criteria for validity, consistency, and reproducibility and shows moderate responsiveness to treatment (Patrick et al. 2000). A recent Dutch translation has been validated, as well as the English language version.

MIDAS is a brief, self-administered questionnaire designed to quantify headache-related disability over a 3-month period. The MIDAS score has been shown to have moderately high test–retest reliability in headache sufferers and is correlated with clinical judgment regarding the need for medical care (Stewart et al. 2000). This instrument incorporates sums from several measures of days lost from functioning, or with significant headache-related impairment. It may be difficult to compare scores for employed versus unemployed patients since some questions specifically address days lost or impaired at work. The distribution of scores in a treatment group may be skewed or bimodal rather than normally distributed, with a subset of highly impaired patients with high scores. In such cases, analysis of changes in MIDAS scores requires non-parametric statistical tests.

The HIT and HIT-6 are validated and reliable measures of the effect that headaches have on patients' physical, social, and emotional functioning (Pryse-Phillips 2002). HIT was designed for administration electronically (on the internet at www.headachetest.com and www.headachetest.com) and as a paper-based form known as HIT-6; it is useful for not only migraine, but also other headache disorders (Dowson 2001). It should be noted that various versions of the HIT measure the disability associated with specific headaches, and not the overall level of disability during a given time period. For example, a patient may experience a significant reduction in the frequency of headaches, but still suffer significant disability when headaches occur. The improvement in function associated with reduced headache days may not be reflected on the HIT.

The MSQ consists of 16 questions that measure aspects of functioning and well-being most affected by migraine (Jhingran et al. 1998). Three scales are scored from the MSQ: (1) role function – restrictive (the degree to which performance of normal daily activities is restricted by migraine); (2) role function – preventative (the degree to which performance of normal daily activities is prevented by migraine); and (3) emotional function (capturing the emotional impact of migraine). The MSQ has been validated and all three MSQ scales were shown to be highly responsive to the effect of sumatriptan treatment on migraine-associated HRQoL in three studies (Kosinski et al. 2003).

Since the IHS guidelines were published in 2000, considerable development has occurred in HRQoL instruments for headache and migraine. The instruments are becoming more widely accepted, and newer instruments seem to have greater responsiveness to change, a feature required for their use in demonstrating benefits of treatment. While no single instrument has yet been recognized as the gold standard in migraine HRQoL assessment, ongoing psychometric and clinical testing on the MIDAS (Stewart et al. 2003) and MSQ (Kosinski et al. 2003) suggest that these instruments may become more widely used in future clinical trials and population-based studies.

Measures of comorbid conditions

Migraine is associated with both psychiatric and non-psychiatric comorbid conditions, including sleep disturbance, anxiety, and depression among others (Breslau et al. 1994; Low and Merikangas 2003). These associated conditions are often appropriate targets for intervention (Lake 2001; Sheftell and Atlas 2002), and the relationship between improvement in one condition to the other is of significant interest (Saper et al. 2001a). In clinical studies of patients with frequent severe and disabling headaches, it may be appropriate to include secondary measures of changes in these conditions using visual analog rating scales (Saper et al. 2001b), frequency measures (e.g., nights with disturbed sleep) (Lake et al. 1993), or standardized measures such as the Beck Depression Inventory II or Hamilton Rating Scales for Anxiety and Depression (Saper et al. 2001a).

CHRONIC TENSION-TYPE HEADACHE PROPHYLAXIS

The measurement approaches to tension-type headache in its episodic form are nearly identical to those for episodic migraine as described above. Similarly, CTTH prevention is measured in the same way as chronic migraine. In fact, cases of pure CTTH without migraine or migrainous ("probably migraine") headaches are extremely rare (Saper et al. 2002b).

PROPHYLAXIS OF EPISODIC CLUSTER HEADACHE

The IHS published guidelines (Lipton et al. 1995) recommend, as primary endpoint, the frequency of attacks per specified unit time (usually 1 week) measured during treatment after a specified period (to allow treatment effect to develop) following dosage stabilization. However, it is important to note this approach has had little empirical testing, because there have been few trials of preventive treatment in cluster headache (Monstad et al. 1995; Leone et al. 1996; Leone et al. 2000; Saper et al. 2002a).

CONCLUSION

A variety of measurement approaches are used to assess efficacy of treatment in clinical trials of headache disorders. Distinct approaches are used based on whether therapy is aimed at relief of acute attacks or prevention of headaches. Furthermore, different measures are needed for measurement of episodic headache disorders versus chronic headache disorders (chronic migraine, chronic tension-type headache, chronic daily headache). Characteristics of the headache disorders also require adaptations to the approaches with regard to timing, severity, and nature of associated symptoms. The majority of methodologic work has been in developing outcome measures for migraine because it is common and significant; however, further work is needed in subsets of patients with chronic migraine because, although less common, it is particularly debilitating.

REFERENCES

Adelman JU, Sharfman M, Johnson R, et al. Impact of oral sumatriptan on workplace productivity, health-related quality of life, healthcare use, and patient satisfaction with medication in nurses with migraine. Am J Manag Care 1996; 2:1407–1416.

Bates D, Ashford E, Dawson R, et al. Subcutaneous sumatriptan during the migraine aura. Neurology 1994; 44:1587–1592.

Bigal ME, Rapoport AM, Sheftell FD, et al. Transformed migraine and medication overuse in a tertiary headache centre: clinical characteristics and treatment outcomes. Cephalalgia 2004; 24:483–490.

Breslau N, Merikangas K, Bowden CL. Comorbidity of migraine and major affective disorders. Neurology 1994; 44:S17–S22.

Classification Subcommittee of the International Headache Society. International classification of headache disorders, 2nd edition. Cephalalgia 2004; 24(suppl 1):1–160.

Cohen JA, Beall D, Miller DW, et al. Subcutaneous sumatriptan for the treatment of migraine: humanistic, economic, and clinical consequences. Fam Med 1996; 28:171–177.

Dahlof C, Bouchard J, Cortelli P, et al. A multinational investigation of the impact of subcutaneous sumatriptan: II. Health-related quality of life. Pharmacoeconomics 1997; 11(suppl 1):24–34.

Dowson AJ. Assessing the impact of migraine. Curr Med Res Opin 2001; 17:298–309.

Grazzi L, Andrasik F, D'Amico D, et al. Behavioral and pharmacologic treatment of transformed migraine with analgesic overuse: outcome at 3 years. Headache 2002; 42:483–490.

Hartmaier SL, Santanello NC, Epstein RS, et al. Validation of a new quality of life questionnaire for acute migraine headache. Headache 1995; 35:330–337.

Headache Classification Committee: Olesen J, Bousser M-C, Diener H-C, et al. New appendix criteria open for a broader concept of chronic migraine. Cephalalgia 2006; 26:742–746.

Jacobson GP, Ramadan NM, Aggarwal SK, et al. The Henry Ford Hospital Headache Disability Inventory (HDI). Neurology 1994; 44:837–842.

Jacobson GP, Ramadan NM, Norris L, et al. Headache disability inventory (HDI): short-term test–retest reliability and spouse perceptions. Headache 1995; 35:534–539.

Jhingran P, Cady RK, Rubino J, et al. Improvements in health-related quality of life with sumatriptan treatment for migraine. J Fam Practice 1996; 42:36–42.

Jhingran P, Osterhaus JT, Miller DW, et al. Development and validation of the Migraine Specific Quality of Life Questionnaire. Headache 1998; 38:295–302.

Katsarava Z, Limmroth V, Finke M, et al. Rates and predictors for relapse in medication overuse headache: a 1-year prospective study. Neurology 2003; 60:1682–1683.

Keele KD. The pain chart. Lancet 1948; 2:6–8.

Kosinski M, Bjorner JB, Ware JE Jr, et al. The responsiveness of headache impact scales scored using "classical" and "modern" psychometric methods: a re-analysis of three clinical trials. Quality Life Res 2003; 12:903–912.

Lake AE III. Behavioral and nonpharmacologic treatments of headache. Med Clin North Am 2001; 85:1055–1075.

Lake AE III, Saper JR. Chronic headache: new advances in treatment strategies. Neurology 2002; 59(5 suppl 2): S8–13.

Lake AE, Saper JR. Chronic migraine with daily pain is more treatment resistant than chronic migraine with non-daily pain [abstract]. Headache 2003; 43:573.

Lake AE III, Saper JR, Madden SF, et al. Comprehensive inpatient treatment for intractable migraine: a prospective long-term outcome study. Headache 1993; 33:55–62.

Langemark M, Olesen J. Effervescent ASA versus solid ASA in the treatment of tension headache. A double-blind, placebo controlled study. Headache 1987; 27:90–95.

Leone M, D'Amico D, Moschiano F, et al. Melatonin versus placebo in the prophylaxis of cluster headache: a double-blind pilot study with parallel groups. Cephalalgia 1996; 16:494–496.

Leone M, D'Amico D, Frediani F, et al. Verapamil in the prophylaxis of episodic cluster headache: a double-blind study versus placebo. Neurology 2000; 54:1382–1385.

Lipton RB, Micieli G, Russell D, et al. Guidelines for controlled trials of drugs in cluster headache. Cephalalgia 1995; 15:452–462.

Lipton RB, Stewart WF, Diamond S, et al. Prevalence and burden of migraine in the United States: data from the American Migraine Study II. Headache 2001; 41:646–657.

Lofland JH, Johnson NE, Batenhorts AS, et al. Changes in resource use and outcomes for patients with migraine treated with sumatriptan. Arch Intern Med 1999; 159:857–863.

Low NC, Merikangas KR. The comorbidity of migraine. CNS Spectr 2003; 8:433–444.

Massiou H, Tzourio C, el Amrani M, et al. Verbal scales in the acute treatment of migraine: semantic categories and clinical relevance. Cephalalgia 1997; 17:37–39.

Monstad I, Krabbe A, Micieli G, et al. Preemptive oral treatment with sumatriptan during a cluster period. Headache 1995; 35:607–613.

Monzon MJ, Lainez MJ. Quality of life in migraine and chronic daily headache patients. Cephalalgia 1998; 18:638–643.

O'Brien B, Goeree R, Streiner D. Prevalence of migraine headache in Canada: a population-based survey. Int J Epidemiol 1994; 23:1020–1026.

Oral Sumatriptan and Aspirin-plus-Metoclopramide Comparative Study Group. A study to compare oral sumatriptan with oral aspirin plus oral metoclopramide in the acute treatment of migraine. Eur Neurol 1992; 32:177–184.

Patrick DL, Hurst BC, Hughes J. Further development and testing of the migraine-specific quality of life (MSQOL) measure. Headache 2000; 40:550–560.

Penzien D, Johnson C, Seville J, et al. Interrelationships among daily and global self-report measures of headache. Headache Quart 1994; 5:8–14.

Pfaffenrath V, Isler H. Evaluation of the nosology of chronic tension-type headache. Cephalalgia 1993; (suppl 12): 60–62.

Pryse-Phillips W. Evaluating migraine disability: the headache impact test instrument in context. Canad J Neurol Sci 2002; 29(suppl 2):S11–S15.

Rasmussen BK. Migraine and tension-type headache in a general population: psychosocial factors. Int J Epidemiol 1992; 21:1138–1143.

Rasmussen BK. Epidemiology of headache. Cephalalgia 2001; 21:774–777.

Santanello NC, Polis AB, Hartmaier SL, et al. Improvement in migraine-specific quality of life in a clinical trial of rizatriptan. Cephalalgia 1997; 17:867–872.

Saper JR, Lake AE III, Madden SF, et al. Comprehensive/tertiary care for headache: a 6-month outcome study. Headache 1999; 39:249–263.

Saper JR, Lake AE III, Tepper SJ. Nefazodone for chronic daily headache prophylaxis: an open-label study. Headache 2001a; 41:465–474.

Saper JR, Winner PK, Lake AE III. An open-label dose-titration study of the efficacy and tolerability of tizanidine hydrochloride tablets in the prophylaxis of chronic daily headache. Headache 2001b; 41:357–368.

Saper JR, Klapper J, Mathew NT, et al. Intranasal civamide for the treatment of episodic cluster headaches. Arch Neurol 2002a; 59:990–994.

Saper JR, Lake AE III, Cantrell DT, et al. Chronic daily headache prophylaxis with tizanidine: a double-blind, placebo-controlled, multicenter outcome study. Headache 2002b; 42:470–482.

Scher AI, Stewart WF, Liberman J, et al. Prevalence of frequent headache in a population sample. Headache 1998; 38:497–506.

Schoenen J. Guidelines for trials of drug treatments in tension-type headache, 1st edition. International Headache Society Committee on Clinical Trials. Cephalalgia 1995; 15:165–179.

Sheftell FD, Atlas SJ. Migraine and psychiatric comorbidity: from theory and hypotheses to clinical application. Headache 2002; 42:934–944.

Silberstein SD. Practice parameter: evidence-based guidelines for migraine headache (an evidence-based review): report of the Quality Standards Subcommittee of the American Academy of Neurology. Neurology 2000; 55:754–762.

Solomon GD. Evolution of the measurement of quality of life in migraine. Neurology 1997; 48:S10–S15.

Solomon GD, Skobieranda FG, Genzen JR. Quality of life assessment among migraine patients treated with sumatriptan. Headache 1995; 35:449–454.

Steiner TJ, Tfelt-Hansen P, McCrory DC. Headache disorders. In: du Souich P, Erill S, Orme M (eds). The IUPHAR Compendium of Basic Principles for Pharmacological Research in Humans. International Union of Basic and Clinical Pharmacology, Irvine, CA, 2004:183–211.

Stewart WF, Lipton RB, Celentano DD, et al. Prevalence of migraine headache in the United States. Relation to age, income, race, and other sociodemographic factors. JAMA 1992; 267:64–69.

Stewart WF, Lipton RB, Simon D, et al. Validity of an illness severity measure for headache in a population sample of migraine sufferers. Pain 1999; 79:291–301.

Stewart WF, Lipton RB, Kolodner KB, et al. Validity of the Migraine Disability Assessment (MIDAS) score in comparison to a diary-based measure in a population sample of migraine sufferers. Pain 2000; 88:41–52.

Stewart WF, Lipton RB, Kolodner K. Migraine disability assessment (MIDAS) score: relation to headache frequency, pain intensity, and headache symptoms. Headache 2003; 43:258–265.

Tfelt-Hansen P, Block G, Dahlof C, et al. International Headache Society Clinical Trials Subcommittee Guidelines for controlled trials of drugs in migraine: second edition. Cephalalgia 2000; 20:765–786.

Turner-Bowker DM, Bayliss MS, Ware JE Jr, et al. Usefulness of the SF-8 Health Survey for comparing the impact of migraine and other conditions. Quality Life Res 2003; 12:1003–1012.

Von Korff M, Stewart WF, Simon DJ, et al. Migraine and reduced work performance: a population-based diary study. Neurology 1998; 50:1741–1745.

Wagner TH, Patrick DL, Galer BS, et al. A new instrument to assess the long-term quality of life effects from migraine: development and psychometric testing of the MSQOL. Headache 1996; 36:484–492.

World Health Organization. The World Health Report 2001. WHO, Geneva, 2001.

CHAPTER 15

Measurement instruments for CRPS

Roberto S.G.M. Perez • Maurice J.M.M. Giezeman

INTRODUCTION

Complex regional pain syndrome (CRPS) is a painful complaint characterized by a variety of autonomic and sensory disturbances in the affected area (usually a limb), and dysfunction, which often lead to limitations in daily activities and role fulfillment of the affected person in society. Since the first descriptions of CRPS (Michell et al. 1864), then known under various names such as reflex sympathetic dystrophy, algodystrophy or posttraumatic dystrophy, many signs and symptoms have been attributed to this syndrome. Bonica (1990) was one of the first to standardize criteria for CRPS, and in recent years Veldman et al. (1993), the IASP (Stanton-Hicks et al. 1995) and Bruehl et al. (1999) have formulated criteria for the diagnosis of CRPS (Table 15.2). In these recent criteria sets, no laboratory tests have been included and the diagnosis "CRPS" is made only on the basis of symptoms and signs.

Different sets of diagnostic criteria are being used side by side in literature (van de Beek et al. 2002; Reinders et al. 2002). As there appears to be no gold standard for its diagnosis, there can be no reference of measurement either. This is even more compelling because of the multifactorial nature of CRPS, which usually requires treatment by specialists of several disciplines.

Though efforts have been made to standardize the criteria upon which CRPS is diagnosed, no uniform measurement or grading method has been proposed. Outcome measures in CRPS have, therefore, been diverse, and even identical phenomena have been measured in different ways.

In the next section, we will evaluate how different aspects of CRPS have been measured in literature. Subsequently, clinimetric properties of those instruments which have been evaluated for the use in CRPS patients will be described. Measurement instruments will be described according to their International Classification of Functioning, Disability and Health (ICF) domain, i.e., impairment, function and participation level (see Chapter 11), in keeping with the problems patients can encounter with this disease. Finally, an attempt will be made to synthesize recommendations for further studies.

METHODS

Articles were retrieved from a PubMed search, supplemented with articles from our personal library. Publications were sought in which complex regional pain

Table 15.1 List of abbreviations. Only those abbreviations appearing in multiple parts of the chapter are listed

AROM	Active range of motion
CRPS	Complex regional pain syndrome
DASH	Disability of Arm, Shoulder and Hand questionnaire
FFT	Foot Function Test board
GRS	Grip strength
HRQL	Health-related quality of life
ISS	Impairment level Sum Score
MPQ	McGill Pain Questionnaire
NHP	Nottingham Health Profile
NPS	Neuropathic Pain Scale
NRS	Numeric Rating Scale
NWC-t	Number of Words Chosen total (in McGill Pain Questionnaire)
QRSD	Questionnaire Rising and Sitting Down
RSQ	Radboud Skills Questionnaire
SDD	Smallest detectable difference
SF-36	Short Form 36
SHS	Shoulder hand syndrome
SIP	Sickness Impact Profile
ULAM	Upper Limb Activity Monitor
VAS	Visual Analogue Scale
VRS	Verbal Rating Scale
WSQ	Walking Stairs Questionnaire

syndrome type I (CRPS I) therapy was evaluated, or studies in which measurement instruments were evaluated for CRPS. Search strings were "complex regional pain syndrome" or "causalgia" or "reflex sympathetic dystrophy." These were combined with "therapy" and limited to human clinical trials. Another search combined the search terms with "measurement." Excluded were articles not written in the English, German, French, Dutch or Italian language, as well as case reports and reviews.

With regard to the therapeutic effects 102 articles were found published between 1980 and 2003 meeting the criteria mentioned above (Williame 1980; Chuinard et al. 1981; Farcot et al. 1981; Glynn et al. 1981; Kozin et al. 1981; Taoussanis 1981; Bruxelle and Menkes 1982; Christensen et al. 1982; Delcambre et al. 1982;

Friez et al. 1982; Nedjar and Ficat 1982; Perrigot et al. 1982; Bonelli et al. 1983; Cherot and Amor 1983; Driessen et al. 1983; Poplawski et al. 1983; Bounameaux et al. 1984; Prough et al. 1985; Reginster and Franchimont 1985; Gobelet et al. 1986; Horton and Gerster 1986; Mayer et al. 1986; Goris et al. 1987; Nuti et al. 1987; Rico et al. 1987; Kettler and Abrams 1988; Sherry 1988; Hanna and Peat 1989; Jeandel et al. 1989; Reiestadt et al. 1989; Rocco et al. 1989; Blanchard et al. 1990; Eulry et al. 1990; Farcot et al. 1990; Bickerstaff and Kanis 1991; Eulry et al. 1991; Kissling et al. 1991; Riou et al. 1991; Gobelet et al. 1992; Hord et al. 1992; Sawicki et al. 1992; Fialka et al. 1993; Field et al. 1993a,b; Glynn and Casale 1993; Langendijk et al. 1993; Mudun et al. 1993; Rauck et al. 1993; Ahn et al. 1994; Bonezzi et al. 1994; Braus et al. 1994; Chaise et al. 1994; Geertzen et al. 1994; Verdugo et al. 1994; Connelly et al. 1995; Dielissen et al. 1995; Gschwind et al. 1995; Jadad et al. 1995; Maillefert et al. 1995; Ramamurthy and Hoffman 1995; Grundberg 1996; Hamamci et al. 1996; Hassenbusch et al. 1996; Kaplan et al. 1996; Zuurmond et al. 1996; Adami et al. 1997; Cortet et al. 1997; Laroche et al. 1997; Muizelaar et al. 1997; Calvillo et al. 1998; Kumar et al. 1998; Malik et al. 1998; Muramatsu et al. 1998; Price et al. 1998; Robbins et al. 1998; Zyluk 1998; Hennart et al. 1999; Korpan et al. 1999; Linchitz and Raheb 1999; Maillefert et al. 1999; Rovetta et al. 1999; Sherry et al. 1999; Smeets et al. 1999; Wu et al. 1999; Zollinger et al. 1999; Azad et al. 2000; Bannink et al. 2000; Kemler et al. 2000a; Oerlemans et al. 2000b; Uher et al. 2000; van Hilten et al. 2000; Varenna et al. 2000; Wallace et al. 2000; Harke et al. 2001; Kondo et al. 2001; Kubalek et al. 2001; Marx et al. 2001; Cazeneuve et al. 2002; Lee et al. 2002; Livingstone and Atkins 2002; Serpell 2002; Perez et al. 2003b). The search contained 49 (48%) pre-experimental designs, 16 (16%) quasi-experimental designs and 37 (36%) true-experimental designs. Pharmaceutical interventions were evaluated in 90 (88%) studies, which were combined with physical or occupational therapy in 6 (6%) cases. Surgical interventions were evaluated in 5 (5%) studies, and physical or occupational therapy in 12 (12%) cases. Overall, pain was used as an outcome measure in most reports (75; 74%) (Table 15.3). Thirteen (13%) studies measured functional impairment, seven evaluated quality of life. In all, 31 different outcome parameters were evaluated, and 84 different measurement instruments or methods of measurement were used (Table 15.4). In the 102 studies, a total of 352 outcome measures were determined.

Twenty-four studies (Davidoff et al. 1988; Atkins and Kanis 1989; Bryan et al. 1991; Bruehl et al. 1996; Galer and Jensen 1997; Geertzen et al.1998a,b,c; Oerlemans et al. 1998; Oerlemans et al. 1999a,b,c; Kemler et al. 2000b,c,d; Oerlemans et al. 2000a; Perez et al. 2001; Forouzanfar et al. 2002; Perez et al. 2002a,b;

Table 15.2 Diagnostic criteria for CRPS I

CRPS I criteria according to Veldman:
1. Presence of four out of five symptoms:
   unexplainable diffuse pain
   difference in color relative to the other extremity
   diffuse edema
   difference in skin temperature relative to the other extremity
   limitation in active range of motion
2. Appearance or increase of above mentioned symptoms due to exercise
3. Presence of these symptoms in an area larger than and primarily distal to the primary lesion

CRPS I criteria according to the IASP:
1. Presence of an initiating noxious event or a cause of immobilization
2. Continuing pain, allodynia or hyperalgesia, with which the pain is disproportionate to any inciting event and is not limited to the area of an individual peripheral nerve
3. Evidence at any time of edema, skin blood flow abnormality, or abnormal sudomotor activity in the painful area since the inciting event
4. Conditions which could otherwise account for the level of pain and dysfunction should be excluded. Note: criteria 2–4 have to be met

Modified CRPS I criteria according to Bruehl:
1. Continuing disproportionate pain
2. Must report at least one symptom in each of the four following categories:
   sensory: hyperesthesia
   vasomotor: temperature asymmetry and/or skin color changes and/or skin color asymmetry
   sudomotor/edema: edema and/or sweating changes and/or sweating asymmetry
   motor/trophic: decreased range of motion and/or motor dysfunction (weakness, tremor, dystonia) and/or trophic changes (hair, nail, skin)
3. Must display at least one sign in two or more of the following categories:
   sensory: evidence of hyperalgesia (to pinprick) and/or allodynia (to light touch)
   vasomotor: evidence of temperature asymmetry and/or skin color changes and/or skin color asymmetry
   sudomotor/edema: evidence of edema and/or sweating changes and/or sweating asymmetry
   motor/trophic: decreased range of motion and/or motor dysfunction (weakness, tremor, dystonia) and/or trophic changes (hair, nail, skin)

Schasfoort et al. 2002; Wasner et al. 2002; van de Vusse et al. 2003; Perez et al. 2005) were found that specifically evaluate measurement instruments for the use in CRPS patients. The other studies evaluated measures on impairment level in 18 cases and on disability level in 4 cases. Two studies evaluated the use of health-related quality of life (HRQL) charts for CRPS patients.

EVALUATION OF CRPS TREATMENT: WHICH MEASUREMENT INSTRUMENTS HAVE BEEN APPLIED?

Treatment outcome has been measured in various ways, depending on the intervention, pathophysiologic and diagnostic perspective of the researchers. Seventy-two studies evaluated multiple parameters. For a substantial part of these measurement instruments general information regarding their reliability and validity is lacking. Of the 352 times instruments

were reported in the studies, reference to or description of clinimetric properties was provided in only 105 (30%) of cases. Many studies used some kind of self-report (90 cases) in the form of a categorical scale, describing either the patients' or the physicians' rating of severity or change. Evaluation of global improvement often comprised the evaluation of different features, which were combined into one categorical scale. As the constituting features were not explicitly described in the majority of these studies, these features were not included as separate entities in the present description.

The categorical ranges described varied from 2-point scores (presence–absence, or improved–not improved) to 10-point scores. In a number of cases the various categories were poorly described.

IMPAIRMENT LEVEL

Most studies have evaluated aspects of body functions and structures. On this ICF domain, features such as

Table 15.3 Summary of parameters measured in listed studies

Parameter	Measurement instrument	Times used
Pain (75 studies)	VAS	42
	VRS	12
	NRS	10
	MPQ	7
	Other	24
Vasomotor changes (51 studies)	Skin color	7
	Temperature difference	19
	Edema	28
	Plethysmography	4
	Other	15
Trophic changes (15 studies)	Changes of skin, nail or hair growth	7
	Bone mineralization	14
ROM measurement (32 studies)	Goniometer	14
	Grip strength	17
	Subjective	8
	Other	2
Disability (14 studies)	ADL	6
	Function	7
	General activities	3
	Other	4

Totals in the second column may be larger than the number of studies, since some studies included more than one parameter.

pain, sensory abnormalities, vasomotor and trophic changes, and limitations in range of motion or motor disturbances have been studied.

With regard to *pain*, the visual analogue scale (VAS) was used in 42 studies, a verbal rating scale (VRS) in 12 cases, and a numeric rating scale (NRS) in 10 cases. Different categorical scales were used for the latter two measurement types, ranging from 3- to 100-point scores for the VRS as well as the NRS. The McGill Pain Questionnaire (MPQ) was applied in 7 cases. A large group of studies (24) used other types of pain measurements including dolorimetry (3 studies), the duration of pain (relief) (4 studies) and the Oxford Pain Chart in one case. Pain presence–absence was registered in 5 cases, and the remaining studies used some kind of categorical scale for which it was unclear whether numeric or verbal rating scales were used.

For *vasomotor changes*, color and temperature difference, edema, and changes in blood flow were used to measure therapeutic improvements. Differences in skin color (6 studies) were measured predominantly by physicians' assessment (5 cases). Two studies used tele-thermography to quantify difference in skin color. Temperature difference was assessed in 19 studies, in which most studies used IR thermometers (7 studies) or other

forms of thermography (7 studies). Three studies used physicians' assessment as a way of establishing temperature differences, and in 2 other studies the way of measurement was unspecified.

Edema was measured in 28 studies, in which water displacement was used as a measurement tool in 5 studies. Circumference measurements were performed in 8 studies, of which one included ring size. The majority, however, used physicians' or patients' assessments (13 studies) to quantify volume differences with categorical scales ranging from two to four points. Changes in blood flow were measured by plethysmography in 4 cases, and the use of laser Doppler and scintigraphy in one study each. Blood pressure was evaluated in 3 studies, although this was performed for guiding treatment in 2 cases. Two studies used a cold stress test to study vasomotor stability. To that purpose, 8 studies used some form of self-report or questionnaire.

Trophic changes, such as alterations of hair, nails, skin, muscle and bone, were used 18 times as outcome parameters in 15 studies. Changes in skin, nails, muscle and hair growth were evaluated by physicians' assessment in 7 cases, 2 studies without specifying which trophic changes were evaluated. Bone mineralization, which is used by some as a diagnostic tool, was measured by scintigraphy in 8 studies and x-ray in 6 studies. One study provided no information on the method of bone mineralization measurement.

Limitations in range of motion and *motor disturbances* were measured in 32 studies. Universal goniometers were used in 14 studies, but self-reports by the patient (5 studies, including 2- to 4-point scales) and by the physician (12 studies, reviewing finger opposition and 2- to 5-point categorical scales) were used as well.

For motor disturbances, grip strength was evaluated in 8 studies, using a dynamometer, vigorimeter, or self-constructed instruments. Furthermore, a VAS for measuring dystonia was used in one study. Coordination was evaluated in one study for lower extremity CRPS by measuring joint timing with electrogoniometers during gait. Other motor disturbances such as tremor and involuntary movement were not specifically measured in this sample of studies.

Sensory disturbances are included in the Bruehl criteria (Table 15.2), but have not been included in previous CRPS criteria. The presence of sensory changes reflects the neuropathic character of the disease. In only 7 studies, sensory testing was performed. Allodynia was determined 5 times, hyperalgesia or hyperesthesia the same number of times. Three of these studies (Harke et al. 2001; Lee et al. 2002; Serpell 2002) appeared after the proposal of research diagnostic criteria for CRPS by Bruehl et al. (1999).

FUNCTIONING

Only a small number of studies performed measurements of patients' functioning. Concepts measured

Table 15.4 Parameters and measurement instruments in CRPS

Study	N	Concepts measured (instruments used)	Clin. ref. provided
Williamme et al. 1980	10	Global improvement (3-point cat. scale)	None
Chuinard et al. 1981	25	Temperature (IR); Global improvement (3-point cat. scale)	None
Farcot et al. 1981	35	Pain (2-point cat. scale); Blood flow (laser doppler, ice response)	None
Glynn et al. 1981	28	Pain (VAS); Temperature (thermistor); Blood flow (plethysmography, ice response); Hyperhydrosis (cobald blue sweat test)	Partial
Kozin et al. 1981	55	Pain (4-point cat. scale); Edema (ring size); Bone mineralization (radiography, scintigraphy); Grip strength (n.s.)	Partial
Taoussanis 1981	126	Pain (3-point cat. scale); Edema (3-point cat. scale); Bone mineralization (n.s.)	None
Bruxelle J & Menkes CJ. 1982	9	Blood flow (bloodpressure); Global improvement (cat. scale)	None
Christensen et al. 1982	23	Global improvement (20-point cat. scale)	None
Delcambre et al. 1982	91	Global improvement (4-point cat. scale)	None
Friez et al. 1982	55	Pain (NRS); ROM (duration limitation); Global improvement (duration recovery); Vasomotor change (duration recovery)	None
Nedjar C, Ficat C. 1982	43	Pain (4-point cat. scale); Edema (n.s.); ROM (n.s.); Global improvement (4-point cat. scale)	None
Perrigot et al. 1982	90	Global improvement (3-point cat. scale)	None
Bonelli et al. 1983	19	Pain (VAS); Allodynia (2-point cat. scale); Edema (4-point cat. scale); Temperature (skin probe); ROM (4-point cat. scale); Hyperalgesia (2-point cat. scale); Thropic change (4-point cat. scale); Blood flow (plethysmography)	Partial
Cherot A, Amor B. 1983	93	Pain (VAS); Edema (3-point cat. scale); Global improvement (2-point cat. scale)	None
Driessen et al. 1983	20	Pain (VAS); Edema (circumference); Hyperesthesia, hyperalgesia (pinprick); Atrophy of skin, nails, hair (cat. scale); Bone mineralization (radiography); Global improvement (4-point cat. scale)	None
Poplawski et al. 1983	126	Pain (3-point cat. scale); AROM (3-point cat. scale); Bone mineralization (radiography)	None
Bounameaux et al. 1984	9	Pain (NRS); ROM (4-point cat. scale); Temperature (thermometer probe); Blood flow (plethysmography)	None
Prough et al. 1985	31	Pain (duration); Blood flow (cold stress test); Global improvement (3-point scale)	None
Reginster JY, Franchimont P. 1985	8	Side effects	None
Gobelet et al. 1986	24	Pain (n.s.); Edema (n.s.); ROM (n.s.); Fitness for work (3-point cat. scale)	None
Horton & Gerster 1986	25	No clear description	None
Mayer et al. 1986	15	Global improvement (3-point cat. scale)	None
Goris et al. 1987	21	AROM (n.s.); Global improvement (2-point cat. scale)	None

(Continued)

Table 15.4 Parameters and measurement instruments in CRPS—Cont'd

Study	N	Concepts measured (instruments used)	Clin. ref. provided
Nuti et al. 1987	12	Pain (4-point cat. scale); Bone mineralization (scintigraphy); Blood and urine analysis	Partial
Rico et al. 1987	26	Bone mineralization (scintigraphy)	Yes
Kettler RE, Abram SE. 1988	6	Pain (VAS, duration relief); Temperature (temperature probe); Blood pressure; Medication use; Side effects	None
Vattimo et al. 1988	8	Bone mineralization (scintigraphy); Blood flow (scintigraphy)	None
Hanna MH, Peat SJ. 1989	16	Pain (VRS); Blood pressure; Side effects	None
Jeandel et al. 1989	25	Pain (VAS); ROM (cat. scale); Global improvement (4-point cat. scale)	None
Reiestadt et al. 1989	7	Pain (VAS, VRS)	None
Rocco et al. 1989	12	Pain (VAS, NRS, VRS); Temperature (electronic thermometer)	None
Blanchard et al. 1990	21	Pain (VAS, duration relief); Blood pressure	None
Eulry et al. 1990	199	Pain (VAS); Bone mineralization (scintigraphy); Global improvement (Guidel. Fr. Rheum. A.)	Yes
Farcot et al. 1990	81	Pain (NRS); Edema (circumference); AROM (finger opposition, n.s.); Disability (hand function)	Partial
Bickerstaff DR, Kanis JA. 1991	40	Pain (dolorimetry, 2-point cat. scale); ROM (2-point cat. scale); Edema (water displacement, 2-point cat. scale); Grip strength (own instrument); Vasomotor change (2-point cat. scale)	Partial
Eulry et al. 1991	103	Pain (VAS); Global improvement (Guidel. Fr. Rheum. A.)	Yes
Kissling et al. 1991	18	Disability (cat. scale); No clear description	Partial
Riou et al. 1991	91	No clear description	None
Gobelet et al. 1992	66	Pain (NRS); Edema (4-point cat. scale); ROM (4-point cat. scale); Fitness for work (4-point cat. scale); Side effects	Partial
Hord et al. 1992	12	Pain (VAS); Temperature (skin thermometer)	None
Sawicki et al. 1992	12	Blood analysis	Yes
Fialka et al. 1993	14	Pain (VAS)	None
Field et al. 1993a	20	Pain (dolorimetry); Edema (arthrocyrcameter); AROM (goniometer); Global improvement (VAS); Grip strength (dynamometer); Vasomotor change (questionnaire)	Yes
Field et al. 1993b	17	Pain (dolorimetry); Edema (arthrocyrcameter); Temperature (thermograph); AROM (goniometer); Grip strength (dynamometer)	Partial
Glynn C, Casale R. 1993	6	Pain (VAS, 2-point cat. scale); Sympathetic function (IGR/SSR); Blood flow (plethysmography)	None
Langendijk et al. 1993	37	Pain (VAS)	None
Mundun et al. 1993	14	Bone mineralization (scintigraphy); Blood analysis	Partial
Rauck et al. 1993	26	Pain (VAS, MPQ)	None
Ahn et al. 1994	9	Global improvement (2-point cat. scale)	None
Bonezzi et al. 1994	100	Pain (NRS); Skin color (tele-thermography); Side effects	None

Table 15.4 Parameters and measurement instruments in CRPS—Cont'd

Study	N	Concepts measured (instruments used)	Clin. ref. provided
Braus et al. 1994	36	Composite score (SHS criteria for pain, edema and ROM)	Yes
Chiase et al. 1994	195	Pain (VAS); Edema (circumference); AROM (opposition fingers); Hyperhydrosis (cat. scale); Global improvement (2-point cat. scale)	None
Geertzen et al. 1994	26	Pain (VAS); Color (3-point cat. scale); Edema (3-point cat. scale); AROM (opposition fingers); Disability (VAS); Psychology (Dutch Personality Q., SCL-90, State Trait Anxiety Inv., Life Evants Q.)	None
Verdugo et al. 1994	100	Pain (NRS); Hyperalgesia (QST)	None
Connelly et al. 1995	61	Pain (duration relief); Global improvement (2-point cat. scale)	None
Dielissen et al. 1995	28	Pain (cat. scale); Temperature (cat. scale); ROM (cat. scale)	None
Gschwind et al. 1995	71	Pain (NRS); Color (tele-thermography); Edema (cat. scale); ROM (cat. scale)	None
Jadad et al. 1995	9	Pain (VAS, NRS, Oxford Pain Chart); Global improvement (5-point cat. scale)	Partial
Maillefert et al. 1995	11	Pain (VAS); Global improvement (4-point cat. scale)	None
Ramamurthy S, Hoffman J. 1995	60	Pain (MPQ); Temperature (n.s.); AROM (n.s.); Blood pressure; Global improvement (10-point cat. scale); Blood & urine analysis	None
Grundberg et al. 1996	39	ROM (n.s.); Grip strength (n.s.)	None
Hamamci et al. 1996	41	Pain (VAS); Edema (4-point cat. scale); AROM (goniometer)	None
Hassenbusch et al. 1996	30	Pain (VRS); Thropic change (cat. scale); Medication use; Disability (general activity, 6-point cat. scale); Motor change (cat. scale); Vasomotor change (cat. scale); Global improvement (cat. scale)	None
Kaplan et al. 1996	53	Pain (cat. scale); Global improvement (cat. scale)	None
Zuurmond et al. 1996	32	Pain (VAS); Global improvement (5-point scale)	Partial
Adami et al. 1997	20	Pain (VAS); Edema (circumference); ROM (4-point cat. scale); Bone mineralization (radiography)	None
Cortet et al. 1997	23	Pain (VAS, VRS); Global improvement (4-point cat. scale)	None
Laroche et al. 1997	72	Global improvement (5-point cat. scale)	None
Muizelaar et al. 1997	59	Pain (cat. scale); ROM (cat. scale); Medication use; Fitness for work	None
Calvillo et al. 1998	36	Pain (VAS); Medication use; HRQL (n.s.)	None
Kumar et al. 1998	12	Pain (VAS, MPQ)	None
Malik et al. 1998	5	Pain (VAS); Temperature (skin tapes); Grip strength (dynamometer)	None
Muramatsu et al. 1998	17	Pain (cat. scale); Color (cat. scale); Edema (cat. scale); AROM (cat. scale)	Partial
Price et al. 1998	7	Pain (VAS); Allodynia (Von Frey monofilaments, cotton wool)	Yes
Robbins et al. 1998	22	Pain (VRS)	None

(Continued)

Table 15.4 Parameters and measurement instruments in CRPS—Cont'd

Study	N	Concepts measured (instruments used)	Clin. ref. provided
Zyluk 1998	36	Pain (2-point cat. scale); Color (2-point cat. scale); Edema (2-point cat. scale); Temperature (2-point cat. scale); ROM (2-point cat. scale); Hyperhydrosis (2-point cat. scale)	None
Hennart et al. 1999	32	Pain (cat. scale); Edema (cat. scale); ROM (cat. scale); Blood flow (cat. scale)	None
Korpan et al. 1999	14	Pain (VAS); Edema (electro optical); Temperature (IR); AROM (goniometer); Disability (VAS)	Partial
Linchitz RM, Raheb JC. 1999	5	Pain (VAS); Side effects	None
Maillefert et al. 1999	35	Pain (VAS); Global improvement (cat. scale)	None
Rovetta et al. 1999	14	Pain (VAS); AROM (goniometer, inclinometer)	None
Sherry et al. 1999	103	Pain (VAS, VRS); Color (cat. scale); Temperature (cat. scale); Hyperhydrosis (cat. scale)	None
Smeets et al. 1999	28	Global severity, global improvement (5-point scale); HRQL (cat. scales)	None
Wu et al. 1999	26	Pain (VAS); Color (cat. scale); Temperature (thermistor); AROM (cat. scale); Atrophy muscle (cat. scale); Psychology (Beck Depr. Inv., Cong.-Som. Anxiety Q.); Medication use	Partial
Zollinger et al. 1999	123	Occurrence CRPS (Veldman's criteria)	None
Azad et al. 2000	9	Pain (VAS); Grip strength (vigorimeter); Side effects	None
Bannink et al. 2000	15	Pain (VRS); Edema (water displacement); Temperature (IR); Disability (QRSD & WSQ); HRQL (COOP/WONCA, SF-36, EuroQol)	None
Kemler et al. 2000	36	Pain (VAS, MPQ); AROM (goniometer); Disability (Jebsen-Taylor test, foot function test); Global improvement (6-point cat. scale); HRQL (NHP, EuroQol, SIP); Psychology (SR Depress. Scale); side effects	Yes
Oerlemans et al. 2000	135	Pain (VAS, MPQ); Edema (water displacement); Temperature (IR); AROM (goniometer); Compound score (ISS); Disability (Radboud dexterity test, RSQ, Greentest); HRQL (SIP)	Yes
Uher et al. 2000	35	Pain (VRS); Edema (circumference); Temperature (IR); AROM (goniometer); Bone mineralization (radiography, scintigraphy)	Partial
Van Hilten et al. 2000	7	Motor problems (VAS-dystonia); Side effects	None
Varenna et al. 2000	32	Pain (VAS); Edema (4-point cat. scale); Global improvement (efficacy verbal scale); Global severity (Clin. Global Ass. Scale); Blood and urine analyses	Partial
Wallace et al. 2000	16	Pain (VAS); Allodynia (Von Frey monofilaments); Hyperalgesia (QST); Side effects	Partial
Harke et al. 2001	7	Pain (NRS); Blood analysis, side effects	None
Kubalek et al. 2001	29	Pain (2-point cat. scale); Disability (2-point cat. scale)	None
Kondo et al. 2001	152	Edema (circumference); Occurrence CRPS (SHS-criteria)	None
Marx et al. 2001	10	Vasomotor change (questionnaire); HRQL (SF-36)	Yes
Cazeneuve et al. 2002	195	Bone mineralization (radiography, scintigraphy)	None

Table 15.4 Parameters and measurement instruments in CRPS—Cont'd

Study	N	Concepts measured (instruments used)	Clin. ref. provided
Lee et al. 2002	28	Pain (VAS, VRS); Allodynia (11-point cat. scale); Disability (standardized gait analysis and walking stairs); HRQL (SF-36); Psychology (Rev. Ch. Man. Anxiety Score, Child Depress. Inv., Child Health Q.)	Partial
Livingstone JA, Atkins RM. 2002	57	Pain (VRS); Edema (water displacement); Grip strength (dynamometer)	Yes
Serpell 2002	85	Allodynia (VAS); Hyperalgesia (VAS); Global improvement (Clin. and Pat. Global Impr. Change)	Partial
Perez et al. 2003	145	Pain (VAS, MPQ); Edema (water displacement); Temperature (IR); AROM (goniometer); Compound score (ISS); Disability (RSQ, Greentest, WSQ and QRSD); HRQL (COOP/WONCA, SF-36, EuroQol); Side effects	Yes

Column "N" indicates number of patients studied. Column "Concepts measured" indicates parameters studied, the measurement instrument put between parentheses; "n.s." = not stated; "Clin. ref. provided" indicates whether the study provided information on or references to the validation of the measurement instruments used.

included ADL skills (6 studies), hand or foot function (7 studies), general activity assessment (3 studies), fitness for work (3 studies) and functional impairment (VAS, one study). ADL skills were assessed by the Radboud Skills Questionnaire in 2 studies, the Questionnaire Rising and Sitting Down and Walking Stairs Questionnaire in two studies, and a VAS for daily activities in one study. One study reported to use a standardized walking stairs observational test. Hand function was evaluated by means of a hand function test in 4 studies, 3 of which used a standardized dexterity test (Greentest, Jebsen-Taylor, Radboud dexterity test). One standardized foot function test was described in this study sample. General activity was assessed on 2- to 6-point categorical scales. Likewise, for measurement of working capacity 3- or 4-point scales were used.

PARTICIPATION

With regard to patients' participation, health-related quality of life was assessed using the COOP/WONCA charts (2 studies), the Short Form 36 (SF-36, 4 studies), the Euroqol (2 studies), the Sickness Impact Profile (SIP, 2 studies) and Nottingham Health Profile (NHP, one study). One study reported to have used a categorical scale based on the SIP.

A remaining category, which evaluated personal factors in CRPS, consists of studies evaluating side effects (10 studies), usually in an unspecified manner. Psychological assessment was performed in 5 studies, using the Self Rating Depression Scale, the Child Health Questionnaire, Child Depression Inventory, the Dutch Personality Questionnaire, the Beck Depression Inventory, the Cognitive-somatic Anxiety

Questionnaire, the Social Life Events Questionnaire, and the Symptoms Check List-90. Laboratory evaluation of blood and urine was performed for treatment guidance in 5 studies. Three studies evaluated the occurrence of CRPS, using Veldman's and SHS criteria as primary outcome measures.

WHICH MEASUREMENT INSTRUMENTS HAVE BEEN EVALUATED?

As was shown in the previous paragraph, a large variety of measurement instruments have been used to assess outcomes of interventions in CRPS I research. However, the number of measurement instruments which have been evaluated for the use in CRPS-related research is limited. Possible explanations of this finding are that the evaluation of clinimetric aspects of various instruments has been performed in other conditions than CRPS, but also that there is limited interest for psychometric research compared to intervention-based research. Furthermore, publication and editorial bias, limiting the amount of published information, could lead to an underestimation of the information about the quality of measurement instruments. In this section, measurement instruments for which validity and/or reliability have been assessed for CRPS patients will be described.

IMPAIRMENTS

In this domain, instruments for measurement of pain, sensory abnormalities, temperature, volume differences, limitations in range of motion and motor disturbances were assessed.

Pain

For measurement of *pain*, the VAS, MPQ, Neuropathic Pain Scale, a dolorimeter and an algometer have been evaluated. The VAS is a reliable and valid instrument for measuring pain intensity (Carlsson 1983; Davidoff et al. 1988), given that patients are well instructed in the use. In a study performed in our institution (Perez et al. 2003b), the reliability of current pain VAS was evaluated in lower extremity CRPS I patients. Patients filled out two subsequent (0–100 cm) VAS scores for current pain. In 40 patients, no significant differences were found between both scores (Independent samples t test: $p = 0.871$). Subsequently, a VAS for pain during or after exercise based on the preceding few days was filled out. The VAS during exercise was significantly higher than that for current pain (mean (SD) respectively 79.1 (21.5) mm and 20.9 (20.4) mm; independent samples t test: $p < 0.001$), which is in accordance with the assumption that pain increases with exercise in CRPS I patients (Veldman et al. 1993). Oerlemans et al. (1998) have found comparable results for upper extremity CRPS I patients (momentary pain: mean (SD) 32 (27) mm; pain during exercise: 73 (22) mm). Furthermore, in a study including 54 CRPS I patients, Forouzanfar et al. (2002) found a high correlation ($r = 0.81$–095) and agreement (mean difference (SD) −0.13 (.067) to 0.03 (0.92)) for single measurement of recalled VAS-pain over the previous week compared to repeated measurement of VAS-pain 3 times daily during that same week.

The diagnostic value of the VAS as a single indicator has been evaluated by Perez et al. (2001). The best combination of sensitivity (SE) and specificity (SP) (SE + SP = 156) for diagnosing CRPS I was found at a cut off value of 3 cm on a 10 cm scale.

The McGill Pain Questionnaire (MPQ) (Melzack 1975) is considered to be a reliable and valid tool to measure pain in a variety of complaints (Cohen et al. 1989; Lowe et al. 1991; Mognini et al. 2000). Regarding the MPQ expressed as the Number of Words Chosen total (NWC-t), average word scores reported in CRPS I literature vary from 8 to 15. In a study performed in our institution (Perez et al. 2003b), we found a mean score of 14.6 (SD: 4.0) words for lower extremity CRPS I, which is in agreement with the results found by Oerlemans et al. (1998) (mean: 15 (SD: 9) words) in an upper extremity CRPS I patient sample. For diagnostic evaluation, the McGill as a single parameter showed a high value for the combination of sensitivity and specificity (SE + SP = 141) at a cut off value of 6 words (Perez et al. 2001). The MPQ has been translated and validated for different languages (see also Chapter 5).

Galer and Jensen (1997) evaluated the Neuropathic Pain Scale (NPS; see Chapter 5 for patients with neuropathic pain, including a sample of 69 CRPS patients). The scale consists of 10 descriptors or items, describing "intense," "sharp," "hot," "dull," "cold," "sensitive," "itchy," "deep" and "surface" pain. Low correlation coefficients between items were found ($r = 0.05$–0.68), indicating minimal overlap. Four items ("sharp," "cold," "sensitive" and "itchy") out of 10 NPS descriptors were capable of discriminating significantly between diagnostic groups, and all items appear to be sensitive to treatment effects.

A dolorimeter, an instrument for measuring pressure pain or tenderness, was evaluated by Atkins et al. (1989) with respect to reproducibility and construct validity in 12 CRPS and 12 healthy controls. They found the reproducibility as expressed by the coefficient of variation to be moderate, and higher on the affected than on the unaffected side for the CRPS sample. No information with respect to reproducibility in healthy subjects was provided. The dolorimetry values were lower for the affected side than for the unaffected side in CRPS I patients. This difference was not found in healthy subjects. However, consistent and significant differences were found between different sites in the hand for healthy subjects. Also, the construction of the dolorimeter does not seem to allow for pressure exertion by the researchers in a reliable fashion.

Bryan et al. (1991) have assessed the use of a device similar to the dolorimeter for diagnostic purposes in 33 CRPS patients. The algometer, a rubber-tipped clamp with which pressure can be exhibited in a controlled fashion, was found to distinguish between the impaired and unimpaired side, showing higher pressure-pain thresholds on the unaffected side (ratio affected:unaffected = 0.70–0.95). However, no information concerning the actual diagnostic value was presented, and the algometer was reported to be accurate in only 73% in lower limb CRPS.

Sensory abnormalities

Repeatability and sensitivity levels of thermal thresholds for assessment of *sensory abnormalities* were studied by Kemler et al. (2000b). With an electronic heat or cold conductor, warm and cold detection thresholds were measured in 53 CRPS patients, using either a method of level (MLE) or method of limit (MLI) measurement protocol. MLE uses predetermined temperature levels and stimulus duration; the MLI exposes a subject to a stimulus of increasing temperature, measuring the reaction time to perceived onset of the temperature stimulus. Sensitivity was found to be equal for both measurement protocols; no significant differences were found in prevalence of abnormality (warm or cold hypoesthesia) detected by MLE of MLI protocol. However, limited levels of agreement were found between both measurement protocols (mean detection differences: warm perception 1.0–2.3°C; cold perception 0.4–3.1°C), and the coefficients of repeatability (CR) were significantly better for MLE (range 1.0–2.0) than for MLI (range 1.7–5.0) for both sensations in upper extremity CRPS. These findings, together with the possible occurrence of reaction time artifacts for MLI, led the authors to propose MLE as the preferred method for measuring temperature threshold for upper extremity CRPS I. No preference was proposed for these measurements for lower extremity CRPS.

Temperature abnormalities

The measurement qualities of instruments measuring *temperature* abnormalities were evaluated for infrared thermography (IR). For CRPS I patients, mean difference ranges between affected and unaffected extremities up to 2.9°C have been reported (Wasner et al. 1999). Oerlemans et al. (1999a) established a normal mean difference between the dorsal aspects of both hands of 0.30°C for healthy subjects using tympanic IR. This range is in agreement with findings by Bruehl et al. (1996), who found a difference of at least 0.4°C to distinguish between CRPS I and non-CRPS I in 63% of cases. Our findings (Perez et al. 2001), showing highest values for sensitivity and specificity combined at the same cut off point of 0.4°C, underline Bruehl's data. Also, Wasner et al. (2002) found skin temperature differences during exercise to distinguish adequately between CRPS, healthy subjects and other extremity pain syndromes with a high sensitivity (SE = 76%) and specificity (SP = 93%). However, sensitivity under resting conditions was found to be poor (SE = 32%). Oerlemans et al. (1999c) found no significant correlation between IR and subjective assessment of temperature by the patient, which they ascribed to possible altered perception by the patient due to CRPS. Although no data with respect to the reliability of temperature measurements for CRPS can be found, data regarding unimpaired subjects, the stability of the measurement instrument applied, and the diagnostic properties of this type of measurement suggest IR to be an adequate tool for assessment of temperature differences in CRPS.

Volume differences

The merits of *volume* difference measurements, using water displacement volumeters, was evaluated in two studies. In both studies, the goal of the study was to assess the validity of physicians' judgments compared to measurement by water displacement volumeters. In a study with 131 upper extremity CRPS I patients, Oerlemans et al. (1999b) found agreement between objective and subjective assessments, where low volume differences were found for patients reported by the physician to have no edema (mean 17 ml), and higher values for those patients reported to have edema (mean 37 ml). Perez et al. (2005), in 131 CRPS I outpatients, found comparable results (edema: mean 46.4 ml; absent volume differences 18.8 ml). However, for those patients reported by the physician to have

smaller volumes of the affected extremity, on average we found the affected extremity to be more voluminous than the unimpaired extremity (mean 12.7 ml). Furthermore, physicians were unable to adequately judge the severity of volume differences on a 4-point scale.

Though this lack of agreement provides little information with respect to the validity of water displacement volumeters, it does stress the necessity for valid volume measurement of CRPS, since subjective measurement does not correspond with objective findings.

In a small sample with healthy subjects, we found the variability between 3 subsequent volumetric measurements to be low (coefficient of variation 0.66–1.20%), indicating good test–retest reliability (Perez et al. 2003a). Nevertheless, we found relatively low sensitivity and specificity values of volumetric measurement by water displacement (SE + SP = 119) when used as a single parameter to diagnose CRPS I (Perez et al. 2001).

Active range of motion

Difference in *active range of motion* (AROM) was assessed by Geertzen et al. (1998c) using hand held goniometers and inclinometers. They investigated the interrater reliability and the sensitivity of a measurement by calculating the smallest detectable difference (SDD) for different joint measurements in 29 CRPS patients. Geertzen et al. found SDDs to range from 9.6 degrees (elbow flexion) to 28.7 degrees (shoulder external rotation) for the affected extremity. The interobserver agreement ranged from moderate to very good ($r = 0.55$–0.96) for the affected side. The most important sources of variation were observer and patient-observer interaction which, they concluded, could be countered by using a rigid measurement protocol as well as extensive training in the use of the measurement instruments or reducing the number of observers.

Our study showed a high combination of sensitivity and specificity (SE + SP = 147) for diagnosing CRPS using hand held goniometers as a single diagnostic parameter (Perez et al. 2001).

Motor disturbances

Instruments for measuring *motor disturbances* have been evaluated in 3 studies. Grip strength was evaluated by Geertzen et al. (1998b) and Perez et al. (2005). Geertzen et al. found good to very good inter observer correlations ($r = 0.78$–0.98) for measurement of full grip, pinch grip and three point grip using hand held dynamometers in 29 CRPS patients. On average, they found lower values for the affected side (range 55.9–84.2 N) compared to the unaffected side (range 66.7–123.1 N). However, the SDDs were considerable (range affected: 26.9–70.5 N) relative to the average grip strength values found. As for range of motion measurements, observer and patient–observer variations, as well as a random error, were found to be the major sources of variation. In our study (Perez et al. 2005), the relationships between grip strength, the severity of pain and AROM were evaluated in patients with CRPS I of one upper extremity participating in an RCT. At different time points, highest correlations were found between grip strength and AROM (r range 0.529–0.772), followed by grip strength and VAS-pain (r range 0.39–0.59) and grip strength and McGill-NWCT (r range 0.24–0.41) respectively, which shows that AROM appears to have a stronger relationship with GRS than pain, and may have a larger influence on grip strength than pain, in these CRPS I patients.

Myometers, measuring strength of foot dorsiflexors and plantarflexors, were evaluated by Kemler et al. (2000c) in 20 CRPS I patients. These tests correlated well with a foot function test (see below), but poor to moderately with other performance tests (NHP, SIP, Timed Up and Go, Three Minute Walk; $r = -0.04$ to 0.43).

Compound scores

A distinct category for evaluation at impairment level is formed by *Compound Scores*, including the Impairment level Sum Score (ISS). The ISS is an adaptation of an evaluation protocol proposed by Davidoff et al. (1998), which included (1) measurement of joint pain by palpation (4-point scale), (2) pain by VAS and MPQ, (3) volumetric measurement by water displacement, (4) measurement of active range of motion by goniometer and finger-hand distance, and (5) skin temperature measurement, for which no instrument was described. With 17 CRPS patients, the authors found significant but moderate correlations between VAS and joint pain, MPQ, AROM, and limb volume ($r = 0.16$–0.51). Furthermore, a significant but fair correlation was found between the MPQ and AROM ($r = 0.15$), but no correlation was found between skin temperature and other indices.

Oerlemans et al. (1998) adapted Davidoff's measurements for use in upper extremity CRPS I patients. The ISS measures the concepts pain (VAS and McGill), temperature (IR thermography), volume (water displacement volumeters) and AROM (universal goniometers), which are converted into a compound score ranging from 5 to 50 (50 indicating the highest impairment). Oerlemans et al. assessed the internal consistency, concurrent validity and responsiveness of the ISS in 45 upper extremity CRPS patients, and found the internal consistency to be moderate (Cronbach's alpha $= 0.42$), a good concurrent validity as expressed by the correlation between the physician's grading of CRPS and the ISS (3-point categorical scale) ($r = 0.69$–0.74), and adequate responsiveness when changes of the ISS were compared to overt decrease of signs and symptoms as established by the physician. The moderate internal consistency of the ISS was explained by the heterogeneous character of the score. The ISS was

subsequently adapted for use in lower extremity CRPS (Perez et al. 2003a), and was tested with respect to the concurrent validity and responsiveness in 18 lower extremity CRPS patients. The concurrent validity proved to be adequate, as the magnitude of the ISS corresponded with the severity of CRPS according to the physician (4-point categorical scale). Also, the responsiveness of the ISS was addressed by comparing the change in the ISS with the change in the complaint as reported by the patients. For patients reporting amelioration, a decrease of the ISS was observed (mean difference -6.8 points), and for patients reporting deterioration an increase of the ISS was found (mean $+3.8$ points). Difference values of the ISS were close to zero (mean -0.9) for patients reporting no change, which indicated adequate responsiveness. However, a shortcoming of the ISS is that it cannot be used properly in patients with an impaired contralateral extremity, as most of the constituting indices of the ISS are measured in comparison to the contralateral limb.

Diagnostic criteria

Besides playing a vital role in defining the research population addressed in a particular study, diagnostic criteria for CRPS I have been used as outcome measures for determining treatment effect in several studies (Zollinger et al. 1999; Kondo et al. 2001). The properties of Veldman's and the IASP's and Bruehl's criteria have been subject to clinimetric testing. Veldman's diagnostic criteria (see Table 15.2) have been evaluated with respect to the inter-rater reliability of this diagnosis and the constituting symptoms for making the diagnosis (Perez et al. 2002a). The inter-rater reliability was evaluated in 37 outpatients presumed to have CRPS I by 3 observers: 1 consultant anesthesiologist and 2 resident anesthesiologists. The inter-rater reliability for diagnosing CRPS I was good for the majority of observer combinations. The percentage of agreement (Po) for the absence or presence of CRPS I was good (88–100%). Cohen's kappa values ranged from 0.60 to 0.86. The agreement for the mean symptom score ranged from 70.2 to 88.6%; kappa values for individual symptoms were lower and showed more variation. However, the inter-rater reliability for the assessment of the severity of CRPS (Po $= 55$–63%; kappa $= 0.38$–0.42) and its symptoms (Po $= 43.6$–54%) was found to be poor, indicating the necessity for adequate measurement instruments.

The IASP's diagnostic criteria formulated in 1994 (Stanton-Hicks et al. 1995) were evaluated with respect to their diagnostic properties by Bruehl et al. (1999). This study, including 117 CRPS patients, revealed that the criteria discriminated well between CRPS and non-CRPS neuropathic pain patients ($n = 34$). However, the specificity of these diagnostic criteria was low, and a positive diagnosis of CRPS I was likely to be correct in just 40% of cases. Based on these findings, modifications were suggested, adding a decision rule to the criteria, requiring at least two (observed) signs and four (reported) symptoms (see Table 15.2). These modifications increased the sensitivity to 83% and the specificity to 88%.

Bruehl's adaptations of the IASP criteria were recently tested by van de Vusse et al. (2003). In this study, 25 chronic CRPS patients were examined by six physicians (3 anesthesiologists, 2 surgeons and one neurologist). According to the researchers, physicians' agreement of individual signs and symptoms varied greatly (Po = 72–97%; kappa = 0.21–0.86). However, agreement with respect to the final diagnosis of CRPS was poor (kappa = 0.20). Applying the IASP criteria, kappa values were slightly higher (kappa = 0.29) and results were fair when Bruehl's criteria were used (kappa = 0.38). Use of Bruehl's criteria, however, resulted in markedly lower frequency of CRPS compared to physicians' own diagnosis (43 and 73% respectively). The latter is in agreement with our data that showed partial agreement between Veldman's and Bruehl's criteria (Po = 69%) in 44 outpatients with presumed CRPS (Perez et al. 2000). In this sample, occurrence of CRPS using Veldman's criteria was 57%, and 34% for Bruehl's criteria.

FUNCTIONING

Assessment of instruments for evaluation of functions has been performed in 4 studies, 2 of which evaluated disability measurement for the upper extremity (Oerlemans et al. 2000a; Schasfoort et al. 2002), and 2 for the lower (Kemler et al. 2000c; Perez et al. 2002b).

Radboud Skills Questionnaire

The inter-observer and test–retest reliability of the Radboud Skills Questionnaire (RSQ) for upper extremity skills was measured in 54 CRPS I patients by Oerlemans et al. (2000a). The test–retest reliability was good, showing low coefficients of variation (median = 2.3–4.5%). The median inter-observer variability proved to be higher, but was again adequate (median 6.6%). Moderate to good inter-questionnaire agreements were found between the RSQ and the Disabilities of Arm Shoulder and Hand Questionnaire (DASH) (Veehof et al. 2002) (r = 0.74), and the Sickness Impact Profile (SIP) (Bruin et al. 1992) (r = 0.48–0.53) by Schasfoort et al. (2002).

Upper Limb Activity Monitor

The Upper Limb Activity Monitor (ULAM) (Schasfoort et al. 2002) is proposed as a reliable measurement instrument for upper extremity activity limitations. The ULAM, which is in essence an accelerometer, is used to measure the amount of activity exhibited by a patient during the day. Using video scores as a reference, the ULAM data were found to be in agreement with rehabilitation-related activity profiles. Furthermore,

a comparison was made between 10 chronic CRPS patients and 10 healthy controls, in which the ULAM was able to distinguish between healthy and impaired subjects, although less so during standing and sitting. Correlations between the ULAM and skills questionnaires were moderate (RSQ: 0.41–0.48; DASH: 0.53–0.57).

Walking Stairs Questionnaire and Questionnaire Rising and Sitting Down

For the lower extremity, the Walking Stairs Questionnaire (WSQ) and the Questionnaire Rising and Sitting Down (QRSD) were tested in 21 CRPS I patients (Perez et al. 2002b). The test–retest reliability for the administration of the questionnaires was fair to good for all scales of both questionnaires. Correlation coefficients ranged from 0.79 to 0.90 for the WSQ, and 0.85 and 0.89 for the QRSD, which were significant for all categories. The intra class correlations (ICC) were good for all categories (range WSQ: 0.78–0.87; QRSD: 0.84–0.87). For patients reporting amelioration of their complaints, positive values were found between subsequent measurements (range 0–0.97), close to zero for patients reporting no changes (range −0.03 to 0.50) and predominantly negative for those reporting worsening of the complaints (range −2.00 to 0.18).

Foot Function Test Board

The Foot Function Test Board (FFT) is another skills instrument constructed to be used in CRPS I patients. Kemler et al. (2000c) compared this test between 86 healthy subjects and 20 CRPS I patients. High (r = 0.85–0.99) inter- and intra-rater reliability were found for the healthy sample. The test is able to distinguish between healthy and CRPS patients (p < 0.001), is applicable for non-ambulant patients as well as ambulant patients, and was able to distinguish between crutch dependent and non-crutch dependent patients (p < 0.001). Correlations between the FFT and other performance tests (NHP, SIP, Timed Up and Go, Three Minute Walk) were, however, predominantly poor (r = 0.02–0.30), except for the correlation with more impairment oriented myometers (r = 0.73–0.77).

PARTICIPATION

For participation, the SIP (de Bruin et al. 1992), NHP (Erdman et al. 1993), the SF-36 (Brazier 1993), COOP/WONCA (van Weel 1993) and Euroqol (EuroQol-group 1990) have been evaluated for use in CRPS patients. Kemler et al. (2000d) evaluated the use of the SIP, the NHP and the EuroQol in a sample of 54 CRPS patients. Comparisons were made with norm values reported in literature, and whether or not these HRQL instruments were able to discriminate between subgroups of patients. Kemler et al. found the charts to discriminate between CRPS and normative values of healthy subjects and patients with migraine and diabetes, although the values were not statistically compared. Furthermore, the NHP and EuroQol were found to adequately assess HRQL for both upper and lower extremity CRPS, whereas the SIP provided better results for patients with lower extremity CRPS. Hoeksema et al. (2003) showed that the SF-36, COOP/WONCA and EuroQol discriminated equally well compared to normative values of healthy and migraine patients reported in literature. Except for the sub-items Overall Health (COOP/WONCA) and Anxiety/Depression (EuroQol), significant differences (all $p < 0.001$) were found between a sample of 145 CRPS patients and normative values derived from a sample of 575 subjects (Essink-bot et al. 1997). Influence of gender, affected extremity (upper or lower) and duration of

CRPS were found, but the influence of these prognostic factors was not consistent between the HRQL measurements.

PROPOSAL FOR MEASUREMENT INSTRUMENTS

IMPAIRMENT LEVEL

From previous paragraphs it has become clear that many concepts and many outcome measures have been used in evaluating treatment effects. However, considering the occurrence of various signs (see Table 15.5) as described by Veldman et al. (1993), ranking of more or less frequently occurring signs might be helpful in choosing measurement instruments for CRPS. In addition, in the most recently proposed diagnostic criteria (Table 15.2) not all signs have been included. Symptoms considered to be cardinal features of CRPS by previous authors do not presently play a decisive role in the diagnostic process.

Since no laboratory test or combination of tests assesses the presence of CRPS, it is not possible to quantify the severity of CRPS on the basis of such a test. Therefore, only signs can be used as parameters to quantify changes in CRPS I. Based on the frequency of signs occurring in CRPS (Table 15.5), measurement instruments should focus on the evaluation of pain, volume and temperature differences, color changes, limitations in (active) range of motion and paresis. However, the research diagnostic criteria proposed by Bruehl et al. (1999) include the assessment of sensory disturbances such as hyperesthesia, allodynia and hyperalgesia, sudomotor and trophic dysfunction as well. One could argue that in order to be in line with internationally accepted diagnostic criteria, these features should be evaluated systematically too. This would lead to the following set of concepts to be measured and proposed measurement instruments.

Pain

Pain is an important parameter in all pain syndromes, but up till now there is no means of objectively measuring its magnitude. Because of this, many measurement instruments have been developed.

Often used pain measures are Visual Analogue Scale (VAS), Verbal Rating Scale (VRS), Numerical Rating Scale (NRS) and McGill Pain Questionnaire (MPQ). The VAS, VRS and NRS are unidimensional and address the intensity of pain; the MPQ is a scale in which the affect of pain can be specified. Other pain intensity measures include picture scales, the Pain-O-Meter (POM) and the Descriptor Differential Scale of Pain Intensity (DDS-I) or Affect (DDS-A) (Gracely and Kwilosz 1988).

All these pain intensity scales are based on self-assessment and are therefore relatively easy to

Table 15.5 Signs and symptoms reported in CRPS

Sign or symptom	Overall incidence (%)
Inflammatory	
Pain	93
Color difference	92
Edema	69
Temperature difference	92
Limited movement	88
Neurologic	
Hyperesthesia	76
Hyperpathy	79
Incoordination	54
Tremor	49
Involuntary movements	36
Muscle spasm	25
Paresis	95
Atrophy	
Skin	40
Nails	27
Muscle	55
Bone	38
Sympathetic	
Hyperhidrosis	47
Changed hair growth	55
Changed nail growth	60

Adapted from Veldman et al. (1993).

administer. They express pain as a (single) number, which allows for numerical treatment. Implicitly, linear behavior of the pain scales is assumed in such a process. This may be true for the VAS, but has not been proved for other pain scales (Price et al. 1994). The relevance hereof that the magnitude of a given pain reduction on e.g. the NRS may be dependent on the initial pain scores has recently been demonstrated in studies of acute pain (Cepeda et al. 2003; Farrar et al. 2003; Forouzanfar et al. 2003).

Taking a pain score deserves some attention. A single pain score at one instant during the day does not accurately reflect the average pain over a whole day. Therefore more than one pain measurement should be taken within a limited period. It seems advisable to perform repeated measurements over several days as proposed by Jensen et al. (1993, 1999). Forouzanfar et al. (2002) have reported comparable results for summary VAS-pain scores in comparison with repeated measurement of pain.

It is still a matter of debate how much a clinically meaningful reduction of pain would be, and whether this is independent of the baseline pain score (Jensen et al. 1993, 1999; Cepeda et al. 2003; Farrar et al. 2003). In general, a pain reduction of about 30% or 2 points on a 10-point scale seems to be a significant pain reduction, though the absolute difference may be dependent on the baseline score (Cepeda et al. 2003).

Another question remains as to how many pain scales should be used. A pain score might be more meaningful when analyzed on two or more different scales, including an intensity and affective scale. Jensen et al. (1993), however, proposed that, for large studies, a single 0–10 scale would suffice. For smaller studies, which is often the case in CRPS research, composite scales are more stable and reliable to detect treatment effects.

Considering the validity and reliability results found in studies evaluating the clinimetric properties of these concepts, and the diagnostic properties of both measurement instruments, the VAS for measurement of pain intensity, and the MPQ for affective aspects of pain, appear to be adequate candidates for evaluation of CRPS I. As an alternative for the assessment of pain type from a neuropathic perspective, the NPS provides a valid measurement instrument.

Vasomotor abnormalities

Skin temperature is easily and noninvasively measured. Both infrared measuring devices and thermistors are often used. Measurements are influenced by room temperature; therefore a standardized environment is preferable. No patient cooperation is needed. Temperature measurements are technically well validated (Oerlemans et al. 1999a). The temperature is assumed to be a good measure for perfusion of an extremity. Though perfusion can be influenced by many factors,

in studies of CRPS it is often used as a measure of sympathetic activity. As a single parameter, temperature differences as measured by an IR thermometer show a high sensitivity and specificity at a cutoff value of $0.4°C$ (Bruehl et al. 1996; Wasner et al. 2002).

Color difference can be noticed by the human eye, but is hard to quantify. Many problems, especially technical ones, arise when measuring the color of an extremity. One has to deal with, among others, light temperature, sensitivity of photosensitive material or light-sensitive cells, nonlinear behavior of film and receptors. To our knowledge, there is no clinical available system to quantify color changes for the study of CRPS.

Edema and sudomotor problems

The volume of an extremity can be measured by a volumeter, which exhibits a high test–retest reliability and a high accuracy in (healthy) subjects (Perez et al. 2003a). The volumeter measures volume displacement of an extremity, which is placed in a fluid-filled container in a standardized way. Volumeters are easy to use and require a minimum of instruction. The measurement of volume is influenced by water and room temperature, but this is of minor importance between 20 and $35°C$ (Oerlemans et al. 1998). Measured volume is also influenced by the way an extremity is placed in the container. This does not seem to be a major problem when placement of the extremity is standardized and only within-subject comparisons are made.

Although change of volume can also be calculated from the change in circumference of an extremity or part of it, this is considered an inaccurate method. Problems occur with the location of measurement, the tightness of the measurement device, and the fact that circumference change is proportional only to the square root of volume changes.

It seems more appropriate, therefore, to use fluid volumeters to measure volume differences in CRPS patients. However, one should take into account that for diagnostic purposes the combined value of sensitivity and specificity of water displacement based volume assessments is rather low, when used as a single parameter to diagnose CRPS.

Sudomotor tests like quantitative sudomotor axon reflex tests, sweat output tests and sympathetic skin response, and vasomotor measurements, the latter usually via temperature measurements, are meant to give an impression of the function of the autonomic nerve fibers in peripheral neuropathies (Dotson 1997). It is also possible to record evoked potentials and to perform microneurography, by which the function of individual nerve fibers of fascicles can be recorded. Although sudomotor features such as the presence of hyperhydrosis have been added as a diagnostic feature in Bruehl's research diagnostic criteria

(Bruehl et al. 1999), actual measurement of this symptom has been limited in CRPS I research. As for the value of measurement instruments for this feature, diagnostic as well as evaluative properties in CRPS have yet to be established.

Motor and throphic abnormalities

The range of motion is usually determined by visual estimation along a goniometer or an inclinometer, although electronic measurement devices have been described as well (Geertzen et al. 1998; Jordan et al. 2001). In this way the active range of motion (AROM), i.e., the angle between maximum active extension and flexion of a joint, can be measured. Although electronic measurement devices can possibly be more accurate, costs involved and complex measurement procedures may limit a broad application of these types of measurement instruments. As universal goniometers are relatively easy to use, and provide direct and easily comprehensible data, this type of measurement provides a good alternative. However, as was described by Geertzen et al. (1998c), a number of factors, such as inter-observer and observer–patient interaction, influence the reliability of goniometric measurements. A rigid measurement protocol, describing positioning of patients, instructions to patients and exact localization of measurement points, is therefore necessary. Using such a rigid protocol, the diagnostic value of goniometric measurement has been proven (Perez et al. 2001).

For motor disturbances, measurement emphasis in CRPS research has been focused on measurement of grip strength. As Geertzen et al. (1998b) pointed out, grip strength measurement with dynamometers is subject to a number of biases. Again, using a rigid measurement protocol could possibly counter these problems. Other motor abnormalities have had less attention. The frequency and amplitude of a tremor can be measured electronically using accelerometers. There are, however, no studies on CRPS using this method. Coordinative disturbances, such as involuntary movements, muscle spasm and paresis, are generally assessed subjectively in the clinical setting. The latter also holds true for measurement of trophic changes. Measurement of growth abnormalities of skin, nails, hair and muscle have been reported descriptively, usually based on physicians' or patients' reports. Whether or not these features will be quantifiable is doubtful.

Sensory abnormalities

Although other sensory abnormalities besides pain frequently occur in CRPS patients, not many efforts have been made to quantify these features in CRPS. Tools for the evaluation of hyper- and hypoesthesia, as well as allodynia and hyperalgesia, are available, usually gathered under the name of quantitative sensory testing (QST). Well known and often performed are the cold or heat (stress) tests and Von Frey monofilament testing, which allow for quantification of the severity of sensory abnormalities. Warm and cold perception thresholds, as well as hot and cold stress limits, can be established with simple measures, such as test tubes filled with hot or cold water, but probably more reliably so with electronic devices. As Kemler et al. (2000b) have shown that thermal thresholds discriminate between affected and unaffected extremities in CRPS with respect to the detection of warm or cold hypoesthesia, this method of QST appears to be valid to assess this sensory feature. Whether or not this measurement method can be used to measure other sensory features, and whether the magnitude of the outcomes corresponds with the severity of the complaints, remains to be studied.

Von Frey monofilaments, also known as the Semmes-Weinstein test, can be used to establish a patient's sensitivity to touch. Presence of hypo- as well as hyperesthesia and allodynia can be quantified using a standardized set of nylon monofilaments and a consistent testing procedure. Although these instruments have been used in CRPS research (Rommel et al. 1999), its clinimetric properties have not been assessed specifically for CRPS. Although Rommel et al. (2000) found Von Frey testing to discriminate between CRPS patients with or without generalized sensory deficits, validity and reliability features of this test have yet to be established in CRPS I. Implications for diagnosis and treatment evaluation, therefore, remain to be settled.

FUNCTION

Problems in coping with daily activities and performing functional skills have been established in CRPS (Geertzen et al. 1998a). It is surprising, therefore, that only a limited number of studies have evaluated the level of disability experienced by CRPS I patients. However, measurement instruments aimed at establishing problems at this level of observation have been evaluated for use in CRPS I patients. The RSQ, for functional problems related to the upper extremity, and the QRSD and WSQ, for lower extremity limitations, appear to be valid and reliable instruments for use in CRPS I patients. These questionnaires are available in the English language (contact Dr. Perez).

Clinimetric properties of the DASH have to be determined for upper extremity CRPS, although good correlations have been found with the RSQ (Schasfoort et al. 2002). The DASH has been translated into many languages and is a well-validated measure of arm function as perceived by the patient. It addresses the domains physical function, symptoms, and social or role function. Since it is a self-administered questionnaire, it can be easily administered. Therefore, the DASH may be a good candidate for evaluation for upper limb function when validity in CRPS is established.

Performance tests can be used to quantify specific functional skills. However, for CRPS patients, only the Foot Function Test (Kemler et al. 2000c) has been evaluated for use in CRPS I patients. Although this test seems to perform adequately, it is questionable whether certain components of the test actually measure functional aspects. For instance, one could argue if sliding one's foot forwards and backwards or sideways can be regarded as a functional activity of the lower extremity. Valid and reliable tests quantifying activities such as walking, walking stairs and rising and sitting down should therefore be developed to deal with this problem. For functional assessment of upper extremity CRPS, the Greentest and the Jebsen-Taylor test (Oerlemans et al. 2000b; Kemler et al. 2000a; Perez et al. 2003b) were used in CRPS I research. Clinimetric properties of these instruments have not yet been evaluated in a CRPS setting. Although both instruments appear to evaluate valid functional activities (i.e., handling objects using different grips) the sensitivity of these instruments for minor functional problems remains to be established. To quantify the amount of activity exhibited by the upper extremity, the ULAM (Schasfoort et al. 2002) provides good results. However, as this electronic activity monitor cannot measure which activity is performed, or how the activity is performed, further functional assessment remains necessary.

In conclusion, especially for the lower limb, reliable function tests for use in CRPS are still lacking. For the upper limb, a small number of tests and questionnaires are available for use in CRPS.

PARTICIPATION LEVEL

Measurement of health-related quality of life using generic questionnaires has increased in recent years. As a consequence, (population-based) data for a variety of illnesses are available, making cross-population comparison possible. For CRPS research, the NHP, EuroQol, COOP/WONCA and SF-36 have been reported to accurately discriminate between CRPS and healthy subjects or patients with other chronic illnesses (Kemler et al. 2000d; Hoeksema et al. 2003). Therefore, these measurement instruments appear to be the best option for determining general health-related problems in CRPS. At this point, however, no information with respect to the best performing instrument can be found. Furthermore, relationships between these HRQL outcome measures and the severity of CRPS have yet to be established.

CONCLUSION

Choosing measurement instruments for evaluating CRPS is complex for a number of reasons. First of all, CRPS is a multidimensional complaint, showing its effect on impairment, disability and handicap level.

Secondly, on impairment level, CRPS patients can exhibit a great variety of symptoms, which results in a heterogeneous patient population. Furthermore, not all symptoms may be equally important from the perspective of the patients, and the intervention to be tested may not influence all symptoms equally. The overall treatment effect should therefore be taken into consideration, since specific treatments can target specific problems associated with CRPS. Another point of discussion is the reactive nature of CRPS. As the complaint tends to worsen with (over)use of a limb, a measurement instrument should not put too much burden on the patient.

Considering the measurement instruments used for CRPS research so far, it is clear that a substantial part of the instruments used in studies lack proper reference to their psychometric properties. Surely, a portion of the studies will have relied on reliability and validity of instruments established for other patient groups and fields of research. Nevertheless, a large number of studies used self-invented instruments without providing information with regard to the stability of these instruments. Of the large number of measurement instruments available, only a minority has been assessed for use in CRPS patients. Within this group of evaluated instruments, different ways of testing the reliability and validity have been performed, making it difficult to compare their quality.

Furthermore, another problem arises when one takes into account the fact that different diagnostic criteria were used, possibly leading to biased findings with regard to the psychometric properties.

Considering these problems, the following issues need to be addressed when choosing measurement instruments:

1. CRPS should be assessed on different levels of observation.
2. No single index will suffice to characterize change of CRPS on impairment level.
3. Presumed treatment effect should be taken into account, leading to primary and secondary outcome measures.
4. Multiple diagnostic criteria are used for establishing the presence of CRPS, all of which face specific problems with respect to the reliability, and none of which can be considered a gold standard as frame of reference (i.e., a discriminative test establishing the pathophysiologic mechanism) is lacking.

Taking these issues into account, we conclude that in order to adequately measure CRPS on impairment level, a compound measurement instrument is needed which addresses the multidimensional nature of CRPS, and which reflects current diagnostic criteria. It should also be "decomposable," making it possible to evaluate the constituting parts separately. On disability level, instruments should be used which are in line with the functional activities performed in daily living, and which do not lead to (permanent) worsening of symptoms. Finally on handicap level, instruments should make comparisons with other populations possible, but should be sensitive enough to be able to discriminate between CRPS and other illnesses.

Therefore, we suggest the use of the ISS on impairment level, the RSQ and the QRSD and WSQ on function level, and COOP/WONCA, SF-36 or Euro-Qol for health-related quality of life assessment in CRPS research.

On impairment level, the ISS provides a compound measure with adequate validity and reliability, for which its constituting parts (VAS, McGill, IR-thermography, water displacement volumetry and goniometric AROM measurement) can be analyzed separately depending on the primary effect to be expected. Provided that the measurements are performed according to protocol, they are easy to administer without much patient burden. However, as a specific neuropathic component is lacking in the ISS, this compound score should be supplemented with instruments providing information on sensory abnormalities in order to be in line with diagnostic criteria. The NPS, or forms of QST, could be applied to that goal. For the latter, however, further clinimetric evaluation in CRPS patients is necessary.

The problem with compound measures is the fact that, until now, no information exists on the relative importance of each symptom for a patient. A change in such a measure may thus not reflect the patient's perception of change. For example, in the ISS all symptoms are equally important. A 5-point reduction of ISS can be accomplished by a 5-point reduction of any parameter, a 1-point reduction of each parameter or another combination. All these situations may be interpreted differently by a patient. Weighing each contributing factor may provide a better correlation with the perceived change. Future studies should focus on such weight factors.

For measuring functions, the RSQ for upper extremity CRPS, and QRSD and WSQ for lower extremity CRPS, are reliable instruments for assessment of functional problems. These instruments, being questionnaires, place little strain on a patient and can therefore be used for measurement of severe cases of CRPS as well.

For evaluation of health-related quality of life, the COOP/WONCA, SF-36 and EuroQol discriminate well between CRPS and patients with other illnesses and healthy subjects. Due to their generic nature and the extensive use of these charts in other patient populations, a broad range of comparisons can be made with other populations.

For all these outcome measures, except for the ISS as a whole, information concerning the relative weight of their constituting symptoms of indices is lacking.

Therefore, future research should assess the relationship between the severity of measured signs and symptoms, functional limitations and general health indices, and the severity of CRPS as expressed by the patient as well as the physician. In this way, valid measures can be obtained, ensuring reliable as well as valid measurement of CRPS.

Finally, the CPRS society is waiting for the elucidation of the pathophysiologic substrate of CRPS. Once this is known, a biochemical test, reflecting the etiology of the syndrome, might be developed which can be used to quantify the severity of CRPS.

REFERENCES

Adami S, Fossaluzza V, Gatti D, et al. Bisphosphonate therapy of reflex sympathetic dystrophy syndrome. Ann Rheum Dis 1997; 56:201–204.

Ahn SS, Machleder HI, Concepcion B, et al. Thoracoscopic cervicodorsal sympathectomy: preliminary results. J Vasc Surg 1994; 20:511–517.

Atkins RM, Kanis JA. The use of dolorimetry in the assessment of post-traumatic algodystrophy of the hand. Br J Rheumatol 1989; 28:404–409.

Azad SC, Beyer A, Romer AW, Galle-Rod A, Peter K, Schops P. Continuous axillary brachial plexus analgesia with low dose morphine in patients with complex regional pain syndromes. Eur J Anaesthesiol 2000; 17:185–188.

Bannink IHM, Vranken JH, Perez RS, et al. Treatment of CRPS type I with intravenous mannitol as an oxygen radical scavenger. Eur J Anaesthesiol 2000; 19(suppl):183.

Bickerstaff DR, Kanis JA. The use of nasal calcitonin in the treatment of post-traumatic algodystrophy. Br J Rheumatol 1991; 30:291–294.

Blanchard J, Ramamurthy S, Walsh N, et al. Intravenous regional sympatholysis: a double-blind comparison of guanethidine, reserpine, and normal saline. J Pain Sympt Manage 1990; 5:357–361.

Bonelli S, Conoscente F, Movilia PG, et al. Regional intravenous guanethidine vs. stellate ganglion block in reflex sympathetic dystrophies: a randomized trial. Pain 1983; 16:297–307.

Bonezzi C, Miotti D, Bettaglio R, et al. Electromotive administration of guanethidine for treatment of reflex sympathetic dystrophy: a pilot study in eight patients. J Pain Sympt Manage 1994; 9:39–43.

Bonica JJ. Causalgia and other reflex sympathetic dystrophies. In: Bonica JJ (ed). The Management of Pain. Lea & Febiger, Philadelphia, PA, 1990:220–243.

Bounameaux HM, Hellemans H, Verhaeghe R. Ketanserin in chronic sympathetic dystrophy. An acute controlled trial. Clin Rheumatol 1984; 3:556–557.

Braus DF, Krauss JK, Strobel J. The shoulder-hand syndrome after stroke: a prospective clinical trial. Ann Neurol 1994; 36:728–733.

Brazier J. The SF-36 health survey questionnaire: a tool for economists. Health Econ 1993; 2:213–215.

Bruehl S, Lubenow TR, Nath H, et al. Validation of thermography in the diagnosis of reflex sympathetic dystrophy. Clin J Pain 1996; 12:316–325.

Bruehl S, Harden RN, Galer BS, et al. External validation of IASP diagnostic criteria for Complex Regional Pain Syndrome and proposed research diagnostic criteria.

International Association for the Study of Pain. Pain 1999; 81:147–154.

Bruxelle J, Menkes CJ. [Treatment of algodystrophy by regional block with intravenous guanethidine]. Rev Rhum Mal Osteoartic 1982; 49:867–869.

Bryan AS, Klenerman L, Bowsher D. The diagnosis of reflex sympathetic dystrophy using an algometer. J Bone Joint Surg Br 1991; 73:644–646.

Calvillo O, Racz G, Didie J, et al. Neuroaugmentation in the treatment of complex regional pain syndrome of the upper extremity. Acta Orthop Belg 1998; 64:57–63.

Carlsson AM. Assessment of chronic pain: I. Aspects of the reliability and validity of the visual analogue scale. Pain 1983; 16:87–101.

Cazeneuve JF, Leborgne JM, Kermad K, et al. [Vitamin C and prevention of reflex sympathetic dystrophy following surgical management of distal radius fractures]. Acta Orthop Belg 2002; 68:481–484.

Chaise F, Guest M, Bellemere P, et al. [The efficacy of naftidrofuryl on unexpected autonomic symptoms following carpal tunnel surgery]. Ann Chir Main Memb Super 1994; 13:214–221.

Cherot A, Amor B. [Treatment of algodystrophy. A randomized study of 95 cases with 3 treatments: Calsyn 100, Visken, Grisefuline and Penthonium]. Rev Rhum Mal Osteoartic 1983; 50:95–97.

Christensen K, Jensen EM, Noer I. The reflex dystrophy syndrome response to treatment with systemic corticosteroids. Acta Chir Scand 1982; 148:653–655.

Chuinard RG, Dabezies EJ, Gould JS, et al. Intravenous reserpine for treatment of reflex sympathetic dystrophy. South Med J 1981; 74:1481–1484.

Cohen MM, Tate RB. Using the McGill Pain Questionnaire to study common postoperative complications. Pain 1989; 39:275–279.

Connelly NR, Reuben S, Brull SJ. Intravenous regional anesthesia with ketorolac-lidocaine for the management of sympathetically-mediated pain. Yale J Biol Med 1995; 68(3–4):95–99.

Cortet B, Flipo RM, Coquerelle P, et al. Treatment of severe, recalcitrant reflex sympathetic dystrophy: assessment of efficacy and safety of the second generation bisphosphonate pamidronate. Clin Rheumatol 1997; 16:51–56.

Davidoff G, Morey K, Amann M, et al. Pain measurement in reflex sympathetic dystrophy syndrome. Pain 1988; 32:27–34.

de Bruin AF, de Witte LP, Stevens F, et al. Sickness Impact Profile: the state of the art of a generic functional status measure. Soc Sci Med 1992; 35(8):1003–1014.

Delcambre B, Duquesnoy B, Baudens G, et al. [Treatment of algodystrophies]. Rev Rhum Mal Osteoartic 1982; 49:849–856.

Dielissen PW, Claassen AT, Veldman PH, et al. Amputation for reflex sympathetic dystrophy. J Bone Joint Surg Br 1995; 77:270–273.

Dotson RM. Clinical neurophysiology laboratory tests to assess the nociceptive system in humans. J Clin Neurophysiol 1997; 14:32–45.

Driessen JJ, van der WC, Nicolai JP, et al. Clinical effects of regional intravenous guanethidine (Ismelin) in reflex sympathetic dystrophy. Acta Anaesthesiol Scand 1983; 27:505–509.

Erdman RA, Passchier J, Kooijman M, et al. The Dutch version of the Nottingham Health Profile: investigations of psychometric aspects. Psychol Rep 1993; 72(3 Pt 1): 1027–1035.

Essink-Bot ML, Krabbe PF, Bonsel GJ, et al. An empirical comparison of four generic health status measures. The Nottingham Health Profile, the Medical Outcomes Study 36-item Short-Form Health Survey, the COOP/WONCA charts, and the EuroQol instrument. Med Care 1997; 35:522–537.

Eulry F, Aczel F, Vasseur P, et al. [Treatment and evolution of algodystrophy of the foot. Retrospective study of 199 cases]. Ann Med Interne (Paris) 1990; 141:20–25.

Eulry F, Alliaume C, Vasseur P, et al. [Treatment of algodystrophy by regional sympathetic blocks with guanethidine (410 blocks in 98 patients). Preliminary results]. Rev Rhum Mal Osteoartic 1991; 58:219–221.

EuroQol-group. EuroQol: a new facility for the measurement of health-related quality of life. The EuroQol Group. Health Policy 1990; 16:199–208.

Farcot JM, Mangin P, Laugner B, et al. Le bloc sympathique periferique par l'anesthesie locale intraveineuse a la guanethidine dans les syndromes algodystrophiques. Anesth Anal Rean 1981; 38:383–385.

Farcot JM, Grasser C, Foucher G, et al. [Local intravenous treatment of algodystrophy of the hand: buflomedil versus guanethidine, long term follow-up]. Ann Chir Main Memb Super 1990; 9:296–304.

Farrar JT, Berlin JA, Strom BL. Clinically important changes in acute pain outcome measures: a validation study. J Pain Symptom Manage 2003; 25:406–411.

Fialka V, Resch KL, Ritter-Dietrich D, et al. Acupuncture for reflex sympathetic dystrophy. Arch Intern Med 1993; 153:661–665.

Field J, Atkins RM. Effect of guanethidine on the natural history of post-traumatic algodystrophy. Ann Rheum Dis 1993; 52:467–469.

Field J, Monk C, Atkins RM. Objective improvements in algodystrophy following regional intravenous guanethidine. J Hand Surg Br 1993; 18:339–342.

Forouzanfar T, Kemler M, Kessels AG, et al. Comparison of multiple against single pain intensity measurements in complex regional pain syndrome type I: analysis of 54 patients. Clin J Pain 2002; 18:234–237.

Forouzanfar T, Weber WE, Kemler M, et al. What is a meaningful pain reduction in patients with complex regional pain syndrome type 1? Clin J Pain 2003; 19:281–285.

Friez L, Pere G, Breuillard P, et al. [Comparison of treatment with griseofulvin, beta blockers and calcitonin in 55 cases of post-traumatic algoneurodystrophies]. Rev Rhum Mal Osteoartic 1982; 49:857–860.

Galer BS, Jensen MP. Development and preliminary validation of a pain measure specific to neuropathic pain: the Neuropathic Pain Scale. Neurology 1997; 48:332–338.

Geertzen JH, de Bruijn H, Bruijn-Kofman AT, et al. Reflex sympathetic dystrophy: early treatment and psychological aspects. Arch Phys Med Rehabil 1994; 75:442–446.

Geertzen JH, Dijkstra PU, van Sonderen ELP, et al. Relationship between impairments, disability and handicap in reflex sympathetic dystrophy patients: a long-term follow-up study. Clin Rehabil 1998a; 12:402–412.

Geertzen JH, Dijkstra PU, Stewart RE, et al. Variation in measurements of grip strength. A study in reflex sympathetic dystrophy patients. Acta Orthop Scand Suppl 1998b; 279:4–11.

Geertzen JH, Dijkstra PU, Stewart RE, et al. Variation in measurements of range of motion: a study in reflex sympathetic dystrophy patients. Clin Rehabil 1998c; 12:254–264.

Glynn C, Casale R. Morphine injected around the stellate ganglion does not modulate the sympathetic nervous system nor does it provide pain relief. Pain 1993; 53:33–37.

Glynn CJ, Basedow RW, Walsh JA. Pain relief following post-ganglionic sympathetic blockade with I.V. guanethidine. Br J Anaesth 1981; 53:1297–1302.

Gobelet C, Meier JL, Schaffner W, et al. Calcitonin and reflex sympathetic dystrophy syndrome. Clin Rheumatol 1986; 5:382–388.

Gobelet C, Waldburger M, Meier JL. The effect of adding calcitonin to physical treatment on reflex sympathetic dystrophy. Pain 1992; 48:171–175.

Goris RJ, Dongen LM, Winters HA. Are toxic oxygen radicals involved in the pathogenesis of reflex sympathetic dystrophy? Free Radic Res Commun 1987; 3:13–18.

Gracely RH, Kwilosz DM. The Descriptor Differential Scale: applying psychophysical principles to clinical pain assessment. Pain 1988; 35:279–288.

Grundberg AB. Reflex sympathetic dystrophy: treatment with long-acting intramuscular corticosteroids. J Hand Surg Am 1996; 21:667–670.

Gschwind C, Fricker R, Lacher G, et al. Does peri-operative guanethidine prevent reflex sympathetic dystrophy? J Hand Surg Br 1995; 20:773–775.

Hamamci N, Dursun E, Ural C, et al. Calcitonin treatment in reflex sympathetic dystrophy: a preliminary study. Br J Clin Pract 1996; 50(7):373–375.

Hanna MH, Peat SJ. Ketanserin in reflex sympathetic dystrophy. A double-blind placebo controlled cross-over trial. Pain 1989; 38:145–150.

Harke H, Gretenkort P, Ladleif HU, et al. The response of neuropathic pain and pain in complex regional pain syndrome I to carbamazepine and sustained-release morphine in patients pretreated with spinal cord stimulation: a double-blinded randomized study. Anesth Analg 2001; 92:488–495.

Hassenbusch SJ, Stanton-Hicks M, Schoppa D, et al. Long-term results of peripheral nerve stimulation for reflex sympathetic dystrophy. J Neurosurg 1996; 84:415–423.

Hennart D, Leon M, Sylin P, et al. Sympathetic nerve blocks in refractory sympathetic dystrophy syndrome. Acta Orthop Belg 1999; 65:83–85.

Hoeksema M, Perez RS, Zuurmond WA, et al. [Quality of life in CRPS I]. Ned Tijdschr Anesth 2003; 16(suppl):48.

Hord AH, Rooks MD, Stephens BO, et al. Intravenous regional bretylium and lidocaine for treatment of reflex sympathetic dystrophy: a randomized, double-blind study. Anesth Analg 1992; 74:818–821.

Horton P, Gerster JC. [Algodystrophy in relation to previous barbiturate therapy. Study of 25 cases]. Schweiz Rundsch Med Prax 1986; 75:4–6.

Jadad AR, Carroll D, Glynn CJ, et al. Intravenous regional sympathetic blockade for pain relief in reflex sympathetic dystrophy: a systematic review and a randomized, double-

blind crossover study. J Pain Sympt Manage 1995; 10:13–20.

Jeandel P, Prigent D, Gilette B, et al. [Treatment of reflex algoneurodystrophies by sympathetic blockade with gua-nethidine]. Ann Med Interne (Paris) 1989; 140:166–168.

Jensen MP, McFarland CA. Increasing the reliability and validity of pain intensity measurement in chronic pain. Pain 1993; 55:195–203.

Jensen MP, Turner JA, Romano JM, et al. Comparative reliability and validity of chronic pain intensity measures. Pain 1999; 83:157–162.

Jordan K, Dziedzic K, Mullis R, et al. The development of three-dimensional range of motion measurement systems for clinical practice. Rheumatology 2001; 40:1081–1084.

Kaplan R, Claudio M, Kepes E, et al. Intravenous guanethidine in patients with reflex sympathetic dystrophy. Acta Anaesthesiol Scand 1996; 40:1216–1222.

Kemler MA, de Vet HC. An objective and standardized test of foot function: normative values and validation in patients with reflex sympathetic dystrophy. Arch Phys Med Rehabil 2000a; 81:1401–1407.

Kemler MA, de Vet HC. Health-related quality of life in chronic refractory reflex sympathetic dystrophy (complex regional pain syndrome type I). J Pain Sympt Manage 2000b; 20:68–76.

Kemler MA, Barendse GA, van Kleef M, et al. Spinal cord stimulation in patients with chronic reflex sympathetic dystrophy. N Engl J Med 2000a; 343:618–624.

Kemler MA, Schouten HJ, Gracely RH. Diagnosing sensory abnormalities with either normal values or values from contralateral skin: comparison of two approaches in complex regional pain syndrome I. Anesthesiology 2000b; 93:718–727.

Kettler RE, Abram SE. Intravenous regional droperidol in the management of reflex sympathetic dystrophy: a double-blind, placebo-controlled, crossover study. Anesthesiology 1988; 69:933–936.

Kissling RO, Boelsch AC, Sager M, et al. [Prevention of recurrence of Sudeck's disease with calcitonin]. Rev Chir Orthop Reparatrice 1991; 77:562–567.

Kondo I, Hosokawa K, Soma M, et al. Protocol to prevent shoulder-hand syndrome after stroke. Arch Phys Med Rehabil 2001; 82:1619–1623.

Korpan MI, Dezu Y, Schneider B, et al. Acupuncture in the treatment of posttraumatic pain syndrome. Acta Orthop Belg 1999; 65:197–201.

Kozin F, Ryan LM, Carerra GF, et al. The reflex sympathetic dystrophy syndrome (RSDS): III. Scintigraphic studies, further evidence for the therapeutic efficacy of systemic corticosteroids, and proposed diagnostic criteria. Am J Med 1981; 70:23–30.

Kubalek I, Fain O, Paries J, et al. Treatment of reflex sympathetic dystrophy with pamidronate: 29 cases. Rheumatology (Oxford) 2001; 40:1394–1397.

Kumar K, Toth C, Nath RK, et al. Epidural spinal cord stimulation for treatment of chronic pain: some predictors of success. A 15-year experience. Surg Neurol 1998; 50:110–120.

Langendijk PN, Zuurmond WW, van Apeldoorn HA, et al. [Good results of treatment of reflex sympathetic dystrophy with a 50% dimethylsulfoxide cream]. Ned Tijdschr Geneeskd 1993; 137:500–503.

Laroche M, Redon-Dumolard A, Moulinier L, et al. Phosphate excretion in reflex sympathetic dystrophy syndrome before and after a single infusion of pamidronate. Rev Rhum Engl Ed 1997; 64:172–176.

Lee BH, Scharff L, Sethna NF, et al. Physical therapy and cognitive-behavioral treatment for complex regional pain syndromes. J Pediatr 2002; 141:135–140.

Linchitz RM, Raheb JC. Subcutaneous infusion of lidocaine provides effective pain relief for CRPS patients. Clin J Pain 1999; 15:67–72.

Livingstone JA, Atkins RM. Intravenous regional guanethidine blockade in the treatment of post-traumatic complex regional pain syndrome type 1 (algodystrophy) of the hand. J Bone Joint Surg Br 2002; 84:380–386.

Lowe NK, Walker SN, MacCallum RC. Confirming the theoretical structure of the McGill Pain Questionnaire in acute clinical pain. Pain 1991; 46:53–60.

Maillefert JF, Chatard C, Owen S, et al. Treatment of refractory reflex sympathetic dystrophy with pamidronate. Ann Rheum Dis 1995; 54:687.

Maillefert JF, Cortet B, Aho S. Pooled results from 2 trials evaluating biphosphonates in reflex sympathetic dystrophy. J Rheumatol 1999; 26:1856–1857.

Malik VK, Inchiosa M-AJ, Mustafa K, et al. Intravenous regional phenoxybenzamine in the treatment of reflex sympathetic dystrophy. Anesthesiology 1998; 88:823–827.

Marx C, Wiedersheim P, Michel BA, et al. Preventing recurrence of reflex sympathetic dystrophy in patients requiring an operative intervention at the site of dystrophy after surgery. Clin Rheumatol 2001; 20:114–118.

Mayer M, Strosche H, Bachmann H. [Therapy of algodystrophy (Sudeck disease) with naftidrofuryl hydrogen oxalate (NH)]. Unfallchirurg 1986; 89:117–120.

Melzack R. The McGill Pain Questionnaire: major properties and scoring methods. Pain 1975; 1:277–299.

Michell SW, Moorehouse GR, Keen WW. Gunshot Wounds and Other Injuries of Nerves. JB Lippincott, Philadelphia, PA, 1864.

Mongini F, Italiano M, Raviola F, et al. The McGill Pain Questionnaire in patients with TMJ pain and with facial pain as a somatoform disorder. Cranio 2000; 18:249–256.

Mudun A, Bursali A, Oklu T, et al. Scintigraphic evaluation of the effectiveness of intranasal calcitonin therapy in Sudeck's atrophy. Nucl Med Commun 1993; 14:805–809.

Muizelaar JP, Kleyer M, Hertogs IA, et al. Complex regional pain syndrome (reflex sympathetic dystrophy and causalgia): management with the calcium channel blocker nifedipine and/or the alpha-sympathetic blocker phenoxybenzamine in 59 patients. Clin Neurol Neurosurg 1997; 99:26–30.

Muramatsu K, Kawai S, Akino T, et al. Treatment of chronic regional pain syndrome using manipulation therapy and regional anesthesia. J Trauma 1998; 44:189–192.

Nedjar C, Ficat C. [Importance of intravenous reserpine in the treatment of reflex sympathetic dystrophy]. Agressologie 1982; 23:317–320.

Nuti R, Vattimo A, Martini G, et al. Carbocalcitonin treatment in Sudeck's atrophy. Clin Orthop 1987; 215:217–222.

Oerlemans HM, Goris RJ, Oostendorp RA. Impairment level sumscore in reflex sympathetic dystrophy of one upper extremity. Arch Phys Med Rehabil 1998; 79:979–990.

Oerlemans HM, Graff MJ, Dijkstra-Hekkink JB, et al. Reliability and normal values for measuring the skin temperature of the hand with an infrared tympanic thermometer: a pilot study. J Hand Ther 1999a; 12:284–290.

Oerlemans HM, Oostendorp RA, de Boo T, et al. Signs and symptoms in complex regional pain syndrome type I/reflex sympathetic dystrophy: judgment of the physician versus objective measurement. Clin J Pain 1999b; 15:224–232.

Oerlemans HM, Perez RS, Oostendorp RA, et al. Objective and subjective assessments of temperature differences between the hands in reflex sympathetic dystrophy. Clin Rehabil 1999c; 13(5):430–438.

Oerlemans HM, Cup EH, de Boo T, et al. The Radboud skills questionnaire: construction and reliability in patients with reflex sympathetic dystrophy of one upper extremity. Disabil Rehabil 2000a; 22:233–245.

Oerlemans HM, Oostendorp RA, de Boo T, et al. Adjuvant physical therapy versus occupational therapy in patients with reflex sympathetic dystrophy/complex regional pain syndrome type I. Arch Phys Med Rehabil 2000b; 81:49–56.

Perez RS, Bauer M, Zuurmond WA, et al. Signs and symptoms of complex regional pain syndrome type I: consequences for diagnosis. Eur J Anaesthesiol 2000; 18(suppl):128.

Perez RS, Burm PE, Rijnsburger ER, et al. Predictive value of pain, temperature, volume and range of motion in complex regional pain syndrome type I. Anesthesiology 2001; 95(suppl):A803.

Perez RS, Burm PE, Zuurmond WW, et al. Interrater reliability of diagnosing complex regional pain syndrome type I. Acta Anaesthesiol Scand 2002a; 46:447–450.

Perez RS, Roorda LD, Zuurmond WW, et al. Measuring perceived activity limitations in lower extremity Complex Regional Pain Syndrome type 1 (CRPS I): test-retest reliability of two questionnaires. Clin Rehabil 2002b; 16:454–460.

Perez RS, Greuters S, Zuurmond WA, et al. Grip strength in Complex Regional Pain Syndrome type I: relationships with pain and active range of motion. Eur J Anaesthesiol 2003a; 20(suppl):A707.

Perez RS, Oerlemans HM, Zuurmond W, et al. Impairment level SumScore for lower extremity Complex Regional Pain Syndrome type I. Disabil Rehabil 2003b; 25:984–991.

Perez RS, Burm PE, Zuurmond WA, et al. Physicians' assessments versus measured symptoms of Complex Regional Pain Syndrome type 1 (RSD): presence and severity. Clin J Pain 2005; 21:272–276.

Perrigot M, Bergego C, Hocini A, et al. [Algodystrophic syndrome in hemiplegia. Clinical and therapeutic study]. Ann Med Interne (Paris) 1982; 133:544–548.

Poplawski ZJ, Wiley AM, Murray JF. Post-traumatic dystrophy of the extremities. J Bone Joint Surg Am 1983; 65:642–655.

Price DD, Bush FM, Long S, et al. A comparison of pain measurement characteristics of mechanical visual analogue and simple numerical rating scales. Pain 1994; 56:217–226.

Price DD, Long S, Wilsey B, et al. Analysis of peak magnitude and duration of analgesia produced by local anesthetics injected into sympathetic ganglia of complex regional pain syndrome patients. Clin J Pain 1998; 14:216–226.

Prough DS, McLeskey CH, Poehling GG, et al. Efficacy of oral nifedipine in the treatment of reflex sympathetic dystrophy. Anesthesiology 1985; 62:796–799.

Ramamurthy S, Hoffman J. Intravenous regional guanethidine in the treatment of reflex sympathetic dystrophy/causalgia: a randomized, double-blind study. Guanethidine Study Group. Anesth Analg 1995; 81:718–723.

Rauck RL, Eisenach JC, Jackson K, et al. Epidural clonidine treatment for refractory reflex sympathetic dystrophy. Anesthesiology 1993; 79:1163–1169.

Reginster JY, Franchimont P. Side effects of synthetic salmon calcitonin given by intranasal spray compared with intramuscular injection. Clin Exp Rheumatol 1985; 3:155–157.

Reiestad F, McIlvaine WB, Kvalheim L, et al. Interpleural analgesia in treatment of upper extremity reflex sympathetic dystrophy. Anesth Analg 1989; 69:671–673.

Reinders MF, Geertzen JH, Dijkstra PU. Complex regional pain syndrome type I: use of the International Association for the Study of Pain diagnostic criteria defined in 1994. Clin J Pain 2002; 18:207–215.

Rico H, Merono E, Gomez-Castresana F, et al. Scintigraphic evaluation of reflex sympathetic dystrophy: comparative study of the course of the disease under two therapeutic regimens. Clin Rheumatol 1987; 6:233–237.

Riou C, Daoudi Y, Langlais F, et al. [Can algodystrophy be prevented by thyrocalcitonin?]. Rev Chir Orthop Reparatrice Appar Mot 1991; 77:208–210.

Robbins WR, Staats PS, Levine J, et al. Treatment of intractable pain with topical large-dose capsaicin: preliminary report. Anesth Analg 1998; 86:579–583.

Rocco AG, Kaul AF, Reisman RM, et al. A comparison of regional intravenous guanethidine and reserpine in reflex sympathetic dystrophy. A controlled, randomized, double-blind crossover study. Clin J Pain 1989; 5:205–209.

Rommel O, Gehling M, Dertwinkel R, et al. Hemisensory impairment in patients with complex regional pain syndrome. Pain 1999; 80:95–101.

Rovetta G, Baratto L, Monteforte P. Low dose gabapentin for shoulder-hand syndrome induced by phenobarbital: a three-month study. Drugs Exp Clin Res 1999; 25:185–191.

Sawicki A, Szulc P, Sobczyk T, et al. Influence of calcitonin treatment on the osteocalcin concentration in the algodystrophy of bone. Clin Rheumatol 1992; 11:346–350.

Schasfoort FC, Bussmann JB, Stam HJ. Ambulatory measurement of upper limb usage and mobility-related activities during normal daily life with an upper limb-activity monitor: a feasibility study. Med Biol Eng Comput 2002; 40:173–182.

Serpell MG. Gabapentin in neuropathic pain syndromes: a randomised, double-blind, placebo-controlled trial. Pain 2002; 99:557–566.

Sherry DD, Weisman R. Psychologic aspects of childhood reflex neurovascular dystrophy. Pediatrics 1988; 81:572–578.

Sherry DD, Wallace CA, Kelley C, et al. Short- and long-term outcomes of children with complex regional pain syndrome type I treated with exercise therapy. Clin J Pain 1999; 15:218–223.

Smeets PM, van den Wildenberg FA, Crebolder HF, et al. [Prospective study of 46 mannitol infusions at home with 28 patients with Reflex sympathetic dystrophy]. Ned Tijschr Pijn Pijnbestr 1999; 19:25–33.

Stanton-Hicks M, Janig W, Hassenbusch S, et al. Reflex sympathetic dystrophy: changing concepts and taxonomy. Pain 1995; 6:127–133.

Taoussanis K. [Treatment of Sudeck's syndrome with calcitonin]. Med Welt 1981; 32(37):1375–1377.

Uher EM, Vacariu G, Schneider B, et al. [Comparison of manual lymph drainage with physical therapy in complex regional pain syndrome, type I. A comparative randomized controlled therapy study]. Wien Klin Wochenschr 2000; 112:133–137.

van de Beek WJ, Schwartzman RJ, van Nes SI, et al. Diagnostic criteria used in studies of reflex sympathetic dystrophy. Neurology 2002; 58:522–526.

van de Vusse AC, Stomp-van den Berg SG, de Vet HC, et al. Interobserver reliability of diagnosis in patients with complex regional pain syndrome. Eur J Pain 2003; 7:259–265.

van Hilten BJ, van de Beek WJ, Hoff JI, et al. Intrathecal baclofen for the treatment of dystonia in patients with reflex sympathetic dystrophy. N Engl J Med 2000; 343:625–630.

van Weel C. Functional status in primary care: COOP/WONCA charts. Disabil Rehabil 1993; 15:96–101.

Varenna M, Zucchi F, Ghiringhelli D, et al. Intravenous clodronate in the treatment of reflex sympathetic dystrophy syndrome. A randomized, double blind, placebo controlled study. J Rheumatol 2000; 27:1477–1483.

Veehof MM, Sleegers EJ, van Veldhoven NH, et al. Psychometric qualities of the Dutch language version of the Disabilities of the Arm, Shoulder, and Hand questionnaire (DASH-DLV). J Hand Ther 2002; 15:347–354.

Veldman PH, Reynen HM, Arntz IE, et al. Signs and symptoms of reflex sympathetic dystrophy: prospective study of 829 patients. Lancet 1993; 342:1012–1016.

Verdugo RJ, Campero M, Ochoa JL. Phentolamine sympathetic block in painful polyneuropathies: II. Further questioning of the concept of "sympathetically maintained pain." Neurology 1994; 44:1010–1014.

Wallace MS, Ridgeway BM, Leung AY, et al. Concentration-effect relationship of intravenous lidocaine on the allodynia of complex regional pain syndrome types I and II. Anesthesiology 2000; 92:75–83.

Wasner G, Heckmann K, Maier C, et al. Vascular abnormalities in acute reflex sympathetic dystrophy (CRPS I): complete inhibition of sympathetic nerve activity with recovery. Arch Neurol 1999; 56:613–620.

Wasner G, Schattschneider J, Baron R. Skin temperature side differences: a diagnostic tool for CRPS? Pain 2002; 98:19–26.

Williame E. [Treatment of reflex sympathetic dystrophy by calcitonine (author's transl)]. Rev Med Brux 1980; 1:457–461.

Wu WH, Bandilla E, Ciccone DS, et al. Effects of qigong on late-stage complex regional pain syndrome. Altern Ther Health Med 1999; 5:45–54.

Zollinger PE, Tuinebreijer WE, Kreis RW, et al. Effect of vitamin C on frequency of reflex sympathetic dystrophy in wrist fractures: a randomised trial. Lancet 1999; 354:2025–2028.

Zuurmond WW, Langendijk PN, Bezemer PD, et al. Treatment of acute reflex sympathetic dystrophy with DMSO 50% in a fatty cream. Acta Anaesthesiol Scand 1996; 40:364–367.

Zyluk A. Results of the treatment of posttraumatic reflex sympathetic dystrophy of the upper extremity with regional intravenous blocks of methylprednisolone and lidocaine. Acta Orthop Belg 1998; 64:452–456.

FURTHER READING

Cepeda MS, Lau J, Carr DB. Defining the therapeutic role of local anesthetic sympathetic blockade in complex regional pain syndrome: a narrative and systematic review. Clin J Pain 2002; 18:216–233.

Perez RS, Zuurmond WW, Bezemer PD, et al. The treatment of complex regional pain syndrome type I with free radical scavengers: a randomized controlled study. Pain 2003c; 102:297–307.

Rommel O, Malin JP, Zenz M, et al. Quantitative sensory testing, neurophysiological and psychological examination in patients with complex regional pain syndrome and hemisensory deficits. Pain 2001; 93:279–293.

CHAPTER 16

Arthritis pain, outcomes, and evidence

Vijay N. Joish • Keri L. Fakata • Arthur G. Lipman

INTRODUCTION

The *International Classification of Functioning, Disability, and Health* (ICF) identifies three levels of human functioning: functioning at the level of (1) body or body part, (2) the whole person, and (3) the whole person in a social context. The arthritides are a group of over 100 heterogeneous diseases that all involve joint inflammation. The most common clinical arthritides are osteoarthritis (OA) and rheumatoid arthritis (RA), both of which commonly affect individuals at one or more of these levels, i.e., impairments, activity limitations, and participation restrictions. Assessment measures for these diseases also may be classified according to these three levels.

IMPAIRMENT MEASUREMENT (BODILY FUNCTIONS AND STRUCTURE)

Several traditional outcomes measures have been used in clinical trials to evaluate the impact of therapeutic interventions on the arthritides. Examples of traditional outcomes measures are listed in Table 16.1. The use of such traditional measures can be problematic when comparing the results of clinical trials due to inconsistencies in traditional outcomes used among trials. Some traditional outcomes overlap similar assessments such as swollen joint counts and joint swelling score, decreasing the sensitivity of the measures. Investigators have attempted to define traditional outcomes that provide sensitivity to change and consistency of use in clinical trials.

Anderson and colleagues (1989) evaluated traditional outcomes utilized in three large multicenter trials on disease modifying antirheumatic drugs (DMARDs). These authors utilized adjusted t-statistics to evaluate traditional outcome measures. They considered measures sensitive that exceeded the value of 2.0, i.e., the value required for significance for a single test in a trial of usual size. They found the tender joint count (t-3.58) most sensitive to change and therefore determined that it could be the sole measurement for the disease activity in joints, erythrocyte sedimentation rate (ESR, t-3.30) was the most sensitive laboratory assessment, grip strength (t-2.13) was most sensitive for functional ability, and physician assessment (t-2.86) was most sensitive for general assessment measures (Anderson et al. 1989).

Table 16.1 Traditional outcome measures

Joint tenderness count
Joint tenderness score
Joint swelling count
Joint swelling score
Proximal interphalangeal joint circumference
Grip strength
50-feet walking time
Pain (VAS)
Duration of morning stiffness
Patient assessment of disease activity (VAS)
Physician assessment of disease activity (VAS)
Functional class assessment
ESR
Hemoglobin
Platelet count
Radiography

In another attempt to identify core measurements for conducting clinical trials in RA, representatives of the ACR and the Outcome Measures in Arthritis Clinical Trials (OMERACT) group met in 1992 to define a core set of measures with construct, face, content, criterion, and discriminate validity. Today, the most common measure of functional ability is the ACR revised criteria for classification of functional status in RA. This core set of values can be found in Table 16.2 (Felson et al. 1993). When the ACR core set is utilized in a trial, a baseline value is assessed for each patient and changes in the patient's condition are reported as a percentage of the baseline score. There are several percentage response criteria levels at which improvement in clinical trials are assessed. These are referred to as the ACR 20%, 50%, 70%, and 90%. The current recommended ACR threshold for improvement is 20%; however, that percentage improvement is frequently being replaced by higher response criteria levels (50%, 70%). Boers et al. (2001) have posited that the amount of improvement is dependent on whether the underlying ACR measure has a score that increases or decreases on improvement. For example, some core measurements are scaled to show an increased value for improvement that could result in a patient achieving over 100% improvement. However, a few are scaled to show a decreased value for improvement for which the maximum response could only be 100% (Boers et al. 2001). These authors evaluated data from the Dutch arthritis multidrug study entitled Combinatietherapie Bij Rheumatoïde Arthritis (COBRA) that involved 155 patients and suggest that it may be beneficial to recode scores that reflect a decrease in value for improvement especially when using high percentages of improvement. Felson et al. (1998) questioned whether improvement of more than 20% in core set parameters should be required before patients are characterized as improved in RA clinical trials. To this purpose they evaluated the discriminate validity of ACR percentages of improvement in 6 controlled clinical trials of RA treatment and found that discriminate validity decreased as the expected percentage of improvement increased. They concluded that (1) adopting a definition of efficacy in RA trials that requires 50 or 70% improvement in core set parameters would likely compromise statistical power and make it more difficult to distinguish between 2 treatments with different efficacy; and (2) ACR 20 should continue to be the primary measure of efficacy in RA trials, with higher thresholds for improvement being determined and reported as secondary efficacy measures.

Table 16.2 ACR core set of disease activity measurements

Measure	*Assessment*
Tender joint count	68 joints (tender versus not tender)
Swollen joint count	66 joints (swollen versus not swollen)
Patient assessment of pain	VAS (10 cm) or Likert scale
Patient global assessment of disease activity	VAS (10 cm) or Likert scale
Physician global assessment of disease activity	VAS (10 cm) or Likert scale
Patient assessment of physical function	AIMS, HAQ, Quality of Well Being, MHIQ, etc.
Acute phase reactant	ESR, CRP
Radiography	$\geq$1 year trial evaluating a DMARD

SIMPLIFIED DISEASE ACTIVITY INDEX FOR RHEUMATOID ARTHRITIS (SDAI-RA)

The Simplified Disease Activity Index for Rheumatoid Arthritis (SDAI-RA) (Smolen et al. 2003) is a clinical assessment tool constructed for everyday use in the busy clinical setting to evaluate disease activity. Complicated analytic procedures limit the usefulness of some other core measure sets in the clinic setting. The SDAI-RA simply requires calculating the sum of 5 outcome parameters. These are: 1, tender joint count; 2, swollen joint count based on a 28-joint assessment; 3, patient and 4, physician global assessment of disease activity as a 0–10 cm visual analogue scale (VAS); and 5, C-reactive protein (CPR-mg/dL). The SDAI-RA was evaluated for validity by analysis of its activity in leflunomide studies. It was statistically significantly associated with other measures of functional ability such as Health Assessment Questionnaire (HAQ) (Pincus et al. 1983) and Disease Activity Score 28 (DAS 28) (van der Heijde et al. 1990), and demonstrated change proportional to the ACR percentages of improvement, supporting sensitivity to change and convergent validity.

EUROPEAN LEAGUE AGAINST RHEUMATISM RESPONSE CRITERIA (EULAR)

While the ACR measures percentage improvement representing patient change, it does not assess absolute disease activity. The European League Against Rheumatism (EULAR) developed a core set of criteria using 28 joint counts that addresses both patient change and disease activity. The disease activity score (DAS) is a multiple regression analysis (van der Heijde et al. 1990) comprising swollen joint count, ESR, patient global assessment of disease activity, and the Ritchie Articular Index. Changes greater than 1.2 from baseline constitutes a good response, changes between 0.6 and 1.2 indicate a moderate response, and changes equal to or smaller than 0.6 indicate no response. There is a high level of agreement between the ACR and the EULAR measures in clinical trials with comparable validity, especially discriminate validity (van Gestel et al. 1998).

RHEUMATOID ARTHRITIS DISEASE ACTIVITY INDEX (RADAI)

The Rheumatoid Arthritis Disease Activity Index (RADAI) is an augmented form of the Rapid Assessment of Disease Activity in Rheumatology (RADAR) in order to provide a global score for use in clinical and epidemiologic studies. The RADAI implemented a numeric rating scale instead of a visual analog scale for 4 of the RADAR disease activity questions including arthritis activity over the last 6 months, arthritis activity today, arthritis pain today, and morning stiffness today. The fifth question on the RADAI asked patients to numerically rate pain in extremity areas instead of

select joints for example. Patients were to rate their pain in their shoulder, instead of referring to the separate joints as the RADAR did. The RADAI also left out the rating of tenderness in joints, because it is addressed separately in the use of a mannequin where patients were to mark on the mannequin areas that represented their swollen and tender joints. The RADAI self-administered questionnaire was validated in 55 consecutive RA patients. This tool was found to have high internal consistency and correlated well with physician assessment ($r = 0.54$, $p < 0.01$), swollen joint count ($r = 0.54$, $p < 0.01$), and C-reactive protein ($r = 0.43$, $p < 0.01$) with a Cronbach's alpha of 0.91. It still needs to be determined if the RADAI is responsive to clinical change; because RADAI is a measurement of inflammatory disease activity, it may be useful in other arthrides. It is not recommended to use this tool to make individual clinical decisions.

SELF-ADMINISTERED JOINT COUNT (SAJC)

The Self-Administered Joint Count (SAJC) (Escalante 1998) is another assessment method for use in busy clinical settings. The SAJC allows the practitioner time to evaluate other disease-related issues. This method uses an anatomical joint mannequin, allowing patients to self-assess painful or swollen joints. Large circles on the mannequin represent 40 separate joints. The temporomandibular, sternoclavicular, acromioclavicular, and the hip joints are not indicated to lessen the confusion about the location of joints on the mannequin. Escalante evaluated the SAJC in two patient samples. One data set included 110 consecutive RA patients seen in a referral RA clinic for which the author of the SAJC performed observer assessments. The second sample included 240 consecutive outpatients enrolled in a longitudinal outcomes study in rheumatology clinics and a veterans administration hospital. The instruments utilized for outcomes and observer assessments in this study varied slightly from those used in the first sample. Test–retest reliability of the SAJC was excellent ($r = 0.89$), as was its agreement with the observer-assessed tender joint counts ($r = 0.78$). The SAJC was significantly correlated ($p \leq 0.01$) to pain on a 10-point scale ($r = 0.33$), the McGill Pain Questionnaire ($r = 0.27$), the pain subscale of the Arthritis Impact Measurement Scales (AIMS) ($r = 0.32$), the duration of morning stiffness ($r = 0.27$), and to the AIMS subscales of physical function ($r = 0.20$), impact ($r = 0.31$), and global health ($r = 0.29$). However, there was significant variability when individual joints were assessed. Patients may have had difficulty with anatomical orientation and the author recommends that the orientation be specified when using the SAJC in clinical settings. Patients also had difficulty assessing swollen joints with the SAJC. That may be more indicative of the destructive disease process. The SAJC may allow clinicians more time to concentrate on swollen joints which may be a better indicator of joint destruction processes.

ACTIVITY

CLASSIFICATION OF GLOBAL FUNCTIONAL STATUS IN RHEUMATOID ARTHRITIS

In 1988, the ACR appointed subcommittee evaluated the Steinbrocker criteria for functional activity in RA and to revise it. The subcommittee felt that the Steinbrocker criteria had several shortcomings: (1) the absence of guidelines for use, (2) lack of prior validation studies, and (3) clinical experience found that the vast majority of patients fell within functional class II which states that functional capacity is adequate to conduct normal activities despite handicap of discomfort or limited mobility of one or more joints. The goal of the committee was to revise the guidelines to provide functional status classification in the clinic setting, and to use to determine work disability. The revised criteria are represented in Table 16.3. The new revised criteria were validated by 6 of the subcommittee members that identified RA patients within their clinical practice. The new criteria were evaluated in 325 RA patients. Both old and revised criteria were evaluated in each patient. Over 75% of patients were classified as Steinbrocker class II, and 90% in classes II and III were, as there was a trend of more uniform distribution pattern of patients with regards to functional classes associated with the revised criteria. There was still a significant percentage of patients (80%) falling into functional classes II and III with the revised criteria; however, more than 10% of patients were considered class I and more than 5% of patients fell into class IV. The revised criteria

proved to be more sensitive to severity of disability; 27% of patients that were characterized as Steinbrocker class III fell into class IV with the revised criteria. The ACR recommends that quantitative measures of physical disability should be used in conjunction with the revised global functional status classification in order to yield the most accurate assessment of patients at a single time point as well as over a number of visits.

FIBROMYALGIA IMPACT QUESTIONNAIRE (FIQ)

The Fibromyalgia Impact Questionnaire (FIQ) is a self-administered, symptom/functioning instrument developed to measure fibromyalgia patient status, progress, and outcomes in adults (Burckhardt et al. 1991). Originally developed in American English, the FIQ has been translated into at least 11 languages. The FIQ contains items that measure physical functioning, i.e., symptoms of pain, fatigue, morning tiredness, stiffness, job difficulty, depression, and anxiety along with days of work missed and overall well-being in the past week. The first 11 items are summed into the physical function score. Each item is rated on a four-point Likert-type scale. Initial assessment of the psychometric properties indicated that it has sufficient evidence of reliability and validity. The FIQ is a brief 20-item instrument and takes less than 5 minutes to complete.

GLOBAL OUTCOME MEASURES (HEALTH STATUS AND HEALTH-RELATED QUALITY OF LIFE)

Health status questionnaires, also called health-related quality of life (HRQoL) instruments, have been developed and validated for use across various rheumatic disorders, e.g., the Arthritis Impact Measurement Scales (AIMS), as well as some that are specific for particular rheumatic diseases, e.g., the Knee Injury and Osteoarthritis Outcomes Score (KOOS) (Roos et al. 1998). Several types of health status or HRQoL instruments available are listed in Table 16.4.

ARTHRITIS IMPACT MEASUREMENT SCALES (AIMS)

The Arthritis Impact Measurement Scales (AIMS) is a HRQoL instrument intended to measure change in global health, pain, mobility, and social function in patients with arthritis (Meenan et al. 1980). The AIMS was originally developed in English and now is available in more than 15 languages and has been validated in various ethnic populations. It is a self-administered instrument and available in three versions: AIMS, AIMS2, and AIMS2-SF.

The AIMS evaluates five components: physical activity, social role and activity, pain, depression, and anxiety. A lower score on the AIMS indicates a better

Table 16.3 Revised ACR criteria for classification of functional status in RA*

Class I	Completely able to perform usual activities of daily living (self-care, vocational, and avocational)
Class II	Able to perform usual self-care and vocational activities, but limited in avocational activities
Class III	Able to perform usual self-care activities, but limited in vocational and avocational activities
Class IV	Limited in ability to perform usual self-care, vocational, and avocational activities

*Usual self-care activities include dressing, feeding, bathing, grooming, and toileting. Avocational (recreational and/or leisure) and vocational (work, school, homemaking) activities are patient-desired and age- and sex-specific.

Table 16.4 Health status or health-related quality-of-life measures commonly used in arthritis patients

Questionnaire	Number of items	Dimensions covered (number of items)	Time recall
Arthritis Impact Measurement Scales (AIMS)	AIMS: 66 AIMS2: 78 AIMS2-SF: 26	Mobility level Walking and bending Hand and finger function Arm function Self-care Household tasks Social activities Support from family and friends Arthritis pain Work Level of tension Mood	During the past month
Health Assessment Questionnaire (HAQ)	HAQ Disability Index: 20, Pain Scale: 1, Global Health Status: 1	Dressing and grooming Arising Eating Walking Hygiene Reach Grip Activities	The past week
Short-Form Health Survey and Arthritis-Specific Health Index (SF-36 ASHI)	36	Physical functioning Role: physical Bodily pain General health Vitality Social functioning Role: emotional Mental health	Last week (acute version) 4 weeks (standard version)
McMaster-Toronto Arthritis patient function preference questionnaire (MACTAR)	19	Overall health Activities of daily living Social functioning Emotional functioning	The last 2 weeks
Western Ontario and McMaster Universities Osteoarthritis Index (WOMAC)	24	Pain Stiffness Physical function	48 hours
Knee Injury and Osteoarthritis Outcomes Score (KOOS)	42	Pain Other symptoms Activities of daily living functions Sport and recreation function Knee-related quality of life	Last week
Western Ontario Osteoarthritis of the Shoulder index (WOOS)	19	Physical symptoms (6 items) Sports/recreation/work (5 items) Lifestyle (5 items) Emotions (3 items)	Last week

(Continued)

Table 16.4 Health status or health-related quality-of-life measures commonly used in arthritis patients—Cont'd

Questionnaire	Number of items	Dimensions covered (number of items)	Time recall
Fibromyalgia Impact Questionnaire (FIQ)	20	Physical functioning (11 items) Well-being (1 item) Work related (2 items) Pain (1 item) Fatigue/sleep (2 items) Stiffness (1 item) Psychological symptoms (2 items)	During the past week
Quality of Life-Rheumatoid Arthritis Scale (QOL-RA Scale)	6	Positive and negative aspects of life with rheumatoid arthritis	Not specified
Osteoporosis Assessment Questionnaire (OPAQ)	OPAQ 1.0: 79 OPAQ 2.0: 54 + 18 optional weighting questions OPAQ SV: 34	Physical: Mobility Walking Flexibility Self-care Household Transfers Work Psychological: Fear of falls Tension Mood Body image Independence Symptoms: Back pain Pain Sleep Fatigue Social: Social activity Social support	The past 2 weeks
Quality of Life Questionnaire of the European Foundation for Osteoporosis (QUALEFFO)	48	Pain ADL Jobs around the house Moving Leisure/social activities General health perception Mood	The last week/the present time
Osteoporosis Quality of Life Questionnaire (OQLQ)	30	Symptoms Physical function Activities of daily living Emotional function Leisure	Not reported
Short Osteoporosis Quality of Life Questionnaire (ECOS-16)	16	Physical functioning (5 items) Illness-related fears (2 items) Psychosocial functioning (4 items) Pain (5 items)	The last week

HRQoL. The original version of the AIMS requires approximately 20 to 30 minutes to complete and is complicated to score. Accordingly, a revised version, the AIMS2, was developed, to overcome some of the original instrument's shortcomings (Meenan et al. 1992). The AIMS scale items were revised and three new scales were added to evaluate arm function, work, and social support. Sections were added to assess satisfaction with function, attribution of problems to arthritis, and self-designation of priority areas for improvement. Measurement performance was tested in 408 subjects. Internal consistency coefficients for the 12 scales were Cronbach's alpha 0.72–0.96 (Meenan et al. 1992). Test–retest reliability was 0.78–0.94 (Meenan et al. 1992). The AIMS2 is the most comprehensive of all disease-specific health status instruments for arthritis and specially developed for use in clinical research.

The average time to complete the AIMS2 instrument exceeds 20 minutes. Thus, the AIMS2-Short Form (AIMS2-SF) was developed as a 2-page derivative of AIMS2 (Guillemin et al. 1997). Psychometric properties of the AIMS2-SF and AIMS2 were compared using data from a cohort of 127 rheumatoid arthritis patients who completed the AIMS2 twice prior to the initiation of methotrexate treatment and 3 months' post-initiation of methotrexate treatment. Factor analysis showed preservation of the 5-component structure. Convergent validity (Physical and Symptom components with clinical variables: $r = 0.24$–0.59), test–retest reproducibility (intraclass correlation coefficient > 0.7), and sensitivity to change at 3 months (standardized response mean 0.36–0.8, except Social Interaction component [0.08]) were very close to the values for the original AIMS2.

An AIMS version for the geriatric population called the GERI-AIMS was developed to control for comorbid conditions that are commonly found in older patients (Hughes et al. 1991). An analysis of scores obtained on 438 elderly persons indicated that more than half of the total disability measured by the generic GERI-AIMS scores was related to arthritis. The GERI-AIMS scales had standardized-item alpha levels greater than 0.70 and correlated well with clinical measures of arthritis severity.

The AIMS-2 is available from: Dr. Meenan, Boston University School of Medicine, Dept. of Public Health, Boston, MA, USA.

HEALTH ASSESSMENT QUESTIONNAIRE (HAQ)

The Health Assessment Questionnaire (HAQ) is the most widely used RA tool throughout the world to assess clinical status, evaluate effectiveness of clinical and observational trials, and to define physical function (Bruce et al. 2003). It is an ACR-sanctioned instrument. The HAQ assesses difficulty in performing ADLs (Fries et al. 1980). Available versions of the HAQ are described below. The full version collects data on five generic patient-centered health dimensions: disability; pain and discomfort, adverse treatment effects, dollar costs of treatment, and postponement of death. Additionally, the full HAQ also assesses drug toxicity including data on drug, dosage, time on drug, specific side effects, degree of severity, importance to the patient, subsequent drug course, and direct and indirect cost data.

The most commonly used form of the HAQ is a 24-question, 2-page instrument that rates disability in ADLs and in instrumental activities of daily living (IADL) of 8 domains as listed in Table 16.1. This version is commonly referred as "the HAQ" and contains the HAQ Disability Index (HAQ-DI), the HAQ visual analog (VAS) pain scale, and the VAS patient global health scale. Disability is measured on a four point scale with scores ranging from zero indicating no difficulty to three representing inability to function. The highest score in each domain determines the category score. Scores are averaged to achieve the patient's Disability Index. The HAQ-DI indicates the extent of the respondent's functional ability, is sensitive to change, and is a good predictor of future disability and costs (Bruce et al. 2003). The HAQ pain scale is designed to assess the presence or absence of arthritis-related pain and its severity. It consists of a doubly anchored, horizontal VAS, that is scored from 0 (no pain) to three or 100 (severe pain). The HAQ pain scale is designed to obtain data relative to the presence or absence of arthritis-related pain and its severity. The HAQ index is very responsive to change and the suggested minimal clinical importance difference of 0.22 or 0.10 (Ramey et al. 1995). The HAQ-DI, HAQ-pain scale, and global health status scale have been validated in numerous studies and disciplines and translated or culturally adapted into more than 60 different languages. The HAQ-DI and pain scale usually take about five minutes, whereas the full HAQ takes approximately 20 to 30 minutes to complete.

The Modified Health Assessment Questionnaire (MHAQ) is a shortened version of the HAQ functional scale plus questions concerning perceived patient satisfaction regarding the ADL, along with perceived change in degree of difficulty (Pincus et al. 1983). In order to add additional questions while maintaining the length of the questionnaire in a format suitable in routine care, the number of ADL questions included in the MHAQ was reduced from 20 to 8. Recent studies comparing the original HAQ functional ability scale to the MHAQ have indicated that the MHAQ does not describe the full range of disability as well as the HAQ (Stucki et al. 1995; Wolfe 2001). Thus, although the format of the MHAQ has the advantage of eliciting a "satisfaction" score, limitations in its sensitivity to detect clinical improvement in patients with relatively little difficulty in activities of daily living (ceiling effect) may not justify the use of this particular version of shorter questionnaire in certain clinical settings.

A multidimensional HAQ (MDHAQ) was developed to overcome "floor effects" of the HAQ and MHAQ in which patients may report normal scores although they experience meaningful functional limitations. In addition psychological items, designed to screen efficiently for psychological distress in routine care, were added (Pincus et al. 1999).

In order to encompass key psychosocial variables, which are clinical determinants and outcomes in rheumatic disease, the Clinical Health Assessment Questionnaire (CLINHAQ) was developed (Wolfe 1997). The CLINHAQ is an aggregate of various instruments which assesses such surrogate psychosocial variables via visual analog scales for pain, fatigue, and sleep disturbance, the helplessness subscale of the Rheumatology Attitudes index, a self-report measure of satisfaction with health, and the AIMS anxiety and depression scales. It also contains the HAQ-DI, a pain diagram, and assessment of global severity, which can be completed in 5 minutes by almost all clinic patients.

Neumann et al. (2000) tested the Hebrew version of the CLINHAQ on a sample of 90 women with fibromyalgia (FM). Construct validity was tested by correlating the CLINHAQ items with measures of symptom severity, count of tender point, tenderness thresholds, physical functioning measured by FIQ, and with a score of QoL. Test–retest reliability coefficients ranged from 0.82 to 0.99, and Cronbach's alpha coefficients from 0.725 to 0.929. Significant moderate to high correlations were obtained between most subscales of CLINHAQ and measures of physical functioning, quality of life and severity of FM symptoms.

The HAQ with its instructions can be downloaded from: http://aramis.stanford.edu/HAQ.html (accessed May 12, 2004).

SHORT-FORM HEALTH SURVEY AND ARTHRITIS-SPECIFIC HEALTH INDEX (SF-36 AND ASHI)

The Medical Outcomes Study Short Form (SF-36) is the most widely used generic instrument to assess HRQoL in the general as well as disease populations (Ware et al. 1992; see also Chapter 1). An arthritis-specific health index (ASHI) for the SF-36 Health Survey was developed by studying its responsiveness to changes in clinical indicators of arthritis severity (Ware et al. 1999). In this instrument the items are the same as in the original SF-36, but it involves a different scoring algorithm. The ASHI appears to be more valid than the eight SF-36 scales and physical- and mental-component summary measures for purposes of distinguishing between treated and untreated patients and between clinical responders and nonresponders (Keller et al.

1999). Thus, the generic SF-36 health profile, which has already been shown to be useful in comparing arthritis with other diseases and treatments, can also be scored specifically to make it more useful in studies of osteoarthritis and rheumatoid arthritis. Additionally, the feasibility of improving the validity of the SF-36 through the use of arthritis-specific scoring also retains the option of generic scoring, which makes it possible to also compare results across diseases and treatments.

MCMASTER-TORONTO ARTHRITIS PATIENT FUNCTION PREFERENCE QUESTIONNAIRE (MACTAR)

The McMaster-Toronto Arthritis patient function preference questionnaire (MACTAR) is a functional index that was developed to assess change in impaired activities selected by each patient in a baseline interview, and change in rheumatoid arthritis (RA) disease activity (Tugwell et al. 1987). Patients are interviewed by trained interviewers and these interviews can last up to 15 minutes. Patients are asked to describe limitation in activities including self-care, household, work and leisure activities, social roles, and sexuality. Although the validity of the MACTAR has been established, its use is not favorable in standard clinical trials and practice due to its cost and resource limitations (Verhoeven et al. 2000).

WESTERN ONTARIO AND MCMASTER UNIVERSITIES OSTEOARTHRITIS INDEX (WOMAC)

The Western Ontario and McMaster Universities Arthritis Index (WOMAC) is a self-administered instrument designed to assess osteoarthritis-related disability in the hip and/or knee (Bellamy 1982). It is a 24-item, disease-specific outcome instrument that assesses pain, stiffness, and physical function. The latest version of the instrument (WOMAC™ 3.1) is available in 65 alternative language forms, and in most languages is available in both 5-point Likert and 100 mm Visual Analogue format. Likert scores range from 0 to 4, with higher scores reflecting more pain, stiffness and lower physical function (Brazier et al. 1999). The scores on the VAS version are usually normalized on a 100 mm (10 cm) VAS. It takes less than 5 minutes to complete, making it easy to use in clinical practice, and it is available in both paper and computer formats (Bellamy et al. 1997). The WOMAC™ 3.1 has been linguistically validated and is widely used in the evaluation of knee and hip osteoarthritis (Thumboo et al. 2001). Reliability coefficients (i.e., Cronbach's alpha, and Kendall's tau c statistic) exceeded 0.80 on both VAS and Likert scales (Bellamy et al. 1988). Construct validity was assessed by showing statistically significant ($p < 0.05$) Pearson's correlation coefficients on both Likert and VAS responses between test items on pain, stiffness and physical function indices with Lequesne-Pain, Lequesne-Stiffness, and Lequesne-Physical Function components on the Doyle Index. Finally, all 24 WOMAC items achieved statistical significance with p values ≤ 0.005 (Wilcoxon's test or Student's t test) after six weeks of treatment, establishing the responsiveness of WOMAC items (Bellamy et al. 1988).

More information on this instrument and on where to order the instrument and its User Guide can be obtained at: http://www.womac.org/womac/ (accessed May 12, 2004).

KNEE INJURY AND OSTEOARTHRITIS OUTCOMES SCORE (KOOS)

The Knee Injury and Osteoarthritis Outcomes Score (KOOS) HRQoL instrument, an extension of the WOMAC, was originally developed and validated in the Swedish language (Roos et al. 1998a) for younger and more active patients to assess short- and long-term patient-relevant outcomes following knee injury (Roos et al. 1998b). It is a 42-item self-administered questionnaire that takes approximately 10 minutes to complete, and available in eight languages including American English. The KOOS assesses five outcomes: pain, symptoms, activities of daily living, sport and recreation function, and knee-related quality of life. The five outcomes are scored separately on a 5-point Likert scale and range from 0 (no problems) to 4 (extreme problems). The scores are then transformed to a 0–100 scale, with zero representing extreme knee problems and 100 representing no knee problems to accord with common orthopedic scales (Barber et al. 1990) and generic measures (Ware et al. 1992).

The KOOS questionnaire, scoring guide and more information can be obtained from: http://www.koos.nu/ (accessed May 12, 2004).

WESTERN ONTARIO OSTEOARTHRITIS OF THE SHOULDER (WOOS) INDEX

The Western Ontario Osteoarthritis of the Shoulder (WOOS) index is a 19-item, self-administered, disease-specific HRQoL instrument developed to assess quality of life in clinical trials involving patients with osteoarthritis of the shoulder (Lo et al. 2001). It is intended to be used in patients greater than nine years of age and takes approximately 10 minutes to complete. Responses are measured on a VAS. A global score is computed that ranges from 0 to 1900. A lower score is indicative of better HRQoL. The instrument is validated and more responsive than other shoulder measurement tools, such as a global health status measure and range of motion, and is available in English, French, Spanish, and German languages.

QUALITY OF LIFE-RHEUMATOID ARTHRITIS (QOL-RA) SCALE

The Quality of Life-Rheumatoid Arthritis (QOL-RA) Scale is a disease-specific, HRQoL instrument developed to assess global quality of life based on positive and negative aspects of life in women with RA (Padilla et al. 1998). The 6-item questionnaire asks respondents to make separate ratings of their quality of life focusing on physical abilities, help received from family and friends, arthritis pain, tension, overall health, and overall arthritis impact. The responses are scored on a 10-point Likert scale ranging from 1 (very poor) to 10 (excellent). It was originally developed in American English and now also exists in Spanish for USA use as well (Danao et al. 2001). It can be self-administered or interviewer-administered by telephone or face to face and takes only two to four minutes to complete.

OSTEOPOROSIS ASSESSMENT QUESTIONNAIRE (OPAQ)

The Osteoporosis Assessment Questionnaire (OPAQ) is a HRQoL instrument developed to assess osteoporosis patients (Silverman et al. 1993). It was originally developed in American English and now also exists in Dutch, Brazilian Portuguese, Russian, and Spanish. The OPAQ 1.0 can be self-administered or interviewer-administered, whereas the OPAQ 2.0 and Short Version (SV) have only been used as self-administered instruments. The original version (OPAQ 1.0) has 79 items, 18 domains, and 4 dimensions as well as a global summary and a measure of patient satisfaction of each domain. The OPAQ is a reliable, consistent, and valid instrument able to distinguish a hierarchy of functional loss in disease states in osteoporosis (Randell et al. 1998).

QUALITY OF LIFE QUESTIONNAIRE OF THE EUROPEAN FOUNDATION FOR OSTEOPOROSIS (QUALEFFO)

The Quality of Life Questionnaire of the European Foundation for Osteoporosis (QUALEFFO) is a self-administered HRQoL instrument developed to measure quality of life for patients with vertebral osteoporosis (Lips et al. 1996). It is available in more than 10 languages. The instrument is meant for use in clinical trials and originally consisted of 48 items and 6 visual analogue scales. The questions concern the domains of pain, ADLs, jobs around the house, moving, leisure and social activities, general health perception and mood. Each domain score and total QUALEFFO scores are expressed on a 100-point scale, with 0 corresponding to the best HRQoL. In a follow-up validation study seven questions were removed from the instrument because of low response rate, linguistic ambiguities, or redundancy.

The QUALEFFO now consists of 41 items (Lips et al. 1999).

The QUALEFFO can be downloaded from: http://www.osteofound.org/publications/quality_of_life/index.html after signing a user agreement (accessed May 12, 2004).

OSTEOPOROSIS QUALITY OF LIFE QUESTIONNAIRE (OQLQ)

The Osteoporosis Quality of Life Questionnaire (OQLQ) is an instrument for measuring HRQoL for women with osteoporosis and back pain caused by vertebral fractures related to osteoporosis (Osteoporosis Quality of Life Study Group 1997). It has 30 items distributed across five domains: symptoms, physical function, ADL, emotional function, and leisure. A shortened osteoporosis OQLQ, called the mini-OQLQ, has been recently derived from the longer 30-item OQLQ, (four to nine items per domain) by choosing the two items with the highest impact in each of five domains, and has shown to demonstrate good discriminative and adequate evaluative properties (Cook et al. 1999). The mini-OQLQ is extremely effective because it is self-administered and quickly completed.

SHORT OSTEOPOROSIS QUALITY OF LIFE QUESTIONNAIRE (ECOS-16)

The short osteoporosis HRQoL questionnaire (ECOS-16) is a Spanish quality of life instrument developed to assess HRQoL among older female patients with osteoporosis (Badia et al. 2000). The 16-item questionnaire is derived from OQLQ (4 items) and the QUALEFFO (12 items) and takes less than 15 minutes to complete. The ECOS-16 is a relatively new instrument and requires further empirical validation (Badia et al. 2002).

PEDIATRIC HRQOL INSTRUMENTS

Functional status and health status measures have been developed for application in children with rheumatic diseases (Dufy et al. 1997). A brief description of the instruments is given below. Traditionally, the term juvenile rheumatoid arthritis (JRA) has been used. Recognizing that this form of pediatric arthritis is really quite different than RA, alternative names for the disease have been adopted in more recent years. There is not yet a consensus about the preferred term in the USA. The British term juvenile chronic arthritis (JCA) is now more commonly used to describe the disease.

In 1993 a nominal group of 16 members convened to establish a core set of outcome variables that would be valid, non-redundant and reliable measures for JRA to be used in clinical trials. After an extensive literature review and data derived from the DMARD clinical trial databank of the Pediatric Rheumatology Collaborative Study Group (PRCSG), the 16-expert panel decided on 6 core variables. The core variables are (1) functional disability, (2) MD global assessment of disease activity,(3) parent or patient global assessment for disease activity, (4) active joint count, (5) limited range of motion joint count, and (6) ESR. These 6 core variables underwent prospective validation as described below (Giannini 1994).

A total of 198 questionnaires were mailed out and 140 were returned from 88 European practitioners and 52 North American practitioners. The same 6 variables achieved the highest scores in the larger survey. The results of the survey indicated that improvement should be classified as 30% improvement within any given variable for all variables except functional ability which was 35%. The 6 outcome variables were assessed for multicollinearity with $r > 0.7$ considered to be evidence of redundancy. Only that number of active joints, and joints with limited range of motion, were considered to be collinear $r > 0.82$. The PRCSG data bank demonstrated $r > 0.65$ for the change in number of joints with limited range of motion, and number of active joints. This demonstrated that the core set of variables were correlated with not being excessively redundant. The advisory committee then proceeded to define the definition of improvement for the use of the 6 outcome variables. This was achieved in 1996 in Pavia, Italy, with the attendants of 21 pediatric rheumatologists with the goals to rate 72 paper patient profiles from an open label, uncontrolled trial of methotrexate conducted by the Italian Pediatric Rheumatology Study Group as clinically improved or not improved using the nominal group technique. The percent of false positive and false negative rates, chi square, sensitivity and specificity for each definition of improvement was judged by physician consensus. Another goal was to observe the ability of the definitions of improvement to discriminate between active agent and placebo using existing trial data. Two additional goals of this advisory committee were to decide upon the remaining definitions of improvement with the highest face validity, and finally to obtain the best definition for improvement. The definition for improvement for the 6 selected outcome variables is at least 30% improvement from baseline in 3 of any 6 variables in the core set, with no more than 1 of the remaining variables worsening by more than 30% (Giannini 1997).

CHILDHOOD ARTHRITIS IMPACT MEASUREMENT SCALES (CHAIMS)

In order to measure functional status, Coulton and colleagues applied and validated selected components of the AIMS in a sample of children with either active or inactive JRA (Coulton et al. 1987). These sets of scales have come to be known as the Childhood Arthritis Impact Measurement Scales (CHAIMS) and assess functional status in JRA patients in two dimensions – revised physical disability dimension; and the pain dimension. The original physical disability dimension consisted of the household activities scale, and was excluded from the CHAIMS in addition to scales in other dimensions. Possible scores ranged from 0 to 10 for each scale and dimension, with zero indicating no and ten indicating maximum disability. The psychometric properties of the instrument have not shown to be good except for the pain dimension that showed good reliability and convergent validity.

CHILDHOOD HEALTH ASSESSMENT QUESTIONNAIRE (CHAQ)

The Childhood Health Assessment Questionnaire (CHAQ) consists of 3 modules (Huber et al. 2001). The first is a generic childhood health questionnaire that measures physical functioning, bodily pain, general health perceptions, mental health, general behavior, self-esteem, parent influence on emotions, parent influence on time, family limitations, and cohesions. The second is a JRA generic or specific scale which evaluates gross motor function, fine motor functioning, ADLs, activity in family, friends and play, with the latter assessment adding school days missed, disability in school, symptoms of JRA (acute, chronic), and pain. The third module contains patient characteristics. The modules appear complex, but can be filled out in the clinic setting in 15 minutes by parents or patients aged 13 years or over (Duffy et al. 2000).

JUVENILE ARTHRITIS FUNCTIONAL ASSESSMENT SCALE (JAFAS) AND REPORT

The Juvenile Arthritis Functional Assessment Scale (JAFAS) is a disability assessment tool developed for, and validated in, patients with JRA (Lovell et al. 1989). Standards for this 10-item tool were developed using the scores of 63 normal school children as controls and comparing these results with those of 71 age-matched 7- to 16-year-old JRA patients. The JRA patients scored statistically significantly higher on the scale, which also demonstrated excellent internal and convergent validity and internal reliability (Lovell et al. 1989). The test is easily administered in 10 minutes by a physical or occupational therapist in a clinical or office setting.

Two questionnaires were developed for measuring disability due to juvenile rheumatoid arthritis (JRA), one based on patient (7–18 years) reports and one on parent reports. These questionnaires were termed the Juvenile Arthritis Functional Assessment Report for Children (JAFAR-C) and for Parents (JAFAR-P) (Howe et al. 1991). Respondents rated the patient's recent ability to perform 23 activities. The JAFAR appears to be a convenient, reliable, and valid measure of disability in patients with JRA.

JUVENILE ARTHRITIS SELF-REPORT INDEX (JASI)

The Juvenile Arthritis Self-report Index (JASI) is a 100-item functional status index for individuals with JRA, ages 8–18 years. The JASI assesses a variety of daily living and functional mobility tasks in children who have JRA (Wright et al. 1994). Part I of the JASI consists of 100 functional items divided into 5 activity categories: self-care, domestic, mobility, school, and extracurricular activities, and is rated on a 7-point difficulty scale. Part II is a priority function section within which the child identifies and scores important activities for improvement. The reliability and validity of JASI are excellent and research is under way to evaluate responsiveness to change and develop shorter JRA functional measures to determine differences in sensitivity (Wright et al. 1996).

JUVENILE ARTHRITIS QUALITY OF LIFE QUESTIONNAIRE (JAQQ)

The Juvenile Arthritis Quality of Life Questionnaire (JAQQ) is a disease-specific measure of HRQoL for application in children with JRA and juvenile spondyloarthritides. This 74-item questionnaire contains 4 dimensions: gross motor function (17 items), fine motor function (16 items), psychosocial function (22 items), and general symptoms (19 items). Responses are rated on a 7-point Likert scale and the instrument has been developed and validated in English and French versions (Duffy et al. 1997).

CHILDHOOD ARTHRITIS HEALTH PROFILE (CAHP)

The Childhood Arthritis Health Profile (CAHP) is a self-administered parent report consisting of three modules: generic health status measures, JRA specific health status measures and patient characteristics (Tucker et al. 1995). The CAHP has been shown to have good internal reliability, with inter-item correlations within scales ranging from 0.84 to 0.97. The discriminant validity of the CAHP was published in abstract form where differences in the JRA-specific scales were compared with clinician-rated disease severity and activity. Significant differences were seen across disease severity and activity for gross motor function, fine motor function, usual role activities affected by JRA, and school functioning, confirming the discriminant ability of the CAHP (Tucker et al. 1996).

CONCLUSION

Patients' ability to carry out activities of daily living (ADLs) is greatly influenced by their physical and psychological status and by the environment and society in which they live (Thompson 1988). The American

College of Rheumatology (ACR) recommends assessing patient-reported quality of life outcomes in addition to the traditional clinical assessments to be a part of disease activity measurements (Lubeck 2003). Great efforts have been made to develop robust, generalizable, standardized measures of functional ability, quality of life and health outcomes to provide some homogeneity in the measures assessed in arthritis trials. This chapter provides an overview of assessment instruments used in clinical trials and practice to evaluate the impact of interventions on HRQoL in patients with arthritis. As more robust interventions for arthritis are investigated, a higher threshold for improvement is desirable to help define optimal therapy, especially in this era of managed care and increasingly expensive treatment modalities.

REFERENCES

Anderson JJ, Felson DT, Meenan RF, et al. Which traditional measures should be used in rheumatoid arthritis clinical trials? Arthritis Rheum 1989; 32:1093–1099.

Badia X, Prieto L, Roset M, et al. Development of the ECOS-16 clinical questionnaire for the assessment of the quality of life in patients with osteoporosis. Med Clin 2000; 114:68–75.

Badia X, Prieto L, Roset M, et al. Development of a short osteoporosis quality of life questionnaire by equating items from two existing instruments. J Clin Epidemiol 2002; 55:32–40.

Barber SD, Noyes FR, Manine RE, et al. Quantitative assessment of functional limitations in normal and anterior cruciate ligament-deficient knees. Clin Orthop 1990:204–214.

Bellamy N. Osteoarthritis: an evaluative index for clinical trials. MSc thesis, McMaster University, Hamilton, Canada, 1982.

Bellamy N, Buchanan WW, Goldsmith CH, et al. Validation study of WOMAC: a health status instrument for measuring clinically important patient relevant outcomes to antirheumatic drug therapy in patients with osteoarthritis of the hip or knee. J Rheumatol 1988; 15:1833–1840.

Bellamy N, Campbell J, Stevens J, et al. Validation study of a computerized version of the Western Ontario and McMaster Universities VA3.0 Osteoarthritis Index. J Rheumatol 1997; 24:2413–2415.

Boers M, Verhoeven AC, van der Linden S. American College of Rheumatology criteria for improvement in rheumatoid arthritis should only be calculated from scores that decrease on improvement. Arthritis Rheum 2001; 44:1052–1055.

Brazier JE, Harper R, Munro J, et al. Generic and condition-specific outcome measures for people with OA of the knee. Rheumatology 1999; 38:870–879.

Bruce B, Fries JF. The Stanford Health Assessment Questionnaire: a review of its history, issues, progress, and documentation. J Rheumatol 2003; 30:167–178.

Burckhardt CS, Clark SR, Bennett RM. The fibromyalgia impact questionnaire: development and validation. J Rheumatol 1991; 18:728–733.

Cook DJ, Guyatt GH, Adachi JD, et al. Development and validation of the mini-osteoporosis quality of life questionnaire (OQLQ) in osteoporotic women with back pain due to vertebral fractures. Osteoporosis Quality of Life Study Group. Osteoporos Int 1999; 10:207–213.

Coulton CJ, Zborowsky E, Lipton J, et al. Assessment of the reliability and validity of the arthritis impact measurement scales for children with juvenile arthritis. Arthritis Rheum 1987; 30:819–824.

Danao LL, Padilla GV, Johnson DA. An English and Spanish quality of life measure for rheumatoid arthritis. Arthritis Rheum 2001; 45:167–173.

Duffy CM, Duffy KN. Health assessment in the rheumatic diseases of childhood. Curr Opin Rheumatol 1997; 9:440–447.

Duffy CM, Tucker L, Burgos-Vargas R. Update on functional assessment tools. J Rheumatol 2000; 27:11–14.

Escalante A. What do self-administered joint counts tell us about patients with rheumatoid arthritis? Arthritis Care Res 1998; 11:280–290.

Felson DT, Anderson JJ, Boers M, et al. The American College of Rheumatology preliminary core set of disease activity measures for rheumatoid arthritis clinical trials. The Committee on Outcome Measures in Rheumatoid Arthritis Clinical Trials. Arthritis Rheum 1993; 36:729–740.

Felson DT, Anderson JJ, Lange ML, et al. Should improvement in rheumatoid arthritis clinical trials be defined as fifty percent or seventy percent improvement in core set measures, rather than twenty percent? Arthritis Rheum 1998; 41:1564–1570.

Fries JF, Spitz P, Kraines RG, et al. Measurement of patient outcome in arthritis. Arthritis Rheum 1980; 23:137–145.

Guillemin F, Coste J, Pouchot J, et al. The AIMS2-SF: a short form of the Arthritis Impact Measurement Scales 2. French Quality of Life in Rheumatology Group. Arthritis Rheum 1997; 40:1267–1274.

Howe S, Levinson J, Shear E, et al. Development of a disability measurement tool for juvenile rheumatoid arthritis. The Juvenile Arthritis Functional Assessment Report for Children and their Parents. Arthritis Rheum 1991; 34:873–880.

Huber AM, Hicks JE, Lachenbruch PA, et al. Juvenile Dermatomyositis Disease Activity Collaborative Study Group. Validation of the Childhood Health Assessment Questionnaire in the juvenile idiopathic myopathies. Juvenile Dermatomyositis Disease Activity Collaborative Study Group. J Rheumatol 2001; 28:1106–1111.

Hughes SL, Edelman P, Chang RW, et al. The GERI-AIMS. Reliability and validity of the arthritis impact measurement scales adapted for elderly respondents. Arthritis Rheum 1991; 34:856–865.

Keller SD, Ware JE Jr, Hatoum HT, et al. The SF-36 Arthritis-Specific Health Index (ASHI): II. Tests of validity in four clinical trials. Med Care 1999; 37:MS51–MS60.

Lips P, Agnusdei D, Caulin F, et al. The development of a European questionnaire for quality of life in patients with vertebral osteoporosis. Scand J Rheumatol 1996; 103:84–85.

Lips P, Cooper C, Agnusdei D, et al. Quality of life in patients with vertebral fractures: validation of the Quality of Life Questionnaire of the European Foundation for Osteoporosis (QUALEFFO). Osteoporos Int 1999; 10:150–160.

Lo IK, Griffin S, Kirkley A. The development of a disease-specific quality of life measurement tool for osteoarthritis of the shoulder: the Western Ontario Osteoarthritis of the Shoulder (WOOS) index. Osteoarthritis Cartilage 2001; 9:771–778.

Lovell DJ, Howe S, Shear E, et al. Development of a disability measurement tool for juvenile rheumatoid arthritis. The Juvenile Arthritis Functional Assessment Scale. Arthritis Rheum 1989; 32:1390–1395.

Lubeck DP. The cost of musculoskeletal disease: health needs assessment and health economics. Best Practice Res Clin Rheumato 2003; 17:529–539.

Meenan RF, Gertman PM, Mason JH. Measuring health status in arthritis. The arthritis impact measurement scales. Arthritis Rheum 1980; 23:146–152.

Meenan RF, Mason JH, Anderson JJ, et al. AIMS2. The content and properties of a revised and expanded Arthritis Impact Measurement Scales Health Status Questionnaire. Arthritis Rheum 1992; 35:1–10.

Osteoporosis Quality of Life Study Group. Measuring quality of life in women with osteoporosis. Osteoporos Int 1997; 7:478–487.

Padilla GV, Berkanovic E, Louie J, et al. Quality of life – Rheumatoid Arthritis Scale. Quality of Life Newsletter 1998; 20:11–12.

Pincus T, Summey JA, Soraci SA Jr, et al. Assessment of patient satisfaction in activities of daily living using a modified Stanford Health Assessment Questionnaire. Arthritis Rheum 1983; 26:1346–1353.

Pincus T, Swearingen C, Wolfe F. Toward a multidimensional Health Assessment Questionnaire (MDHAQ): assessment of advanced activities of daily living and psychological status in the patient-friendly health assessment questionnaire format. Arthritis Rheum 1999; 42:2220–2230.

Ramey D, Fries J, Singh G. The Health Assessment Questionnaire 1995: status and review. In: Spilker B (ed). Quality of Life and Pharmacoeconomics in Clinical Trials. Lippincott-Raven, Philadelphia, PA, 1995:227–237.

Randell AG, Bhalerao N, Nguyen TV, et al. Quality of life in osteoporosis: reliability, consistency, and validity of the Osteoporosis Assessment Questionnaire. J Rheumatol 1998; 25:1171–1179.

Roos EM, Roos HP, Ekdahl C, et al. Knee injury and Osteoarthritis Outcome Score (KOOS) – validation of a Swedish version. Scand J Med Sci Sports 1998a; 8:439–448.

Roos EM, Roos HP, Lohmander LS, et al. Knee Injury and Osteoarthritis Outcome Score (KOOS): development of a self-administered outcome measure. J Orthop Sports Phys Ther 1998b; 28:88–96.

Silverman SL, Mason J, Grennwald M. The Osteoporosis Assessment Questionnaire (OPAQ): a reliable and valid self-assessment measure of quality of life in osteoporosis. J Bone Miner Res 1993; 8:S343.

Smolen JS, Breedveld FC, Schiff MH, et al. A simplified disease activity index for rheumatoid arthritis for use in clinical practice. Rheumatology (Oxford) 2003; 42:244–257.

Thompson PW. Functional outcome in rheumatoid arthritis. Br J Rheumatol 1988; 27:37–43.

Thumboo J, Chew LH, Soh CH. Validation of the Western Ontario and McMaster University Osteoarthritis Index in Asians with osteoarthritis in Singapore. Osteoarthritis Cartilage 2001; 9:440–446.

Tucker LB, De Nardo BA, Abetz LN. The Childhood Arthritis Health Profile (CHAP): validity and reliability of the condition specific scales. Arthritis Rheum 1995; 38:S57.

Tucker LB, De Nardo BA, Schaller JG. The Childhood Arthritis Health Profile: correlation of juvenile-rheumatoid arthritis specific scales with disease severity and activity. Arthritis Rheum 1996; 39:S57.

Tugwell P, Bombardier C, Buchanan WW, et al. The MACTAR Patient Preference Disability Questionnaire: an individualized functional priority approach for assessing improvement in physical disability in clinical trials in rheumatoid arthritis. J Rheumatol 1987; 14:446–451.

van der Heijde DM, van 't Hof MA, van Riel PL, et al. Judging disease activity in clinical practice in rheumatoid arthritis: first step in the development of a disease activity score. Ann Rheum Dis 1990; 49:916–920.

Verhoeven AC, Boers M, van der Liden S. Validity of the MACTAR questionnaire as a functional index in a rheumatoid arthritis clinical trial. The McMaster Toronto Arthritis. J Rheumatol 2000; 27:2801–2809.

Ware JE Jr, Sherbourne CD. The MOS 36-item short-form health survey (SF-36): I. Conceptual framework and item selection. Med Care 1992; 30:473–483.

Ware JE Jr, Keller SD, Hatoum HT, et al. The SF-36 Arthritis-Specific Health Index (ASHI): I. Development and cross-validation of scoring algorithms. Med Care 1999; 37: MS40–MS50.

Wolfe F. Practical issues in psychosocial measures. J Rheumatol 1997; 24:990–993.

Wolfe F. Which HAQ is best? A comparison of the HAQ, MHAQ and RA-HAQ, a difficult 8 item HAQ (DHAQ), and a rescored 20 item HAQ (HAQ20): analyses in 2491 rheumatoid arthritis patients following leflunomide initiation. J Rheumatol 2001; 28:982–989.

Wright FV, Law M, Crombie V, et al. Development of a self-report functional status index for juvenile rheumatoid arthritis. J Rheumatol 1994; 21:536–544.

Wright FV, Kimber JL, Law M, et al. The Juvenile Arthritis Functional Status Index (JASI): a validation study. J Rheumatol 1996; 23:1066–1079.

FURTHER READING

Duffy CM, Arsenault L, Duffy KN, et al. The Juvenile Arthritis Quality of Life Questionnaire: development of a new responsive index for juvenile rheumatoid arthritis and juvenile spondyloarthritides. J Rheumatol 1997; 24:738–746.

Hawley DJ. Functional ability, health status, and quality of life. In: Wegener ST, Belza BL, Gall EP (eds). Clinical Care in the Rheumatic Diseases. American College of Rheumatology, 1996:53–59.

Hochberg MC, Chang RW, Dwosh I, et al. The American College of Rheumatology 1991 revised criteria for the classification of global functional status in rheumatoid arthritis. Arthritis Rheum 1992; 35:498–502.

Stucki G, Liang MH, Stucki S, et al. A self-administered Rheumatoid Arthritis Disease Activity Index (RADAI) for epidemiologic research: psychometric properties and correlation with parameters of disease activity. Arthritis Rheum 1995a; 38:795–798.

Stucki G, Stucki S, Bruhlmann P, et al. Ceiling effects of the Health Assessment Questionnaire and its modified version in some ambulatory rheumatoid arthritis patients. Ann Rheum Dis 1995b; 54:461–465.

van Gestel AM, Anderson JJ, van Riel PL, et al. ACR and EULAR improvement criteria have comparable validity in rheumatoid arthritis trials. American College of Rheumatology European League of Associations for Rheumatology. J Rheumatol 1999; 26:705–711.

CHAPTER 17

Measuring functional status in patients with chronic musculoskeletal pain

Harriët Wittink • Erwin van Wegen

INTRODUCTION: THE PROBLEM OF MUSCULOSKELETAL PAIN

Worldwide, musculoskeletal conditions are the most common causes of severe long-term pain and physical disability. Chronic musculoskeletal pain (CMP) represents a significant burden to all sectors of the population, with pain interfering with the ability to perform activities of daily living (ADL: washing, dressing, grooming and eating) and instrumental activities of daily living (IADL: walking, shopping, getting to work). In older adults activity limitations may progressively lead to loss of independence, while in the working age musculoskeletal impairments are the most common causes for reduced work performance, sick days and work disability. The consequences in terms of the health status and suffering of patients and their families, for employers in terms of lost productivity during work and sick days and for society as a whole in terms of welfare benefits and health care costs are enormous. For example: a recent study (Stewart et al. 2003) found that the prevalence of arthritis, back pain, headache, and other musculoskeletal conditions was 52.7% among the workforce. Overall, 12.7% of the workforce lost an average of 4.6 hours of productive time in a 2 week period. The cost due to lost productivity time in the USA because of these common pain conditions to employers was estimated at $61.2 billion a year.

Musculoskeletal pain encompasses all pain in muscle, connective tissue, bone and joints due to disease, injury or trauma. There are more than 150 different musculoskeletal disorders, all of which share symptoms of pain and/or inflammation and can involve limitation of motion, disability and even death (Lidgren 2003). Joint diseases account for more than half of all chronic conditions in persons aged 60 years and over. Back pain is the most frequent cause of limitation of activity in the young and middle aged, one of the commonest reasons for medical consultation, the most frequent occupational injury and the second leading cause of sick leave (Lidgren 2003). With the aging population the incidence and prevalence of CMP is expected to rise exponentially with a concomitant escalation of treatment costs. The burden of musculoskeletal pain (MP) has been recognized by the United Nations and the World Health Organization (WHO) by endorsing the Bone and Joint Decade 2000–2010. The goal for the Bone and Joint Decade is to improve the health-related quality of life for people with musculoskeletal disorders throughout the world.

The prevalence of MP is difficult to estimate because there appears to be no agreement on what to measure between medical specialists, medical specialties and the general public and between cultures and languages (Picavet and Hazes 2003). MP has been measured across a number of diseases, by site of pain, by wide spread or local pain, by varying time frames (e.g., "in the past year," "lasting more than one week," or "for at least 5 consecutive days"), by patient self report and/or physician assessment. Disease specific surveys have gathered data on osteoporosis, osteoarthritis (OA), rheumatoid arthritis (RA), fibromyalgia, repetitive strain injury, capsulitis and tendonitis, whereas site specific surveys have included back and neck pain, and shoulder, knee and/or elbow pain. The prevalence of many of these conditions increase markedly by age and many are affected by lifestyle factors such as obesity and lack of physical activity (Woolf and Pfleger 2003). For these largely chronic non-fatal conditions, disability assessment is more important than mortality figures, and the WHO-revised classification of effects of health conditions, the International Classification of Functioning, Disability and Health (ICF), provides a framework to describe the consequences of MP and factors that may influence them. A WHO scientific group meeting considered *pain*, *mobility*, and *independence* to be the most relevant domains for musculoskeletal conditions, and it identified the need for simpler instruments usable in all populations to monitor these aspects (Woolf and Akesson 2001).

Diagnostic and intervention codes, currently used in health administrative records, reveal nothing about the outcome of the health care system that is meaningful to patients' lives. The impact of a disease, injury or trauma on a person's life can be understood by measuring the capacity to carry out the full range of actions, activities and tasks required to fully engage in all areas of human life (Ustun et al. 2003b). The outcome of health care interventions should therefore be measured in terms of functional status. The importance of the measurement of functional ability was underscored by a report by the National Committee on Vital and Health Statistics (NCVHS) in 2001 in which was stated "without functional status information, the researchers, policymakers and others who are already using administrative data have at best a rough idea of how people, individually and collectively, are doing and at worst they are making erroneous assumptions and decisions."

Musculoskeletal conditions are a diverse group with regard to pathophysiology but are linked anatomically by their association with pain and impaired function. Moreover, the pain and physical disability brought about by musculoskeletal conditions affects social functioning and mental health, further diminishing the patient's quality of life (Woolf and Pfleger 2003).

Because they cover an area of such fundamental concern in health care, there has been a proliferation of scales that measure physical activity levels, functional limitations and participation restrictions. The available measurement methods serve a variety of purposes: some apply to particular diseases, while others are broadly applicable; there are research instruments, screening tests, and clinical rating scales; some methods are designed for severely ill inpatients, while others are for outpatients with lower levels of limitations, or for the general population with no limitations. Physical activity questionnaires, for instance, measure type, frequency, intensity and duration of occupational, household and leisure time activities. These questionnaires are mostly used for epidemiologic studies interested in assessing typical or long-term physical activity due to its potential association with diseases. Some of these instruments are starting to emerge in studies on (C)MP (Verbunt et al. 2005).

Many self-report instruments have been developed, some generic, others disease specific, and there is evidence of good reliability and validity for a number of them. In validation studies, estimates of physical activity or functional limitations made by a questionnaire are compared with those measured by a more accurate method, ideally a gold standard. Unfortunately there are no perfect measures of physical activity or activity limitations. Comparison measures include both "subjective" measures (based on self report) and "objective" measures (based on direct measurement). Self-report measures can be self-administered or interviewer administered, both in person or on the telephone. Objective measures include functional capacity tasks, markers of movement (accelerometers), and observed or videotaped activity (direct observation). Self reported status often involves outcomes of most relevance and importance to patients and their loved ones because they capture patient experience and perspective (Patrick and Chiang 2000). Objective measurements may have more meaning to clinicians in terms of formulating a treatment plan. In CMP relatively few comparison studies have been performed between self report and objective measures. The studies that are available seem to indicate a gap between self report and objective measurement (Verbunt et al. 2001). It is not clear as yet whether this gap reflects different measurement methods and measurement error, a difference between the patient's perception and objective reality of their ability to function or whether the different measurement methods tap into different domains of functioning.

A recent review on reporting on reliability and validity of outcome measures in medical rehabilitation research found that the 171 papers identified included 651 outcome measures. Some type of reliability data was provided for 20.1% of these measures; for validity this was 6.9% (Dijkers et al. 2002). Physical impairments were the most common class of outcomes

(60%), while functional assessment comprised 12% of the outcome measures. The WHO report on the burden of musculoskeletal conditions at the start of a new millennium (2003) identifies 147 instruments for the measurement of MP for which some reliability and validity data exist. Garratt et al. (2002) in their systematic review of self-report instruments found 147 dimension specific instruments for physical function. It is therefore a daunting and virtually impossible task to cover all functional assessment instruments in a single chapter. It is not the intention of this chapter to be all-inclusive, but rather to give an overview of frequently used instruments that measure functional ability and functional limitations from self-report to objective assessment methods.

As Chapter 16 discusses instruments applicable for osteoarthritis and rheumatoid arthritis as well as fibromyalgia and osteoporosis, we will focus on neck and back pain when discussing disease-specific instruments as these conditions belong to the most prevalent and costly of CMP. For disease-specific instruments on shoulder pain and dysfunction, see the recent review by Bot et al. (2004).

We performed a systematic search using the search terms "outcome measure, outcome assessment, questionnaire, or measurement" with "musculoskeletal pain, back pain or neck pain" in PubMed, Medline, CINAHL and PsychLit in an attempt to be as comprehensive as possible within the constraints of a single chapter. Citations were supplemented by the authors' personal databases, hand searches of *Spine* and current textbooks on rating scales and questionnaires.

DEFINITION OF FUNCTION

While it is understood that CMP has a major impact of people's ability to function we are faced with two fundamental problems, namely how is "function" defined and how do we best measure it?

The literature as a whole suffers from imprecise terminology and function is no exception. Terms used include physical functioning, functional ability, physical ability, physical activity, activity, capacity, performance, activity level, functional status, functional limitations, physical inability, activity restrictions and physical functional status. The words capacity, performance and ability, but also physical (body functions and structure, such as muscle strength, range of motion and coordination) and functional (activities such as walking, sitting and standing), are being used interchangeably. In order for clinicians and researchers to understand each other a common language with clear definitions of terms is imperative (Wittink 2005).

Nagi (1991) described the pathway to diminished physical functioning as a series of four steps. The initial step in this pathway is the onset of disease states, followed by the physiologic manifestation of disease in multiple systems, leading to functional limitations, such as difficulty walking, grasping, climbing stairs, and, ultimately, the onset of disability, described as the inability to fulfill roles. Halter and Reuben (2001) have proposed a useful model to describe how the "building blocks" of functioning are integrated to form a hierarchy of ability. These building blocks include strength, balance, coordination, flexibility, and endurance. At the most basic level of integration, these elements are coordinated to execute specific physical movements such as rolling over, sitting up, standing, walking, and gripping. In the second integration level, these movements are coordinated into more specific goal-oriented functional tasks (e.g., instrumental activities of daily living), such as dressing, bathing, feeding, writing, and climbing stairs. At the highest level of integration, the goal-oriented functional tasks are coordinated with cognitive and affective resources and integrated into behaviors aimed at fulfilling societal roles and recreational activities, the so-called advanced activities of daily living (AADL) (Reuben and Solomon 1989). At this level, function is often determined by personal choice rather than by physical capacity.

The International Classification of Functioning, Disability and Health (ICF) (World Health Organization 2001) provides a biopsychosocial model that identifies three concepts described from the perspective of body systems, the individual and society. For the definitions within the model see Table 17.1.

Each component of the ICF can be expressed in either neutral or negative terms. Disability is the ICF umbrella term for impairment, activity limitation and participation restrictions. Non-problematic or neutral aspects of health and health-related states can be summarized under the umbrella term functioning (refers to all Body Functions, Activities and Participation). Although the WHO has stated that it is difficult to distinguish between the Activities and Participation domains, there is evidence that conceptualizing activity as being at the person level and participation at the societal level can separate these concepts (Rogers et al. 2000a,b; Jette et al. 2003). Contextual factors are provided within the ICF framework, consisting of environmental factors and personal factors.

Qualifiers for the Activities and Participation classification make it possible to clearly separate the patient's inherent capacity to perform actions within a domain and performance in his or her actual environmental context (Ustun et al. 2003a). Capacity refers to what a person can do in a standardized environment, while performance refers to what persons actually do in their own environment. From a rehabilitation perspective the gap between capacity and performance, i.e., the difference between what a person can do and what a person actually does, is of particular use for treatment planning and outcome assessment. Figure 17.1

Table 17.1 Definitions of the ICF domains and measurements

Functional status domain	Definition	Measurement
Body Function and Structure	Physiologic functions of body systems or anatomical elements, such as organs, limbs and their components. This includes: static and dynamic muscular strength, flexibility of the joints and surrounding tissues, coordination, muscular and cardiovascular endurance, etc.	Physiologic measurements such as VO2max, maximal heart rate
Impairments	Limitations in functions of body systems or anatomical elements	CT scan, MRI, x-rays, physiologic parameters, ROM, strength
Activity	Execution of specific tasks or actions by an individual	ADL and IADL self-report (frequency questions, capacity questions such as "can you?" and performance questions, such as "do you?") pertaining to specific functional tasks (individual based)
Activity limitation	Difficulties an individual may have in executing activities	Individual based self-report (limitation or interference questions)
Participation	Involvement in life situation with emphasis on the person's involvement in society	AADL self-report (frequency questions, capacity questions such as "can you?" and performance questions, such as "do you?") pertaining to functional activities in a social context
Participation restriction	Restriction in involvement in life situation	Social context based self-report (limitation or interference questions)
Activity and Participation Capacity	The highest probable level of functioning that a person may reach in a given domain at a given moment in a standardized or uniform environment	Externally observable functional test in standardized environment, such as functional capacity testing
Activity and Participation Performance	Describes what a person does in his or her current environment (ICF), in usual or current environment, and thus describes the person's functioning as observed or reported in the person's real-life environment with the existing facilitators and barriers (Stucki et al. 2002)	Accelerometry, videotaping
Environmental factors	Physical, social and attitudinal environment in which people live and conduct their lives	Self-report on significant others, work environment, etc.
Personal factors	E.g., fear-avoidance, coping, catastrophizing	Self-report on worry, fear, bothersomeness or "harm" items

represents the conceptual model as applied to patients with chronic pain.

Having formulated a hypothetical conceptual framework, the next problem is what and how to measure. Most of the self-administered instruments typically focus on performance, i.e., patients' perception of what they do (activities and participation). Questions tend to include the following categories:

Can you? Or: are you capable of/able to? (capacity question)

Do you? (performance question)

How often do you do a particular task/social activity? (frequency question)

Does your health (pain, stiffness, fatigue) interfere with what you do and how much? (interference or limitation question)

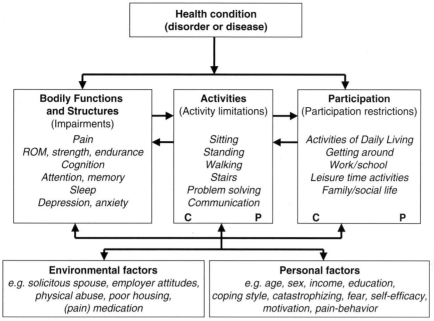

Figure 17.1 An ICF model as applied to patients with chronic pain (C = capacity; P = participation).

Do you have difficulty with a particular task? (effort question)

Do you need help doing it and how much? (assistance or dependence question).

Personal factor questions include:

Does it bother you that you are limited in these activities? (meaning of interference or limitation question)

Do you avoid activities? (fear of movement, fear of pain question).

McDowell and Newell (1996) believe that capacity oriented questions tend to exaggerate the healthiness of the respondent, whereas performance questions provide a more realistic assessment of the actual disability. Since capacity and performance questions tap into different domains of the ICF Activities and Participation domains they are both important and should not be substituted for the other. In practical terms, the distinction has been blurred and some questionnaires use "difficulty," "trouble" and "avoid" in the same scale. Limitation or interference questions as seen in the SF-36 Physical Functioning scale such as "does your health limit you doing a particular task?" with responses ranging from "yes, limited a lot" to "no, not limited at all" reflect activity limitations and participation restrictions. The Multidimensional Personality Inventory (MPI) activity scale includes frequency questions such as "how often do you…wash dishes/play cards/go grocery shopping, etc?" with responses ranging from "very often" to "never." A recent paper showed very little overlap between these two scales (Wittink et al. 2004),

supporting that, although both scales measure functional status, they measure different aspects of the functional activities domain. The lack of overlap begs the question whether these scales can be combined in, for instance, a meta-analysis.

Functional status is a patient-referenced concept and it is different for each individual, with some patients making higher demands on function than others (Beurskens et al. 1995). With the wide range of physical capacities and functional activity levels in the population the patient is presumed to "calibrate" the instrument individually (Salen et al. 1994). For instance, a young construction worker will have a different concept of a "heavy lift" than an eighty year old. In limitation questionnaires each patient will rate questions about functional status from his or her own internal standard of what their "normal" level of functioning was. Thus, functional status, or for that matter any self report instrument, is filtered by the subjective perceptions and expectations of the individual patient (Testa and Simonson 1996). This equally goes for expectations of improvement in functional status. Questionnaires may not be suited to detect change, either because of ambiguity in wording, the way scales are constructed (dichotomous versus multileveled), timing, or even mode of administration (Epstein 2000). For instance, if yes/no options are used, the effect of an intervention that reduced, but did not eliminate, difficulty with a functional task could not be detected (Greenough and Fraser 1992). Furthermore, respondents may be at the ceiling or floor of a given scale and have nowhere to go in terms of measurement of change (Epstein 2000). Guyatt et al. (1987) defined responsiveness as the ability of a scale to detect minimally clinically important differences (MCID). Liang (2000) defined responsiveness as "the ability of an instrument to measure a meaningful or important change in a clinical state," as opposed to sensitivity which is the "ability of an instrument to measure change in a state irrespective of whether it is relevant and/or meaningful to the decision maker." With this definition responsiveness equates to longitudinal construct validity.

When a questionnaire can detect change, however, one patient may find a small change clinically important, while for another patient a large change in that scale is not clinically important. If one starts out with excellent functioning, even a small decrement might cause a large change in expected functioning. For instance, an ankle distortion can completely disable an athlete, but may interfere with walking "a little bit" for the majority of people. Individuals at lower initial levels might find the same decrement negligible, or just the opposite might be true (Testa 2000). Consequently, minimally clinically important differences are difficult to interpret as the operative range that defines the MCID is typically not constant over the full range of the scale.

Patient-based outcomes are usually classified as generic or disease specific. Generic measures are designed to be applicable to patients across populations and different types of conditions. Normative data may exist to allow for comparison with the "healthy" population. The hallmark of a disease specific instrument is the attribution of symptoms and limitations to a specific disease or condition. In this chapter this means the attribution of limitations in functional activities to back or neck pain. Both generic and disease specific instruments can be one-dimensional (measure one domain or construct, such as functional status) or multidimensional (measure multiple domains, such as symptoms (e.g., pain), functional status, mental health and social functioning). Most self-report instruments are – intentioned or not – multidimensional in nature (see also Table 17.2).

GENERIC INSTRUMENTS

The first measurements of ADL were observer ratings, introduced by Karnofsky in 1948. The Karnofsky measure (see Chapter 23) is still used today, mostly in hospital settings and in very sick patients. One of the first self-report measures was developed by Katz and colleagues (1963), reflecting an assessment of difficulties in performing what were referred to as "Activities of Daily Living" (e.g., dressing, eating, toileting, transferring from a bed to a chair, bathing, dressing and maintaining continence).

McDowell and Newell (1996), in their outstanding guide to measuring health, report to have found more than 50 ADL scales in the literature, but review seven due to the lack of reliability and validity of many of the scales. The ADL scales in general are generic, applicable to severely impaired inpatients and nursing home residents and include the Barthel Index (Mahoney et al. 1958) (see Instrument), the Index of Independence in Activities of Daily Living, or Index of ADL (Katz and Akpom 1976), the Physical Self-Maintenance Scale (Lawton and Brody 1969) and the Functional Status Rating System (Forer and Miller 1980). The type of questionnaire to choose depends on the target population. ADL questionnaires were devised quite specifically for inpatient rehabilitation use and include severe dysfunctions (toileting, continence and feeding). ADL scales are therefore not able to identify low levels of disability, nor minor changes in level of disability. Community ambulating patients are likely to score at the ceiling of these scales and thus need scales with more complex items, such as walking, doing stairs, getting outside, cooking, shopping, housework and transportation (i.e., IADL scales). The following instruments are IADL-based instruments that can be used in a wide range of patients with musculoskeletal pain.

PAIN DISABILITY INDEX (PDI)

The Pain Disability Index (PDI) (Pollard 1984; Tait et al. 1987) is composed of 7 calibrated visual analogue scales, divided into tenths. It measures the impact of average pain on each of 7 areas of normal daily activities:

1. Family and home responsibilities: activities related to home and family
2. Recreation: hobbies, sports and other leisure time activities
3. Social activity: participation with friends and acquaintances other than family members
4. Occupation: activities partly or directly related to working including housework or volunteering
5. Sexual behavior: frequency and quality of sex life
6. Self-care: personal maintenance and independent daily living (bathing, dressing, etc.)
7. Life-support activity: basic life-supporting behaviors (eating, sleeping, breathing, etc.)

The response scale ranges from 0 (not limited at all) to 10 (completely limited). Response recall is unclear. The total score ranges from 0 to 70, with a higher score indicating more disability. Test–retest reliability in 20 patients (time interval 1 week) was ICC = 0.91, PDI factor 1 ICC = 0.87, and PDI factor 2 ICC = 0.73, respectively (Gronblad et al. 1993). Test–retest reliability is fair after 2 months ($r = 0.44$) (Tait et al. 1990). The internal consistency is high (alpha = 0.86; Tait et al. 1987). The scale is able to discriminate between

Table 17.2 Generic health status instruments and functional limitations

	Short Form-36 (SF-36)	Nottingham Health Profile (NHP)	Sickness Impact Profile (SIP)	EuroQol (EQ-5D)
Response recall	"Now"	"At the moment"	"Today"	(none given)
Response items	3 "Yes, limited a lot" "No, not limited at all"	2 Yes/No statements	2 Yes/No statements	2 Yes/No statements
Domain	Physical Functioning	Physical Ability	Physical domain	Mobility Self-care Usual activities
Number of items	10	8	Ambulation 10 Mobility 10 Body care and movement 23	9
Cronbach's alpha	>0.90	>0.80	>0.80	N/A
Test–retest reliability	$R > 0.8$	ICC = 0.95	$R = 0.97$ (interviewer) $R = 0.87$ (self-completed)	ICC = 0.69–0.94
Activities				
Getting up			X	
Bending, kneeling	X	X	X	
Eating (use a knife, drink from a cup)				
Standing		X	X	
Walking	X	X	X	X
Running	X			
Stairs	X	X	X	
Reaching		X		
Gripping (door handle, jar, holding a pencil)			X	
Lifting or carrying	X			
Participation				
Self-care (washing and dressing)	X	X	X	X
Mobility (leaving the house)			X	
Housekeeping	X	X	X	
Sports	X	X		
Usual activities				X

inpatients and outpatients. Patients with high PDI scores reported more psychological distress ($P < 0.001$), more severe pain characteristics ($P < 0.001$), and more restriction of activities ($P < 0.001$) than patients with low PDI scores, findings supportive of the construct validity of the measure. Further construct validity was supported by high correlations with the ODI ($r = 0.83$) (Gronblad et al. 1993). A multiple regression showed that a linear combination of 9 variables predicted PDI scores ($R = 0.74$): time spent in bed, psychosomatic symptoms, stopping activities because of pain, work status, pain duration, usual pain intensity, quality of life, pain extent, and education (Tait et al. 1987). Factor analysis revealed 2 factors: The first factor seemed to include more discretionary, less obligatory activities. The second factor included activities more basic to daily living and survival (Tait et al. 1987). Partial correlation controlling for pain intensity demonstrated PDI factor 1 and was significantly related to depression, employment status, and medication usage (Jerome and Gross 1991). A one-factor solution for the PDI was found in a large sample of patients with chronic pain ($N = 1059$). Normative data were generated from this sample (Chibnall and Tait 1994).

DISABILITY RATING INDEX (DRI)

The Disability Rating Index (DRI) (Salen et al. 1994) is a questionnaire that includes functional activities only, with the exception of the last question (participation question). It contains 12 items (see Instrument).

It is constructed as a self-administered form, where the patients mark on a 100 mm visual analogue scale in accordance to their presumed ability to "manage the following activities." The anchor points are without difficulty (0) and not at all (100). The 12 items are divided into three sections: 1–4, common basic activities of daily life; 5–8, more demanding physical activities; and 9–12, work-related or more vigorous activities. The questions are arranged in increasing order of physical demand, particularly with reference to low back pain. This arrangement also helps the health personnel to interpret the consistency of the answers and roughly indicates the severity of the self-reported disability without measurement or calculation (Salen et al. 1994). It takes 2–4 minutes to fill out. A test–retest correlation of $r = 0.95$ (1 day interval) was achieved for the whole DRI, $r = 0.70$–0.92 for the 12 different items in neck, shoulder and back pain patients and $r = 0.92$ and $r = 0.46$–0.96 for patients with arthritis and multiple sclerosis. Inter-rater reliability was $r = 0.99$ and intra-rater reliability was $r = 0.98$. Internal consistency was alpha $= 0.84$ in the neck, shoulder and low back pain group.

The DRI was able to discriminate between different disability categories, but had poor to fair construct validity when compared to the Oswestry Disability Index (ICC $= 0.38$), the Functional Status Questionnaire (ICC $= 0.46$) and observer's assessment of performance of the 12 items (ICC $= 0.48$). However, the correlation between the DRI with the patient's perception of his/her functional ability was 0.69. Responsiveness was measured by percent improvement in a sample of arthritis patients ($N = 19$) before and after operation (mean 92 days) and was reported by the authors to be excellent. No further support for the reliability, validity and responsiveness of this instrument could be found in the current literature.

HEALTH ASSESSMENT QUESTIONNAIRE-DISABILITY INDEX (HAQ-DI)

The Health Assessment Questionnaire (HAQ) was originally developed in 1978 by Fries and colleagues at Stanford University (Fries et al. 1980, 1982). It has been applied to a large range of musculoskeletal diseases, in adults and children (Childhood Health Assessment Questionnaire or CHAQ), is culturally adapted in a number of languages and is supported by a bibliography of more than 500 references (Bruce and Fries 2003b). The HAQ is discussed in some detail in Chapter 16, but of interest to this chapter is the HAQ Disability Index (HAQ-DI). The HAQ-DI contains 20 items in 8 domains of functioning, which represent a comprehensive set of functional activities: dressing, rising, eating, walking, hygiene, grip, reach and usual activities. The HAQ-DI is usually self administered but can also be given face to face in a clinical setting or in a telephone interview format by trained assessors. It can be completed in 5 minutes. Response recall is "over the past week." The items are in capacity format and ask whether the respondent is "able to…," with 4 response items ranging from "Without any difficulty" to "Unable to do." According to the manual, the DI score can be calculated using either a so-called standard method or an alternative method. In the standard method the eight category scores are corrected using the section on aid and devices at the bottom of the questionnaire. Whenever aid by others or the use of devices is required to perform a certain activity, the corresponding category score (range 0–3, 0 = best, 3 = worst) is increased to 2 when that score was 0 or 1. In the alternative method no correction for aid and devices is made and the eight category scales are averaged into an overall HAQ-DI score on a scale from 0 (no disability) to 3 (completely disabled). Scores of 0–1 are generally considered to represent mild to moderate difficulty, 1–2 moderate to severe difficulty and 2–3 severe to very severe difficulty. Zandbelt et al. (2001) suggest for the sake of international uniformity that the HAQ or any validated translation should be used and calculated in a standard way, including correcting for the use of aid and devices and taking the maximum within each category as the category score.

Average scores that have been reported in population based studies are 0.49 and in osteo arthritis and rheumatoid arthritis patients 0.8 and 1.2, respectively (Bruce and Fries 2003b).

Test–retest correlations confirming reproducibility range from $r = 0.87$ (Fries and Spitz 1990) to 0.98 (Fries et al. 1982), and correlations between interview and questionnaire formats have ranged from 0.85 to 0.95. Inter-item correlations were modest, ranging from 0.51 to 0.81 (Fries et al. 1980). Internal consistency for the entire instrument was alpha = 0.94 (Milligan et al. 1993). Validity was confirmed in numerous studies. Liang et al. (1985) compared responses of 50 patients with arthritis on 5 different instruments. The correlation of the HAQ with the Arthritis Impact Measurement Scale (AIMS) was 0.84 and was 0.78 with the SIP, 0.75 with the Functional Status Index (FSI) and 0.60 with the Quality of Well-being scale. Another study found a correlation of 0.91 between the HAQ-DI and the AIMS (Brown et al. 1984). There is consensus that the HAQ-DI possesses face and content validity. Correlations between questionnaire or interview scores and task performance have ranged from 0.71 to 0.95, indicating criterion validity. The construct/convergent validity, predictive validity, and sensitivity to change have also been established in numerous observational studies and clinical trials (Ramey et al. 1996). The minimal clinically important difference is reported to range between 0.10 and 0.22 points (Bruce and Fries 2003a,b).

A number of translations/adaptations are available through the MAPI Institute (website: http://www.mapi-research-inst.com). Independent translations in a number of languages also exist. The entire HAQ with instructions for scoring can be downloaded from the internet at http://aramis.stanford.edu/HAQ.html (accessed May 15, 2007).

SHORT MUSCULOSKELETAL FUNCTIONAL ASSESSMENT (SMFA)

According to Beaton and Schemitsch (2003) the Musculoskeletal Functional Assessment (MFA) (Martin et al. 1996a) is one of the most used measures in the orthopedic literature. A 46-item questionnaire, the Short Musculoskeletal Functional Assessment (SMFA) (Swiontkowski et al. 1999), was developed as an extension of the work to develop the longer 101-item MFA and was specifically designed to detect differences in the status of patients with MSP that are commonly seen in community practices. The SMFA questionnaire consists of the dysfunction index, which has 34 items for the assessment of patient function, and the bother index, which has 12 items for the assessment of how much patients are bothered by functional problems. The dysfunction index has two subscales: 25 items assess the amount of difficulty that patients have when performing certain functions and 9 items assess how

often the patients have difficulty when performing certain functions. Each item has a 5-point response format ranging from 1 point for good function to 5 for poor function.

The bother index allows patients to assess how much they are bothered by problems in broad functional areas, such as recreation and leisure, sleep and rest, work and family. Each item has a 5-point response format ranging from 1 point (not at all bothered) to 5 (extremely bothered).

The scores on the dysfunction index and the bother index are calculated by summing the responses to the items and then transforming the scores so that they range from 0 to 100, with higher scores indicating poorer function. Response recall is "this week" and questions are phrased in terms of difficulty or problems with daily activities and bothered by problems because "of your injury or arthritis."

Validity, reliability and responsiveness of the SMFA was assessed in a sample of 420 patients who had musculoskeletal disease or injury, recruited from 18 sites across the USA.

Test–retest reliability (one to two weeks) was ICC = 0.93 for the dysfunction index and ICC = 0.88 for the bother index. Internal consistency was alpha = 0.95 and 0.96 for the baseline and follow-up data of the dysfunction index and alpha = 0.92 and 0.95 for the bother index. The mean (SD) scores for the SMFA in patients with a wide range of musculoskeletal problems was 27.3 (16.9) for dysfunction index ($N + 420$) and 31.2 (20.8) for the bother index ($N = 396$).

Content validity was supported by the absence of floor or ceiling effects and non-skew distributed scores across the entire range. Convergent validity was supported by significant correlations with walking speed and grip strength and the dysfunction scale alone was significantly correlated to range of motion of the wrist and ankle. The SMFA indexes were significantly related to all SF-36 domains. Patients with good health status scored significantly higher on the SMFA than patients with poor or fair health status, supporting discriminant validity of the SMFA. The values for the Receiver Operating Characteristics of the dysfunction index were 0.90 and 0.84 for sensitivity and specificity and the area under the curve was 0.94. For the bother index, values for sensitivity and specificity were 0.87 and 0.84, respectively, and the area under the curve was 0.94.

Responsiveness, as measured by the standardized response means, ranged from moderate (0.76) to large (-1.14) for patients with changes in health status. The SMFA is reliable, valid and responsive in Swedish (SMFA-Swe), German (SMFA-D) and Brazilian-Portuguese (SMFA-BR) translations.

HEALTH STATUS INSTRUMENTS

Health-related quality of life or health status is increasingly used as an outcome in clinical trials, outcomes research and research on quality of care. All health status instruments include a measure of physical functioning. The most frequently used health status instrument in the literature is the Short Form-36 (SF-36), with almost 6000 citations in Medline alone. The most frequently *evaluated* health status instruments in the general literature (Garratt et al. 2002) are the SF-36, the Nottingham Health Profile (NHP) and the Sickness Impact Profile (SIP). These three measures have been evaluated across numerous patient populations, have been translated into many languages and have population norms available. These questionnaires include a wide range of physical activities (see Table 17.2). Whereas the SIP measures changes in performance as a consequence of sickness, the NHP measures current performance. The SF-36 measures limitation of activities because of "your health."

Other well-known health status instruments such as the COOP charts (Nelson et al. 1987) for primary care practice or the Duke Health Profile (Parkerson et al. 1990) sample functional activities in much less detail. For example, only one of the eight COOP charts refers to functional activities (daily activities), while another chart questions physical fitness. The 17-item Duke Health Profile includes 2 items on functional activities: "walking up a flight of stairs" and "running the length of a football field."

In a cross-sectional comparison of health status measures in injured workers (Beaton et al. 1996), that included the SF-36, NHP, Duke Health Profile, the SIP and the Ontario Health Survey (OHS), the NHP and the OHS were found to have the highest ceiling effects. The SIP also had high ceiling effects and had the highest respondent burden. The NHP was able to best discriminate between respondents with different self-rated health, overcoming the high ceiling effects. The SF-36 was the second most discriminating. There was moderate to good convergent validity between the instruments except for the OHS. Bronfort and Bouter (1999) compared the SF-36 and the COOP charts for use in patients with chronic low back pain. Comparisons between improved and nonimproved patients for the COOP charts and SF-36, using pain as an external criterion (EC), yielded differences which translated into large effect sizes (0.8 and 0.7) ($P = 0.0008$ and 0.003). Using disability as EC, differences of moderate effect size were found (0.5 and 0.6) ($P = 0.02$ and 0.002). The ROC curve calculations using pain as EC resulted in areas under the curve of 0.76 (95% CI: 0.64, 0.88) for the COOP charts, and 0.74 (95% CI: 0.60, 0.88) for the SF-36. The corresponding areas using disability as EC were 0.67 (95% CI: 0.55, 0.79) and 0.72 (95% CI: 0.60, 0.84). The best cut-off point in both instruments for differentiating between improved and non-improved patients was approximately six percentage points.

It is generally recommended to use both a generic and disease specific instrument to adequately assess the impact of a disease or a symptom, such as pain. Considerable overlap between a generic and a disease specific instrument may exist, however (Wittink et al. 2004), unduly imposing a large respondent burden when using both.

The validity of using the SF-36 in the LBP population is supported by its highly statistically significant ($p < 0.001$) correlations with the Oswestry Disability Index and Low Back Pain disability domains (Grevitt et al. 1997). Walsh et al. (2003) evaluated the responsiveness of the Oswestry Disability Index, MODEMS scales, and all scales and summary scales of the SF-36 for patients with low back pain/leg symptoms ($N = 970$). They concluded that for studies of patients with low back problems, the general SF-36 may be a sufficient measure of health status and patient function, without the need for additional condition-specific instruments. Pain scales appeared to be the most responsive measures in patients with low back pain. Conversely, Taylor et al. (1999) reported that although the disease specific questionnaires showed the greatest overall responsiveness, the SF-36 PF scale was more sensitive to change than either the Oswestry or the Low Back Outcome Score for patients with back pain whose status improved or remained unchanged.

Fanuele et al. (2000) used the Physical Component Summary scale (PCS) of the SF-36 to quantify the effect spinal diagnoses have on patients' functional status compared to other common comorbidities and to quantify the effects of comorbidities on physical functional status in patients with spine disorders. They found that the PCS score in patients with spinal problems was lower or similar to patients with congestive heart failure, chronic obstructive disease, lupus, primary total hip replacement, total knee replacement and glenohumeral joint disease.

Several "enhanced" SF-36 scales have recently been developed. Relevant to this chapter are the Treatment of Outcomes in Pain Survey (TOPS) (Rogers et al. 2000a,b), a (chronic) pain-specific tool, the Index of Physical Functional Health (FHS) (Hart and Wright 2002), applicable to a range of musculoskeletal conditions, and a low back-specific version of the SF-36 Physical Functioning scale (Davidson et al. 2004), that includes 4 questions from the Oswestry Disability Index and 4 questions from the Roland-Morris Disability questionnaire. While the TOPS incorporates the entire SF-36, the FSH and the back-specific SF-36 Physical Functioning scale incorporate the SF-36 Physical Functioning scale only. The advantage of these instruments is that while they have greater sensitivity to the impact of a disease upon health status, the generic scale(s) can still be used to compare the burden of the disease in question to that of other diseases.

TREATMENT OF OUTCOMES IN PAIN SURVEY (TOPS)

Because, when applied to individual patients, the SF-36 lacked measurement reliability for assessment of treatment outcomes, lacked sensitivity to upper extremity or facial pathology, and failed to separate limitations of work versus everyday activity, colleagues at the New England Medical Center in Boston conducted a two-part study to develop an outcomes instrument suitable for measurement of change in individual patients with chronic pain. A disease attribution approach (Rogers et al. 2000a,b) was employed to construct a condition-specific, "enhanced" SF-36 instrument which was named the Treatment of Outcomes in Pain Survey (TOPS). This approach, in which items from a previously validated generic instrument are rewritten with a specific disease attribution, has been used in other patient populations (Wagner et al. 1997; Ren et al. 1998). The instrument was developed using a large sample of patients with chronic pain attending an inter disciplinary pain program ($N = 1230$).

A novel group of scales derived from responses to 61 questions or 120 items (which include the SF-36) proved sufficiently reliable for routine follow-up of individual patients during treatment for chronic pain. This new "Treatment of Outcomes in Pain Survey" (TOPS) allows assessment of individual patient outcomes, and aggregate or individual clinician performance during interdisciplinary treatment of chronic pain.

In addition to the SF-36, this instrument contains demographic data and 14 scales of which 7 fit into the Nagi framework (Nagi 1991). The other 7 scales are considered to be mediating factors between the domains of pain, functional limitation and disability. The 7 main scales include pain symptom, perceived and objective family disability, work limitations, objective work disability, and upper and lower body limitations. Cronbach's alphas of these scales range from 0.70 for objective work disability to 0.92 for lower body functioning and 0.93 for perceived family/social disability. The mediating scales include fear-avoidance, passive coping, life control and solicitous responses. The pain context dimensions have internal consistencies ranging from alpha = 0.69 for Fear-Avoidance to alpha = 0.84 for Life Control. In addition, 2 scales measure patient satisfaction with care and outcomes. The final scale is the Total Pain Experience scale, which is a composite of pain intensity, pain interference, physical functioning and disability.

For evaluating a single patient, the TOPS Pain Symptom, Perceived Family/Social Disability, and Total Pain Experience scales are considerably more sensitive to individual change than the SF-36 BP scale. Their increased sensitivity can be attributed to their greater measurement reliability. For example, Cronbach's alpha equals 0.93 for Total Pain Experience compared with 0.84 for the SF-36 BP scale. The TOPS scales also provide a clearer and more clinically relevant set of concepts for the pain clinician who may have objectives apart from a simple reduction in pain intensity, such as the reduction of suffering or the reduction of disability in spite of pain.

Content validity was supported by a number of validation studies (Rogers et al. 2000b). Discriminant validity success ranged from 98 to 100%. Effect sizes ranged for individual patients from ES = 0.04 for Objective Work Disability (i.e., patients who are receiving disability benefits) to ES = 0.33 for Pain Symptom. For Total Pain Experience the ES was -0.37. Standard error as a percentage of the SD, as a measurement of change in the individual patient, ranged from 0.33 for Total Pain Experience to 0.78 for Fear-Avoidance. In addition to its utility as an outcomes research tool, the TOPS is sensitive enough to document clinical changes in individual patients, making it a useful assessment tool for clinicians. The instrument was translated and validated in English for the UK, French, Canadian French, German, Italian, Polish and Spanish.

THE WORLD HEALTH ORGANIZATION DISABILITY ASSESSMENT SCHEDULE II (WHODAS II)

The WHODAS II is a new measure of functioning and disability that is conceptually compatible with WHO's recent revisions to the International Classification of Functioning and Disability (ICF) (World Health Organization 2001). The WHODAS II is a tool for measuring level of functioning/disability across a variety of conditions and treatment interventions. It assesses functioning/disability at the individual level instead of the disorder-specific level. As a result, the total impact of co-morbid conditions (e.g., depression and diabetes) is straightforward to assess.

The domains of functioning assessed by the WHODAS II are:

- Understanding and communicating
- Getting around
- Self-care
- Getting along with others
- Household and work activities
- Participation in society (from http://www.who.int/icidh/whodas/index.html (accessed May 15, 2007).

Although the original instrument has 36 items, shorter instruments are available (12 or 6 items). Available versions include self-administered, interviewer-administered, and proxy-reported.

In a sample of primary care patients with depression ($n = 73$) and back pain ($n = 76$) the WHODAS II had an internal consistency of Cronbach's alpha of 0.95 for the total score, ranging from alpha = 0.65 for self-care to alpha = 0.91 for work and household activities (Chwastiak and Von Korff 2003). Tests of convergent validity of the WHODAS II with the SF-36 and the Roland Morris Disability Questionnaire (RDQ) produced correlations of moderate to large sizes. In the back pain sample the WHODAS II total score was highly correlated with the RDQ ($r = 0.75$) and moderately correlated with the SF-36 pain score ($r = -0.55$). The physical functioning subscale of the WHODAS II was highly correlated with the SF-36 physical functioning scale ($r = -0.77$). The mean (SD) WHODAS II score was 27.14 (17.1) and 22.75 (13.49) in depressed and back pain patients, respectively. Responsiveness was calculated by effect sizes. The WHODAS II total score had a moderate effect size (ES) in patients with depression (ES = 0.65) and low back pain (ES = 0.60). The mean (SD) WHODAS II score was 23.9 (SD 15.5) in a sample of patients with ankylosing spondylitis. Scores on the WHODAS II were significantly correlated with all disease specific questionnaires measured (all $p < 0.001$). The WHODAS II ($n = 31$) showed a comparable short term responsiveness score (Standardized Response Mean 0.41; Effect Size 0.39). In regression analysis these short term changes on the WHODAS II were significantly associated with changes in functioning (van Tubergen et al. 2003).

THE MULTIDIMENSIONAL PAIN INVENTORY (MPI)

The Multidimensional Pain Inventory (MPI; formerly the West Haven-Yale Multidimensional Pain Inventory or WHYMPI) was developed by Kerns et al. (1985). Based on a survey of pain centers, the McGill Pain Questionnaire along with the MPI were reported to be among the top five pain-specific assessment instruments used to evaluate patients with chronic pain.

The MPI is a 64 item, self-report questionnaire comprising three parts and 12 subscales. The first two parts are related to patients' appraisals of pain and its impact upon different domains of their lives, and patients' perceptions of the responses of significant others to their distress and suffering. The third part assesses how frequently patients perform 18 common daily activities.

Test–retest reliability (2 weeks) ranged between $r = 0.62$ for distracting responses to 0.91 for household chores ($N = 60$) (Kerns et al. 1985) and from $r = 0.69$ for life control to 0.94 for household chores in the Dutch language MPI (MPI-DLV)(Lousberg et al. 1999).

Internal consistency ranges from Cronbach alpha 0.70 for outdoor activities to 0.90 for interference.

Using cluster-analytic and multivariate classification methods, three homogeneous subgroups of chronic pain patient have been identified and replicated across a wide range of medical diagnoses (back pain, temporomandibular disorders, headache). The three groups' distinct profiles were labeled "dysfunctional," "interpersonally distressed" and "adaptive coper."

Burton et al. (1999) suggested that a psychometric battery consisting of the MPI and the Brief Pain Inventory was useful for both identifying problem areas that might impede treatment of chronic pain patients and for assessing treatment outcome. Moreover, the MPI has been shown to be predictive of chronicity of pain following acute symptom onset (Epker and Gatchel 2000; Olsson et al. 2002). The MPI has demonstrated reliability and validity in patients with chronic low back pain (Turk and Rudy 1990).

A recent study (Wittink et al. 2004) compared the redundancy, reliability, validity, and sensitivity to change among the SF-36, Oswestry Disability Index (ODI; see later in this chapter), and MPI on a cross-sectional sample of $N = 424$, with a follow-up sample of $N = 87$ of patients with chronic pain, seen in an interdisciplinary pain clinic. Cronbach's alphas ranged from 0.69 to 0.92 for the MPI, from 0.79 to 0.91 for the SF-36 and was 0.86 for the ODI. Three concepts overlapped between the SF-36 and the MPI: pain, interference/social functioning, and mental health. Both the SF-36 and the MPI contributed unique scales (e.g., the MPI "significant other" scales; R^2 range 0.03–0.16). The MPI Pain Severity, Interference and Outdoor Work Activities were the most sensitive to change with effect sizes ranging from -0.42 for Interference to 0.38 for Outdoor Work.

The MPI is used widely, and has been translated into Spanish, Portuguese, French, Swedish, Dutch and Italian.

ACTIVITY AVOIDANCE TOOLS

Moderate to strong associations have been identified between coping responses, pain severity, psychological well-being and physical functioning (Jensen et al. 1991). Fear avoidance beliefs correlated significantly with self-reported disability in activities of daily living and work loss (Waddell et al. 1993) and were shown to be a significant predictor of chronic pain (Vlaeyen and Linton 2000) in patients with musculoskeletal disorders. Fear-avoidance beliefs about work were significant predictors of 4-week disability and work status even after controlling for initial levels of pain intensity, physical impairment, and disability, and the type of therapy received in a sample of patients with acute low back pain (Fritz et al. 2001). Catastrophizing was shown to predict depression (Turner et al. 2000), perception of pain (Hassett et al. 2000), lower self-efficacy for pain, lower spousal ratings of self-efficacy for control of fatigue or mood symptoms (Keefe et al. 1997), and disability (Martin et al. 1996b).

Two questionnaires relate to avoidance of functional activities: the Fear-Avoidance Beliefs Questionnaire (FABQ) and the Tampa Scale of Kinesiophobia (TSK). The Pain Catastrophizing Scale does not contain questions about functional activities and is discussed further in Chapter 19 on mental health. Although the Pain Anxiety Symptoms Scale (PASS) (McCracken et al. 1992) is frequently mentioned as a measure of fear avoidance, it does not, in fact, contain any items pertaining to functional activities and will therefore not be discussed in this chapter.

Concurrent validity of the FABQ and the TSK has been examined in a sample of patients with acute back pain (Swinkels-Meewisse et al. 2003). Pearson's rho between the TSK and the FABQ work scale was $r = 0.33$ at initial measurement and $r = 0.38$ at repeat measurement (24 hours later). Pearson's rho between the TSK and the FABQ physical activity scale was $r = 0.39$ at initial measurement and $r = 0.59$ at repeat measurement. Crombez et al. (1999) also found moderate correlations between the TSK, the FABQ physical activity subscale ($r = 0.57$ and 0.76) and the FABQ work subscale ($r = 0.53$ and 0.56).

The moderate correlation between the two instruments suggests that they may be tapping into different domains. Swinkels-Meewisse et al. (2003) suggest that the TSK may be aimed more at measuring a fear of (re) injury, whereas the FABQ measures more a fear of pain directly, caused by physical activities or work.

THE FEAR AVOIDANCE BELIEFS QUESTIONNAIRE (FABQ)

The Fear Avoidance Beliefs Questionnaire (FABQ) is a 16 item instrument developed by Waddell et al. (1993). It contains 16 items in two subscales: 7 items on fear avoidance beliefs about the relationship between low back pain and work and 4 items on fear avoidance beliefs about physical activity in general. Five of the 16 items are not scored for fear avoidance beliefs. Items are scored on a 7-point Likert scale with item responses ranging from 0 (strongly disagree) to 6 (strongly agree). The total score of the FABQ work scale ranges from 0 to 42 and the total score of the FABQ physical activities scale ranges from 0 to 24. In both subscales higher scores represent more fear.

Test–retest reliability had a kappa equal to 0.74 ($N = 26$) in a sample of patients with chronic back pain. Test–retest reliability in terms of Pearson's rho ranging between $r = 0.87$ for all 16 items (Pfingsten et al. 2000) to $r = 0.95$ and 0.88 (Waddell et al. 1993) have been reported. Internal consistency for the work subscale ranges from Cronbach alpha = 0.84–0.92 and internal consistency for the physical activity subscale ranges from Cronbach alpha = 0.52–0.77 (Waddell et al. 1993; Vendrig et al. 1998; Crombez et al. 1999).

In validating the German translation ($N = 302$) of the FABQ, Pfingsten et al. (2000) found a different factor structure than was found for the English version. Whereas the factor "physical activity" (8.9% of the variance) remained the same as in the English version, the second factor of the original version split into two: one related to "work as cause of pain" (43.4% of the variance) and the other to patients' assumptions of their probable return to work (11.8% of the variance). Both work-related subscales showed a good internal consistency (alpha = 0.89, resp. alpha = 0.94), whereas the consistency of subscale 3, "physical activity," was only modest (alpha = 0.64).

In a recent study (Swinkels-Meewisse et al. 2003) on the reliability and validity of the FABQ in a sample of patients ($N = 176$) with acute back pain, test–retest reliability (24 hours) was $r = 0.64$ and 0.80 for the FABQ physical activity and work scales, respectively. Internal consistency was Cronbach's alpha = 0.70 for the physical activity subscale and alpha = 0.82 for the work subscale. The mean (SD) FABQ physical activity score was 14.1 (5.5) and 13.4 (5.8) for baseline and retest, respectively, and was 14.4 (10.1) and 14.7 (10.3) for the FABQ work subscale.

Fritz and George (2002) studied a group of patients with acute, work-related LBP and demonstrated that FABQ work scale scores greater than 34 were associated with an increased risk of not returning to work (positive likelihood ratio = 3.33, 95% CI = 1.65, 6.77) and work scale scores of less than 29 were associated with a decreased risk of not returning to work (negative likelihood ratio = 0.08, 95% CI = 0.01, 0.54). Grotle et al. (2006) confirmed that the FABQ-Work predicts pain and disability at 12 months in patients with acute back pain. In combination with non-organic signs the FABQ predicts prolonged disability in neck pain (Landers et al. 2007). The FABQ has been translated into Spanish, Norwegian, German, French and Dutch.

TAMPA SCALE FOR KINESIOPHOBIA

The Tampa Scale for Kinesiophobia (TSK) (Kori et al. 1990) is a 17-item questionnaire which aims to identify fear of (re) injury due to movement or activities. Items are scored on a 4-point Likert scale with 4 item responses ranging from 1 (strongly disagree) to 4 (strongly agree). The total score is the sum of the 17 items, in which each 4th question is scored in reverse. The total score ranges from 17 to 68 with higher scores representing more fear. Most of the psychometric research on the TSK has been done on the Dutch version of the TSK (Vlaeyen et al. 1995; Crombez et al. 1999; Swinkels-Meewisse et al. 2003; Goubert et al. 2004). An 11 item English version of the Tampa Scale for Kinesiophobia was developed on a sample of patients with chronic back pain. This TSK-11 possessed similar psychometric properties to the original TSK and offers the advantage of brevity (Woby et al. 2005). More research is needed on other groups of patients with chronic pain for the TSK-11.

The internal consistency of the TSK ranges from Cronbach's alpha = 0.68–0.80 (Vlaeyen et al. 1995; Crombez et al. 1999). Swinkels-Meewisse et al. (2003) reported on the reliability and validity of the TSK-Dutch Version (TSK-DV) in a sample of patients ($N = 176$) with acute back pain; test–retest reliability (24 hours) was $r = 0.78$. The internal consistency was alpha = 0.70 at the initial measurement and alpha = 0.76 at the second measurement 24 hours later. The mean (SD) TSK score was 36.3 (6.8) and 36.0 (7.4) at baseline and retest 24 hours later. Similar mean scores were found by Vlaeyen et al. (1995), who designated patients with TSK scores under 37 "confronters" and more than 37 "avoiders." The TSK discriminated well between avoiders and confronters during a behavioral performance task.

Confirmatory factor analysis of the TSK-DV in a sample of 188 patients with back pain and 89 patients with fibromyalgia showed that a 2-factor structure provided the best fit of the data in both patient samples. The authors (Goubert et al. 2004) recommend using the version of the TSK without the reversed key items in both clinical practice and future research. The two factors were named "Harm" and "Fear-Avoidance." The internal consistency of the TSK without the reverse key items was reported as alpha = 0.80 in patients with chronic back pain and alpha = 0.82 in patients with fibromyalgia. The internal consistency of the "Harm" subscale was alpha = 0.70 for both patient samples and was alpha = 0.73 and 0.76 for the "Fear-Avoidance" subscale in patients with chronic back pain and patients with fibromyalgia, respectively. In this study the mean (SD) TSK score was reported as 31.6 (7.2) for chronic back pain patients ($N = 188$) and 30.2 (7.5) for patients with fibromyalgia ($N = 89$).

The relationship of kinesiophobia with activities and participation is controversial. Heuts et al. (2004) found that level of pain and level of pain-related fear were significantly associated with functional limitations in patients with osteoarthritis. Reneman et al. (2003), however, were unable to find a relationship between a lifting task and kinesiophobia in a sample of patients with chronic back pain. Similarly, a recent study showed a lack of correlation between kinesiophobia (TSK-Dutch Version) and exercise capacity, activity limitations, or participation restrictions, in patients with CFS who were experiencing widespread muscle or joint pain (Nijs et al. 2004).

DISEASE-SPECIFIC OUTCOMES MEASURES (BACK AND NECK PAIN)

Disease-specific instruments reflect particular limitations or restrictions associated with specific disease states. These instruments are designed to be sensitive in determining the effects of treatment upon or the spontaneous

longitudinal course of a single disease or condition. A large variety of disease-specific measures have been developed for almost every imaginable condition. In 1994, Ruta wrote that he was aware of "only three measures designed specifically to assess health status in patients with low back pain that are not restricted to measurement of impairment alone" (Ruta et al. 1994). Not surprising then that a number of (older) disease-specific instruments such as the Waddell Disability Index and the Million Visual Analogue Scale also include measures of impairment. Scales have proliferated since then. Although the construction of the scales and their psychometric analysis has become much more advanced, the choice of items has remained largely the same (see Table 17.3) and addresses those functional activities thought to be affected by back pain.

A number of reviews of back-specific questionnaires have been published (Beurskens et al. 1995; Taylor et al. 1999; Kopec 2000; Garratt et al. 2001; Resnik and Dobrzykowski 2003; Schaufele and Boden 2003) and increasingly studies are designed for the specific purpose of evaluating and comparing psychometric properties of questionnaires (Roland and Fairbank 2000; Bombardier et al. 2001; Fritz and Irrgang 2001). For instance, Davidson and Keating (2002) compared the modified Oswestry Disability Index (ODI), Roland Disability Questionnaire (RDQ), Quebec Back Pain Disability Scale (QBPDS), the Waddell Disability Index and the SF-36 in a sample of patients ($n = 106$) undergoing physical therapy for back pain. Patients with low back pain completed the questionnaires during initial consultation with a physical therapist and again 6 weeks later. Test–retest reliability (Intraclass Correlation Coefficients or ICCs) was examined for a group of 47 subjects who were classified as "unchanged" and a subgroup of 16 subjects who were self-rated as "about the same." Responsiveness was compared using standardized response means, receiver operating characteristic curves, and the proportions of subjects who changed by at least as much as the minimum detectable change (MDC) (90% confidence interval of the standard error for repeated measures). None of the scales were more responsive than any other. Measurements obtained with the modified ODI, the SF-36 Physical Functioning scale, and the Quebec Back Pain Disability Scale were the most reliable and had sufficient width scale to reliably detect improvement or worsening in most subjects. The Waddell Disability Index, RDQ and the Role Limitations-Physical and Bodily Pain scales of the SF-36 were not recommended for clinical application. Riddle and Stratford (2002) responded that of the 13 other studies that investigated the reliability of the RDQ the ICC correlations ranged from ICC = 0.66 to ICC = 0.96 and that therefore their findings should be interpreted with caution.

Deyo et al. (1998) proposed a standardized set of clinical outcomes measures in patients with low back

Table 17.3 Back pain specific instruments and functional items

	ABPS	BPFS	FRI	HAQ-DI	LBOS	LBRS	Million	ODI	QBPDS	RDQ	Waddell
Impairments											
Pain intensity	X		X		X	X	X	X			X
Frequency of pain			X							X	
Change in pain							X	X			
Sleeping/resting	X	X	X		X	X	X	X	X	X	X
Pain medication	X				X	X	X				X
Spine ROM						X	X				X
Straight leg raise							X				X
Activities											
Eating				X						X	
Turning (over)/twisting							X		X	X	X
Getting up (chair/bed)				X		X			X	X	
Putting on socks/shoes		X				X			X	X	X
Sitting	X	X			X		X	X	X	X	X
Standing	X	X	X				X	X	X	X	X
Reaching				X					X		
Walking	X	X	X	X	X	X	X	X	X	X	X
Running						X			X		
Stairs		X				X			X	X	
Bending/kneeling/stooping	X	X		X		X			X	X	
Lifting		X	X	X					X	X	X
Carrying				X		X			X		
Participation											
Self-care (washing and dressing)	X		X	X	X			X		X	
Travel/drive		X	X		X	X			X	X	X
Housekeeping	X	X				X			X		
Work	X	X	X		X	X	X	X			
(usual) Social life/recreation/sports	X	X	X	X	X	X	X	X			X
Activities around the house		X			X					X	
Sexual activity	X				X						X

ABPS = Aberdeen Back Pain Scale; BPFS = Back Pain Functional Scale; FRI = Functional Rating Index; HAQ-DI = Health Assessment Questionnaire-Disability Index; LBOS = Low Back Outcome Scale; LBRS = Low Back Pain Rating Scale; Million = Million Visual Analogue Scale; ODI = Oswestry Disability Index; QBPDS = Quebec Back Pain Disability Scale; RDQ = Roland-Morris Disability Questionnaire; Waddell = Waddell Disability Index.

pain (LBP). A six-item set was proposed, which is sufficiently brief that it could be used in routine care settings for quality improvement and for research purposes. An expanded outcome set, which would provide more precise measurement for research purposes, includes measures of severity and frequency of symptoms, either the Roland or the Oswestry Disability Scale, either the SF-12 or the EuroQol measure of general health status, a question about satisfaction with symptoms, three types of "disability days," and an optional single item on overall satisfaction with medical care (Deyo et al. 1998). Recommendations from this Cochrane group were updated in 2000 (Bombardier 2000) and it was agreed that a core set of measures would include the following five domains: back specific function, generic health status, pain, work disability and patient satisfaction. As no back specific instrument appears clearly superior to another the authors suggest use of one of the two most commonly used disease-specific tools for back pain: the Oswestry Disability Index (ODI) or the Roland-Morris Disability Questionnaire (RDQ). The ODI and RDQ scores are highly correlated, with similar test–retest reliability and internal consistency. Floor and ceiling effects determine the choice of instruments. A greater proportion of patients score in the top half of the distribution of RDQ scores than in the top half of the ODI scores. The ODI is therefore recommended in patients who are likely to have persistent severe disability and the RDQ in patients who are likely to have relatively little disability (Roland and Fairbank 2000).

The WHO recommendations for epidemiologic survey or other group survey outcome measures appropriate to *all* cultures include the history of the complaint and the physical examination as central outcome measures. The only additional measure considered useful was a modified Schober test of spinal mobility. Studies were carried out on 6 continents to ascertain their applicability; other favorite examination techniques failed universality. In addition, for the purpose of studies, severity of pain should be measured with a visual analogue scale (VAS in a single line). The Oswestry Disability Index, modified Zung and modified somatic perception questionnaire were considered appropriate measurements after 21 other commonly-used assessments were found to lack universality. In addition Waddell disability indices for chronic disability and physical impairment (Ehrlich and Khaltaev 1999) were recommended.

Much less information is available on disease specific outcome measures for neck pain. We identified one systematic review (Pietrobon et al. 2002), but were unable to find recommendations regarding which outcome measures to use. In parallel with Deyo's (1998) and Bombardier's (2000) recommendations for back pain, a core set of measures could include the following five domains: neck specific function, generic health

status, pain, work disability and patient satisfaction. Significantly fewer disease specific instruments for neck pain exist than for back pain. A nice approach for determining which items should be included in a neck specific questionnaire was illustrated by Hoving et al. (2003) who performed a cross-sectional study of 71 patients with varying severity and duration of whiplash-associated disorders (WAD). Patients were asked to identify their own problems that had arisen as a result of the whiplash-type injury, using an interviewer administered instrument that asks the patient as those that they would most like to see improve as a result of therapy. Items that showed a high prevalence (identified by more than 25% of patients) included "work for wages" (52.1%), "fatigued during the day" (50.7%), "participation in sports" (47.9%), "depression" (43.7%), "drive a car" (43.7%), "socialize with friends" (33.8%), "sleep through the night" (31.0%), "frustration" (31.0%) and "anger" (28.2%). Three of these nine problems are specifically included in the NDI (work, driving, and sleeping) and four are included in the Northwick Park Neck Pain Questionnaire (NPQ) (work, driving, sleeping, and social activities).

The Neck Disability Index has been used more frequently than the other existing instruments and appears reliable and valid. Various new instruments have been developed in recent years that show promise. We have included several of these in this chapter, with the caveat that they need to be validated in other studies.

BACK PAIN-SPECIFIC INSTRUMENTS

Table 17.4 provides an overview of the reliability and validity of the back-specific instruments discussed in this chapter. References for the content of the overview can be found in the text below. The instruments are presented in alphabetical order.

ABERDEEN BACK PAIN SCALE (ABPS)

The Aberdeen Back Pain Scale (ABPS) (Ruta et al. 1994), also called the Clinical Back Pain Questionnaire, was devised from questions commonly used in the assessment of patients with low back pain. The 19 items include duration of pain, duration of analgesia, effect of lying down, areas of pain, areas of weakness and loss of feeling, bending, sleep, work, confinement to bed, sex life, leisure and self-care. Response recall is "in the last two weeks." The items are either a forced choice (mark one box) or a multiple choice format (check all boxes that apply). The choices are summed and rescaled to produce a back pain severity score between 0 and 100, where 0 equals no back pain and 100 the most severe back pain severity score. Test–retest reliability in patients who did not report changes in

Table 17.4 Overview of reliability, validity and responsiveness of the instruments in this chapter

Instrument	Time to complete (min)	Items, domains	Reliability, test–retest	Reliability, Cronbach's alpha	Validity, concurrent	Minimal detectable change
Aberdeen Low Back Scale	10	19	$R = 0.94$, 2 weeks	0.80	RDQ, EQ-5	SRM = 0.6
Back Pain Functional Scale	5	12	ICC = 0.88, 48 hours	0.93	RDQ	3.9 points
Disability Rating Index	2–4	12 items 3 domains	NR	0.84	Poor to fair ODI	NR
Functional Rating Index	1	10	ICC = 0.99, 1–11 days	0.92	SF-36 Physical Functioning scale	SRM = 1.24
Health Assessment Questionnaire – Disability Index	5	20 items 4 domains	$R = 0.87$, 2 weeks $R = 0.95$, 1 week $R = 0.98$, 6 months	0.94	WOMAC, AIMS, SIP	0.10–0.22
Low Back Outcome Score	NR	13	84% agreement, 1 week	0.85	Waddell, ODI	NR
Low Back Pain Rating Scale	15	25 items 4 domains	NR	NR	NR	NR
Million Visual Analogue Scale	10	15	$R = 0.97$, same day	NR	NR	NR
Oswestry Disability Index	5	10	$R = 0.99$, over 24 hours ICC = 0.94, 1–14 days ICC = 0.84, 6 weeks	0.71–0.87	RDQ, PDI, LBOS, Waddell, Quebec	5.2–16.3 points
Pain Disability Index	NR	7	ICC = 0.91, 1 week	0.86	ODI	NR
Quebec Back Pain Disability Scale	5	20	ICC = 0.93, 1–14 days ICC = 0.84, 6 weeks	0.96	RDQ, ODI, SF-36	15–19 points

(Continued)

Table 17.4 Overview of reliability, validity and responsiveness of the instruments in this chapter—Cont'd

Instrument	Time to complete (min)	Items, domains	Reliability, test-retest	Reliability, Cronbach's alpha	Validity, concurrent	Minimal detectable change
Roland-Morris Disability Questionnaire	5	24	ICC = 0.91, same day ICC = 0.93, 1–14 days ICC = 0.86, 3–6 weeks ICC = 0.53, 6 weeks	0.84–0.93	ODI, SF-36, SIP	2–9.5 points
Short Musculoskeletal Functional Assessment	NR	46 items 2 domains	ICC = 0.88–0.93, 2 weeks	0.92–0.95	SF-36	SRM 1.14–0.76
Treatment Outcomes of Pain Survey	20	120 items 16 domains	NR	0.70–0.92	Patient diary	ES 0.04–0.33
Waddell Disability Index	NR	9	ICC = 0.74, 6 weeks	0.76	ODI, LBOS	2.8 points
WODAS II	NR	36 items 6 domains	NR	0.65–0.91	SF-36, RDQ	ES = 0.39–0.65

NR = not reported; SRM = standardized response mean; ES = effect size.

health after 2 weeks was $r = 0.94$, and the internal consistency was alpha = 0.80 ($N = 568$).

Garratt et al. (2001) compared the ABPS, the RDQ and the EQ-5D in 187 patients with low back pain who were randomized either to an exercise program or to usual care. The ABPS and the RDQ were highly correlated ($r = 0.68$) and a good correlation was found between the EQ-5D and the RDQ ($r = 0.50$). The ABPS was more powerful than the EQ-5D and the RDQ at discriminating between groups of patients in relation to medication variables and between patients' ability to do housework and sports. The ABPS was able to discriminate between different levels of severity of low back pain and between those who take analgesics versus those who do not. The ABPS was also strongly associated with the presence of other medical conditions. The ABPS had moderate correlations with the SF-36. The mean ABPS score for patients who were prescribed analgesics in the past 6 months was 30.89 ($N = 68$); for those who were not prescribed analgesics the mean score was 24.76 (N = 95) (no SD given) (Garratt et al. 2001). The standardized response mean was -0.62 ($N = 273$) (Ruta et al. 1994). The standardized response mean for patients with back pain more than 4 weeks and less than 6 months who were unchanged after one year was -8.18 (9.13) (Garratt et al. 2001).

Williams et al. (2001) extended the ABPS to create a set of interlocking outcome measures for the neck, upper and lower back.

The instrument is in the public domain and can be used free of charge.

BACK PAIN FUNCTIONAL SCALE (BPFS)

The Back Pain Functional Scale (BPFS) (Stratford et al. 2000) is based on the World Health Organization's model of impairment, disability and handicap. The BPFS has 12 items, each scored on a 0–5 point scale. Adjectives with approximately equal interval properties define the scale points. Item recall is "today" and the items are phrased in terms of "do you have difficulty..." with the response option ranging from unable to perform activity (0) to no difficulty (5). The total score ranges from 0 (lowest functional level) to 60 (highest functional level).

The aim in the development of the BPFS was to create a self-report functional status measure appropriate for clinical practice and clinical research. Guiding principles were that the measure should be based on the WHO's model of impairment, disability and handicap, have sound psychometric properties, take less than 5 min to complete and take less than 30 seconds to score. Items were derived from existing literature, patient and clinician input.

Test–retest reliability (48 hours) was ICC = 0.88 ($N = 28$) and internal consistency was alpha = 0.93 ($N = 77$). Inter-item correlation ranged from 0.61

(standing one hour) to 0.80 (usual work). Mean (SD) score in a sample of patients with back pain was 34.1 (13.0).

Construct validity was supported by a high correlation with the RDQ ($r = 0.79$). There was also a high correlation between the change scores of the BPFS and the RDQ ($r = 0.82$). The BPFS was able to differentiate among levels of work status, smoking status, location of symptoms and educational level (Stratford et al. 2000).

The standardized Standard Error of Measurement (SEM) for the BPFS was 6.5% (95% CI 5.2–8.8), while the SEM was 3.9 (95% CI 3.1–5.3) points.

LOW BACK OUTCOME SCORE (LBOS)

The Low Back Outcome Score (LBOS) (Greenough and Fraser 1992; Greenough 1993) is a 13-item questionnaire intended as a comprehensive rating system for patients with low back pain. It includes questions about current pain, employment, domestic and sports activities, use of medication and medical services, rest, sex life and daily activities. Each item has 4 graded responses that are weighted. Pain and active activities are weighted more than treatments and rest required. The scale is scored from 0 to 75 with increasing disability representing a reduction in score.

Overall agreement for test–retest reliability (one week) was 84%, and the reliability coefficient (K) reached a range of 0.51 to 0.86 ($p < 0.05$). Internal consistency was alpha = 0.85 (Holt et al. 2002). Good concurrent validity was found with the Waddell Disability Index ($r = -0.74$) and the ODI ($r = -0.87$). The Low Back Outcome Score is able to discriminate between employed and unemployed patients (Greenough 1993).

LOW BACK PAIN RATING SCALE (LBPRS)

The Low Back Pain Rating Scale was developed by Manniche et al. (1994) and validated in 58 patients following first-time discectomy. It can be used, with slight modification, in office and telephone interviews, as well as in postal questionnaires. The scale consists of 4 domains: back pain, leg pain, disability and physical impairment. The pain intensity scale uses a 0–11 point scale and consists of 3 questions that are scored for back pain and leg pain separately and includes: 1, pain at the time of examination; 2, the worst low back pain within the past 2 weeks; and 3, the average level of pain within the past 2 weeks. It takes about 15 minutes to complete.

The disability domain is measured by a questionnaire containing 15 questions about functional activities, social life and work. Ten of the questions are phrased "because of low back pain." Response options are 0 (yes), 1 (can be a problem) and 2 (no), giving a total score of 0–30 points, with higher scores indicating greater disability.

The physical impairment scale consists of 3 tests (a back muscle endurance test, a back mobility test and a mobility test) and the use of analgesics. This scale is omitted if the instrument is self-administered. The components are weighted as follows: 60 points for pain, 30 points for disability and 40 points for physical impairment. The total score ranges from 0 to 130 points with higher scores indicating higher disability.

Inter-rater agreement was 97.7%. Construct validity was determined by factor analysis and criteria validity by partial correlation to the Doctor's Global Assessment and Patient Global Assessment.

MILLION VISUAL ANALOGUE SCALE

The Million Visual Analogue Scale (Million et al. 1982) is an instrument that combines a 15-item questionnaire with 10 objective assessments of spinal-related impairment. The questionnaire response items are 100 mm visual analogue scales relating to pain severity, night pain, relief from pain medication, stiffness in the back, pain and discomfort when walking, standing still, twisting, sitting, lying down, overall lifestyle and work. In the original study questions were asked in a standardized way with the patients making their ratings using a modified slide rule by moving an arrow along a 100 mm line.

The inter-observer (2 observers) reproducibility was $r = 0.92$ and intraobserver agreement was 0.97 (same day) (Million et al. 1982). Test–retest reliability was $r = 0.97$. No internal consistency or validity measures were reported.

The objective assessments include straight leg raising left and right, lumbar extension and flexion in degrees and cm, and lateral flexion left and right in degrees and cm. Intraobserver agreement (same day) on these measures was $r = 0.99$ ($N = 19$).

OSWESTRY DISABILITY INDEX (ODI)

There are at least 5 different versions of the Oswestry Disability Index (ODI) in English (Fairbank et al. 1980) and 9 in other languages (Fairbank and Pynsent 2000). In the original version pain was assessed in terms of analgesic intake. Because this represented difficulties for those who did not take pain medication, the question was replaced with one about "pain severity," modifying the Oswestry slightly. Hudson-Cook et al. (1989) designed the revised Oswestry questionnaire in a study by the Medical Research Council group. They changed the wording of all sections and replacing the sex life question with a question about the patient's interpretation about his or her own changing pain pattern. The Oswestry versions 1.0 and 2.0 were found to be equally reliable and valid (Hudson-Cook et al. 1989). The ODI version 1.0 has excellent test–retest reliability ($r = 0.99$) (24 hours) (Fairbank et al. 1980), ICC = 0.83 (1 week) (Gronblad et al. 1993).

The internal reliability was alpha = 0.71 for version 1.0 (Strong et al. 1994). The reliability of version 2.0 was alpha = 0.76 (Fisher and Johnson 1997) and 0.87 (Kopec et al. 1996). Version 2.0 is recommended for use by the original author (Fairbank) over version 1.0 as it specifically asks for "pain today," a format that patients prefer (Fairbank and Pynsent 2000).

The ODI consists of 10 sections that include pain intensity, personal care, lifting, walking, sitting, standing, sleeping, sex and social life and traveling. Each section is scored on a 6-point scale (0–5), with 0 representing no limitation and 5 representing maximal limitation. The subscales combined add up to a maximum score of 50. The score is then doubled and interpreted as a percentage of patient perceived disability (the higher the score, the greater the disability). If items are missing the percentage score is calculated as follows: (total score)/[5 × (number of answered questions)] × 100. The mean (SD) ODI score is 27 (5.8–23.6) for primary back pain patients ($N = 2166$) and 43.3 (10–21) in patients with chronic low back pain ($N = 1530$) (Roland and Fairbank 2000).

The ODI has been correlated with impairments such as pain as scored on a visual analogue scale (VAS) ($r = 0.62$) (Gronblad et al. 1993) and to the presence or absence of relaxation in back muscles during flexion in CLBP patients ($p < 0.001$) (Triano and Schultz 1987). A moderate correlation ($r = -0.52$) was found between the Isernhagen Work Systems Functional Capacity Evaluation (FCE) and the ODI (Reneman et al. 2002). Correlations of the ODI with the Low Back Outcome Scale ($r = -0.87$) (Greenough and Fraser 1992), the Pain Disability Index ($r = 0.83$) (Gronblad et al. 1993) and the RDQ ($r = 066-0.72$) (Leclaire et al. 1997) are good. Correlations with the Waddell Disability Scores ($p < 0.001$) and Waddell Impairment Rating ($p < 0.05$) were significant (r not reported) (Greenough and Fraser 1992). Significant correlations were reported between the SF-36 domains and the ODI with the Mental Health scale having the lowest correlation (Grevitt et al. 1997), and between the ODI and the Quebec Back Pain Disability Scale (Fritz and Irrgang 2001). Thus, construct validity of the ODQ was confirmed.

The ODI was able to differentiate between employed and unemployed subjects in a sample of subjects with LBP seeking workers' compensation (Sanderson et al. 1995). The ODQ was also able to differentiate between compensation LBP patients seeking or not seeking compensation (Greenough and Fraser 1992), confirming discriminant validity of this measure.

The ODI has been used to validate a number of back pain specific outcomes tools (Gronblad et al. 1993, 1994; Ruta et al. 1994) and has been mined for questions by the designers of other instruments such as the Neck Disability Index and the Northwick Park Neck Pain Questionnaire.

The Minimally Clinically Important Difference of the ODI has been reported as 5.2 (Suarez-Almazor et al. 2000), 6.0 (Fritz and Irrgang 2001), 7.0 (Walsh et al. 2003), 10.0 (Hagg et al. 2003) and 16.3 (Taylor et al. 1999). The receiver operating characteristic was 0.76, in a sample of patients that was not severely affected by pain (Beurskens et al. 1996).

The ODI has been used to a more limited extent with other pain complaints, such as fibromyalgia (Turk et al. 1996). A recent study validated the ODI for the general (chronic) pain population (Wittink et al. 2004). ODI version 1.0 questions were rephrased to ask about "pain" instead of "back pain." The mean (SD) ODI score ($N = 424$) was 45.16 (19.6). Internal consistency was Cronbach's alpha = 0.86. The ODI had an effect size of -0.39 and a standard error of 0.81. Significant overlap was found between the ODI, the SF-36 and the Multidimensional Pain Inventory.

The copy of the instrument in this book is version 2.0, a modification of the original version.

QUEBEC BACK PAIN DISABILITY SCALE

The Quebec Back Pain Disability Scale (QBPDS) (Kopec et al. 1995, 1996) was constructed to be a multi-purpose questionnaire that could be used in outcome trials, for monitoring the progress of patients participating in treatment or rehabilitation trials and for comparing different groups of patients with back pain. Disability was operationalized in the WHO term of "any restriction or lack of ability to perform an activity in a manner or within the range considered normal for a human being" (World Health Organization 1980). The content of the QBPDS was developed in several stages, including a literature review, two studies seeking the opinions of patients and experts, pilot testing, and a longitudinal study of back pain patients ($N = 242$). Forty-eight disability items were extensively studied using standard methods such as test–retest reliability, item-total correlations, and factor analysis, as well as item response theory. Items that were highly effective in discriminating between different levels of disability were selected for the final, reduced 20 item scale. The items refer to specific, simple activities and cover sleeping and resting, sitting, standing, walking, movement, bending and stooping and handling large or heavy objects. For each item there is a 6 point difficulty scale, ranging from 0 (not difficult at all) to 5 (extremely difficult). The total score is the sum of all items and ranges from 0 to 100. The questionnaire takes about 5 minutes to fill out. Test–retest reliability was ICC = 0.92 (4 days). Test–retest correlations of the individual items ranged from 0.65 to 0.91 and Cronbach's alpha for the total scale was 0.96. For the Dutch adaptation of the Quebec Back Pain Disability Scale Pearson and intraclass correlation coefficients for test–retest reliability were 0.90. Cronbach's alpha was 0.95 (Schoppink

et al. 1996). Fritz and Irrgang (2001) warn that the QBPDS shows diminished reliability (ICC = 0.55, 95% CI 0.20–0.78) in the scale when applied in patients ($N = 23$) with acute back pain.

Patients diagnosed with non-specific CLBP referred to the outpatient department of a university hospital in the Netherlands scored a mean of 37.8 (15.7) points (Reneman et al. 2002) and acute back pain patients scored a mean (SD) of 49.3 (Fritz and Irrgang 2001). The QBPDS was compared with the RDQ ($r = 0.77$), ODI ($r = 0.80$) and the SF-36 Physical Functioning scale ($r = 0.72$) and a 7-point pain scale ($r = 0.54$) supporting concurrent validity (Kopec et al. 1995). The scale was able to discriminate between groups of subjects with different levels of disability, specifically between males and females, use of medication, yes/no, compensation status, yes/no, and work absence, yes/no. Significant changes in disability over time, and differences in change scores between patients that were expected to differ in the direction of change, were found. Overall the scale performed as well as the standard measures and was more responsive than the SF-36 Physical Functioning scale. Fritz and Irrgang (2001) compared the QBPDS to the modified ODI in acute back pain patients ($N = 67$) and found that the modified ODI showed higher test–retest reliability and responsiveness than the QBPDS. Minimal detectable change (90% confidence interval) = 15 points (Davidson et al. 2004). The MCID calculated from the ROC curve using the cut-off point nearest to the upper left-hand corner of the graph was 15 points for the QBPDS, sensitivity 82%, specificity 83% (Fritz and Irrgang 2001) in acute LBP patients. The MCIC of the QBPDS was estimated between 17.5 to 32.9 points and 8.5 to 24.6 points for (sub)acute and chronic patients with low back pain (van der Roer et al. 2006)

ROLAND-MORRIS DISABILITY QUESTIONNAIRE (RDQ)

The Roland-Morris Disability Questionnaire (RDQ-24) (Roland and Morris 1983a,b), also called the St. Thomas questionnaire, was derived from the Sickness Impact Profile (SIP). The generic SIP was constructed to be disease-specific by adding "because of my back pain" to each item. Twenty-four yes/no items were selected from the SIP by the original authors because they related specifically to physical functions that were likely to be affected by low back pain. These items include walking, bending over, sitting, lying down, dressing, sleeping, self care and activities of daily living. Response recall is "today." The RDQ can be administered as self report, by computer or telephone. The RDQ takes about 5 min. to complete.

There are several other versions of the RDQ: the modified RDQ (MRDQ) (Patrick et al. 1995) and the short RDQ (RM-18) (Stratford and Binkley 1997).

The two modified versions of the RDQ are not substantially different from the RDQ with regard to reproducibility or responsiveness in patients post lumbar disc surgery (Ostelo et al. 2004).

The scoring of the RDQ is achieved by adding the equally weighted number of positive responses. A score can vary from 0 (no disability) to 24 (severe disability).

Test–retest reliability ranges from ICC = 0.66 to ICC = 0.96 (Riddle and Stratford 2002). ICC values lower than this were found ranging from ICC = 0.42 to 0.66 (Davidson and Keating 2002; Patrick et al. 1995). Most studies with ICC values of ≥ 0.75 used an interval of 1–14 days, whereas for the studies with an ICC of lower than 0.75 an interval of 6 weeks or more was used (Brouwer et al. 2004). Cronbach's alpha for the scale has been estimated between alpha = 0.84 and 0.93 (Roland and Fairbank 2000). The RDQ correlates well with the SF-36 physical subscales, the SIP (Jensen et al. 1992; Patrick et al. 1995) and pain ratings (Beurskens et al. 1996), the Quebec Back Pain Disability Scale (Kopec et al. 1996) and the ODI (Stratford et al. 1994; Leclaire et al. 1997; Davidson and Keating 2002).

The RDQ is reliable and valid in assessing dysfunction of chronic pain patients with pain in other sites than the low back as well as those with back pain (Jensen et al. 1992). The RDQ has a good correlation with the SIP physical domain ($r = 0.85$), and moderate correlations with the Beck Depression Inventory ($r = 0.47$) and the McGill Pain Questionnaire ($r = 0.27$) (Jensen et al. 1992).

Studies have determined the cutoff score for change of the RDQ ranging from 2 to 9.5 points (Deyo and Centor 1986; Beurskens et al. 1995; Patrick et al. 1995; Stratford et al. 1996; Brouwer et al. 2004). Stratford et al. (1998) suggest that the minimum clinically important change in scores is 1–2 points for patients with little disability, 7–8 points for patients reporting high levels of disability and 5 points in unselected patients. The RDQ is available in 12 languages, and translations are available from the author (mroland@man.ac.uk).

WADDELL DISABILITY INDEX

The Waddell Disability Index (Waddell and Main 1984) originally was an interview and physical examination-based index. The interview focused on 9 basic physical activities of daily living commonly restricted by back pain, with the emphasis on loss of function rather than pain. Questions were phrased in terms of "have you reduced or do you now avoid, or now require help with, this activity?" Response recall was "since the onset of your back pain." Each of these items has yes or no responses. See instrument for included items (the instructions for completion of the instrument were added by the authors of this chapter).

Although initially not reported in self-report form, a questionnaire was derived from the original article

and published in 1994 (Delitto 1994). The total score ranges from 0 to 9. Internal consistency of these items is alpha = 0.76. Inter-observer agreement for individual items ranged from 73% agreement for sitting one half hour to 90% for help with footwear. Test–retest reliability is not reported for the total score, but individual items have test–retest correlations of $r = 0.73$–0.90 (Patrick et al. 1995). Correlations ($r = 0.70$) with the Oswestry provide evidence of construct validity. The disability scale is accompanied by a physical impairment scale which includes pain pattern (back pain versus back and referred leg versus root pain), recurring or chronic pain, previous fracture, previous back surgery and root compression. In addition lumbar flexion is measured in cm. and straight leg raising left and right. These impairments are added up to approximate a total body impairment of a maximum of 40%, representing the worst possible back problem. Percent agreement between examiners for the impairment tests ranged from 77% (root compression signs) to 100% (previous back surgery) (Waddell and Main 1984). In a comparison of 5 back specific instruments (Davidson et al. 2004) the Waddell Disability Index had a test–retest reliability (6 weeks, in patients that self-rated "unchanged") of ICC = 0.74, the standard error of measurement (SEM) was 1.2 and the minimally detectable change (MDC) was 2.8. Davidson and Keating (2002) report that the potential clinical utility of the Waddell Disability Index is diminished by the relatively large MDC and a lack of scale width, as 21% of their sample ($N = 106$) scored less than 3 points and 20% more than 6 points at the initial measurement.

NECK AND BACK PAIN-SPECIFIC MEASUREMENTS

FUNCTIONAL RATING INDEX

The Functional Rating Index (FRI) (Feise and Michael 2001) combines the content of the ODI and the NDI in a format that reduces the administrative burden. The FRI instrument contains 10 items that measure pain and function of the spinal musculoskeletal system: eight refer to activities of daily living that might be adversely affected by a spinal condition; two refer to different attributes of pain. The FRI requires about one minute for a patient to complete, and about 20 seconds for a health care worker to score. This instrument can be used with cervical, thoracic or lumbar conditions, which reduces the need for multiple instruments for spine-related conditions. Response recall is "right now" and item responses are scored on a 5-point scale with higher scores indicating more dysfunction or pain. The instrument can be scored by item, or the items can be summed. When all 10 items are completed the FRI score is calculated as (total score/40) × 100%.

Test–retest reliability was ICC = 0.99 (N = 51). Cronbach's alpha was 0.92 for all variables with the individual items scoring either alpha = 0.91 or 0.92 (N = 51). Validity was supported by strong correlations with the SF-12 Physical Component Score (r = 0.76) and a weak correlation with the SF-12 Mental Health Component Score (r = 0.36). The overall standardized response mean was 1.24 (N = 36). The mean (SD) score of the FRI was 47.9 (22.1) in a sample of 139 patients with lumbar, thoracic and neck pain. The reliability, validity and responsiveness of this instrument need yet to be confirmed in other studies.

NECK PAIN-SPECIFIC INSTRUMENTS

NECK DISABILITY INDEX (NDI)

The Neck Disability Index (NDI) (Vernon and Mior 1991), also called the Vernon neck disability index, is a tool derived from the ODI with permission from the original author (Fairbank et al. 1980). It contains 10 items, which include pain intensity, personal care, lifting, reading, headaches, concentration, work, driving, sleeping and recreation. Each item has 6 response items expressing progressive levels of functional capability. The NDI is scored the same as the ODI by summing the responses (range 0–50) and multiplying by 2 to achieve a percentage score. When an item is missing, the average of the other items is substituted. Test–retest reliability (N = 17) is r = 0.89 and the internal consistency of the entire instrument is alpha = 0.80, with each of the questions having an alpha > 0.75 (Vernon and Mior 1991). Hains et al. (1998) also confirmed good psychometric properties (Cronbach alpha of 0.92) of the instrument as did Riddle and Stratford (1998). Riddle and Stratford (1998) reported a ceiling effect, however, suggesting that the NDI may not be able to detect differences in the very to completely disabled range. Furthermore, the NDI appears to be susceptible to missing data on the "driving" item among elderly patients and the reading item among patients of low educational status. Face and content validity were demonstrated in several studies (Hains et al. 1998; Vernon and Mior 1991). The NDI consists of one factor – "physical disability" – although NDI scores correlate well with SF-36 mental component scores (Riddle and Stratford 1998) as well. In fact, Riddle and Stratford found substantial overlap between the NDI and the SF-36 and concluded that the use of both measures, therefore, is probably not necessary. Concurrent validity was supported by a correlation of r = 0.7 with the McGill Pain Questionnaire (Vernon and Mior 1991). The minimum detectable score and the minimal clinically important difference amount to the same figure: 5 NDI points.

Nederhand et al. (2004) reported that by using a combination of the baseline NDI and TSK, it appears to be possible to predict chronic disability with a probability of 54.3% (95% confidence interval [CI], 35.2–72.3%) after entering the NDI (cutoff = 15 points) as a first test, and with a probability of 83.3% (95% CI, 70.3–91.3%) after entering the TSK (cutoff = 40 points) in a second test, in a sample of acute neck pain patients (N = 82).

NECK PAIN AND DISABILITY SCALE

The Neck Pain and Disability Scale (NPAD) (Wheeler et al. 1999) was developed based on the Million Visual Analogue Scale. It has 20 items, each with a VAS scale graded from 0 (normal function) to 5 (the worst possible situation your pain problem has taken you). Response recall is not specified. The questionnaire has 4 domains: neck problems, pain intensity, effect of neck pain on emotion and cognition and degree to which neck pain interferes with life activities. The questionnaire takes less than 5 min. to complete. Test–retest reliability was good (r = 0.97) in a sample of 28 patients with neck pain (Goolkasian et al. 2002). Internal reliability (N = 100) is alpha = 0.93. No internal consistency for each of the domains was reported.

Construct validity was supported by good correlations with the ODI (r = 0.78) and the PDI (r = 0.80). Pain intensity was significantly ($p < 0.01$) correlated with the total NPAD score (r = 0.55) and with each of the four effects of neck pain represented in the NPAD subdomains (r = 0.42–0.63) (Clair et al. 2004). The NPAD is able to discriminate between patients with neck pain and normal controls and between patients with neck pain and patients with lower back and leg pain. NPAD changes were correlated with changes in muscle tenderness as measured by pressure algometry, and with changes in performance on the NDI and PDI (Goolkasian et al. 2002).

The NPAD showed a large treatment effect size (ES = 1.4) after 16 weeks of intervention. When subdivided into factor scores, factor 2 (pain intensity, ES = 1.68) and factor 4 (interference in life events, ES = 1.45) yielded the largest treatment effects.

Contact authors for use at pagoolka@email.uncc.edu.

THE NORTHWICK PARK NECK PAIN QUESTIONNAIRE (NPQ)

Like the NDI, the Northwick Questionnaire (Leak et al. 1994) is based on the ODI. The NPQ consists of nine items including pain intensity, duration of symptoms, pins and needles or numbness at night, pain affecting sleep, effect on social life, carrying, reading/watching television (TV), working/housework, and driving. For each item, there are five potential responses describing a greater degree of difficulty ranging from 0 (no difficulty) to 4 (severe difficulty). An overall percentage

NDQ score is calculated by adding together the scores for each item (0–36) and calculating a percentage (total score/36 × 100%). If items are not applicable, the total potential score is reduced (e.g., one item not applicable, total score out of 32).

Test–retest reliability was kappa = 0.62 (3 days) and was reported as ICC = 0.84 (24 hours) in the French translation (Wlodyka-Demaille et al. 2002). Internal consistency is α = 0.79 (Sim et al. 2006). The item "duration of symptoms" had the highest item score (mean score, 3.0; SD, 1.3), followed by carrying (mean score, 2.0; SD, 1.0). The mean score for most other items in the NPQ were between 1.4 and 1.7 with the exception of pins and needles or numbness in the arms at night (mean score, 0.7; SD, 0.8) (Hoving et al. 2003). The NPQ has been validated in patients complaining of neck pain attending a rheumatology clinic in the UK where mean scores for each item were shown to correlate with intensity of pain (Leak et al. 1994). Construct validity in patients with whiplash associated dysfunction is supported by good correlations between the NDI and NPQ (r = 0.88, p < 0.01) (Hoving et al. 2003). The MCID for the NPQ was determined as a 25% reduction in score from baseline together with a patient's global rating of their neck pain of at least "better." (Sim et al. 2006)

THE COPENHAGEN NECK FUNCTIONAL DISABILITY SCALE

The Copenhagen Neck Functional Disability Scale (CNFDS) (Jordan et al. 1998) is a 15-item questionnaire related to neck dysfunction. Response items include "Yes," "Occasionally" and "No." The instrument takes about 10 minutes to complete. Test–retest reliability (24 hours) was r = 0.99 and r = 0.98 (2 days). Internal reliability for the entire questionnaire is Cronbach's alpha = 0.90. Construct validity was demonstrated by high correlations with pain scores (r = 0.83) and the patient's global assessment (r = 0.89). Moderate correlations were found for the doctor's global assessment (Jordan et al. 1998).

FUNCTIONAL CAPACITY AND PERFORMANCE TESTING

Functional performance of daily activities can be assessed by several different methods, for example by using questionnaires or diaries. Questionnaires are easily administered, often easily scored and can yield important information with relatively little time investment. These measurement instruments have the advantage that they can measure several aspects of activity. The underlying principle for self report validity is that individuals' perception of their functional ability is highly related to their actual physical performance. In terms of rehabilitation assessment and treatment, it is important to know what patients' actual performance is in daily life, as a number of studies noted that chronic pain patients' self reported levels of physical activity were significantly lower than those observed or measured objectively. Affective states are known to influence self reported well-being or pain. Depression appears to play a role in this discrepancy (Casten et al. 2000; Wittink et al. 2001, 2003) and pain-related factors such as fear avoidance, pain threshold, pain expectancy, pain at exertion and pain catastrophizing may also play a role. For instance, Verbunt et al. (2001) recently measured the activity levels of patients suffering from CLBP and matched healthy controls continuously for 2 weeks using a triaxial accelerometer. The results demonstrated that the mean activity levels of the patients, who had rated their disability as substantial, did not differ significantly from the controls.

In addition, questionnaires are unable to measure quality of movement, such as how long it takes a person to perform a task, whether and how much movement is compensated, whether rests are necessary and if pain behavior is present. These factors are deemed important in the development of a treatment plan and in assessing the outcome of treatment by health professionals. Patients may not be aware of a change in their motor behavior and thus not report it. Solutions were therefore sought to quantify and qualify functional capacity and performance. In ICF language functional *capacity* tests measure functional (standardized) tasks in a laboratory environment to determine the patient's ability or capacity to complete these tasks. Standardized testing can be performed using several different techniques, either in the laboratory using for instance an advanced motion analysis system, or in a clinical setting or home environment using functional capacity tests (e.g., Bussmann et al. 1998a,b; Bussmann and Stam 1998). Functional *performance*, however, refers to the actual activity pattern in everyday life, which does not necessarily reflect physical capacity (for example, when tested with a 10-meter walk test a subject could walk 10 meters in 5 seconds, but may never actually do so or even attain a speed of 2 m/s in daily life). Therefore, to inform, improve and evaluate rehabilitation treatment strategies of patients living with (chronic) illness, their mobility or activities in everyday life should be evaluated or monitored in the daily living environment (Veltink et al. 1996; Bussmann and Stam 1998). Since the personal environment is where existing disabilities limit functional activity, it is important to know about existing methods that can be applied to assess functional performance and mobility in normal daily functioning.

FUNCTIONAL CAPACITY TESTS

Standardized functional tests have been developed, such as the 50 foot walk test, the 5 and 10 minute walking test, stair climb, reach and sit to stand tests, which reflect common basic functional tasks. Typically these tasks set criteria of time and/or distance and/or number of repetitions in a given timeframe. These tests can be administered under controlled conditions in order to have an objective measure of a patient's ability to perform simple tasks. While in the literature functional capacity tests refer to work-related tasks (Reneman and Wittink 2007), non-work-related functional tests have been called physical performance, functional performance, physical ability, and functional assessment tests. Most authors refer to performance testing. This terminology is based on the definition of capacity as the maximum level of *physical* performance, defined by the limits of the anatomical, physiologic and psychological systems of the person, and is measured in terms of maximal oxygen uptake (VO2max), maximal heart rate, and maximal muscle strength and endurance testing. In this context performance is defined as capacity as modified by individual behavioral attitudes, in addition to modifications by external factors such as injury, pain and environmental and social stressors (Abdel-Moty et al. 1996). Because of the ICF terminology, we will refer to all tests that measure functional tasks in a standardized environment as functional capacity tests. Unfortunately, affective states appear to influence functional capacity tests as well. Poorer achievement on physical performance testing by patients with chronic low back pain (CLBP) has been linked to fear of injury during movement (Waddell et al. 1993; Vlaeyen et al. 1995; Crombez et al. 1998), depression (Herr et al. 1993), cognitive factors (Schmidt 1985), pain expectations (Crombez et al. 1996; Murphy et al. 1997), pain increase during testing (Murphy et al. 1997; Wittink et al. 2001), disability status (Keefe and Hill 1985), the presence of a solicitous spouse (Jensen et al. 1994) and motivation. It appears that performance testing, however, is less influenced by culture, language and education or depression and disability status than self-report. Self-report measurements and functional capacity-based assessments appear to provide information about related but distinct aspects of functional status and should be used as supplementary measures (Wittink et al. 2003). Because of the tendency of affective states to influence self-report and functional capacity tests, additional measures should evaluate the affective state.

Overall, the correlation between self-report and functional capacity tests is low to moderate. For instance, functional capacity tests in chronic low back pain studies, such as repeated squatting, loaded reach, sit-to-stand, 5 minute walk or 50 foot walk, had no better than moderate correlations with disease-specific instruments (Simmonds et al. 1998). Stratford et al. (2003) report that by combining time, pain and exertion variables into a composite score greater correlation is achieved with the self-report measure. This suggests that using a single dimension in a functional task, such as time, is insufficient to reflect the patient's perception of what it involves to do such a task.

THE PHYSICAL PERFORMANCE TEST (PPT)

The Physical Performance Test (PPT) was developed by Simmonds et al. (1998). The PPT includes a series of 5 tasks in which the time taken or distance reached or walked is measured. The timed tasks include a 50 foot walk at fastest speed, repeated trunk flexion ($\times 10$) and repeated sit to stand tasks ($\times 5$). The distance tests include a 5 minute walk and a loaded reach task. The PPT takes about 20 minutes to administer. Intra-rater reliability ranged from ICC = 0.45 for sit to stand to ICC $\geq$ 0.95 for the 4 other tests. Inter-rater reliability was ICC $\geq$ 0.98 for all tests ($N = 44$ patients with low back pain and 4). Test–retest reliability (2 weeks) ranged from ICC = 0.76 to 0.91. The tests had good discriminant validity between a group of healthy subjects and subjects with low back pain (Simmonds et al. 1998). Two correlated (0.74) factors, speed and coordination and endurance and strength, were derived from the physical performance tasks. Both factors had statistically significant correlations with measures of physical disability, lack of self-efficacy, and negative affect. Both factors had a trivial correlation with a numeric rating of pain intensity (Novy et al. 2002).

Correlations between the individual items of the RDQ and individual tests of the PPT were weak to moderate, as were the correlations between the total RDQ score and the individual tests (Lee et al. 2001). Predicted peak VO2 was moderately correlated to the 5 minute walk test in a sample of chronic back pain patients ($N = 51$) (Cunha et al. 2002).

THE INPUT TESTS

Harding et al. (1994) developed a set of tests designed to cover speed and endurance in walking, stair climbing, standing up from a chair, sit-ups, arm endurance, grip strength, and peak flow. Standard instructions and testing conditions were used by a trained tester on a population of chronic inpatient pain patients before and after a cognitive-behavioral chronic pain management program. Testing took about 45 minutes. The tests included the 10 and 5 minute walk, a 2 minute stair climbing test, a 2 minute stand-up test, sit ups to tolerance, an arm endurance test, grip (kg) and peak flow (L/min). Inter-rater reliability was ICC > 0.98 for all measures. Test–retest reliability ranged from $r = 0.70$ for arm endurance to ICC = 0.99 for the speed walk. The 10 and 5 minute walk correlated strongly ($r = 0.99$), as did the 2 minute and 1 minute stair climb test ($r = 0.98$) and the 1 and 2 minute stand up tests ($r = 0.98$). These shorter tests can thus be substituted when there is lack of time.

BACK PERFORMANCE SCALE (BPS)

The Back Performance Scale (BPS) (Strand et al. 2002; Magnussen et al. 2004) was developed as a test battery of daily physical functioning, including five tests of activities requiring mobility of the trunk, primarily in the sagittal plane. The five activities include the following:

1. Sock test
2. Pick-up test
3. Roll-up test
4. Fingertip to floor test
5. Lift test.

Each test is scored on a 4-point ordinal scale according to observed physical performance. The total score ranges from 0 (no activity limitation) to 16 (major activity limitation).

In a sample of 288 patients with long standing musculoskeletal pain bivariate correlations (rs) of scores among tests ranged from 0.27 to 0.50, and correlations between separate tests and the BPS ranged from 0.63 to 0.73 (Strand et al. 2002). Cronbach's alpha of the BPS was alpha = 0.73. The BPS sum scores discriminated between patients with different return to work status and were higher for back pain than for other musculoskeletal pain. Responsiveness was high (effect size = 1.33) in patients who had changed and low (effect size = 0.31) in patients who had not changed, using return to work as an external indicator of important change. The total BPS was more responsive than its parts, the separate tests.

Inter-tester reliability (N = 32) ranged from kappa = 0.96 for the sock test to kappa = 1.0 for the roll-up and lift test. Test–retest reliability ranged from kappa = 0.55 for the lift test to 0.83 for the roll-up test.

For the BPS sum score inter-tester ICC = 0.99 and test–retest reliability ICC = 0.91.

A moderate correlation between the BPS and the RDQ (r = 0.45) was found supporting concurrent validity. No significant correlation was present between the BPS and the FABQ (r = 0.05).

The mean (SD) sum score of the BPS in patients with long lasting pain (N = 41) was 6.4 (3.8) and 9.6 (2.7) for patients with acute pain (N = 9). Based on the ICC score for test–retest reliability the investigators concluded that a change in BPS sum score should exceed 3.6 to claim that the physical performance has actually changed (Magnussen et al. 2004).

FUNCTIONAL PERFORMANCE MEASUREMENT: ACTIVITY MONITORING

Methods for the measurement of functional performance (what the patient does in daily life) include, for example, techniques based on analysis of observation data (video recordings or observer registration, which is time-consuming and expensive) or so-called actigraphy, which uses actometers, usually worn at about center of mass height. These devices contain motion sensors that can be used to derive activity by for example counting steps (Le Masurier 2004). Recent technological advances have encouraged the development of other, more advanced "activity monitors" that use uniaxial or triaxial accelerometers connected to or embedded in a portable digital data-logger. Today, measurement of daily activity during normal daily life is possible (Bussmann et al. 2001), without the above mentioned disadvantages of other methods. This type of "activity monitoring" allows for the assessment of changes in activity patterns across several days as well as the assessment of changes in the amount of physical activity within a registration period. Another advantage of these ambulatory systems is that the activity registration takes place in the absence of the observer, eliminating observer bias and significantly cutting costs. Gradually, activity monitoring is being used to study movement patterns and activity in patients with pain (Bussmann et al. 1998a,b; Verbunt et al. 2001; Spenkelink et al. 2002; Schasfoort et al. 2004). However, it is beyond the scope of this chapter to provide detailed information regarding methods and results of these studies.

The basics of activity monitors

Ambulatory activity monitors can be of a more simple design using a single uni-, bi- or triaxial accelerometer embedded in a data-logger worn at the waist or the system can be more complex and contain multiple sensors placed on the body at different locations such as the chest, legs and arms (Bussmann et al. 1998a,b, 2001; Zijlstra 2004). In the latter case, the sensors are connected to a portable data recorder via wires. Systems that use a single uniaxial or triaxial accelerometer usually do not provide information regarding the type of activities performed and provide a very global measure of activity or mobility index. To obtain more detailed information regarding the type of activities a more comprehensive combination of sensors is required, enabling the registration of trunk, arm and leg positions and movements (see Figure 17.2). To obtain information regarding basic postures and motion such as lying-down, sitting, standing and walking, a minimum of two accelerometers is required, one on the trunk and one on the leg.

Several systems are available that use multiple accelerometers (for a comprehensive overview of such a system refer to Bussmann et al. 2001). These sensors provide combined information regarding the position of a limb or segment (postures) as well as dynamic movement (motions). Off-line analysis of the obtained time-series of accelerations can thus yield information regarding the type of daily activities. Such analysis can be used to classify postures (static activities such as standing, sitting, lying down) and motions (dynamic of the segment with respect to the gravitational field, while dynamic activities are usually identified from cyclical motion characteristics of the segments (Veltink et al. 1996). This results in quantitative measures such as the relative proportion of time spent performing these activities (duration) during a registration period. Figure 17.3 shows an example of an activity profile. The quantitative data can be downloaded to spreadsheet files and further analyzed. In addition to the quantitative analysis of postures and motions, the accelerometer signal contains qualitative features such as frequency, walking speed, motility, stability over time and phasing which can also be explored (Bussmann et al. 2001; Zijlstra 2004).

Currently, advanced activity monitoring systems also allow for concurrent ambulatory registration of for example ECG, heart-rate, EMG and even oxygen uptake, providing even more detail about daily activities and their underlying physiology.

Several other physiologic measurement techniques to estimate energy expenditure (as an indication of activity levels) are available. Usually some physiologic parameter such as oxygen uptake or heart-rate is used. An alternative but expensive method is to measure the rate of decline in labeled isotopes to determine metabolic rate (the doubly labeled water technique). The doubly labeled water technique is considered the gold standard for measuring energy expenditure under free-living conditions. In combination with basal metabolic rate estimates, it can be used to estimate energy expenditure for up to three weeks (Conway et al. 2002; Livingstone and Black 2003). Major disadvantages of this method in the assessment of functional physical performance are that it is expensive and provides no detail regarding the types of activities performed.

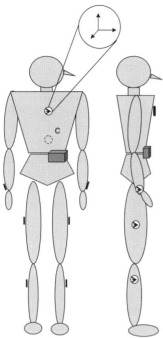

Figure 17.2 Schematic of a possible sensor configuration. Sensors are distributed across the body to record detailed leg, trunk and arm movements. Arm and leg sensors are single axis and applied so that the sensitive axis is along the sagittal plane of motion. The inset shows that the trunk sensor is triaxial, i.e., it has three sensitive axes along the frontal, transverse and sagittal plane (c = approximate center of mass position).

activities such as walking, stair walking, cycling, standing up, sitting down, wheel chair driving). Static activities (postures) can be identified by the orientations

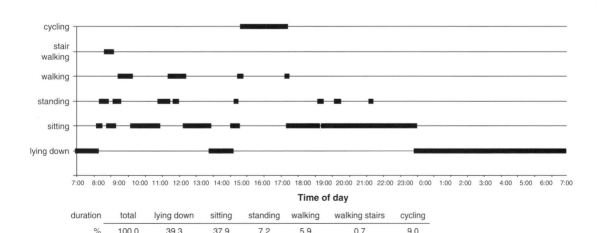

duration	total	lying down	sitting	standing	walking	walking stairs	cycling
%	100.0	39.3	37.9	7.2	5.9	0.7	9.0
hours	24.0	9.5	9.2	1.8	1.4	0.2	2.2

Figure 17.3 Activity profile. Top graph: example data of a 24-hour monitoring session for 6 types of daily activity. Due to figure compression, activities may appear somewhat longer in duration. Visible overlap between activities in the figure is in fact nonexistent. Bottom table: summary statistics for the 6 activities.

Some practical and methodologic considerations of ambulatory activity monitoring

One of the main issues in ambulatory monitoring of functional activities is that the method of measurement should be relatively simple, easy to use, and non-time-consuming (Bussmann et al. 1998a; Bussmann and Stam 1998; Zijlstra 2004). In addition, the system should not interfere with daily activities and be light-weight. Therefore, one of the considerations for monitoring should involve the level of detail required to answer the research questions (i.e., can a single accelerometer on the trunk or leg provide the required activity information or is a more elaborate system necessary with the potential for more detail about types of activities?).

Another related important issue is the duration of monitoring. Due to day-to-day variations in activity patterns there is variability both between similar weekdays and between different weekdays (e.g., van den Berg-Emons et al. 2001). To obtain sufficient statistical power, the number of weekdays and/or the number of subjects will need to be increased due to this inherent variability. Since between-day variability or even between-season variability may differ between patient populations, study designs and interpretations of monitoring data should therefore include considerations regarding possible existing differences in activity patterns. Some knowledge about between-day variability is therefore useful before using activity monitoring in intervention studies.

Current technology allows for detailed ambulatory analysis of postures and motions. Generally speaking, however, the higher the level of detail, the more sensors are needed, which increases the "burden" on the subjects due to increased weight of the data-logging device (including batteries) and the presence of multiple wires and sensors. This can prevent the subject from for example taking a shower, since sensors are semi-permanently attached. Combined with limited battery-life and higher power consumption for advanced monitoring systems, these factors result in a feasible monitoring-period of about two to three days (Bussmann, personal communication).

When lower levels of detail are required, one can make do with a more simple monitoring system (i.e., a single accelerometer, or a step-counter) that can be taken off when needed and is more suited for multiple days (>3) of monitoring. For example, commercially available "sports-watches" are currently able to do straightforward step counting.

Another consideration with activity monitoring is the possible influence of monitoring on the activities performed by the subject. This is called reactivity (Melanson and Freedson 1996; Foerster and Fahrenberg 2000). The mere presence of instrumentation can modify the activity pattern: subjects can either become more active than usual "to make the measurement better" or they can feel hindered by the weight or size of the device, or are "afraid to break something" and refrain from normal activities. Proper instruction of the subject to maintain the usual activity pattern plays an important role here to minimize reactivity effects.

In summary, activity monitoring is being applied more and more in the fields of movement sciences and rehabilitation medicine. Technological developments currently allow for very detailed ambulatory registration of postures and motions in the natural living environment, providing objective and valid measures of activities of daily living. This type of information can be used in the evaluation of pain treatment as well as in the study of pain-related behavior in daily life.

CONCLUSION

Musculoskeletal pain (MP) encompasses all pain in muscle, connective tissue, bone and joints due to disease, injury or trauma. A WHO scientific group meeting considered *pain, mobility,* and *independence to be the most relevant domains for musculoskeletal conditions, and it identified the need for simpler instruments usable in all populations to monitor these aspects.*

This chapter provides an overview of available instruments for measuring functional status. These instruments include both "subjective" measures (based on self-report) and "objective" measures (based on direct measurement). We have included generic instruments that can be used in all populations with (C)MP, but focused on back and neck pain specific instruments to illustrate disease specific instruments because these conditions belong to the most prevalent and costly of (C)MP.

REFERENCES

Abdel-Moty A, Maguire GH, Kaplan SH, et al. Stated versus observed performance levels in patients with chronic low back pain. Occupat Ther Health Care 1996; 10:3–23.

Beaton DE, Schemitsch E. Measures of health-related quality of life and physical function. Clin Orthop 2003; 413:90–105.

Beaton DE, Bombardier C, Hogg-Johnson SA. Measuring health in injured workers: a cross-sectional comparison of five generic health status instruments in workers with musculoskeletal injuries. Am J Ind Med 1996; 29:618–631.

Beurskens AJ, de Vet HC, Koke AJ, et al. Measuring the functional status of patients with low back pain. Assessment of the quality of four disease-specific questionnaires. Spine 1995; 20:1017–1028.

Beurskens AJ, de Vet HC, Koke AJ. Responsiveness of functional status in low back pain: a comparison of different instruments. Pain 1996; 65:71–76.

Bombardier C. Outcome assessments in the evaluation of treatment of spinal disorders: summary and general recommendations. Spine 2000; 25:3100–3103.

Bombardier C, Hayden J, Beaton DE. Minimal clinically important difference. Low back pain: outcome measures. J Rheumatol 2001; 28:431–438.

Bot SD, Terwee CB, van der Windt DA. Clinimetric evaluation of shoulder disability questionnaires: a systematic review of the literature. Ann Rheum Dis 2004; 63:335–341.

Brouwer S, Kuijer W, Dijkstra PU, et al. Reliability and stability of the Roland Morris Disability Questionnaire: intra class correlation and limits of agreement. Disabil Rehabil 2004; 26:162–165.

Brown JH, Kazis LE, Spitz PW, et al. The dimensions of health outcomes: a cross-validated examination of health status measurement. Am J Public Health 1984; 74:159–161.

Bruce B, Fries JF. The Stanford Health Assessment Questionnaire: a review of its history, issues, progress, and documentation. J Rheumatol 2003a; 30:167–178.

Bruce B, Fries JF. The Stanford Health Assessment Questionnaire: dimensions and practical applications. Health Qual Life Outcomes 2003b; 1:20.

Burton HJ, Sline SA, Hargadon R, et al. Assessing patients with chronic pain using the basic personality inventory as a complement to the multidimensional pain inventory. Pain Res Manage 1999; 4:131–129.

Bussmann JB, Stam HJ. Techniques for measurement and assessment of mobility in rehabilitation: a theoretical approach. Clin Rehabil 1998; 12:455–464.

Bussmann JB, Tulen JH, van Herel EC, et al. Quantification of physical activities by means of ambulatory accelerometry: a validation study. Psychophysiology 1998a; 35:488–496.

Bussmann JB, van de Laar YM, Neeleman MP, et al. Ambulatory accelerometry to quantify motor behaviour in patients after failed back surgery: a validation study. Pain 1998b; 74:153–161.

Bussmann JB, Martens WL, Tulen JH, et al. Measuring daily behavior using ambulatory accelerometry: the Activity Monitor. Behav Res Methods Instrum Comput 2001; 33:349–356.

Casten RJ, Rovner BW, Pasternak RE, et al. A comparison of self-reported function assessed before and after depression treatment among depressed geriatric inpatients. Int J Geriatr Psychiatry 2000; 15:813–818.

Chibnall JT, Tait RC. The Pain Disability Index: factor structure and normative data. Arch Phys Med Rehabil 1994; 75:1082–1086.

Chwastiak LA, Von Korff M. Disability in depression and back pain: evaluation of the World Health Organization Disability Assessment Schedule (WHO DAS II) in a primary care setting. J Clin Epidemiol 2003; 56:507–514.

Clair D, Edmondston S, Allison G. Variability in pain intensity, physical and psychological function in non-acute, non-traumatic neck pain. Physiother Res Int 2004; 9:43–54.

Conway JM, Seale JL, Jacobs DR Jr, et al. Comparison of energy expenditure estimates from doubly labeled water, a physical activity questionnaire, and physical activity records. Am J Clin Nutr 2002; 75:519–525.

Crombez G, Vervaet L, Baeyens F, et al. Do pain expectancies cause pain in chronic low back patients? A clinical investigation. Behav Res Ther 1996; 34:919–925.

Crombez G, Vervaet L, Lysens R, et al. Avoidance and confrontation of painful, back-straining movements in chronic back pain patients. Behav Modif 1998; 22:62–77.

Crombez G, Vlaeyen JW, Heuts PH, et al. Pain-related fear is more disabling than pain itself: evidence on the role of pain-related fear in chronic back pain disability. Pain 1999; 80:329–339.

Cunha IT, Simmonds MJ, Protas EJ, et al. Back pain, physical function and estimates of aerobic capacity. What are the relationships among methods and measures? Am J Phys Med Rehabil 2002; 81:913–920.

Davidson M, Keating JL. A comparison of five low back disability questionnaires: reliability and responsiveness. Phys Ther 2002; 82:8–24.

Davidson M, Keating JL, Eyres S. A Low Back-Specific Version of the SF-36 Physical Functioning Scale. Spine 2004; 29:586–594.

Delitto A. Are measures of function and disability important in low back care? Phys Ther 1994; 74:452–462.

Deyo RA, Centor RM. Assessing the responsiveness of functional scales to clinical change: an analogy to diagnostic test performance. J Chronic Dis 1986; 39:897–906.

Deyo RA, Battie M, Beurskens AJ, et al. Outcome measures for low back pain research. A proposal for standardized use. Spine 1998; 23:2003–2013.

Dijkers MP, Kropp GC, Esper RM, et al. Reporting on reliability and validity of outcome measures in medical rehabilitation research. Disabil Rehabil 2002; 24:819–827.

Ehrlich GE, Khaltaev NG. Low Back Pain Initiative. World Health Organization, Geneva, 1999.

Epker J, Gatchel RJ. Prediction of treatment-seeking behavior in acute TMD patients: practical application in clinical settings. J Orofacial Pain 2000; 14:303–309.

Epstein RS. Responsiveness in quality-of-life assessment: nomenclature, determinants, and clinical applications. Med Care 2000; 38(9 suppl):II91–II94.

Fairbank J, Pynsent PB. The Oswestry Disability Index. Spine 2000; 25:2940–2953.

Fairbank J, Couper J, Davies J, et al. The Oswestry Low Back Pain Disability Questionnaire. Physiotherapy 1980; 66:271–273.

Fanuele JC, Birkmyer NJO, Abdu WA, et al. The impact on spinal problems on the health status of patients: have we underestimated the effect? Spine 2000; 25:1509–1514.

Feise RJ, Michael MJ. Functional rating index: a new valid and reliable instrument to measure the magnitude of clinical change in spinal conditions. Spine 2001; 26:78–86.

Fisher K, Johnson M. Validation of the Oswestry low back pain disability questionnaire, its sensitivity as a measure of change following treatment and its relationship with other aspects of the chronic pain experience. Physiother Theory Pract 1997; 13:67–80.

Foerster F, Fahrenberg J. Motion pattern and posture: correctly assessed by calibrated accelerometers. Behav Res Methods Instrum Comput 2000; 32:450–457.

Forer SK, Miller LS. Rehabilitation outcome: comparative analysis of different patient types. Arch Phys Med Rehabil 1980; 61:359–365.

Fries JF, Spitz PW. The hierarchy of patient outcomes. In: Spilker B (ed). Quality of Life Assessments in Clinical Trials. Raven Press, New York, 1990:25–35.

Fries JF, Spitz P, Kraines RG, et al. Measurement of patient outcome in arthritis. Arthritis Rheum 1980; 23:137–145.

Fries JF, Spitz PW, Young DY. The dimensions of health outcomes: the health assessment questionnaire, disability and pain scales. J Rheumatol 1982; 9:789–793.

Fritz JM, George SZ. Identifying psychosocial variables in patients with acute work-related low back pain: the importance of fear-avoidance beliefs. Phys Ther 2002; 82:973–983.

Fritz JM, Irrgang JJ. A comparison of a modified Oswestry Low Back Pain Disability Questionnaire and the Quebec Back Pain Disability Scale. Phys Ther 2001; 81:776–788.

Fritz JM, George SZ, Delitto A. The role of fear-avoidance beliefs in acute low back pain: relationships with current and future disability and work status. Pain 2001; 94:7–15.

Garratt AM, Klaber MJ, Farrin AJ. Responsiveness of generic and specific measures of health outcome in low back pain. Spine 2001; 26:71–77.

Garratt A, Schmidt L, Mackintosh A, et al. Quality of life measurement: bibliographic study of patient assessed health outcome measures. Br Med J 2002; 324:1417.

Goolkasian P, Wheeler AH, Gretz SS. The neck pain and disability scale: test–retest reliability and construct validity. Clin J Pain 2002; 18:245–250.

Goubert L, Crombez G, Van Damme S, et al. Confirmatory factor analysis of the Tampa Scale for Kinesiophobia: invariant two-factor model across low back pain patients and fibromyalgia patients. Clin J Pain 2004; 20:103–110.

Greenough CG. Recovery from low back pain. 1–5 year follow-up of 287 injury-related cases. Acta Orthop Scand Suppl 1993; 254:1–34.

Greenough C, Fraser R. Assessment of outcome in patients with low back pain. Spine 1992; 17:36–41.

Grevitt M, Khazim R, Webb J, et al. The short form-36 health survey questionnaire in spine surgery. J Bone Joint Surg Br 1997; 79:48–52.

Gronblad M, Hupli M, Wennerstrand P, et al. Intercorrelation and test–retest reliability of the Pain Disability Index (PDI) and the Oswestry Disability Questionnaire (ODQ) and their correlation with pain intensity in low back pain patients. Clin J Pain 1993; 9:189–195.

Grotle M, Vollestad NK, Brox JI. Clinical course and impact of fear-avoidance beliefs in low back pain: prospective cohort study of acute and chronic low back pain: II. Spine. 2006 Apr 20; 31(9):1038–1046.

Guyatt G, Walter S, Norman G. Measuring change over time: assessing the usefulness of evaluative instruments. J Chronic Dis 1987; 40:171–178.

Hagg O, Fritzell P, Nordwall A. The clinical importance of changes in outcome scores after treatment for chronic low back pain. Eur Spine J 2003; 12:12–20.

Hains F, Waalen J, Mior S. Psychometric properties of the neck disability index. J Manipul Physiol Therap 1998; 21:75–80.

Halter J, Ruben D. Indicators of function in the geriatric population. Cells and Surveys: Should Biological Measures Be Included in Social Science Research? National Academy Press, Washington, DC, 2001:159–179.

Harding VR, Williams AC, Richardson PH, et al. The development of a battery of measures for assessing physical functioning of chronic pain patients. Pain 1994; 58:367–375.

Hart DL, Wright BD. Development of an index of physical functional health status in rehabilitation. Arch Phys Med Rehabil 2002; 83:655–665.

Hassett AL, Cone JD, Patella SJ, et al. The role of catastrophizing in the pain and depression of women with fibromyalgia syndrome. Arthritis Rheum 2000; 43:2493–2500.

Herr KA, Mobily PR, Smith C. Depression and the experience of chronic back pain: a study of related variables and age differences. Clin J Pain 1993; 9:104–114.

Heuts PH, Vlaeyen JW, Roelofs J, et al. Pain-related fear and daily functioning in patients with osteoarthritis. Pain 2004; 110:228–235.

Holt AE, Shaw NJ, Shetty A, et al. The reliability of the Low Back Outcome Score for back pain. Spine 2002; 27:206–210.

Hoving JL, O'Leary EF, Niere KR, et al. Validity of the neck disability index, Northwick Park neck pain questionnaire, and problem elicitation technique for measuring disability associated with whiplash-associated disorders. Pain 2003; 102:273–281.

Hudson-Cook N, Tomes-Nicholson K, Breen A. A revised Oswestry disability questionnaire. In: Roland OM, Jenner JR (eds). Back Pain: New Approaches to Rehabilitation and Education. Manchester University Press, Manchester, 1989:187–204.

Jensen MP, Turner JA, Romano JM, et al. Coping with chronic pain: a critical review of the literature. Pain 1991; 47:249–283.

Jensen MP, Strom SE, Turner JA, et al. Validity of the Sickness Impact Profile Roland scale as a measure of dysfunction in chronic pain patients. Pain 1992; 50:157–162.

Jensen MP, Turner JA, Romano JM. What is the maximum number of levels needed in pain intensity measurement? Pain 1994; 58:387–392.

Jerome A, Gross RT. Pain disability index: construct and discriminant validity. Arch Phys Med Rehabil 1991; 72:920–922.

Jette AM, Haley SM, Kooyoomjian JT. Are the ICF Activity and Participation dimensions distinct? J Rehabil Med 2003; 35:145–149.

Jordan A, Manniche C, Mosdal C, et al. The Copenhagen Neck Functional Disability Scale: a study of reliability and validity. J Manipul Physiol Ther 1998; 21:520–527.

Katz S, Akpom CA. 12. Index of ADL. Med Care 1976; 14(5 suppl):116–118.

Katz S, Ford AB, Moskowitz RW, et al. Studies of illness in the aged. The index of ADL: a standardized measure of biological and psychosocial function. JAMA 1963; 185:914–919.

Keefe FJ, Hill RW. An objective approach to quantifying pain behavior and gait patterns in low back pain patients. Pain 1985; 21:153–161.

Keefe FJ, Kashikar-Zuck S, Robinson E, et al. Pain coping strategies that predict patients' and spouses' ratings of patients' self-efficacy. Pain 1997; 73:191–199.

Kerns RD, Turk DC, Rudy TE. The West Haven–Yale Multidimensional Pain Inventory (WHYMPI). Pain 1985; 23:345–356.

Kopec JA. Measuring functional outcomes in persons with back pain: a review of back-specific questionnaires. Spine 2000; 25:3110–3114.

Kopec JA, Esdaile JM, Abrahamowicz M, et al. The Quebec Back Pain Disability Scale. Measurement properties. Spine 1995; 20:341–352.

Kopec JA, Esdaile JM, Abrahamowicz M, et al. The Quebec Back Pain Disability Scale: conceptualization and development. J Clin Epidemiol 1996; 49:151–161.

Kori SH, Miller RP, Todd DD. Kinesiophobia: a new view of chronic pain behavior. Pain Manage 1990; Jan/Feb:35–43.

Landers MR, Creger RV, Baker CV, Stutelberg KS. The use of fear-avoidance beliefs and nonorganic signs in predicting prolonged disability in patients with neck pain. Man Ther 2007 Mar 21.

Lawton MP, Brody EM. Assessment of older people: self-maintaining and instrumental activities of daily living. Gerontologist 1969; 9:179–186.

Le Masurier G. Pedometer sensitivity and specificity. Med Sci Sports Exerc 2004; 36:346.

Leak AM, Cooper J, Dyer S, et al. The Northwick Park Neck Pain Questionnaire, devised to measure neck pain and disability. Br J Rheumatol 1994; 33:469–474.

Leclaire R, Blier F, Fortin L, et al. A cross-sectional study comparing the Oswestry and Roland-Morris Functional Disability scales in two populations of patients with low back pain of different levels of severity. Spine 1997; 22:68–71.

Liang MH. Longitudinal construct validity: establishment of clinical meaning in patient evaluative instruments. Med Care 2000; 38(9 suppl):II84–II90.

Liang MH, Larson MG, Cullen KE, et al. Comparative measurement efficiency and sensitivity of five health status instruments for arthritis research. Arthritis Rheum 1985; 28:542–547.

Lidgren L. The Bone and Joint Decade 2000–2010. Bull WHO 2003; 81:629.

Livingstone MB, Black AE. Markers of the validity of reported energy intake. J Nutr 2003; 133(suppl 3): 895S–920S.

Lousberg R, Van B, Groenman NH, et al. Psychometric properties of the Multidimensional Pain Inventory, Dutch language version (MPI-DLV). Behav Res Ther 1999; 37:167–182.

Magnussen L, Strand LI, Lygren H. Reliability and validity of the back performance scale: observing activity limitation in patients with back pain. Spine 2004; 29:903–907.

Mahoney FI, Wood OH, Barthel DW. Rehabilitation of chronically ill patients: the influence of complications on the final goal. South Med 1958; 51:609.

Manniche C, Asmussen K, Lauritsen B, et al. Low Back Pain Rating scale: validation of a tool for assessment of low back pain. Pain 1994; 57:317–326.

Martin DP, Engelberg R, Agel J, et al. Development of a musculoskeletal extremity health status instrument: the Musculoskeletal Function Assessment instrument. J Orthop Res 1996a; 14:173–181.

Martin MY, Bradley LA, Alexander RW, et al. Coping strategies predict disability in patients with primary fibromyalgia. Pain 1996b; 68:45–53.

McCracken LM, Zayfert C, Gross RT. The Pain Anxiety Symptoms Scale: development and validation of a scale to measure fear of pain. Pain 1992; 50:67–73.

McDowell I, Newell C. Measuring Health. A Guide to Rating Scales and Questionnaires. 2nd edn. Oxford University Press, Oxford, 1996.

Melanson EL Jr, Freedson PS. Physical activity assessment: a review of methods. Crit Rev Food Sci Nutr 1996; 36:385–396.

Milligan SE, Hom DL, Ballou SP, et al. An assessment of the Health Assessment Questionnaire functional ability index among women with systemic lupus erythematosus. J Rheumatol 1993; 20:972–976.

Million R, Hall W, Nilsen KH, et al. Assessment of the progress of the back-pain patient 1981 Volvo Award in Clinical Science. Spine 1982; 7:204–212.

Nagi S. Disability concepts revisited: implications for prevention. Disability in America: Toward a New Agenda Toward Prevention. Committee on a National Agenda for the Prevention of Disabilities, Division of Health Promotion and Disease Prevention, Institute of Medicine, National Academy Press, Washington, DC, 1991:309–327.

Nederhand MJ, Ijzerman MJ, Hermens HJ, et al. Predictive value of fear avoidance in developing chronic neck pain disability: consequences for clinical decision making. Arch Phys Med Rehabil 2004; 85:496–501.

Nelson E, Wasson J, Kirk J, et al. Assessment of function in routine clinical practice: description of the COOP Chart method and preliminary findings. J Chronic Dis 1987; 40(suppl 1):55S–69S.

Nijs J, Vanherberghen K, Duquet W, et al. Chronic fatigue syndrome: lack of association between pain-related fear of movement and exercise capacity and disability. Phys Ther 2004; 84:696–705.

Novy DM, Simmonds MJ, Lee CE. Physical performance tasks: what are the underlying constructs? Arch Phys Med Rehabil 2002; 83:44–47.

Olsson I, Bunketorp O, Carlsson SG, et al. Prediction of outcome in Whiplash Associated Disorders using West Haven-Yale Multidimensional Pain Inventory. Clin J Pain 2002; 18:238–244.

Ostelo RW, de Vet HC, Knol DL, et al. 24-item Roland-Morris Disability Questionnaire was preferred out of six functional status questionnaires for post-lumbar disc surgery. J Clin Epidemiol 2004; 57:268–276.

Parkerson GR Jr, Broadhead WE, Tse CK. The Duke Health Profile. A 17-item measure of health and dysfunction. Med Care 1990; 28:1056–1072.

Patrick DL, Chiang YP. Measurement of health outcomes in treatment effectiveness evaluations: conceptual and methodological challenges. Med Care 2000; 38(9 suppl): II14–II25.

Patrick DL, Deyo RA, Atlas SJ, et al. Assessing health-related quality of life in patients with sciatica. Spine 1995; 20:1899–1908.

Pfingsten M, Kroner-Herwig B, Leibing E, et al. Validation of the German version of the Fear-Avoidance Beliefs Questionnaire (FABQ). Eur J Pain 2000; 4:259–266.

Picavet HS, Hazes JM. Prevalence of self reported musculoskeletal diseases is high. Ann Rheum Dis 2003; 62:644–650.

Pietrobon R, Coeytaux RR, Carey TS, et al. Standard scales for measurement of functional outcome for cervical pain or dysfunction: a systematic review. Spine 2002; 27:515–522.

Pollard CA. Preliminary validity study of the pain disability index. Percept Mot Skills 1984; 59:974.

Ramey D, Fries J, Singh G. The Health Assessment Questionnaire 1995: status and review. In: Spilker B (ed). Quality of Life and Pharmacoeconomics in Clinical Trials, 2nd edn. Lippincott-Raven, Philadelphia, PA, 1996:227–237.

Ren XS, Kazis L, Lee A, et al. Comparing generic and disease-specific measures of physical and role functioning: results from the Veterans Health Study. Med Care 1998; 36:155–166.

Reneman MF, Wittink HM. Functional performance evaluation. In: Nordin M, Pope MH, Andersson G (eds). Musculoskeletal Disorders in the Workplace: The Prevention of Disability, 2nd edn. Mosby, Philadelphia, PA, 2007.

Reneman MF, Jorritsma W, Schellekens JM, et al. Concurrent validity of questionnaire and performance-based disability measurements in patients with chronic nonspecific low back pain. J Occup Rehabil 2002; 12:119–129.

Reneman MF, Jorritsma W, Dijkstra SJ, et al. Relationship between kinesiophobia and performance in a functional capacity evaluation. J Occup Rehabil 2003; 13:277–285.

Resnik L, Dobrzykowski E. Guide to outcomes measurement for patients with low back pain syndromes. J Orthop Sports Phys Ther 2003; 33:307–316.

Reuben DB, Solomon DH. Assessment in geriatrics. Of caveats and names. J Am Geriatr Soc 1989; 37:570–572.

Riddle DL, Stratford PW. Use of generic versus region-specific functional status measures on patients with cervical spine disorders. Phys Ther 1998; 78:951–963.

Riddle DL, Stratford PW. Roland-Morris scale reliability. Phys Ther 2002; 82:512–515.

Rogers W, Wittink HM, Wagner A, et al. Assessing individual outcomes during outpatient, multidisciplinary chronic pain treatment by means of an augmented SF-36. Pain Med 2000a; 1:44–54.

Rogers WH, Wittink HM, Ashburn MA, et al. Using the "TOPS": an outcomes instrument for multidisciplinary outpatient pain treatment. Pain Med 2000b; 1:55–67.

Roland M, Fairbank J. The Roland-Morris Disability Questionnaire and the Oswestry Disability Questionnaire. Spine 2000; 25:3115–3124.

Roland M, Morris R. A study of the natural history of back pain: I. Development of a reliable and sensitive measure of disability in low-back pain. Spine 1983a; 8:141–144.

Ruta D, Garratt A, Wardlaw D, et al. Developing a valid and reliable measure of health outcome for patients with low back pain. Spine 1994; 19:1887–1896.

Salen BA, Spangfort EV, Nygren AL, et al. The Disability Rating Index: an instrument for the assessment of disability in clinical settings. J Clin Epidemiol 1994; 47:1423–1435.

Sanderson P, Todd B, Holt G, et al. Compensation, work status and disability in low back pain patients. Spine 1995; 20:554–556.

Schasfoort FC, Bussmann JB, Stam HJ. Impairments and activity limitations in subjects with chronic upper-limb complex regional pain syndrome type I. Arch Phys Med Rehabil 2004; 85:557–566.

Schaufele MK, Boden SD. Outcome research in patients with chronic low back pain. Orthop Clin North Am 2003; 34:231–237.

Schmidt AJ. Cognitive factors in the performance level of chronic low back pain patients. J Psychosom Res 1985; 29:183–189.

Schoppink EM, van Tulder MW, Koes BW, et al. Reliability and validity of the Dutch adaptation of the Quebec Back Pain Disability Scale. Phys Ther 1996; 76:268–275.

Sim J, Jordan K, Lewis M, Hill J, Hay EM, Dziedzic K. Sensitivity to change and internal consistency of the Northwick Park Neck Pain Questionnaire and derivation of a minimal clinically important difference. Clin J Pain. 2006 Nov–Dec; 22(9):820–6.

Simmonds MJ, Olson SL, Jones S, et al. Psychometric characteristics and clinical usefulness of physical performance tests in patients with low back pain. Spine 1998; 23:2412–2421.

Spenkelink CD, Hutten MM, Hermens HJ, et al. Assessment of activities of daily living with an ambulatory monitoring system: a comparative study in patients with chronic low back pain and nonsymptomatic controls. Clin Rehabil 2002; 16:16–26.

Stewart WF, Ricci JA, Chee E, et al. Lost productive work time costs from health conditions in the United States: results from the American Productivity Audit. J Occup Environ Med 2003; 45:1234–1246.

Strand LI, Moe-Nilssen R, Ljunggren AE. Back Performance Scale for the assessment of mobility-related activities in people with back pain. Phys Ther 2002; 82:1213–1223.

Stratford PW, Binkley JM. Measurement properties of the RM-18. A modified version of the Roland-Morris Disability Scale. Spine 1997; 22:2416–2421.

Stratford PW, Binkley J, Solomon P, et al. Assessing change over time in patients with low back pain. Phys Ther 1994; 74:528–533.

Stratford PW, Binkley J, Solomon P, et al. Defining the minimum level of detectable change for the Roland-Morris questionnaire. Phys Ther 1996; 76:359–365.

Stratford PW, Binkley JM, Riddle DL, et al. Sensitivity to change of the Roland-Morris Back Pain Questionnaire: part 1. Phys Ther 1998; 78:1186–1196.

Stratford PW, Binkley JM, Riddle DL. Development and initial validation of the back pain functional scale. Spine 2000; 25:2095–2102.

Stratford PW, Kennedy D, Pagura SM, et al. The relationship between self-report and performance-related measures: questioning the content validity of timed tests. Arthritis Rheum 2003; 49:535–540.

Strong J, Ashton R, Large RG. Function and the patient with chronic low back pain. Clin J Pain 1994; 10:191–196.

Suarez-Almazor ME, Kendall C, Johnson JA, et al. Use of health status measures in patients with low back pain in clinical settings. Comparison of specific, generic and preference-based instruments. Rheumatology (Oxford) 2000; 39:783–790.

Swinkels-Meewisse EJ, Swinkels RA, Verbeek AL, et al. Psychometric properties of the Tampa Scale for kinesiophobia and the fear-avoidance beliefs questionnaire in acute low back pain. Man Ther 2003; 8:29–36.

Swiontkowski MF, Engelberg R, Martin DP, et al. Short musculoskeletal function assessment questionnaire: validity, reliability, and responsiveness. J Bone Joint Surg Am 1999; 81:1245–1260.

Tait RC, Pollard CA, Margolis RB, et al. The Pain Disability Index: psychometric and validity data. Arch Phys Med Rehabil 1987; 68:438–441.

Tait RC, Chibnall JT, Margolis RB. Pain extent: relations with psychological state, pain severity, pain history, and disability. Pain 1990; 41:295–301.

Taylor SJ, Taylor AE, Foy MA, et al. Responsiveness of common outcome measures for patients with low back pain. Spine 1999; 24:1805–1812.

Testa MA. Interpretation of quality-of-life outcomes: issues that affect magnitude and meaning. Med Care 2000; 38(9 suppl):II166–II174.

Testa MA, Simonson DC. Assessment of quality-of-life outcomes. N Engl J Med 1996; 334:835–840.

Triano J, Schultz A. Correlation of objective measure of trunk motion and muscle function with low back disability ratings. Spine 1987; 12:561–565.

Turk DC, Rudy TE. The robustness of an empirically derived taxonomy of chronic pain patients. Pain 1990; 43:27–35.

Turk DC, Okifuji A, Sinclair JD, et al. Pain, disability, and physical functioning in subgroups of patients with fibromyalgia. J Rheumatol 1996; 23:1255–1262.

Turner JA, Jensen MP, Romano JM. Do beliefs, coping, and catastrophizing independently predict functioning in patients with chronic pain? Pain 2000; 85:115–125.

Ustun TB, Chatterji S, Bickenbach J, et al. The International Classification of Functioning, Disability and Health: a new tool for understanding disability and health. Disabil Rehabil 2003a; 25:565–571.

Ustun TB, Chatterji S, Kostansjek N, et al. WHO's ICF and functional status information in health records. Health Care Financ Rev 2003b; 24:77–88.

van den Berg-Emons BH, Bussmann J, Balk A, et al. Level of activities associated with mobility during everyday life in patients with chronic congestive heart failure as measured with an "activity monitor." Phys Ther 2001; 81:1502–1511.

van der Roer N, Ostelo RW, Bekkering GE, van Tulder MW, de Vet HC. Minimal clinically important change for pain intensity, functional status, and general health status in patients with nonspecific low back pain. Spine 2006 Mar 1; 31(5):578–582.

van Tubergen A, Landewe R, Heuft-Dorenbosch L, et al. Assessment of disability with the World Health Organization Disability Assessment Schedule II in patients with ankylosing spondylitis. Ann Rheum Dis 2003; 62:140–145.

Veltink PH, Bussmann HB, de Vries W, et al. Detection of static and dynamic activities using uniaxial accelerometers. IEEE Trans Rehabil Eng 1996; 4:375–385.

Vendrig A, Deutz P, Vink I. Nederlandse vertaling en bewerking van de fear-avoidance beliefs questionnaire. Nederlands Tijdschrift voor Psychologie 1998; 18:11–14.

Verbunt JA, Westerterp KR, van der Heijden GJ, et al. Physical activity in daily life in patients with chronic low back pain. Arch Phys Med Rehabil 2001; 82:726–730.

Verbunt JA, Sieben JM, Seelen HA, et al. Decline in physical activity, disability and pain-related fear in sub-acute low back pain. Eur J Pain 2005; 9:417–425.

Vernon H, Mior S. The Neck Disability Index: a study of reliability and validity. J Manipul Physiol Ther 1991; 14:409–415.

Vlaeyen JW, Linton SJ. Fear-avoidance and its consequences in chronic musculoskeletal pain: a state of the art. Pain 2000; 85:317–332.

Vlaeyen JW, Kole-Snijders AM, Boeren RG, et al. Fear of movement/(re)injury in chronic low back pain and its relation to behavioral performance. Pain 1995; 62:363–372.

Waddell G, Main CJ. Assessment of severity in low-back disorders. Spine 1984; 9:204–208.

Waddell G, Newton M, Henderson I, et al. A Fear-Avoidance Beliefs Questionnaire (FABQ) and the role of fear-avoidance beliefs in chronic low back pain and disability. Pain 1993; 52:157–168.

Wagner AK, Ehrenberg BL, Tran TA, et al. Patient-based health status measurement in clinical practice: a study of its impact on epilepsy patients' care. Qual Life Res 1997; 6:329–341.

Walsh TL, Hanscom B, Lurie JD, et al. Is a condition-specific instrument for patients with low back pain/leg symptoms really necessary? The responsiveness of the Oswestry Disability Index, MODEMS, and the SF-36. Spine 2003; 28:607–615.

Wheeler AH, Goolkasian P, Baird AC, et al. Development of the Neck Pain and Disability Scale. Item analysis, face, and criterion-related validity. Spine 1999; 24:1290–1294.

WHO Scientific Group on the Burden of Musculoskeletal Conditions at the Start of the New Millennium. The burden of musculoskeletal conditions at the start of the new millennium. WHO Tech Rep Ser 2003; 919:i–218, back.

Williams NH, Wilkinson C, Russell IT. Extending the Aberdeen Back Pain Scale to include the whole spine: a set of outcome measures for the neck, upper and lower back. Pain 2001; 94:261–274.

Wittink H. Functional capacity testing in patients with chronic pain. Clin J Pain 2005; 21:197–199.

Wittink H, Rogers W, Gascon C, et al. Relative contribution of mental health and exercise-related pain increment to treadmill test intolerance in patients with chronic low back pain. Spine 2001; 26:2368–2374.

Wittink H, Rogers W, Sukiennik A, et al. Physical functioning: self-report and performance measures are related but distinct. Spine 2003; 28:2407–2413.

Wittink H, Turk DC, Carr DB, et al. Comparison of the redundancy, reliability, and responsiveness to change among SF-36, Oswestry Disability Index, and Multidimensional Pain Inventory. Clin J Pain 2004; 20:133–142.

Wlodyka-Demaille S, Poiraudeau S, Catanzariti JF, et al. French translation and validation of 3 functional disability scales for neck pain. Arch Phys Med Rehabil 2002; 83:376–382.

Woby SR, Roach NK, Urmston M, Watson PJ. Psychometric properties of the TSK-11: a shortened version of the Tampa Scale for Kinesiophobia. Pain 2005 Sep; 117 (1–2):137–144.

Woolf AD, Akesson K. Understanding the burden of musculoskeletal conditions. The burden is huge and not reflected in national health priorities. Br Med J 2001; 322:1079–1080.

Woolf AD, Pfleger B. Burden of major musculoskeletal conditions. Bull WHO 2003; 81:646–656.

World Health Organization. International Classification of Impairments, Disabilities and Handicaps (ICIDH). WHO, Geneva, 1980.

World Health Organization. The International Classification of Functioning, Disability and Health (ICF), 2nd edn. WHO, Marketing and Dissemination, Geneva, 2001.

Zandbelt MM, Welsing PM, van Gestel AM, et al. Health Assessment Questionnaire modifications: is standardisation needed? Ann Rheum Dis 2001; 60:841–845.

Zijlstra W. Assessment of spatio-temporal parameters during unconstrained walking. Eur J Appl Physiol 2004; 92:39–44.

FURTHER READING

To find tools there are multiple websites available: See for instance: http://www.cebp.nl/ then go to tools or http://www.medal.org/visitor/login.aspx (accessed May 15, 2007).

CHAPTER
18

The initiative on methods, measurement, and pain assessment in clinical trials (IMMPACT)

Dennis C. Turk • Robert H. Dworkin

CHRONIC PAIN: MAGNITUDE OF THE PROBLEM

Precise estimates of the prevalence of different pain syndromes in the USA are difficult to ascertain; however, nearly one-half of Americans who seek treatment with a physician report that their primary symptom is pain. This makes pain the single most frequent reason for physician consultation in the USA (Abbott and Fraser 1998). In 2002, over 66 million prescriptions for opioid analgesics (14% of the total of all prescriptions) nonsteroidal anti-inflammatory agents (12.3%), or nonnarcotic analgesics (4.5%) for pain were mentioned in emergency department reports. Back pain alone accounted for over 4 million visits to emergency departments (McCraig and Burt 2002). The United States National Health Interview Survey determined that in the 3-month period prior to the interview, 28% had experienced pain in the lower back, 16% experienced a severe headache, 15% had experienced pain in the neck region, and 4% had experienced pain in the face or jaw (Pleis and Coles 1998). There may be over 30 million people with chronic or recurrent painful conditions. The figures provide a basis for concluding that pain is, in fact, very prevalent.

In addition to being prevalent, pain is very costly to society as well as for the individual. For example, in 1995 and 1996 estimates of the cost of chronic pain (including treatment, lost work days, indemnity) ranged from $150 billion to $215 billion per year (United States Bureau of the Census 1996; National Research Council 2001). When viewing such figures it is easy to overlook the impact that chronic pain has on the lives of individual sufferers. People with conditions such as low back pain, headaches, fibromyalgia with pain, osteoarthritis, and postherpetic neuralgia experience pain that impairs their quality of life, causing significant physical disability and considerable emotional distress.

ESTABLISH THE EFFECTIVENESS OF TREATMENTS

Advances in knowledge of the neurobiology of pain have resulted in an explosion in the number of potentially efficacious treatments. With the development of each new treatment come clinical trials designed to demonstrate its beneficial effects and safety. In discussions of clinical trials, a distinction is often made between efficacy and effectiveness trials, although some clinical trials combine elements of both (see also Chapter 1). Efficacy trials test the hypothesis of whether or not there are beneficial effects of treatment in a group of participants, and the methods and procedures are tightly controlled and standardized. In such studies, threats to the internal validity are minimized. Effectiveness trials, in contrast, are conducted to test the value of a treatment as applied in clinical practice. Typically, in effectiveness trials there is increased participants baseline variability, and there is often less control of methods and procedures. In an effectiveness study, external validity and generalizability are emphasized, and the trial is designed so that conclusions about the value of the treatment as it is actually used in the population can be drawn (Dworkin et al. 2001).

One method that can increase confidence in assessments of both efficacy and effectiveness involves the aggregation of data across different clinical trials of the same treatment. Clinical trials, however, often incorporate idiosyncratic samples, research designs, and outcome measures, that makes synthesis of data on treatment response problematic. Although there are guidelines for conducting meta-analyses, conclusions have been inconsistent when different analyses of the same treatment using meta-analysis and related methods are conducted (e.g., Jadad et al. 1997; Ferreira et al. 2002).

To determine the benefits of treatment, investigators must decide the appropriate endpoints for establishing both the statistical significance and also the clinical importance of the effects of treatment. In a clinical trial of the efficacy or effectiveness of a treatment for chronic pain, pain reduction and safety are necessary outcome variables but they may not be sufficient for a comprehensive evaluation of the overall benefit or harm of treatment. The complexity of chronic pain and its negative impact on diverse aspects of function require the assessment of multiple outcome domains to evaluate treatments comprehensively. A number of considerations are important in deciding which domains should be included in chronic pain clinical trials. The domains should match the purpose of the study, measure positive and negative outcomes of treatment, and be appropriate for the chronic pain syndrome studied and the specific characteristics of the sample (e.g., geriatric participants). Central issues involve the identification of outcome domains that are clinically meaningful and for which there are measures that are responsive and provide a comprehensive yet efficient evaluation of treatment response (Bellamy et al. 1997; Revicki and Ehreth 1997).

Once domains and measures have been selected, investigators must establish criteria not only for the statistical significance of the outcomes but also for their clinical importance (e.g., Jaeschke et al. 1989; Juniper et al. 1994; Farrar et al. 2001). When evaluating clinical importance, consideration must be given to the question of "importance to whom." The importance of different degrees of symptom reduction and of the presence and intensity of adverse effects associated with treatment can vary between and among clinical investigators, patients, and disease conditions (Fischer et al. 1999; Ganz 2002).

When multiple outcome variables are included in a study, investigators must consider how inconsistencies among outcomes will be interpreted. Strategies for classifying participants as responders across multiple endpoints have been suggested (Dougados et al. 2000), and there are also statistical approaches available for analyzing outcomes when multiple measures have been used (e.g., O'Brien 1984; Lehmacher et al. 1991; Legler et al. 1995).

Variability among clinical trials in outcome assessments has impeded evaluations of the efficacy and effectiveness of treatments for chronic pain, and the use of different outcome domains and measures precludes meaningful comparisons among studies. One way to facilitate such evaluations would be through the use of a standard set of outcome domains and measures. Although investigators may wish to augment a core set of measures with others that are specific to the situation or treatment being studied, use of a core set of outcomes among studies would permit comparisons among different samples, treatments, and settings.

Development of a core set of outcome domains and measurement procedures would have important advantages for clinicians and investigators. It would facilitate comparison and pooling of data while leaving investigators free to augment the core set with others of their choice. In addition, a core set of domains and measures would encourage more complete investigation and reporting of relevant outcomes, so that investigators do not simply present a single outcome while ignoring others. Another advantage is that it would encourage development of cooperative multicenter projects, in which different centers agree to assess the core domains and measures, in addition to any measures selected to evaluate specific research questions. Such standardization would simplify the process of designing and reviewing research proposals, manuscripts, and published articles. Finally, published results of clinical trials with common outcomes will allow clinicians to make more informed clinical decisions for each patient regarding the optimal treatment, especially with respect to its risks and benefits.

The Initiative on Methods, Measurement, and Pain Assessment in Clinical Trials (IMMPACT) convened a first meeting to develop consensus recommendations for core outcome domains for chronic pain clinical trials. Other initiatives provide precedents for this undertaking, including OMERACT (Outcome Measures in Rheumatoid Arthritis Clinical Trials; Bellamy et al. 1997) and WHO/ILARS (World Health Organization/International League of

Associations for Rheumatology; Brooks and Hochberg 2001) in rheumatology, EORTC (European Organization for Research and Treatment of Cancer; Aaronson et al. 1993) and the Research Network of the European Association of Palliative Care (Caraceni et al. 2002) in oncology, and an international consortium of back pain researchers (Deyo et al. 1998). Our goal in this chapter is to provide an overview of the IMMPACT process and consensus recommendations. The intended audience is all individuals involved in designing, reviewing, and interpreting clinical trials of treatments for adults with chronic pain.

THE INITIATIVE ON METHODS, MEASUREMENT, AND PAIN ASSESSMENT IN CLINICAL TRIALS (IMMPACT)

IMMPACT is a consortium of professionals from academia, the US Food and Drug Administration, the National Institutes of Health, US Veterans Administration, industry, and consumers. The professional participants are engaged in research, clinical, or administrative activities relevant to the design and evaluation of chronic pain treatment outcomes and they represent anesthesiology, biostatistics, clinical pharmacology, epidemiology, geriatrics, internal medicine, law, neurology, nursing, oncology, outcomes research, patient perspectives, pediatric pain, physical medicine and rehabilitation, psychology, and rheumatology. All participants have research, clinical, or administrative expertise relevant to evaluating chronic pain treatment outcomes or to representing people included in clinical trials. No outside observers are permitted to be present at the consensus meeting. The authors of this chapter have served as the facilitators for each of the consensus meetings described below. Since the inception in November of 2002, there have been six IMMPACT meetings with a seventh planned to meet shortly after the preparation of this chapter.

IMMPACT-I

The first meeting (IMMPACT-I) focused on developing consensus recommendations for core outcome domains for chronic pain clinical trials. Over the past few decades, there has been a growing realization that the traditional outcome domains of symptom reduction and safety are inadequate when evaluating response to treatments for chronic disease states and symptoms that are as subjective as pain. Physical, emotional, and social functioning, and patient satisfaction and perception of improvement have been identified as important targets of intervention when the treatment being evaluated does not cure a disease (discussed below and in Turk et al. 2003).

IMMPACT-II

IMMPACT-II focused on identifying specific instruments that could be used to assess each of the domains identified at IMMPACT-I. There have been recent attempts to recommend outcome measures for specific chronic pain conditions – including osteoarthritis (Bellamy et al. 1997) and low back pain (Naliboff et al. 1985; Deyo et al. 1998) – and several suggestions for chronic pain more generally (e.g., Turk and Rudy 1987; Williams 1988); the latter efforts are more generally directed toward clinical assessment rather than specifically for outcome trials.

A recognized set of experts (Drs. John Farrar, Jennifer Haythornthwaite, Mark Jensen, Nathanial Katz, Robert Kerns, and Dennis Turk) was commissioned to complete comprehensive reviews of available measures for each domain and to make specific recommendations regarding what were the measures with the best available psychometic support and that were responsive to change. These literature reviews focused on measures that could be used in trials of all chronic pain conditions and did not examine measures that were specific to certain types of chronic pain. At the meeting, the authors made brief presentations summarizing their conclusions and recommendations. The IMMPACT-II background materials and slide presentations are available at www.immpact.org/meetings.html. A paper with recommendations regarding specific measures based on the background and consensus of the participants at IMMPACT-II was recently published (Dworkin et al. 2005).

Included among the criteria used in evaluating potential core outcome measures were: (1) appropriateness of the measure's content and conceptual model; (2) reliability; (3) validity; (4) responsiveness; (5) interpretability; (6) precision of scores; (7) respondent and administrator acceptability; (8) burden and feasibility; (9) availability and equivalence of alternative forms and methods of administration (e.g., self-report, interviewer); and (10) availability and equivalence of versions for different cultures and languages (Fitzpatrick et al. 1998; Scientific Advisory Committee of the Medical Outcomes Trust 2002).

Although responsiveness has been defined and assessed in numerous ways, it most often refers to the ability of a measure to detect changes over time, and with respect to clinical trials has also included the ability of a measure to distinguish between treatments (Guyatt et al. 1987; Terwee et al. 2003). Although Hays and Hadorn (1992) have noted that responsiveness is a component of validity, we considered responsiveness a separate attribute of outcome measures because of its pivotal role in clinical trials.

IMMPACT-III

The IMMPACT-III meeting focused on consensus recommendations for criteria and procedures necessary in the development of new outcome measures to be used in clinical trials of treatments for chronic pain. One important conclusion from the IMMPACT-III meeting concerned the need to include patient groups (consumers) in the development process to identify what are important outcomes from their perspective and what content should be included when assessing outcomes in the different domains (Turk et al. 2006). As the result of the meeting, a series of consumer focus groups and surveys are in preparation to identify important outcomes from the perspective of the consumer.

IMMPACT-IV

The IMMPACT-IV meeting addressed the issue of how much change on the recommended measures from the IMMPACT-II meeting is meaningful and important. That is, how much change would have to be detected to judge the change as important and worthwhile in light of the possibility that any treatment makes demands on the consumer and may include adverse events.

CORE OUTCOME DOMAINS AND MEASURES (IMMPACT-I AND IMMPACT-II)

The complexity of chronic pain suggests that multiple domains are relevant when evaluating the effects of treatment. A number of considerations are important in deciding what domains should be considered in any clinical trial. The domains should match the purpose of the study, measure positive and negative outcomes of treatment, and be appropriate for the chronic pain disorder and the population of interest (e.g., geriatric). A central issue is identification of the set of domains that are clinically meaningful and that might be expected to change as a result of treatment (Revicki 1993).

The authors of the IMMPACT-I manuscript recommended that the core outcome domains and measures described below should be *considered* in the design of all clinical trials of the efficacy and effectiveness of treatments for any type of chronic pain. These general recommendations are presented in an effort to promote collection and publication of standardized outcomes, which will improve the design and interpretation of studies of chronic pain treatments. It is not the intention of these recommendations that use of these domains and measures should be considered a *requirement* for approval of applications by regulatory agencies or that treatments must demonstrate statistically significant or clinically important benefits with all of these outcomes to establish evidence of efficacy or effectiveness. There may be circumstances in which use of some or all of these core outcomes will not be appropriate, for example in clinical trials in the cognitively impaired

or in infants and children. These recommendations are most applicable to phase III and IV clinical trials of chronic pain treatments and are made with the assumption that these trials will be conducted in accord with the principles of good clinical practice (International Conference on Harmonization 1996a; United States Department of Health and Human Services 1997).

The IMMPACT-I and -II recommendations are presented in an effort to promote collection and publication of standardized outcomes, which will facilitate improved evidence-based comparisons and meta-analyses of pain treatments. We believe that even the results of clinical trials that do not demonstrate statistically significant treatment effects on all of the recommended core outcome domains described below should still be published (Jadad and Rennie 1998)

PAIN

Although a ubiquitous phenomenon, pain is inherently subjective. The only way to know about someone's pain is by what they say or show by their behavior. Because there is no "objective" method for assessing pain, self-report provides the gold standard in assessments of pain and its characteristics. Pain assessment therefore requires that patients and participants in clinical trials describe their experience from their own perspective. Although different individuals interpret measures of pain in different ways, these interpretations can be expected to remain relatively constant within people over time, providing valid measures of change in pain as a result of treatment (or natural history).

There are many different aspects of pain that can be assessed in a clinical trial. These include intensity; unpleasantness, onset, location, and durability of pain relief; whether pain is intermittent or constant; frequency of pain; qualities of pain (including the distinction between stimulus-evoked and stimulus-independent pain); radiation; use of rescue medications and other rescue treatments; and pain behaviors, including facial expression.

Surrogate endpoints for pain may also be assessed (e.g., physiologic findings, including imaging measures); however, these cannot be considered primary endpoints because of the inherently subjective nature of pain. Most chronic pain clinical trials will also assess pain history, including measures such as age at onset, duration, and exacerbating and alleviating factors, but these variables are more likely to be considered baseline characteristics or covariates.

Pain intensity

For most clinical trials of chronic pain treatments, a measure of pain intensity will provide the primary outcome measure. Each of the commonly used methods of rating pain intensity, including visual analogue scales

(VAS), numerical rating scales (NRS), and verbal rating scales (VRS), appear sufficiently reliable and valid, and no one scale consistently demonstrates greater responsiveness in detecting improvements associated with pain treatment (Jensen and Karoly 2001). However, there are important differences among VAS, NRS, and VRS measures of pain intensity with respect to missing data from failure to complete the measure, patient preference, ease of data recording, and ability to administer the measure by telephone or with electronic diaries.

VRS and NRS measures tend to be preferred over VAS measures by patients, and VAS measures usually demonstrate more missing data than NRS measures. Greater difficulty completing VAS measures is associated with increased age and greater opioid intake, and cognitive impairment has been shown to be associated with inability to complete NRS ratings of pain intensity (Jensen and Karoly 2001). Patients who are unable to complete NRS ratings may be able to complete VRS pain ratings (e.g., none, mild, moderate, severe) (see also Chapter 5). Other measures are available to assess pain in children and those who are unable to communicate (e.g., stroke patients, mentally impaired people) (Hadjistavropoulos et al. 2001).

On the basis of a review of the literature on pain measures prepared for the IMMPACT-II consensus meeting (Jensen 2003) and discussions among the participants, an 11-point (i.e., 0–10) NRS measure of pain intensity is recommended as a core outcome measure in clinical trials of chronic pain treatments. In order to facilitate consistency among studies, we recommend that the specific format of this rating should be the numbers from 0 through 10 presented with the descriptor "no pain" centered below the "0" and "pain as bad as you can imagine" centered below the "10," accompanied by the instruction "Please rate your pain by indicating the number that best describes your pain on average in the last 24 hours" (Cleeland and Ryan 1994). Pain "at its worst" or pain "at its least" could also be included in the assessment. Depending on the specific aims and design of the clinical trial, pain during the past week can also be assessed using the scale described.

There are circumstances in which reliable, valid, and responsive measures of pain intensity that do not use an NRS are routinely used, for example the Western Ontario and McMaster Universities Osteoarthritis Index (WOMAC; Bellamy et al. 1988) VAS ratings in studies of patients with osteoarthritis. These circumstances should be distinguished from those for which no such measures exist and NRS ratings of pain intensity are recommended. Of course, when other measures of pain intensity are used, it may also be valuable to administer NRS ratings to compare with other diseases or treatments.

Investigators should also consider including a VRS measure of pain intensity (none, mild, moderate, severe) as a secondary outcome measure to limit the amount of missing data if study participants have difficulty with the primary NRS measure. Such measures describe the effects of pain treatment in terms of changes in categorical descriptors, which may be more readily interpreted than VAS and NRS ratings, but do not have the interval and ratio scale qualities of VAS and NRS scales.

In addition to analyzing and reporting absolute changes in pain intensity during the clinical trial, it is recommended that the percentages of patients obtaining reductions in pain intensity from baseline of at least 30% be reported when an NRS (or VAS) has been used (Farrar et al. 2001).

Rescue analgesics and concomitant pain treatments

The use of all pain-related treatments during the course of a clinical trial should be assessed, including rescue analgesics and any other concomitant pain treatments. This is a straightforward task in single-dose analgesic trials that prohibit the concurrent use of other medications, but it is more difficult in chronic pain clinical trials that allow concurrent use of pain medications and other treatments for pain (e.g., physical therapy) for weeks or months. Some chronic pain trials have allowed previously used pain medications to be continued throughout the trial, and dosage stabilization is often required before patients are allowed to enroll in such trials. However, when changes in the use of concomitant pain treatments are permitted, they can be considered an outcome measure (e.g., Kieburtz et al. 1998).

Providing patients with access to rescue analgesics makes it easier to include a placebo group in treatment efficacy studies, since patients not obtaining adequate pain relief are provided with an analgesic. However, administration of rescue treatment complicates the interpretation of differences in pain ratings between patients taking placebo and active treatments because of the reduction in pain expected in patients receiving rescue treatment. The use of rescue medications is affected by both patient and provider beliefs, and patients use rescue medications to achieve varying levels of pain relief, and also for a variety of other reasons, including to improve sleep or reduce anxiety, to prevent increased pain resulting from increased activity, and to treat an episode of pain (e.g., headache) unrelated to the clinical trial.

Rescue medication consumption has been used as an outcome measure in clinical trials, with assessments including amount used and time-to-use (e.g., Morrison et al. 1999; Eisenberg et al. 2001). Scales have been developed that allow quantification of medication use in chronic pain patients based on dosage and medication class (Steedman 1992), and composite measures have been proposed that combine rescue medication usage and pain intensity ratings into a single score (Lehmann 1990; Silverman et al. 1993). Although these may be used to compare different treatment groups in clinical trials, the psychometric properties of such composite measures are not well established.

Despite the complex issues involved in the interpretation of rescue medication usage in a clinical trial, in many circumstances patients in a placebo group can be expected to take more of a rescue treatment than patients administered an efficacious investigational treatment. When considered together with pain intensity ratings, the amount of rescue treatment used by patients can therefore provide an important supplemental measure of the efficacy of the treatment being evaluated. Assessments of rescue treatments are recommended as a core outcome in trials where rescue treatment is provided.

Pain quality

Pain is known to have different sensory and affective qualities in addition to its intensity, and measures of these components of pain may be used to more fully describe a patient's pain experience (Melzack and Torgerson 1971; Price et al. 1987). It is possible that the efficacy of pain treatments varies for different pain qualities, and measures of pain quality may therefore identify treatments that are efficacious for certain types of pain but not for overall pain intensity. Assessment of specific pain qualities at baseline also makes it possible to determine whether certain patterns of pain quality moderate the effects of treatment. The Short-Form McGill Pain Questionnaire (Melzack 1987) assesses 15 sensory and affective pain descriptors and its sensory and affective subscales have demonstrated responsivity in clinical trials (e.g., Rowbotham et al. 1998; Dworkin et al. 2003). This questionnaire is recommended for inclusion in clinical trials as a secondary outcome measure to evaluate the effects of pain treatment on specific pain qualities.

Temporal aspects of pain

Measures of the temporal aspects of pain – including variability in intensity; time to onset of meaningful pain relief; durability of pain relief; and frequency, duration, and intensity of pain episodes – have not received adequate attention in pain research. The available evidence indicates that measures of pain frequency have validity and represent a distinct dimension of pain (Jensen and Karoly 2001). Frequency of "breakthrough" pain (i.e., periods of severe pain superimposed on ongoing pain) is an important temporal aspect of pain that has been used as an outcome measure in clinical trials (e.g., Farrar et al. 1998). When appropriate, investigators should consider administering measures of the temporal aspects of pain as secondary outcome measures in clinical trials. The temporal dimensions that should be considered include patients'

reports of the time to onset of meaningful pain relief and its durability as well as the frequency and intensity of episodes of breakthrough pain.

HEALTH-RELATED QUALITY OF LIFE

It has often been assumed that chronic pain is highly associated with alterations in emotional and physical functioning and that reduction in pain will inevitably lead to improvement in function and satisfaction with treatment. This is not necessarily the case, and in many studies pain and functioning are only modestly related. Moreover, changes in pain severity may have only a limited relationship with patients' ratings of improvement and satisfaction (Dougados et al. 2000; Dawson et al. 2002). Such data indicate that even though pain is typically considered the primary outcome in evaluating pain treatments, it is important to consider other outcomes in clinical trials.

In addition to relieving clinical symptoms and prolonging survival, the objectives of healthcare intervention include improvement of functioning (Revicki et al. 2000). Thus, there is a need to assess multiple domains of functioning and well-being, including behavior, mood, and satisfaction (Ware 1984; Revicki 1993) in clinical trials of chronic pain outcomes. *Quality of life* (QOL) is a term that refers to how a person feels and how he or she functions in daily life. Seid et al. (2000) define QOL as involving all aspects of an individual's life, including not only health but also housing, income, environment, work, school, and a safe neighborhood, which are traditionally viewed as beyond the scope of the healthcare system (Guyatt et al. 1993). Perhaps the greatest challenge to researchers who investigate QOL is the lack of a clear definition of the term, which has comprised health status, physical functioning, perceived health status, subjective health, health perceptions, symptoms, and functional disability (Hunt 1997). The use of such a broad approach is problematic not only with respect to instrument development and selection but also when attempting to identify relevant prior research (Deyo and Patrick 1989).

Concerns with the all-encompassing nature of QOL have led a number of investigators to use a more circumscribed construct, *health-related quality of life* (HRQOL). Although HRQOL has been used interchangeably with terms such as health status and functional status, researchers agree that HRQOL is a narrower term than QOL because it does not include aspects of work, environmental conditions, housing, and other variables that are often considered relevant to QOL but that do not involve health directly (Faden and LePlege 1992; Greenfield and Nelson 1992).

HRQOL is a multidimensional construct that includes the physical, psychological, and social domains recognized by the World Health Organization, as well as the impact of disease-specific and treatment-related symptoms on self-perceptions of functioning (Guyatt et al. 1993; Pal 1996; Testa and Simonson 1996). HRQOL refers to those domains that are specifically related to health and that can be potentially influenced by the healthcare system (Varni et al. 1999; Seid et al. 2000), and HRQOL outcomes are especially important for evaluating the impact of treatment on chronic diseases for which cure is not possible and therapy may be prolonged. Moreover, especially when treatment extends over long periods, it is critical to examine whether the benefits of symptom reduction are compromised by reductions in quality of life resulting from adverse effects of treatment.

There is, however, a lack of agreement regarding the specific variables that should be included in assessments of HRQOL, which has important consequences for researchers, especially with respect to study design and instrument development (Gladis et al. 1999). There is a plethora of measures intended to assess QOL and HRQOL (Hunt 1997; Jenkinson and Ziebland 1999), and one compendium of QOL instruments contains more than 1600 pages (Salek 1998). Indeed, it has been argued that the assessment of QOL and HRQOL is problematic because of the lack of clear definitions and shared theoretical frameworks, which makes it difficult to determine whether a given scale is a valid measure (Faden and LePlege 1992; Cella and Bonomi 1995).

Although the lack of consensual definitions of QOL and HRQOL is unfortunate, measures of both of these constructs have demonstrated reliability and validity and are widely used in clinical trials of diverse disorders. The consensus of the IMMPACT group is that two central components of existing HRQOL instruments, physical functioning and emotional functioning, are core domains that should be considered in all clinical trials of the efficacy and effectiveness of chronic pain treatments. This recommendation is supported by the results of studies in which exploratory and confirmatory factor analyses were used to identify the variables needed to comprehensively assess chronic pain patients which suggested that three relatively independent domains – pain severity, physical functioning, and emotional functioning – are required to capture the multidimensionality of the pain experience (De Gagné et al. 1995; Holroyd et al. 1999).

PHYSICAL FUNCTIONING

A major decision to be made in assessing the impact of a treatment on physical functioning involves whether a generic or a disease-specific measure will be used. Disease-specific measures are designed to evaluate the impact of a specific condition (e.g., ability to wear clothing in subjects with postherpetic neuralgia). Such specific effects of a disorder may not be assessed by

a generic measure, and disease-specific measures may therefore be more likely to reveal clinically important improvement or deterioration in function that is a consequence of treatment. In addition, responses on disease-specific measures will generally not reflect the effects of comorbid conditions on physical functioning, which may confound the interpretation of change occurring over the course of a trial when generic measures are used. Generic measures, however, make it possible to compare the physical functioning associated with a given disorder and its treatment with those of different conditions (Dworkin et al. 2001). Thus, the use of disease-specific and generic measures in combination facilitates the achievement of both sets of objectives. Regardless of whether a generic or a specific measure of physical functioning is selected, physical functioning is a core outcome domain in clinical trials of chronic pain treatment efficacy and effectiveness.

Functional status typically refers to the ability to perform particular defined tasks, such as walking a short distance, and social role functioning and participation in social interactions may also be assessed. A major decision to be made in assessing the impact of a treatment on physical functioning involves whether a generic or a disease-specific measure will be used. The tradeoffs between these two approaches have important implications for the interpretation of the results of a trial. Disease-specific measures of disability (e.g., WOMAC; Chapter 16) are designed to evaluate the impact of a specific condition. Specific effects of a disorder may be missed by a generic measure, and disease-specific measures may therefore be more likely to reveal changes in disability that are a consequence of treatment. In addition, responses on disease-specific measures will generally not reflect interference in physical functioning associated with co-morbid conditions, which may confound the interpretation of changes in functioning occurring over the course of a trial when generic measures are used. Generic measures, however, make it possible to compare functioning and public health impacts of a disorder and its treatment with those of different conditions. Regardless of whether an investigator selects a generic or a disease-specific measure, physical functioning is a core outcome domain for clinical trials of pain treatment.

Disease-specific measures may be more responsive to the effects of treatment on function, but generic measures provide information about physical functioning and treatment benefits that can be compared across different conditions and studies (Guyatt et al. 1993; Fowler et al. 1994). Because each of these approaches has strengths, use of both disease-specific measures, when available, and generic measures of physical functioning should be considered in designing chronic pain clinical trials.

On the basis of reviews of the literature on generic and pain-related measures of physical functioning prepared for the IMMPACT-II consensus meeting (Haythornthwaite 2003; Stucki and Cieza 2003) and discussions among the participants, use of a disease-specific measure of physical functioning is recommended in chronic pain clinical trials when a suitable and well-accepted one is available. Examples of such disease-specific measures of physical functioning are the WOMAC (Bellamy et al. 1988) and the Roland and Morris Back Pain Disability Scale (Roland and Morris 1983; Chapter 17). However, disease-specific measures of physical functioning have not been developed and validated for many chronic pain conditions. In clinical trials examining such disorders, use of either the Multidimensional Pain Inventory (MPI; Kerns et al. 1985; Chapter 17) Interference Scale or the Brief Pain Inventory (BPI; Cleeland and Ryan 1994; Cleeland et al. 1996; Chapter 22) pain interference items (i.e., general activity, mood, walking ability, normal work, relations with other people, sleep, enjoyment of life) is recommended. The MPI and BPI interference scales both provide reliable and valid measures of pain interference that have been translated into many languages and studied in diverse chronic pain conditions in multiple countries.

The IMPI and the BPI have distinct advantages and disadvantages, and use of both may be considered when doing so would not impose an undue burden on participants. The MPI Interference Scale does not assess sleep, and if this measure of physical functioning is administered, then use of a measure of sleep is recommended; there are both single-item (Rowbotham et al. 1998) and multiple-item (Peloso et al. 2000; Watson et al. 2003) measures of the impact of pain on sleep that can be used for this purpose. The BPI does include an item assessing pain interference with sleep, but also includes ratings of mood, social relations, and enjoyment of life. These three items may constitute a separate factor measuring affective state that is relatively independent of the remaining items (Cleeland et al. 1996). Few clinical trials, however, have examined BPI factors separately and so administration and analysis of only the three BPI activity items (general activity, walking ability, normal work) as a measure of physical functioning cannot be recommended until data become available.

Regardless of whether a disease-specific measure of physical functioning or the MPI interference scale or the BPI interference items are used in a clinical trial, administration of a generic measure of physical functioning should be considered to obtain data that will allow comparisons with other disorders and that could be used in cost-effectiveness analyses (Thompson 2002; Turk 2002).

The SF-36 Health Survey (Ware and Sherbourne 1992) is the most commonly used generic measure of HRQOL and it has been used in studies of diverse medical and psychiatric disorders and in numerous clinical trials. In patients with chronic pain, scores on this measure are associated with other HRQOL measures, such as the Nottingham Health Profile (Meyer-Rosburg et al. 2001). However, the SF-36 is recommended as a generic measure of physical functioning because its psychometric properties are somewhat superior and much more data are available for comparison with other disorders and treatments. The development of new HRQOL measures is an active area of research and these may offer improvements over the SF-36 and ultimately replace it (e.g., Chwastiak and Von Korff 2003).

In many chronic pain conditions, increased activity is accompanied by increased pain. Some patients limit their physical functioning because of pain, and their response to decreased pain may be to increase their activity until pain increases to their tolerated intensity. Other patients will tolerate increased pain to maintain a desired level of function and their response to decreased pain may be to report less pain as long as their level of function remains satisfactory. Both situations represent true relief of pain but in the first this would be reflected in increased activity with little change in pain and in the second in decreased pain with little change in activity. Although this issue has been addressed in some studies by examining combined measures of activity level and pain intensity to assess outcome (Malec et al. 1981; Peters and Large 1990), additional research on such composite measures is needed.

EMOTIONAL FUNCTIONING

The results of numerous studies suggest that chronic pain is often associated with emotional distress, particularly depression, anxiety, anger, and irritability. In addition, there is considerable co-morbidity between chronic pain and various psychiatric disorders (Sullivan and Turk 2001). The nature of the causal pathways accounting for these relationships is an important question for research on the pathogenesis of chronic pain, but may be less relevant in the clinical trial setting. For example, whether depression causes pain or pain causes depression, a treatment that alleviates both is much desired from a clinical perspective. To explain the mechanisms of treatment effects, however, it would be important to determine whether pain relief is a direct consequence of treatment or is secondary to a treatment-associated improvement in emotional distress. In special cases, testing of such mechanistic hypotheses may need to be included in clinical trials for regulatory or other purposes.

The presence of emotional distress in people with chronic pain presents a challenge when assessing symptoms such as fatigue, reduced activity level, decreased libido, appetite change, sleep disturbance, weight gain or loss, and memory and concentration deficits.

These symptoms are often associated with pain and have also been considered "vegetative" symptoms of depressive disorders. Improvements or deterioration in such symptoms, therefore, can be a result of changes in either pain or emotional distress. Although it is difficult to interpret changes in emotional functioning because of the many factors that contribute, this domain is central in people's assessments of their well-being and satisfaction with life and the authors recommend that it should be considered a core outcome domain in clinical trials of the efficacy or effectiveness of treatments for chronic pain.

On the basis of a review of the literature of measures of emotional functioning prepared for the IMMPACT-II consensus meeting (Kerns 2003) and discussions among the participants, the Beck Depression Inventory (BDI; Beck et al. 1961) and the Profile of Mood States (POMS; McNair et al. 1971) are recommended as core outcome measures of emotional functioning in chronic pain clinical trials. Both the BDI and POMS have well-established reliability and validity in the assessment of symptoms of depression and emotional distress, and they have been used in numerous clinical trials in psychiatry and an increasing number of chronic pain clinical trials (Kerns 2003). In research in psychiatry and chronic pain, the BDI provides a well-accepted criterion of the level of psychological distress in a sample and its response to treatment.

The POMS assesses six mood states – tension-anxiety, depression-dejection, anger-hostility, vigor-activity, fatigue-inertia, and confusion-bewilderment – and also provides a summary measure of total mood disturbance. Although the discriminant validity of the POMS scales in patients with chronic pain has not been adequately documented, it has scales for the three most important dimensions of emotional functioning in chronic pain patients (depression, anxiety, anger) and also assesses three other dimensions that are very relevant to chronic pain and its treatment, including a positive mood scale of vigor-activity. Moreover, the POMS has demonstrated beneficial effects of treatment in some (but not all) recent chronic pain trials (e.g., Rowbotham et al. 1998; Dworkin et al. 2003). For these reasons, administration of both the BDI and the POMS is recommended in chronic pain clinical trials to assess the major aspects of the emotional functioning outcome domain.

As noted above, various symptoms of depression – such as decreased libido, appetite or weight changes, fatigue, and memory and concentration deficits – are also commonly believed to be consequences of chronic pain and the medications used for its treatment (Gallagher and Verma 2004). It is unclear whether the presence of such symptoms in patients with chronic pain (and other medical disorders) should nevertheless be considered evidence of depressed mood, or whether the assessment of mood in these patients should

emphasize symptoms that are less likely to be secondary to physical disorders (Wilson et al. 2001). Because of the evidence that measures of emotional functioning are adequately reliable, valid, and responsive when used in the medically ill (Kerns 2003), the IMMPACT group recommend that the principal analyses of the BDI and POMS in chronic pain clinical trials use the original versions without adjustment for presumed confounding by somatic symptoms. Depending on the specific objective of the clinical trial, supplemental analyses could be conducted to separately examine non-somatic and somatic aspects of emotional functioning.

PATIENT GLOBAL RATING OF IMPROVEMENT AND SATISFACTION

Assessments of individual outcome domains such as pain and physical and emotional functioning may not adequately characterize the clinical trial participant's overall assessment of treatment and the meaningfulness to the patient of any improvement (or worsening). Global evaluations by participants in clinical trials of the benefits of treatment reflect not only the magnitude of the changes in these outcomes but also the personal importance that these outcomes have for participants. Such perceptions of the importance of treatment-associated changes often differ considerably from those of healthcare professionals, and the value and significance of therapeutic changes differ greatly among subjects and are important determinants of their treatment satisfaction.

Many different approaches have been used to assess clinical trial participants' overall evaluation of their benefit from and satisfaction with treatment provided. One of the most common involves assessments of improvement or worsening with treatment, for example the Patient Global Impression of Change (PGIC) scale (Guy 1976) which requires patients to rate changes they have experienced since the beginning of a clinical trial. The Global Improvement item requires the clinician to rate how much the patient's illness has improved or worsened relative to a baseline state. Compared to condition at baseline, a patient's illness is compared to change over time, and rated according to: very much improved; much improved; moderately improved; minimally improved; no change; minimally worse; moderately worse; much worse; or very much worse. Other approaches to the global assessment of treatment response include ratings of participant satisfaction with treatment and global ratings of disease state from which changes from baseline can be calculated. These ratings may differ in the degree of emphasis given to rating the treatment's performance (e.g., degree of response to treatment, helpfulness or usefulness of treatment) versus the patient's feelings about the treatment (e.g., satisfaction, preference).

The use of assessments of participants' overall evaluation of treatment in clinical trials is not without controversy. First, many such assessments are based on rating a single item, and it is not possible to establish the internal consistency of one rating. In addition, global impressions of improvement may fail to detect important changes (e.g., Just et al. 1999). Moreover, the judgment of change requires patients to assess both their present and initial state and then perform what may be an unreliable mental subtraction; because patients may be unable to recall their initial state, their ratings may be based on an "implicit theory" of change beginning with their present state and working backward (Ross 1989). However, if a treatment is associated with severe adverse effects, the patient may not need to remember baseline pain to rate satisfaction with treatment. The role of memory may therefore be greater in rating global impression of change than overall satisfaction with treatment.

Despite the necessity for care in the use of participant global assessments, the results of recent research provide support for their validity. For example, Collins et al. (2001) found that a global rating ("How effective do you think the treatment was?") provided similar evidence of analgesic efficacy as an aggregate measure of relief of acute pain, and Fischer et al. (1999) reported that retrospective measures were not only more responsive to change than serial pain assessments but were also more strongly associated with clinical trial participant satisfaction. These data illustrate that concerns about the influence of memory in evaluating improvement may not always be relevant to the processes by which participants actually evaluate their satisfaction with treatment and assess its benefits.

Ultimately, patients decide whether the positive attributes of a treatment outweigh its negative aspects, and this is an important determinant of whether they adhere to and continue with treatment. Participant ratings of improvement and satisfaction with treatment provide unique information in outcomes assessment in clinical trials because they may allow an integration of the benefits of treatment and adverse events and other costs from within the participant's personal perspective. One such rating should therefore be considered for inclusion in all chronic pain efficacy and effectiveness clinical trials.

Patients' perceptions of change in physical and emotional functioning with treatment may vary considerably from healthcare professionals. Patients' preferences reflect the relative importance that each outcome has for them. The value, significance, and impact of a therapeutic change of a given magnitude may vary considerably for different patients, and be an important determinant of adherence to treatment.

By soliciting patients' preferences, investigators acknowledge the unique values of different outcomes and their aggregate for individual patients. Patients'

values and preferences are what distinguish global ratings from other measures, and such ratings provide sufficient unique information to warrant inclusion in all clinical trials of treatments for chronic pain (Turk et al. 2006).

Many different approaches have been used in clinical trials to assess participants' overall evaluation of their treatment. On the basis of a review of the literature of measures of global outcome prepared for the IMMPACT-II consensus meeting (Farrar 2003) and discussions among the participants, the Patient Global Impression of Change scale (PGIC; Guy 1976) is recommended for use in chronic pain clinical trials as a core outcome measure of global improvement with treatment. This measure is a single-item rating by participants of their improvement with treatment during a clinical trial on a seven-point scale that ranges from "very much improved" to "very much worse" with "no change" as the midpoint.

There has been widespread use of the PGIC in recent chronic pain clinical trials (Dunkl et al. 2002; Farrar et al. 2001), and the data provide a responsive and readily interpretable measure of participants' assessments of the clinical importance of their improvement or worsening over the course of a clinical trial. Impressions of change scores using different verbal outcome categories have also been used to determine the minimally important difference in quality of life measures (Guyatt et al. 2002). Although these measures appear to have validity, additional research is necessary to determine the relative extent to which ratings on the PGIC and similar measures reflect reduced pain, improvement in functioning, side effect burden, or other variables and whether this varies for different people.

Other approaches to the global assessment of treatment response that have been used less frequently than the PGIC in chronic pain trials include ratings of participant satisfaction with treatment, prospectively conducted global ratings of disease state from which changes from baseline can be calculated, and global ratings of specific outcome domains, for example global ratings of improvement in physical functioning or in overall side effect burden (Middel et al. 2001). Single-item ratings of treatment outcome have both advantages and disadvantages when compared to multiple-item scales (Sloan et al. 2002), and additional research will be important to determine the optimal method for obtaining global ratings from patients.

SYMPTOMS AND ADVERSE EVENTS

Most patients will experience some degree of side effect burden with any pharmacologic treatment, and the importance of monitoring adverse events in the evaluation of new drugs has long been recognized and is a component of all clinical trials. Two treatments may be equally effective and their adverse events not significantly different on a statistical basis but patients may view the side effects of a treatment as sufficiently noxious to discontinue or not comply fully with treatment (Anderson et al. 1999).

Therapies, such as the drugs that relieve pain, have a variety of effects, and these can not only cause discomfort but also may potentially impair physical and emotional function and exacerbate comorbid symptoms, which thereby may potentially offset the therapeutic benefit. Max and Laska (1991) have noted that common analgesic adverse events (e.g., gastrointestinal distress, sedation, depression) can limit the dosage that can be realistically prescribed. Moreover, side effect burden plays an important role in treatment adherence. Patients may view adverse events as sufficiently noxious to discontinue treatment or limit dosage, and the overall benefit of treatment may therefore be reduced. The challenge is finding the dosage that maximizes pain relief and functional improvements and minimizes side effects. The onset of new diseases and initiation of new treatments during a clinical trial complicates assessments of symptoms and adverse events. When initiated during a trial, concomitant treatments (e.g., drugs, physical therapy, psychological therapy, nerve blocks) are often protocol violations. Characteristics of the disease are baseline features or covariates when present at the beginning of a trial but are an adverse event when it emerges or worsens.

The usual strategy is to ask patients and clinicians to record the occurrence of any adverse events that might be attributed to the treatment. Several studies (e.g., Anderson and Testa 1994), however, suggest that patients may not acknowledge the presence of many potentially important side effects spontaneously during open-ended inquiry. Although there may be many reasons for the differences (memory, embarrassment), the fact is that important side effects may be missed by the use of open-ended questions. Negative health consequences of treatment using standard lists of symptoms that patients can rate with respect to presence, severity, and importance are an important domain that should be systematically assessed and reported in all clinical trials of treatments for chronic pain. Investigators should consider broad-based measures rather than ones more limited in scope as the latter may underestimate the symptom distress experienced by the patient (Anderson et al. 1999). Moreover, not only should investigators determine the presence of side effects but their severity and importance to the patient.

Assessment of the percentages of clinical trial participants experiencing adverse events based on passive capture is standard in clinical trials; however, assessments of their severity and importance to patients are much less common, although this may provide valuable information. The IMMPACT group recommends that the prospective assessment of symptoms and adverse events relevant to the specific trial is a core outcome domain that should be included in all chronic pain clinical trials, and that the strategy used to assess these events should include patient ratings of their presence, severity, and importance.

Clinical trial protocols should define the method of assessment and the rationale for that approach. In selecting the approach used for ascertaining adverse events and the methods used for recording and coding the terms used to describe these events (e.g., Medical Dictionary for Regulatory Activities, Brown 2003), consideration should be given to the type and purpose of the trial, whether international regulatory requirements dictate certain approaches (International Conference on Harmonization 1995a,b, 1996b), the phase of development or postmarketing, and the total safety experience with the product.

On the basis of a review of the literature on the assessment of symptoms and adverse events prepared for the IMMPACT-II consensus meeting (Katz 2003) and discussions among the participants, the IMMPACT group recommend that "passive capture" of spontaneously reported events and the use of open-ended prompts should be used in chronic pain clinical trials to assess adverse events, ideally supplemented by periodic review of systems beginning at baseline. In describing the results of clinical trials, the incidence of individual adverse events and serious adverse events should be reported by the treatment group, including the percentages of participants who experienced at least one treatment emergent adverse event.

Active capture using structured interviews or questionnaires to assess specific symptoms and adverse events that are relevant to the disorder or treatment being studied will often be more sensitive and more informative than passive capture or general inquiries (Rabkin et al. 1992; Testa et al. 1993; Anderson and Testa 1994). Depending on the objectives of a chronic pain clinical trial, prospective capture of symptoms and adverse events can be conducted at periodic intervals throughout the trial, including baseline and the conclusion of the trial, ideally by the same investigator. The frequency, duration, intensity, distress, importance to the patient, impact on daily function, and causal attribution by investigator and patient of symptoms and adverse events can be assessed (Lingjaerde et al. 1987; Anderson et al. 1999), which will provide information about the clinical importance of safety and tolerability outcomes.

The authors recommend that methods for prospectively investigating symptoms and adverse events relevant to chronic pain and its treatment be vigorously explored. In developing comprehensive strategies to assess these events, consideration should be given to including participant ratings of frequency, severity, importance, and associated distress and also to the possibility that use of such methods might increase the reported incidence of clinically insignificant events.

PATIENT DISPOSITION

The CONSORT (Consolidated Standards of Reporting Trials) guidelines (Begg et al. 1996; Moher et al. 2001) should be adhered to when publishing the results of clinical trials and these guidelines provide a valuable overview of the types of patient disposition data that should be obtained when conducting trials. All potential study participants screened for a clinical trial should be carefully described with respect to the proportion who are ultimately enrolled, and why those who were not enrolled were not included. Detailed information should be provided regarding the extent and reasons for treatment nonadherence, prohibited concomitant medications and all other protocol deviations that may impact the interpretation of the trial results, treatment modification, premature patient withdrawal from the trial, and loss to follow-up. Investigators should report the number of withdrawals related to each of the symptoms and adverse events identified in each of the treatment groups. This detailed characterization of participant disposition is the sixth core domain that should be assessed in all clinical trials of chronic pain treatment efficacy and effectiveness.

To be effective, a treatment must have a beneficial effect on the symptom or disease being treated and the clinical trial participant must adhere to the treatment regimen. The most potent analgesic may demonstrate less than its potential benefit if patients in a clinical trial fail to use the medication in the manner prescribed, are unable to tolerate a fully effective dose, or drop out of the trial due to unacceptable adverse events or inadequate pain relief. Furthermore, the benefit of the treatment being studied may be obscured if participants receive any treatments that are not allowed in the protocol (Turk et al. 2003).

The dosage and duration of all treatments received by participants during the clinical trial must be recorded, not only the treatment being investigated, but also all concomitant treatments. Treatments initiated during the trial often reflect inadequate pain relief or the presence of distressing or uncontrolled adverse events (the use of rescue medications and changes in concomitant medication use may be justifiable as pain outcome measures when specified in the protocol). Assessments of the use of rescue (described above) and prohibited medications and alterations in prescribed treatment due to adverse events and symptoms must be considered in evaluating the results of chronic pain clinical trials.

Significant percentages of patients enrolled in clinical trials prematurely terminate participation in the study. The IMMPACT recommendations are in agreement with the CONSORT statement (Moher et al. 2001) as to the importance of reporting data on patient attrition and loss to follow-up, and emphasize that the reasons for nonadherence be provided and not just the percentage who fail to comply. Patient disposition, premature exit from a trial, nonadherence to treatment, and loss to follow-up form a core domain that should be reported as an outcome in all clinical trials.

Although the CONSORT guidelines (Begg et al. 1996; Altman et al. 2001; Moher et al. 2001) provide a valuable enumeration of the core elements of information on participant disposition that should be recorded when conducting trials, the following additional information should be collected and reported in chronic pain clinical trials if collecting this information is practical: (1) the recruitment process and the percentages of participants enrolled from each recruitment method used; (2) the number of candidate participants who were excluded from participation and the reasons why; (3) the number of candidates who chose not to enter the trial and the reasons why; (4) the use of prohibited concomitant medications and all other protocol deviations that may impact the interpretation of the trial results; (5) the number and reasons for withdrawal from each treatment group, including deaths and patients lost to follow up; and (6) the types, rates, and reasons for nonadherence with treatment in each treatment group.

Dosages and duration of all treatments received by participants during the clinical trial should be recorded, including assessments of the use of rescue, concomitant, and prohibited medications and all alterations in prescribed treatment. Detailed information describing the extent to which each participant adhered to the protocol will make it possible for data analyses to be conducted that examine efficacy in patients who adhered to the protocol. Such *efficacy evaluable* or *per protocol* analyses can sometimes be valuable in interpreting the results of intention-to-treat analyses, although the benefits of comparing randomized groups are lost. Although an important component of patient disposition, withdrawal from a clinical trial due to lack of treatment effectiveness can also be considered an endpoint (e.g., Bensen et al., 1999; Ehrich et al. 1999; International Conference on Harmonization 2001; European Agency for the Evaluation of Medicinal Products 2002).

Although reasons for withdrawal are usually provided in reports of clinical trials, this information is often inadequate. For example, "drop out due to adverse events" may be given as a reason for withdrawal, but this is not informative without tabulation of the specific adverse events associated with the withdrawals. Similarly, "withdrawal of consent" is commonly given as a reason for withdrawals, but this is impossible to interpret without description of the reasons why patients withdrew consent.

There are several factors that may compromise the integrity of the double-blind used in a clinical trial (Even et al. 2000). Participants' and investigators' guesses of which treatment was administered should therefore be assessed, and the reasons for the specific guesses (e.g., medication side effects or pain relief) should also be collected to assist in interpreting any unblinding that may have occurred (Moscucci et al. 1987; Turner et al. 2002).

COMMENTS ON THE CORE DOMAINS

The IMMPACT group believes that investigators designing and conducting clinical trials of chronic pain treatment efficacy and effectiveness should consider each of the six core domains discussed. It is important to emphasize, however, that we are not suggesting that positive results must be obtained for all of the core domains for the treatment to be deemed efficacious. Also we want to emphasize the word *considered*. These core domains and measures should be considered and are not mandatory because it is possible that there are specific trials for which one or more of these domains might not be relevant. In such instances, our recommendation is that investigators should acknowledge that they have considered each outcome domain and provide the rationale when they decide not to include assessment of a particular domain. Of course, there are many supplemental outcome domains that can be included in a chronic pain clinical trial (see next section), and we expect that the core outcome domains will be supplemented by assessment of additional domains that are required to evaluate a specific treatment (or that the investigator wishes to include for exploratory purposes).

The core outcome domains specified in these IMMPACT consensus recommendations – pain, physical functioning, emotional functioning, patient ratings of global improvement and satisfaction with treatment, symptoms and adverse events, and patient disposition – are generally consistent with the recommendations for arthritis clinical trials from OMERACT-III (Bellamy et al. 1997) and the World Health Organization/International Leagues of Associations for Rheumatology (Brooks and Hochberg 2001). Pain, physical function, subject global assessment, and imaging studies are the core outcome domains specified in the OMERACT guidelines, and the first three of these domains are included in the present recommendations.

The statistical power of clinical trials is typically determined for the primary endpoint, and it can therefore be expected that inadequate power may often explain negative results for secondary outcome measures. Conversely, positive results for secondary endpoints in chronic pain trials such as physical and emotional functioning would not necessarily provide adequate demonstration to support additional efficacy claims for such outcomes.

he IMMPACT group acknowledges that there will be circumstances in which one or more of the core outcome measures will not be relevant, and we also expect that these measures will typically be supplemented by other measures that are included for exploratory purposes or to evaluate treatment- or disease-specific issues. Regardless of the measures used, the reasons for selecting each of the specific measures that have been included in a clinical trial should be provided.

There are many decisions that must be made in administering outcome measures in chronic pain trials. For example, whether ratings of pain or the other measures we have discussed are made using retrospective or serial assessments is a very important issue that may have implications for the ability of a measure to detect change (Fischer et al. 1999). These and other decisions will depend on the specific design of the trial, the resources available, and other considerations that are beyond the scope of this chapter.

Although recommending specific core outcome measures, IMMPACT acknowledges the limitations of existing measures and the need to develop improved methods for assessing chronic pain outcomes. Future IMMPACT recommendations will discuss strategies for developing improved measures of chronic pain outcomes (Turk et al. 2006), methods to identify the clinical importance of changes in chronic pain outcome measures, and approaches for combining multiple outcome measures in evaluating treatment efficacy as well as domains and measures for use in acute pain clinical trials.

SUPPLEMENTAL OUTCOME DOMAINS

There are many other outcome domains that can be considered in the design of pain clinical trials depending on the specific research question. Supplemental assessment domains may be included in a clinical trial without a hypothesis that they will change and without the trial having adequate power to test the hypothesis that they will respond to treatment. Other outcome domains that might be used to supplement or complement the core domains include: role functioning (i.e., work and educational activities), interpersonal functioning (i.e. relationships and activities with family, friends, and others), pharmacoeconomic measures and healthcare utilization, biologic markers (e.g., assessments based on quantitative sensory testing, imaging, genetic markers, pharmacogenomics, and skin punch biopsy), coping, clinician or surrogate ratings of global improvement, neuropsychological assessments of cognitive and motor function, suffering and other end-of-life issues (Turk et al. 2003). These supplemental outcome domains might be considered in the design of chronic pain clinical trials.

It would be possible to combine role functioning and interpersonal functioning into a single outcome domain of social functioning in some circumstances. If reliable, valid, and responsive measures of these variables become available, such a combined domain of social functioning might merit consideration as a potential core outcome domain. Depending on the specific clinical trial, suffering and other end-of-life issues could be included within the core outcome domain of emotional functioning.

CONCLUSION

IMMPACT is a process and not an outcome. The topics addressed will require revising as new information becomes available. The composition of IMMPACT is dynamic, with the participation at the meetings varying depending on the focus of the topic being addressed. It is our belief that it is impossible to include all those who have an interest in the topic at a meeting as large numbers inhibit discussion. In an effort to make the information as readily available as possible, the IMMPACT website was developed and efforts for dissemination are facilitated by publication of papers summarizing the thinking and recommendations of the panel in widely available journals.

A number of topics have been proposed as targets for discussion and consensus at IMMPACT meetings. These include use of composite measures and responder analyses in chronic pain clinical trials; the ethical and methodologic aspects of the use of placebos and no-treatment groups in chronic pain research; baseline characteristics, covariates, moderators, mediators, mechanisms; research designs; primary versus secondary endpoints; assessments of side-effects; diversity, cross-cultural issues, pediatric patients, cognitively impaired; physical functioning patient-reported outcomes versus performance measures; early phase II clinical models and human experimental models; surrogate endpoints; pharmacoeconomics; non-pharmacologic treatment approaches; and reporting of clinical trials. These are not listed in any particular order.

Academic, healthcare, and pharmaceutical industry investigators who conduct clinical trials, the government and private organizations that provide funding for many such studies, and the government regulatory agencies that review this research and ultimately approve new therapies for the public all share a commitment to identifying treatments for chronic pain that are more effective and have fewer adverse effects than those currently available. These different groups, however, sometimes have different goals, contrasting ideologies, and separate constituencies with particular interests in clinical trials. Although unsystematic efforts to bring these different individuals together have occurred in various medical specialties, much more can and should be done to enhance mutual understanding and promote creativity in the development and investigation of improved treatment approaches (Klein et al. 2002). The authors hope that IMMPACT and the recommendations described in this chapter will provide an example of the value of such collaborative efforts among academia, government, and industry. The ultimate goal of such efforts should be to advance the science of pain clinical trials and thereby provide improved treatments for patients suffering from pain. Additional information on IMMPACT activities is available at www.immpact.org.

REFERENCES

Aaronson NK, Ahmedzai S, Bergman B, et al. The European Organization for Research and Treatment of Cancer QLQ-C30: a quality-of-life instrument of use in international clinical trials in oncology. J Natl Cancer Inst 1993; 85:365–376.

Abbott FV, Fraser MI. Use and abuse of over-the-counter analgesic agents. J Psychiat Neurosci 1998; 23:13–34.

Altman DG, Schulz KF, Moher D, et al. CONSORT Group. The revised CONSORT statement for reporting randomized trials: explanation and elaboration. Ann Intern Med 2001; 134:663–694.

Anderson RB, Testa MA. Symptom distress checklists as a component of quality of life measurement: comparing prompted reports by patient and physician with concurrent adverse event reports via the physician. Drug Information J 1994; 28:89–114.

Anderson RB, Hollenberg NK, Williams GH. Physical Symptoms Distress Index. A sensitive tool to evaluate the impact of pharmacological agents. Arch Intern Med 1999; 159:693–700.

Beck AT, Ward CH, Mendelson M, et al. An inventory for measuring depression. Arch Gen Psychiatry 1961; 4:561–571.

Begg C, Cho M, Eastwood S, et al. Improving the quality of reporting of randomized controlled trials: the CONSORT statement. JAMA 1996; 276:637–639.

Bellamy N, Buchanan WW, Goldsmith CH, et al. Validation study of WOMAC: a health status instrument for measuring clinically important patient relevant outcomes to antirheumatic drug therapy in patients with osteoarthritis of the hip or knee. J Rheumatol 1988; 15:1833–1840.

Bellamy N, Kirwan J, Boers M, et al. Recommendations for a core set of outcome measures for future phase III clinical trials in knee, hip, and hand osteoarthritis. Consensus development at OMERACT III. J Rheumatol 1997; 24:799–802.

Bensen WG, Fiechtner JJ, McMillen JI, et al. Treatment of osteoarthritis with celecoxib, a cyclooxygenase-2 inhibitor: a randomized controlled trial. Mayo Clinic Proc 1999; 74:1095–1105.

Brooks P, Hochberg M for ILAR and OMERACT. Outcome measures and classification criteria for the rheumatic diseases. A compilation of data from OMERACT (Outcome Measures for Arthritis Clinical Trials), ILAR (International League of Associations for Rheumatology), regional leagues and other groups. Rheumatology 2001; 40:896–906.

Brown EG. Methods and pitfalls in searching drug safety databases utilising the Medical Dictionary for Regulatory Activities (MedDRA). Drug Safety 2003; 26:145–158.

Caraceni A, Cherny N, Fainsinger R, et al. Pain measurement tools and methods in clinical research in palliative care: recommendations of an expert working group of the European Association of Palliative Care. J Pain Sympt Manage 2002; 23:239–255.

Cella D, Bonomi AE. Measuring quality of life: update. Oncology 1995; 1995:47–60.

Chwastiak LA, Von Korff M. Disability in depression and back pain: evaluation of the World Health Organization Disability Assessment Schedule (WHO DAS II) in a primary care setting. J Clin Epidemiol 2003; 56:507–514.

Cleeland CS, Ryan KM. Pain assessment: global use of the Brief Pain Inventory. Ann Acad Med 1994; 23:129–138.

Cleeland CS, Nakamura Y, Mendoza TR, et al. Dimensions of the impact of cancer pain in a four country sample: new information from multidimensional scaling. Pain 1996; 67:267–273.

Collins SL, Edwards J, Moore RA, et al. Seeking a simple measure of analgesia for mega-trials: is a single global assessment good enough? Pain 2001; 91:189–194.

Dawson R, Spross JA, Jablonski ES, et al. Probing the paradox of patients' satisfaction with inadequate pain management. J Pain Sympt Manage 2002; 23:211–220.

De Gagné TA, Mikail SF, D'Eon JL. Confirmatory factor analysis of a 4-factor model of chronic pain evaluation. Pain 1995; 60:195–202.

Deyo RA, Patrick DL. Barriers to the use of health status measures in clinical investigation, patient care, and policy research. Med Care 1989; 30(5 suppl):S176–S180.

Deyo RA, Battie M, Beurskens AHHM, et al. Outcome measures for low back pain research. A proposal for standardized use. Spine 1998; 23:2003–2013.

Dworkin RH, Nagasako EM, Hetzel RD, et al. Assessment of pain and pain-related quality of life in clinical trials. In: Turk DC, Melzack R (eds). Handbook of Pain Assessment, 2nd edn. GuilfordPress, New York, 2001:659–692.

Dworkin RH, Corbin AE, Young JP, et al. Pregabalin for the treatment of postherpetic neuralgia: a randomized, placebo-controlled trial. Neurology 2003; 60:1274–1283.

Dworkin RH, Turk DC, Farrar JT, et al. Core outcome measures for chronic pain clinical trials: IMMPACT recommendations. Pain 2005; 113:9–19.

Ehrich EW, Schnitzer TJ, McIlwain H, et al. Effect of specific COX-2 inhibition in osteoarthritis of the knee: a 6 week double blind, placebo controlled pilot study of rofecoxib. J Rheumatol 1999; 26:2438–2447.

Eisenberg E, Lurie Y, Daoud D, et al. Lamotrigine reduces painful diabetic neuropathy: a randomized controlled study. Neurology 2001; 57:505–509.

European Agency for the Evaluation of Medicinal Products. Note for guidance on clinical investigation of medicinal products for treatment of nociceptive pain, 2002. Available at www.emea.eu.int/pdfs/human/ewp/061200en.pdf (accessed May 12, 2004).

Even C, Siobud-Dorocant E, Dardennes RM. Critical approach to antidepressant trials: blindness protection is necessary, feasible and measurable. Br J Psychiatry 2000; 177:47–51.

Faden R, LePlege A. Assessing quality of life: moral implications for clinical practice. Med Care 1992; 30(5 suppl):MS166–MS175.

Farrar JT, Cleary J, Rauck R, et al. Oral transmucosal fentanyl cirate: randomized, double-blinded, placebo-controlled trial for treatment of breakthrough pain in cancer patients. J Natl Cancer Inst 1998; 90:611–616.

Farrar JT, Young JP, LaMoreaux L, et al. Clinical importance of changes in chronic pain intensity measured on an 11-point numerical pain rating scale. Pain 2001; 94:149–158.

Farrar JT. The global assessment of pain and related symptoms. Presented at the second meeting of the Initiative on Methods, Measurement, and Pain Assessment in Clinical Trials (IMMPACT-II), 2003. Available at www.immpact.org/meetings.html (accessed May 12, 2004).

Ferreira PH, Ferreira ML, Maher CG, et al. Effects of applying different "levels of evidence" criteria on conclusions of Cochrane reviews of interventions for low back pain. J Clin Epidemiol 2002; 55:1126–1129.

Fischer D, Stewart AL, Blich DA, et al. Capturing the patient's view of change as a clinical outcome measure. JAMA 1999; 282:1157–1162.

Fitzpatrick R, Davey C, Buxton MJ, et al. Evaluating patient-based outcome measures for use in clinical trials. Health Technol Assessment 1998; 2(14).

Fowler FJ, Cleary PD, Magaziner J, et al. Methodological issues in measuring patient-reported outcomes: the agenda of the work group on outcomes assessment. Med Care 1994; 32:JS65–JS76.

Gallagher RM, Verma S. Mood and anxiety disorders in chronic pain. In: Dworkin RH, Breitbart WS (eds). Psychosocial Aspects of Pain: A Handbook for Health Care Providers. IASP Press, Seattle, WA, 2004:589–606.

Ganz PA. What outcomes matter to patients. A physician-researcher point of view. Med Care 2002; 40(suppl):III11–III19.

Gladis M, Gosch E, Dishuk N, et al. Quality of life: expanding the scope of clinical significance. J Consult Clin Psychol 1999; 67:320–331.

Greenfield S, Nelson EC. Recent developments and future issues in the use of health status assessment measures in clinical settings. Med Care 1992; 30(5 suppl):MS23–MS41.

Guy W. ECDEU Assessment Manual for Psychopharmacology (DHEW Publication No. ADM 76–338). US Government Printing Office, Washington, DC, 1976.

Guyatt G, Walter S, Norman G. Measuring change over time: assessing the usefulness of evaluative instruments. J Chronic Dis 1987; 40:171–178.

Guyatt GH, Feeney DH, Patrick DL. Measuring health-related quality of life. Ann Intern Med 1993; 118:622–629.

Guyatt GH, Osoba D, Wu AW, et al. Clinical Significance Consensus Meeting Group. Methods to explain the clinical significance of health status measures. Mayo Clin Proc 2002; 77:371–383.

Hays RD, Hadorn D. Responsiveness to change: an aspect of validity, not a separate dimension. Qual Life Res 1992; 1:73–75.

Haythornthwaite JA. The assessment of pain-related physical function for clinical trials in chronic pain. Presented at the second meeting of the Initiative on Methods, Measurement, and Pain Assessment in Clinical Trials (IMMPACT-II), 2003. Available at www.immpact.org/meetings.html (accessed May 12, 2004).

Holroyd KA, Malinoski P, Davis MK, et al. The three dimensions of headache impact: pain, disability and affective distress. Pain 1999; 83:571–578.

Hunt SM. The problem of quality of life. Qual Life Res 1997; 6:205–212.

International Conference on Harmonization. Guideline for industry, E1A: the extent of population exposure to assess clinical safety: for drugs intended for long-term treatment of non-life threatening conditions, 1995a. Available at www.fda.gov/cder/guidance/index.html (accessed May 12, 2004).

International Conference on Harmonization. Guideline for industry, E2A: International Conference on Harmonization. Guideline for industry, E2A: clinical safety data management: definitions and standards for expedited reporting, 1995b. Available at www.fda.gov/cder/guidance/index.htm (accessed May 12, 2004).

International Conference on Harmonization. Guideline for industry, E6: good clinical practice: consolidated guidance, 1996a. Available at www.fda.gov/cder/guidance/index.htm (accessed May 12, 2004).

International Conference on Harmonization. Guideline for industry, E3: structure and content of clinical study reports, 1996b. Available at www.fda.gov/cder/guidance/index.htm (accessed May 12, 2004).

International Conference on Harmonization. Guidance for industry, E10: choice of control group and related issues in clinical trials, 2001. Available at www.fda.gov/cder/guidance/index.htm (accessed May 12, 2004).

Jadad AR, Cook D, Browman GP. When arbitrators disagree: a guide to interpreting discordant systematic reviews of health care interventions. Can Med Assoc J 1997; 156:1411–1416.

Jadad AE, Rennie D. The randomized controlled trial gets a middle-aged checkup. JAMA 1998; 279:319–320.

Jaeschke R, Singer J, Guyatt GH. Measurement of health status: ascertaining the minimal clinically important difference. Control Clin Trials 1989; 10:407–415.

Jenkinson C, Ziebland S. Interpretation of data from health status measures: what do the numbers mean? In: McGee H, O'Boyle C (eds). Individual Quality of Life: Approaches to Conceptualization and Assessment. Psychology Press, 1999:75–85.

Jensen MP, Karoly P. Self-report scales and procedures for assessing pain in adults. In: Turk DC, Melzack R (eds). Handbook of Pain Assessment, 2nd edn. Guilford Press, New York, 2001:15–34.

Jensen MP. The validity and reliability of pain measures for use in clinical trials in adults. Presented at the second meeting of the Initiative on Methods, Measurement, and Pain Assessment in Clinical Trials (IMMPACT-II), 2003. Available at www.immpact.org/meetings.html (accessed May 12, 2004).

Juniper EF, Guyatt GH, Willan A, et al. Determining a minimal important change in a disease-specific quality of life questionnaire. J Clin Epidemiol 1994; 47:81–87.

Just N, Ciccone DS, Bandilla EB, et al. Global impressions versus validated measures of treatment effectiveness in patients with chronic nonmalignant pain. Rehabil Psychol 1999; 44:194–207.

Katz N. The measurement of symptoms and side effects in clinical trials of chronic pain. Presented at the second meeting of the Initiative on Methods, Measurement, and Pain Assessment in Clinical Trials (IMMPACT-II), 2003. Available at www.immpact.org/meetings.html (accessed May 12, 2004).

Kerns RD, Turk DC, Rudy TE. The West Haven-Yale Multidimensional Pain Inventory (WHYMPI). Pain 1985; 23:345–356.

Kerns RD. Assessment of emotional functioning in pain treatment outcome research. Presented at the second meeting of the Initiative on Methods, Measurement, and Pain Assessment in Clinical Trials (IMMPACT-II), 2003.

Available at www.immpact.org/meetings.html (accessed May 12, 2004).

Kieburtz K, Simpson D, Yiannoutsos C, et al. AIDS Clinical Trial Group 242 Protocol Team. A randomized trial of amitriptyline and mexiletine for painful neuropathy in HIV infection. Neurology 1998; 51:1682–1688.

Klein DF, Thase ME, Endicott J, et al. Improving clinical trials. American Society of Clinical Psychopharmcology recommendations. Arch Gen Psychiatry 2002; 59:272–278.

Legler JM, Lefkopoulou M, Ryan LM. Efficiency and power of tests for multiple binary outcomes. J Am Stat Assoc 1995; 90:680–693.

Lehmacher W, Wassmer G, Reitmeir P. Procedures for two-sample comparisons with multiple endpoints controlling the experimentwise error rates. Biometrics 1991; 47:511–521.

Lehmann KA. Patient-controlled analgesia for postoperative pain. In: Benedetti C, Chapman CR, Giron G (eds). Opioid Analgesia: Recent Advances in Systemic Administration. Raven Press, New York, 1990:297–334.

Lingjaerde O, Ahlfors UG, Bech P, et al. The UKU side effect rating scale: a new comprehensive rating scale for psychotropic drugs and a cross-sectional study of side effects in neuroleptic-treated patients. Acta Psychiatr Scand Suppl 1987; 334:1–100.

Malec J, Cayner JJ, Harvey RF, et al. Pain management: long-term follow-up of an inpatient program. Arch Phys Med Rehabil 1981; 62:369–372.

Max MB, Laska EM. Single-dose analgesic comparisons. In: Max M, Portenoy R, Laska E (eds). Advances in Pain Research and Therapy, vol 18. Raven Press, New York, 1991:55–95.

McNair DM, Lorr M, Droppleman LF. Profile of Mood States. Educational and Industrial Testing Service, San Diego, CA, 1971.

Melzack R. The short-form McGill Pain Questionnaire. Pain 1987; 30:191–197.

Meyer-Rosberg K, Burckhardt CS, Huizar K, et al. A comparison of the SF-36 and Nottingham Health Profile in patients with chronic neuropathic pain. Eur J Pain 2001; 5:391–403.

Moher D, Schulz K, Altman DG for the CONSORT Group. The CONSORT Statement: revised recommendations for improving the quality of reports of parallel-group randomized trials. Ann Intern Med 2001; 134:657–662.

Morrison BW, Daniels SE, Kotey P, et al. Rofecoxib, a specific cyclooxygenase-2 inhibitor, in primary dysmenorrhea: a randomized controlled trial. Obstet Gynecol 1999; 94:504–508.

Moscucci M, Byrne L, Weintraub M, et al. Blinding, unblinding, and the placebo effect: an analysis of patients' guesses of treatment assignment in a double-blind clinical trial. Clin Pharmacol Ther 1987; 41:259–265.

Naliboff BD, Cohen MJ, Swanson GA, et al. Comprehensive assessment of chronic low back pain patients and controls: physical abilities, level of activity, psychological adjustment and pain perception. Pain 1985; 23:121–134.

National Research Council. Musculoskeletal Disorders and the Workplace. National Academy Press, Washington, DC, 2001.

O'Brien PC. Procedures for comparing samples with multiple endpoints. Biometrics 1984; 40:1079–1087.

Pal DK. Quality of life assessment in children: a review of conceptual and methodological issues in multidimensional health status measures. J Epidemiol Commun Health 1996; 50:391–396.

Peloso PM, Bellamy N, Bensen W, et al. Double blind randomized placebo control trial of controlled release codeine in the treatment of osteoarthritis of the hip or knee. J Rheumatol 2000; 27:764–771.

Peters JL, Large RG. A randomised control trial evaluating in- and outpatient pain management programmes. Pain 1990; 41:283–293.

Pleis JR, Coles R. Summary health statistics for US adults: National Health Interview Survey. National Center for Health Statistics. Vital Health Statistics 1998; 10(209).

Price DD, Harkins SW, Baker C. Sensory-affective relationships among different types of clinical and experimental pain. Pain 1987; 28:297–307.

Rabkin JG, Markowitz JS, Ocepek-Welikson K, et al. General versus systematic inquiry about emergent clinical events with SAFTEE: implications for clinical research. J Clin Psychopharm 1992; 12:3–10.

Revicki DA. Health care technology assessment and health-related quality of life. In: Banta D, Luce BR (eds). Health Care Technology and its Assessment: An International Perspective. Oxford University Press, New York, 1993:114–131.

Revicki DA, Ehreth JL. Health-related quality of life assessment and planning for the pharmaceutical industry. Clin Ther 1997; 19:1101–1115.

Revicki DA, Osoba D, Fairclough D, et al. Recommendations on health-related quality of life research to support labeling and promotional claims in the United States. Qual Life Res 2000; 9:887–900.

Roland M, Morris R. A study of the natural history of back pain: I. Development of a reliable and sensitive measure of disability in low back pain. Spine 1983; 8:141–144.

Ross M. Relation of implicit theories to the construction of personal histories. Psychol Rev 1989; 96:341–347.

Rowbotham MC, Harden N, Stacey B, et al. Gabapentin Postherpetic Neuralgia Study Group. Gabapentin for the treatment of postherpetic neuralgia: a randomized controlled trial. JAMA 1998; 280:1837–1842.

Salek S. Compendium of Quality of Life Instruments. John Wiley, New York, 1998.

Scientific Advisory Committee of the Medical Outcomes Trust. Assessing health status and quality-of-life instruments: attributes and review criteria. Qual Life Res 2002; 11:193–205.

Seid M, Varni J, Jacobs J. Pediatric health-related quality-of-life measurement technology: intersections between science, managed care, and clinical care. J Clin Psychol Med Settings 2000; 7:17–27.

Silverman DG, O'Connor TZ, Brull SJ. Integrated assessment of pain scores and rescue morphine doses during studies of analgesic efficacy. Anesth Analg 1993; 77:168–170.

Sloan JA, Aaronson N, Cappelleri JC, et al. Clinical Significance Consensus Group. Assessing the clinical significance of single items relative to summated scores. Mayo Clin Proc 2002; 77:479–487.

Steedman SM, Middaugh SJ, Kee WG, et al. Chronic-pain medications: equivalence levels and method of quantifying usage. Clin J Pain 1992; 8:204–214.

Stucki G, Cieza A. HRQL measures in chronic pain trials. Presented at the second meeting of the Initiative on Methods, Measurement, and Pain Assessment in Clinical Trials (IMMPACT-II), 2003. Available at www.immpact.org/meetings.html (accessed May 12, 2004).

Sullivan M, Turk DC. Psychiatric disorders and psychogenic pain. In: Loeser JD, Butler SD, Chapman CR, Turk DC (eds). Bonica's Management of Pain, 3rd edn. Williams & Wilkins, Baltimore, MD, 2001:483–500.

Terwee CB, Dekker FW, Wiersinga WM, et al. On assessing responsiveness of health-related quality of life instruments: guidelines for instrument evaluation. Qual Life Res 2003; 12:349–362.

Testa MA, Anderson RB, Nackley JF, et al. Quality of Life Hypertension Study Group. Quality of life and antihypertensive therapy in men: a comparison of captopril with enalapril. N Engl J Med 1993; 328:907–913.

Testa MA, Simonson DC. Assessment of quality-of-life outcomes. Curr Concepts 1996; 334:835–840.

Thompson D. Toward a pharmacoeconomic model of neuropathic pain. Clin J Pain 2002; 18:366–372.

Turk DC, Rudy TE. Toward a comprehensive assessment of chronic pain patients: a multiaxial approach. Behav Res Ther 1987; 25:237–249.

Turk DC. Clinical effectiveness and cost-effectiveness of treatments for patients with chronic pain. Clin J Pain 2002; 18:355–365.

Turk DC, Dworkin RH, Allen RR, et al. Core outcome domains for chronic pain clinical trials: IMMPACT recommendations. Pain 2003; 106:337–345.

Turk DC, Dworkin RH, Burke et al. Developing patient-reported outcome measures for pain clinical trials. IMMPACT recommendations. Pain 2006; 125:208–215.

Turner JA, Jensen MP, Warms CA, et al. Blinding effectiveness and association of pretreatment expectations with pain improvement in a double-blind randomized controlled trial. Pain 2002; 99:91–99.

United States Department of Health and Human Services Food and Drug Administration (Docket No. 97D-0188): International Conference on Harmonization; guidance on general considerations for clinical trials. Federal Register, 62:66113–66119, 1997. Available at www.fda.gov/cder/guidance/1857fnl.pdf (accessed May 12, 2004).

Varni JW, Seid M, Kurtin PS. Pediatric health-related quality of life measurement technology: a guide for healthcare decision makers. JCOM 1999; 6:33–40.

Ware JE. Methodological consideration in the selection of health status assessment procedures. In: Wenger N, Mattson M, Furberg C, Elinson J (eds). Assessment of Quality of Life in Clinical Trials of Cardiovasular Therapies. La Jacq, Greenwich, CT, 1984:87–111.

Ware JE, Sherbourne CD. The MOS 36-item short-form health survey (SF-36). Med Care 1992; 30:473–483.

Watson CPN, Moulin D, Watt-Watson J, et al. Controlled-release oxycodone relieves neuropathic pain: a randomized controlled trial in diabetic neuropathy. Pain 2003; 105:71–78.

Williams RC. Toward a set of reliable and valid measures for chronic pain assessment and outcome research. Pain 1988; 35:239–251.

Wilson KG, Mikail SF, D'Eon JL, et al. Alternative diagnostic criteria for major depressive disorder in patients with chronic pain. Pain 2001; 91:227–234.

FURTHER READING

Dougados M, LeClaire P, van der Heijde D, et al. A report of the Osteoarthritis Research Society International Standing Committee for Clinical Trials Response Criteria Initiative. Osteoarthritis Cartilage 2002; 8:395–403.

Dunkl PR, Taylor AF, McConnell G, et al. Responsiveness of fibromyalgia clinical trial outcome measures. J Rheumatol 2002; 27:2683–2691.

Hadjistavropoulos T, von Baeyer C, Craig KD. Pain assessment in persons with limited ability to communicate. In: Turk DC, Melzack R (eds). Handbook of Pain Assessment, 2nd edn. Guilford Press, New York, 2001:134–152.

McCraig LF, Burt CW. National Hospital Ambulatory Medical Care Survey: Emergency Department Summary. Advance data from Vital and Health Statistics; no 340. National Center for Health Statistics, Hayattsville, MD, 2002.

Melzack R, Torgerson WS. On the language of pain. Anesthesiology 1991; 34:50–59.

Middel B, Stewart R, Bouma J, et al. How to validate clinically important change in health-related functional status: is the magnitude of the effect size consistently related to magnitude of change as indicated by a global question rating? J Eval Clin Pract 2001; 7:399–410.

Turk DC. Reporting on participant disposition in clinical trials. Presented at the second meeting of the Initiative on Methods, Measurement, and Pain Assessment in Clinical Trials (IMMPACT-II), 2003. Available at www.immpact. org/meetings.html (accessed May 12, 2004).

CHAPTER 19

Mental health outcomes of chronic pain

Michael J.L. Sullivan • Nathalie Gauthier • Isabelle Tremblay

INTRODUCTION

Chronic pain conditions vary in their manner of onset, their expression, trajectory and response to treatment. Current state of knowledge however does not permit fine discriminations among chronic pain conditions with regard to their associations with mental health outcomes. The present chapter will restrict discussion to the mental health outcomes of chronic nonmalignant pain conditions, but will proceed under the assumption that the various conditions subsumed under this general category share similar relations with mental health outcomes. Current approaches to intervention will be described and issues central to current clinical research will be explored. Due to space considerations, the chapter will not provide an exhaustive overview of all possible mental health outcomes of chronic pain. Rather, the focus will be on mental health conditions with high prevalence, and on questions that are current and topical in contemporary clinical research. The mental health disorders examined in the present chapter include depression, post-traumatic stress disorder, generalized anxiety disorder and simple and social phobias. The majority of studies reviewed deal with chronic musculoskeletal pain. However, a number of studies in the present review also deal with other pain conditions such as neuropathic pain, headache, sympathetic dystrophy, and phantom limb pain.

HISTORICAL PERSPECTIVE

The relationship between pain and mental health has a long history. Paradoxically, mental health practice of antiquity was more concerned with the infliction of pain than its alleviation. Demonology dominated early views of mental illness. The archeological record suggests that shaman of the Stone Age bored holes in the skulls of "affected" individuals in order to provide an escape route for evil spirits (Selling 1948). Priests of the middle ages engaged in practices such as exorcism in order to rid the body of the evil spirits that possessed it (White 1896). When unsuccessful, rituals of exorcism were supplemented by flogging, starving, immersion in cold water and other torturous methods. These methods were devised to create such an unpleasant environment within the body that no evil spirit would wish to remain. Torturous techniques were

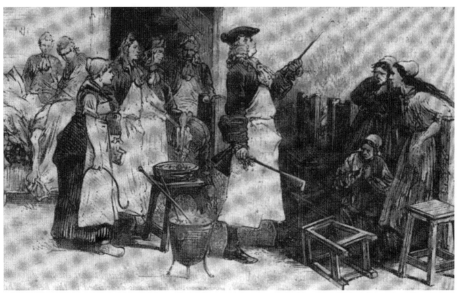

Figure 19.1 "In the insane asylum at Leyden, hot irons were applied to the head to bring patients to their senses. Here, Boerhaave, a medical authority of the time, is threatening hysteric women patients with cauterisation" (White 1896). A woodcut by Figuerier.

later adopted by medical practitioners of mental asylums as useful techniques to calm agitated patients (Figure 19.1).

It is only within the last century that mental health practice has turned its attention toward the treatment of individuals with chronic pain conditions. There remain however vestiges of the conceptual models of antiquity in current conceptualizations of chronic pain. Even certain aspects of demonology have remained central to current explanatory models and methods of intervention for chronic pain. For example, Freudian theory suggests that certain psychological conflicts suppressed from consciousness can find expression as physical symptoms such as pain and disability. Within this framework, analytic and abreactive techniques are used to "free" sufferers from the conflicts trapped within their subconscious minds that are at the root of their pain problems (Breuer and Freud 1893/1957). The notion that some form of noxious agent is locked within the individual with chronic pain and must be released in order to bring about a cure continues to find expression in many domains of mental health practice associated with chronic pain (Szasz 1957; Sternbach 1974; Blumer and Heilbronn 1982; Weintraub 1988).

Despite a century of clinical and theoretical discussions of the relation between pain and mental health, there is a sense that significant advance has not occurred. Advance in our understanding of the links between pain and mental health, and in our ability to effectively treat mental health conditions associated with pain, has been modest. The billions of dollars spent each year on disability-related costs of chronic

pain, and the extensive wait lists of hundreds of pain clinics, speak to the magnitude of the pain problem in our society. The all-too-frequent negligible impact of treatments offered at pain clinics highlights the limits of the tools available to bring about meaningful change in the suffering and disability associated with chronic pain.

The lack of progress in understanding the links between chronic pain and mental health can be attributed to a number of factors. A central issue concerns the lack of consensus on how chronic pain should be conceptualized. In current literature there is still debate about whether chronic pain is a legitimate physical condition or whether it represents the expression of some form of psychological dysfunction (Sternbach 1974; Blumer and Heilbronn 1982; Weintraub 1988; Hodgkiss 1997). Faced with a situation where patients present with physical symptoms with no discernible organic pathology, to the medical practitioner, the "leap to the head" might appear like a reasonable approach to understanding the pain patient. It is not uncommon in medical reports to see reference to terms such as "symptom amplification," "pain magnification" or "functional overlay." These terms reflect assumptions about psychological contributions to presenting physical symptoms that are not based on any objective finding from physical or psychological assessment.

According to the DSM-IV, most chronic pain conditions would meet the criteria for a diagnosis of "Pain Disorder associated with a medical condition." Pain disorder is classified as one of the Somatoform Disorders. The essential feature of somatoform disorders is that psychological conflicts have been transformed into physical symptoms (Ford 1995). The inclusion of chronic pain phenomena within the taxonomy of psychiatric disorders perpetuates the view that mental health issues are at the root of, as opposed to the consequence of, chronic pain and encourages the undesirable clinical practice of diagnosis by exclusion (Weintraub 1988). By requiring that the clinician make a judgment that psychological factors are causally related to the onset of pain implies that a knowledge base exists to accurately discern physical and psychological contributions to the etiology of pain (Howell et al. 2003; Ciamarella et al. 2004). Given that such knowledge base does not currently exist, the diagnosis of pain-related somatoform disorders necessarily proceeds solely on the basis of clinician intuition.

Other obstacles to progress in this area are that many of the psychological variables implicated as causative of chronic pain have been poorly defined, impossible to measure or couched within theoretical frameworks that have minimal value for either conceptualizing or treating chronic pain (Sternbach 1974; Weintraub 1988; Ferrari and Russell 1997). Although the role of unconscious psychological processes in the development of pain cannot be ruled out, the uncritical acceptance of models that appeal to unconscious mental processes in the etiology of pain conditions can have a negative impact on clinical practice and research. For significant advance to take place in the conceptualization and treatment of chronic pain conditions, it will be paramount to focus on theoretical models with clearly testable hypotheses, and on clinical practice that is supported by research.

DEPRESSION

Anecdotal reports on the experience of pain frequently highlight the associated experience of emotional distress. The earliest recorded accounts of pain experience described not only the physical aspects of the condition, but the emotional aspects as well (cf. Fulop-Muller 1938). In many cases, the emotional anguish associated with pain appears as central to experience than the actual injury or pain-related condition.

Migraine is atrocious torment, one of the worst in the world, weakening the nerves, driving one mad, scattering one's thoughts to the winds and impairing the memory. So terrible are these headaches that I can do nothing but lie on the couch and try to dull the pain by sniffing ether.

G. Maupassant (Sur L'eau), 1875

Of all mental health outcomes associated with chronic pain, depression is by far the most prevalent. Community surveys indicate that approximately 20% of individuals with chronic pain symptoms suffer from a diagnosable depressive condition (McWilliams et al. 2003). Much higher rates are seen in specialty pain treatment centers (France et al. 1986). For the clinician working in a specialty pain treatment center, statistics suggest that at least every second patient seen will likely meet diagnostic criteria for a depressive disorder.

Numerous reviews have commented on the high rate of depressive disorders in samples of chronic pain patients (Romano and Turner 1985; Sullivan et al. 1992; Banks and Kerns 1996; Rush et al. 2000). The high levels of comorbidity of pain and depression have prompted considerable debate over the putative mechanisms that might underlie both pain and depression (Blumer and Heilbronn 1982; Turk and Salovey 1984; Dworkin and Gitlin 1991; Fishbain et al. 1997).

The research on the prevalence of depression in chronic pain is reviewed briefly below. Prevalence estimates have been derived from studies that have used structured interviews and standardized diagnostic criteria to assess depressive symptomatology. Studies that have used self-report methods to assess prevalence are not included in this review. Self-report methods of diagnosing depression have been shown to have unacceptably low specificity values thus rendering prevalence estimates difficult to interpret (Bishop et al. 1993).

PREVALENCE OF DEPRESSION IN CHRONIC PAIN PATIENTS

A diagnosis of major depressive disorder (MDD) according to DSM-IV (APA 1994) criteria requires the presence of at least five depressive symptoms (from a list of 9 possible symptoms) that have persisted over a two week period, and represent a change from a previous level of functioning. Depressed mood and a markedly diminished interest of pleasure are considered essential symptoms of MDD such that at least one of these must be present in order to consider a diagnosis. Other depressive symptoms considered for a diagnosis of MDD include: significant weight loss when not dieting or weight gain or decrease or increase in appetite, insomnia or hypersomnia, observable psychomotor agitation or retardation, fatigue or loss of energy, feelings of worthlessness or excessive or inappropriate guilt, diminished ability to think or concentrate, or indecisiveness, and recurrent thoughts of death with or without a specific plan, or a suicide attempt.

For a diagnosis of MDD, presenting symptoms must cause clinically significant distress or impairment in social, occupational, or other areas of functioning and must not be due to the direct physiologic effects of a substance or a general medical condition. The symptoms must not be better accounted for by bereavement and they must not meet criteria for a mixed episode.

As shown in Table 19.1, most studies using standardized criteria to diagnose depression in samples of

Table 19.1 Summary of research on the prevalence of depression in chronic pain

Reference	Sample	Criteria	Findings
Lindsay and Wyckoff (1981)	300 consecutive referrals to pain centers	RDC	87% major depressive disorder
Kramlinger et al. (1983)	100 consecutive admissions to an inpatient pain program	RDC	25% major depressive disorder 39% probable major depressive disorder
Feinmann (1983)	93 consecutive referrals to a surgery department	ICD-IX	35% depressive neurosis
Remick et al. (1983)	68 referrals to a pain clinic	DSM-III	13% major depressive disorder
Katon et al. (1984)	49 patients from a pain service	DSM-III	57% major depressive disorder 8% dysthymic disorder
Turner and Romano (1984)	40 consecutive referrals to a pain clinic	DSM-III	30% major depressive disorder
Katon et al. (1985)	37 admissions to an inpatient pain program	DSM-III	32% major depressive disorder
Krishnan et al. (1985)	71 consecutive referrals to an inpatient pain program	RDC	45% major depressive disorder 11% minor depressive disorder 26% intermittent depressive disorder
Atkinson et al. (1986)	52 consecutive admissions to an inpatient neurosurgery program	RDC	44% major depressive disorder 19% minor depressive disorder
Fishbain et al. (1986)	283 consecutive referrals to a pain clinic	DSM-III	5% major depressive disorder 23% dysthymic disorder 28% adjustment disorder
France et al. (1986)	80 consecutive referrals to a pain clinic	RDC	21% major depressive disorder 54% intermittent depressive disorder 4% minor depressive disorder 3% endogenous depressive disorder
Love (1987)	68 consecutive referrals to a general practice clinic	DSM-III	25% major depressive disorder
Atkinson et al. (1988)	34 consecutive referrals to an orthopedics clinic	DSM-III	15% major depressive disorder
Haythornthwaite et al. (1991)	69 subjects from consecutive admission to an interdisciplinary pain rehabilitation program	RDC	53.6% major depressive disorder
Goldberg et al. (1993)	105 men referred at a management pain center	RDC	41% major depressive disorder 12% minor depressive disorder
Kinney et al. (1993)	90 chronic low back pain (CLBP) patients who presented for a treatment at a rehabilitation center	DSM-III-R (SCID)	46% major depressive disorder 2% bipolar disorder 2% dysthymia
Polatin et al. (1993)	200 chronic pain patients of a functional restoration program	DSM-III-R (SCID)	45% major depressive disorder 2% bipolar disorder 2% dysthymia

Table 19.1 Summary of research on the prevalence of depression in chronic pain—Cont'd

Reference	Sample	Criteria	Findings
Gatchel et al. (1994)	152 patients admitted to a 3-week functional restoration treatment program	DSM-III-R (SCID)	44% major depressive disorder 2% bipolar disorder
Turk et al. (1995)	100 chronic pain patients referred at a multidisciplinary pain center	DSM-III-R	11% major depressive disorder 4% dysthymia 6% depressive disorder NOS
Geisser et al. (1997)	132 consecutive persons with chronic pain referred at a pain management in a medical center	DSM-IV	33% major depressive disorder
Wesley et al. (1999)	200 consecutive chronic back pain patients in a tertiary rehabilitation facility for chronic back pain	DSM-III-R (SCID)	49.5% major depressive disorder
Geisser et al. (2000)	211 consecutive patients with chronic pain referred at a pain management in a medical center	DSM-IV	29.9% major depressive disorder
Wilson et al. (2001)	129 consecutive patients with musculoskeletal pain in a chronic pain clinic	DSM-IV	35.7% major depressive disorder
Wijeratne et al. (2001)	50 patients from a chronic pain outpatient clinic	DSM-IV	34% major depressive disorder
McWilliams et al. (2003)	382 chronic pain participants (arthritis) who participated to the National Comorbidity Survey	DSM-III-R (CIDI)	20.2% major depressive disorder

chronic pain patients have reported prevalence rates between 20 and 50% (Frinman 1983; Kramlinger et al. 1983; Turner and Romano 1984; Katon et al. 1985; Krishnan et al. 1985; Atkinson et al. 1986; France et al. 1986; Love 1987; Goldberg et al. 1993; Kinney et al. 1993; Polatin et al. 1993; Gatchel et al. 1994; Geisser et al. 1997; Wesley et al. 1999; Geisser et al. 2000; Wijeratne et al. 2001; Wilson et al. 2001; McWilliams et al. 2003).

A number of studies have reported rates of MDD in chronic pain samples lower than 20% (Remick et al. 1983; Atkinson et al. 1988; Fishbain et al. 1986; Turk et al. 1995). Other studies have reported rates of MDD in chronic pain samples greater than 50% (Lindsey and Wyckoff 1981; Katon et al. 1984; Haythornthwaite et al. 1991; Bishop et al. 1993). In a review of prevalence rates of depression in chronic low back pain, Sullivan et al. (1992) derived a weighted prevalence rate (adjusted for sample sizes across studies) and suggested that a 21% point prevalence rate might represent the best estimate of MDD associated with chronic pain.

Although self-report measures of depression are not well suited as diagnostic instruments, they can be very useful as screening measures or as measures of improvement associated with treatment (Bishop et al.

1993; Burns et al. 2003; Vowles et al. 2004). The Beck Depression Inventory (Beck et al. 1996) is a self-report measure of depression that is being used with increasing frequency with chronic pain patients (Morley et al. 2002; Burns et al. 2003; Sullivan and Stanish 2003; Turner et al. 2004). The BDI-II consists of 21 items describing various symptoms of depression. The BDI-II has been shown to be a reliable and valid index of depressive symptoms in chronic pain patients and primary care medical patients (Bishop et al. 1993; Arnau et al. 2001; Morley et al. 2002). Other self-report measures of depression that have been used with chronic pain include the Centre for Epidemiologic Studies Depression Scale (CES-D; Radloff 1977), the Zung Self Rating Depression Scale (Zung-D; Zung 1965) and the Hamilton Rating Scale for Depression (HAM-D; Hamilton 1965). Although these different self-report measures share similar psychometric properties, several investigators have discussed the advantages of the BDI due its relatively low proportion of somatic items (Rodin et al. 1991; Sullivan et al. 1992; Bishop et al. 1993).

INTERPRETIVE CHALLENGES

One of the challenges associated with the interpretation of prevalence rates of depression in chronic pain is that most studies have been conducted within specialty clinics. As a result of referral biases that favor an over-representation of individuals with emotional distress, prevalence rates of depression reported in studies of pain clinic samples are likely to be inflated.

Another interpretive difficulty is that symptoms of chronic pain and depression overlap to some degree. For example, symptoms of appetite and sleep disturbance, psychomotor retardation, fatigue or reduced energy are common to both chronic pain and depression. Therefore, criterion contamination complicates the assessment of depression in chronic pain population (Dersh et al. 2002). There have been numerous discussions of strategies that might minimize the potential for inflated prevalence rates of depression (due to symptom overlap) in patients with chronic pain (Rodin et al. 1991; Sullivan et al. 1992; Banks and Kerns 1996; Wilson et al. 2002). It has become clear that prevalence rates will vary significantly as a function of the method used to deal with symptom overlap (Wilson et al. 2002). Given the difficulty in determining, with any degree of reliability, whether a particular symptom should be attributed to chronic pain or depression, several clinical researchers have suggested that current diagnostic symptoms should be used in standard fashion with patients suffering from chronic pain (Rodin et al. 1991; Sullivan et al. 1992; Banks and Kerns 1996).

Although current diagnostic approaches might be associated with higher risk of false positive diagnoses when used with chronic pain patients, elimination of overlapping symptoms, or symptom substitution, risks increasing the rate of false negative diagnoses. The clinical inconvenience of offering treatment to someone who is not clinically depressed (i.e., the consequence of false positive diagnosis) is preferable to not offering treatment to someone who is depressed (i.e., the consequence of false negative diagnosis).

DETERMINANTS OF DEPRESSION IN CHRONIC PAIN

Recent research has tended to appeal primarily to "diathesis stress" formulations in efforts to explain how depression might arise following the development of a pain condition (Banks and Kerns 1996). These models suggest that depressive symptoms might arise when vulnerability factors (i.e., diatheses) interact with vulnerability-relevant contextual factors (i.e., stresses). The "vulnerability-relevant contextual factors" component of the model encompasses all the stresses that might be associated with chronic pain including persistent physical distress, loss of employment, loss of financial security, loss of independence, adversarial relations with third party payers, disrupted family relations, etc. For example, it has been reported that depressive symptoms associated with chronic pain may arise in the context of negative spouse responses to pain (Cano et al.

2000), low social support (Faucett 1994; Trief et al. 1995), marital dissatisfaction (Cano et al. 2000) and low family cohesion (Trief et al. 1995; Nicassio et al. 1995). In the bulk of research conducted to date, the presence of "vulnerability-relevant contextual factors" has been assumed more than it has been measured and there have been few tests of the hypothesized interaction between vulnerability factors and vulnerability-relevant contextual factors (Banks and Kerns 1996; Sullivan et al. 2002).

Considerably more research has aimed at identifying potential intra-individual vulnerability factors. Initial pain intensity and pain frequency have been shown to be concurrently and prospectively associated with elevated depressive symptomatology (Haythornthwaite et al. 1991; Kuch et al. 1993; Magni et al. 1994; Nicassio et al. 1995; Sist et al. 1998; Arnstein et al. 1999; Klinger et al. 1999). Recent investigations have suggested that pain intensity might be indirectly related to depression through mediating factors such as perceived life control, perceived life interference, and attributions (Turk et al. 1995; Maxwell et al. 1998). Given that there is significant stability to depressive symptoms, numerous investigations have noted that a substantive proportion of variance in outcome or follow-up depression is accounted for by initial levels of depression (Keefe et al. 1989; Epping-Jordan et al. 1998; Sullivan et al. 2006).

Several investigations also highlighted the potential contribution of negative cognitions to the development or maintenance of depression. Appraisal-related variables such as perceived disability (Arnstein et al. 1999; Geisser et al. 2000), perceived interference due to pain (Haythornthwaite et al. 1991; Maxwell et al. 1998), perceived inadequacy of problem-solving skills (Kerns et al. 2002) and cognitive distortions (Smith et al. 1994; Maxwell et al. 1998) have been associated with elevations of depressive symptomatology. Factors such as self-efficacy for managing pain (Arnstein et al. 1999; Rabin et al. 2000), self-control (Maxwell et al. 1998) and greater acceptance of pain (McCracken 1998) have been discussed as protective or resilience factors that might decrease susceptibility to depression in individuals with persistent pain.

PAIN CATASTROPHIZING AND DEPRESSION

Numerous investigations have addressed the role of pain catastrophizing as a determinant of depression and other pain-related outcomes (Rosenstiel and Keefe 1983; Sullivan et al. 1990; Affleck et al. 1992; Geisser et al. 2000; Madland et al. 2000; Turner et al. 2001, 2002). Pain catastrophizing has been defined as "a negative cognitive set brought to bear during actual or anticipated pain experience" (Sullivan et al. 2001).

Prior to its emergence in the pain literature, catastrophizing had been discussed primarily within the context of cognitive theories of depression. For example, in the cognitive model of emotional disorders of Beck et al. (1978), catastrophizing is viewed as a "cognitive distortion" that might contribute to the precipitation and maintenance of depressive symptoms. Beck et al. (1978) proposed that "depressive schema" may become activated following the occurrence of negative life events. Once activated, depressive schema were said to give rise to a variety of cognitive distortions including catastrophizing, overgeneralization, personalization, and selective abstraction. In the model of Beck et al. (1978), cognitive errors are expected to bias information processing in such a manner as to increase the likelihood of the development of depressive symptoms. Adapted to pain, the events associated with the onset of pain, or the stresses associated with living with a persistent pain condition, might contribute to the activation of depressive schema in vulnerable individuals (Banks and Kerns 1996).

The Pain Catastrophizing Scale (PCS; Sullivan et al. 1995) is a commonly used measure of pain catastrophizing. The PCS is a 13-item instrument derived from definitions of pain catastrophizing described in the literature (Spanos et al. 1979; Chaves and Brown 1987) as well as items from the catastrophizing subscale of the CSQ (Rosenstiel and Keefe 1983). Factor analysis of the measure revealed 3 correlated factors: rumination ("I can't stop thinking about how much it hurts"), magnification ("I worry that something serious may happen"), and helplessness ("It's awful and I feel that it overwhelms me"). Self-report measures have been developed for assessing catastrophizing in children and adolescents (Gil et al. 1993; Reid et al. 1998; Crombez et al. 2003) as well as in more acute pain situations (Butler et al. 1989). Interview methods have also been used (e.g., Spanos et al. 1979; Chaves and Brown 1987); however, their application to clinical settings has been limited.

The self-report measures of catastrophizing described above have been shown to have good psychometric properties. Coefficients of internal consistency have ranged from 0.76 to 0.87 (Rosenstiel and Keefe 1983; Gil et al. 1993; Sullivan et al. 1995). Test–retest correlations indicate a high level of stability in levels of catastrophizing, in both clinical (Keefe et al. 1989) and nonclinical samples (Sullivan et al. 1995). Most of the self-report measures of catastrophizing can be completed and scored in less than 5 minutes, and thus are easily amenable to inclusion within standard clinical practice.

In light of the strong link between pain catastrophizing and depression, it has been suggested that interventions aimed at reducing pain catastrophizing should be integral components of treatment programs for individuals with persistent pain conditions (Sullivan et al. 2001, 2006; Turner et al. 2001, 2002). In recent years, intervention programs have been developed that specifically target catastrophic thinking associated with pain (Thorn et al. 2002; Burns et al. 2003; Sullivan and Stanish 2003). Results to date suggest that reductions in pain catastrophizing are significant predictors of treatment outcome of pain-disability management programs (Jensen et al. 1994; Burns et al. 2003; Sullivan and Stanish 2003).

The Pain-Disability Prevention Program (PDP) is an example of a community-based risk factor targeted intervention for individuals with high levels of pain and pain-related disability (Sullivan and Stanish 2003; Sullivan, M.J.L. et al. 2005). Through a combination of techniques such a structured activity scheduling, thought monitoring, reinterpretation, problem-solving, and graded activity participation, the PDP program aims to reduce psychological barriers to rehabilitation progress and facilitate return to work (Sullivan and Stanish 2003). In a sample of 257 injured workers who participated in the program, 47% ($N = 113$) were experiencing clinically significant levels of depression (BDI-II > 16) at the time of referral. At the time of treatment termination, the prevalence of depression in the sample was reduced by approximately 50% (i.e., 22% still scored above 16 on the BDI-II). Higher post-treatment levels of depression were associated with failure to return to work. Of the individuals who were still depressed at the end of treatment, only 22% returned to work, compared to 75% of individuals who were not depressed at the end of treatment (Sullivan et al. 2006).

Analyses were conducted to address whether reductions in pain catastrophizing were associated with reductions in depression. Analyses also addressed the differential influence of reductions in the three dimensions of pain catastrophizing (i.e., rumination, magnification, helplessness) on treatment-related reductions in depression. Two regressions were conducted: the first addressing whether early treatment (first 5 weeks of treatment) reductions in pain catastrophizing were associated with treatment-related reductions in depression, and the second addressing whether late treatment (last 5 weeks of treatment) in pain catastrophizing were associated with treatment-related reductions in depression. The results of these analyses are presented in Table 19.2.

The results of the regression analyses reveal that late treatment changes in pain catastrophizing were more strongly associated with treatment-related reductions in depression than early treatment changes in pain catastrophizing. Examination of the beta weights indicates that late treatment changes in helplessness contributed significant unique variance in treatment-related reductions in depression. This association remained significant even when controlling for pre-treatment scores on the helplessness subscale of the PCS. These findings are consistent with those of Burns et al. (2003) who also found that reductions in pain

Table 19.2 Predicting treatment-related reductions in depression

Variable	R	Beta	F change	P	r
Early treatment reductions in pain catastrophizing					
Sex		−0.07			−0.02
Age	0.08	−0.07	0.44 (2, 110)	0.64	−0.08
Rumin		0.01			0.11
Magni		0.06			0.16*
Helps	0.25	0.20	2.3 (3, 107)	0.09	0.22**
Late treatment reductions in pain catastrophizing					
Sex		−0.01			−0.02
Age	0.08	−0.04	0.44 (2, 110)	0.64	−0.08
Rumin		0.11			0.31**
Magni		0.04			0.27**
Helps	0.41	0.29**	6.9 (3, 107)	0.001	0.39**

$N = 113$. PCS subscales: rumin = rumination; magni = magnification; helps = helplessness. Beat weights are from the final regression equation. $*p < 0.05$; $**p < 0.01$.

catastrophizing and helplessness were associated with more positive treatment outcome (see also Vowles et al. 2004).

These and other findings highlight several important aspects of depression associated with chronic pain. First, depression not only impacts negatively on the quality of life of the individual suffering from persistent pain, but there are indications that depression adds to the burden of disability associated with persistent pain. In several investigations, depression has been shown to be a risk factor for chronic disability (Carroll et al. 2003; Waddell et al. 2003).

There is accumulating evidence that interventions that lead to reductions in pain catastrophizing are associated with improvement in depressive symptoms (Turner and Clancy 1986; Jensen et al. 1994; Burns et al. 2003). Reductions in the helplessness dimension of pain catastrophizing appear to contribute most strongly to reductions in depression. Intervention programs that specifically target catastrophic thinking may be the ones associated with the best outcomes.

PHARMACOLOGIC INTERVENTIONS FOR DEPRESSION ASSOCIATED WITH CHRONIC PAIN

The prescription of antidepressant medication in the treatment of chronic pain patients is commonplace. Depressive symptoms however are not always the main target of these interventions. Physicians frequently prescribe antidepressant medication to chronic pain patients for their analgesic effects as opposed to their antidepressant effects. Physicians also prescribe antidepressant medication as a sleeping aid for patients with chronic pain. When used for their analgesic properties, or as a sleeping aid, antidepressants are likely to be prescribed far below therapeutic dose levels required to effectively treat depression (Spiegel et al. 1983; France and Krishnan 1988).

Clinicians will undoubtedly have noted that while the majority of pain patients referred to their clinics have likely been prescribed antidepressant medication, only a minority of patients will be taking antidepressant medication at a dose level likely to ameliorate their depressive symptoms (Sullivan, M.J.L. et al. in press). One of the reasons for the underprescription of therapeutic doses of antidepressants for depression associated with pain is that depression often goes undetected in primary care practice. Patients will not necessarily report depressive symptoms to their physicians, and physicians may not enquire about mental health symptoms. Alternately, physicians may infer that depressive symptoms are a consequence of pain that will be alleviated once the pain has been effectively managed. The unfortunate consequence of both scenarios is that the patient does not receive the treatment that he or she needs (Sullivan et al. 1992).

It has often been noted that pain patients appear to be particularly sensitive to the side effects of antidepressant medication. This view is expressed with sufficient frequency in clinical discussions giving the impression that side-effect sensitivity has been extensively studied in chronic pain. However, a search of the available literature provides little concrete evidence to clarify the relation, if any, between chronic pain and exaggerated reactivity to medication side effects. Clearly this is an area that requires further investigation.

An early review of the literature on the treatment of depression in chronic pain suggested that treatment response to tricyclic antidepressants appeared to be similar in individuals with chronic pain and without chronic pain (Sullivan et al. 1992). This statement however was based on only two controlled trials of antidepressant (tricyclic) medication for the treatment of depression in chronic pain. A recent literature search has revealed that there have not been any new controlled clinical trials of antidepressant medication for depressed chronic pain patients since 1991 (Sullivan et al. 2006, Campbell et al. 2003).

Tricyclics such as doxepin (Sinequan) or amitripyline (Elavil) have significant sedating properties and may be prescribed for chronic pain patients with sleep difficulties or with symptoms of agitation or anxiety (Polatin 1996). Chronic pain patients with marked symptoms of psychomotor retardation or fatigue may be prescribed antidepressants with more activating properties such as fluoxetine (Prozac) or paroxetine (Paxil). Available research has addressed primarily the effects of tricyclic antidepressants on depression and chronic pain; research on the use of more recent heterocyclics in depression and chronic pain is still sparse (Arnold et al. 2004).

Side effects such as dry mouth, early morning sedation, nausea and sexual dysfunction are the most commonly reported by chronic pain patients taking tricyclic antidepressants. Side effects are most pronounced during the first week of treatment, decreasing steadily in intensity over a period of two to three weeks (Polatin 1996). For the majority of depressed chronic pain patients, the side effects are tolerable and considered a viable tradeoff for the reduction in depressive symptoms experienced. For others, side effects may be so intense and antidepressant effects minimal such that continuation of treatment is difficult to justify.

The lack of research on the efficacy of antidepressant medication for the treatment of depression associated with pain is problematic. Questions concerning the relative efficacy of different antidepressant agents for different types of persistent pain conditions need to be addressed in order to guide treatment decisions. In addition, there is little or no information available about the influence of drug interactions, in particular opioids, on the efficacy of antidepressant medication for depressed chronic pain patients (Ciccone et al. 2000, Wasan et al. 2005).

In other areas of clinical research, research suggests that a combination of antidepressant medication and psychological intervention might have advantages over either alone. This may be particularly true in chronic pain conditions. Given that chronic pain and depression are both associated with activity withdrawal, the depressed chronic pain patient may benefit most from multidisciplinary approaches that combine pharmacotherapy, pain management strategies, and activity mobilization strategies (Polatin 1996).

POST-TRAUMATIC STRESS DISORDER

Characteristics of events associated with the onset of a pain disorder have a bearing on the nature of mental health outcomes that might be experienced. Road accidents or occupationally-related traumatic events can expose individuals to stresses that are so severe as to overwhelm their coping resources and leave them struggling to keep their emotional world intact (Asmundson et al. 1998). Incidents characterized by high levels of threat or exposure to horrific or disturbing circumstances can lead to symptoms of post-traumatic stress disorder (PTSD). Diagnoses of PTSD are being made with increasing frequency in individuals with pain conditions associated with traumatic onset (Aghabeigi et al. 1992; Mayou and Bryant 1996; Asmundson et al. 1998; Mayou et al. 2002). Comorbid experience of chronic pain and PTSD appears to be associated with more severe presenting symptomatology than either condition alone (Geisser et al. 1996). Diagnoses of PTSD are also being discussed as a significant obstacle to rehabilitation progress in individuals with persistent pain (Asmundson et al. 1998; Sharp and Harvey 2001).

CASE EXAMPLE

Bob was a 38-year-old truck driver who was involved in a head-on motor vehicle collision. His physical symptoms included persistent neck and shoulder pain, and frequent occipital headaches. These symptoms contributed to some degree of disability, primarily with respect to tolerance for the prolonged postural positioning associated with driving. Bob's emotional symptoms contributed further to his distress and disability. The accident had occurred when an oncoming vehicle swerved into the path of Bob's truck. Unable to maneuver the 18-wheeler to avert the accident, Bob's truck ran over the car. Bob exited his truck and ran to the car which was now lodged just ahead of his rear axle. The couple in the front seat appeared to have died on impact, crushed under the engine which had been pushed into the front seat. A 5-year-old girl in the back seat was still alive but trapped inside the car. Flames erupted from under the car, and Bob watched as the young girl burned to her death.

Bob was seen at the clinic approximately 2 months after his accident. He had been referred by his family physician who became alarmed that Bob's state was steadily deteriorating over time. When he

Continued

CASE EXAMPLE—CONT'D

arrived for his appointment, Bob appeared highly anxious, agitated, tearful, and exhausted. He explained that he had barely slept since his accident. He feared going to sleep because his mind constantly *replayed the scene of the young girl dying in the fire. He blamed himself for the accident, for the deaths of the girl and her parents, and swore that he would never drive again. Other than the taxi ride to and from treatment sessions, Bob did not leave the house; he did not answer the phone, and he did not receive any visitors.*

Bob's ongoing symptoms included an inability to suppress thoughts about the accident, or effectively divert his attention away from thoughts and images associated with the accident. He had recurring dreams of the accident. Bob avoided driving for fear of causing harm to someone else. He rehearsed in his mind endless scenarios where a different decision (e.g., leaving the house 5 minutes later) might have averted the accident. He experienced intense guilt about the life that he had robbed the young girl and her parents. He lost the sense of meaning and purpose of his life, and entertained thoughts of ending his life. He lost all interest in interpersonal relations and social contact. Bob was diagnosed with PTSD.

PREVALENCE OF PTSD ASSOCIATED WITH PAIN

The diagnosis of PTSD is one of the few mental health diagnoses that requires, as an essential symptom, the occurrence of an external event. The majority of mental health diagnoses are made based on symptom profiles that exist within the individual. PTSD however requires that an individual be exposed to an event (i.e., stressor) that is "outside the usual range of human experience" (APA 1994). Criminal acts, wars, natural disasters and motor vehicle accidents are some examples of traumatic events that would satisfy the stressor criterion (Criterion A). The DSM-IV also notes that the individuals' reaction to the stressor must have been one that included intense fear, horror or helplessness (APA 1994).

The symptom domains considered for a diagnosis of PTSD include (1) re-experiencing phenomena, (2) cognitive or behavioral avoidance and (3) physiological hyper-reactivity. Re-experiencing phenomena may include intrusive and recurrent recollections of the event, nightmares, and behaving or feeling as if reliving the traumatic situation. Avoidance phenomena might include efforts to avoid thoughts of the trauma, and persistent avoidance of stimuli associated with the trauma. Avoidance phenomena also include diminished interest in activities, feeling of detachment from others, restricted range of affect and sense of a foreshortened future. Symptoms of physiologic hyper-reactivity might include increased arousal, difficulty falling or staying asleep, irritability, difficulty concentrating and hypervigilance. For a diagnosis of PTSD to be considered, the above symptoms must not have been present before the traumatic event. The duration of the posttraumatic symptoms must be more than 1 month and must be associated with observable disturbance in social, personal, or occupational functioning.

The lifetime prevalence of PTSD in the general population is estimated between 1 and 14% (APA 1994). Prevalence estimates of PTSD among chronic pain patients vary widely across studies. Polatin et al. (1993) recruited 200 chronic low back pain patients to assess the current and lifetime incidence of psychiatric disorders. Among their subjects, only 1% met lifetime prevalence of PTSD and 1% met current PTSD criteria. These results are similar to the lifetime prevalence of PTSD in the general population. In a large population survey, McWilliams et al. (2003) reported point prevalence rate of 10% for individuals with chronic pain compared to 3% in individuals without chronic pain.

Other studies have reported higher prevalence rates, particularly in individuals who were involved in motor vehicle accidents. Chibnall and Duckro (1994) examined 42 patients with chronic post-traumatic headache subsequent to a motor vehicle accident. A diagnosis of PTSD was made for 29.3% of subjects and 19.5% met criteria for partial PTSD. Other studies have shown that the prevalence of PTSD among motor vehicle automobile victims with chronic pain may range between 37 and 75% (Kuch et al. 1985, 1994; Hickling and Blanchard 1992; Hickling et al. 1992; Bryant et al. 1999).

The pattern of findings shows wide variability (1–75%) in the prevalence rates of PTSD associated with chronic pain. Although there are no studies directly addressing the prevalence of PTSD as a function of type of onset, it appears that PTSD symptoms might be more likely in pain conditions associated with traumatic onset as opposed to insidious onset (Geisser et al. 1996). Pain alone is probably not sufficient to give rise to symptoms of PTSD; however, the incident that gave rise to the pain may have characteristics that can lead to PTSD symptoms (Asmundson et al. 1998; Glynn et al. 2003). History of early trauma might heighten the risk of PTSD in individuals who develop pain conditions such as fibromyalgia (Cohen et al. 2002). It has been suggested that pain might contribute to the persistence of PTSD symptoms by acting as a "trigger" for memories of the traumatic incident (Sharp and Harvey 2001; Asmundson et al. 2002; Mayou et al. 2002).

INTERPRETIVE CHALLENGES

As discussed in relation to depression, prevalence rates for PTSD might be inflated in samples drawn from specialty treatment centers. Symptom overlap might also contribute to inflation of prevalence rates. Symptoms of appetite and sleep disturbance, psychomotor retardation, fatigue or reduced energy, and activity avoidance are common to both chronic pain and PTSD. The dangers associated with exclusion of overlapping symptoms, or substitution of symptoms, are the same for PTSD as for depression. As such, adherence to standard diagnostic guidelines with particular attention to differential diagnosis is probably the best clinical practice.

Litigation and compensation might also play a role in the inflation of prevalence rates of PTSD. Since a diagnosis of PTSD requires the experience of a traumatic event, questions of liability for the traumatic event might engender litigation or compensation for losses (Ferrari and Russell 1997; Rainville et al. 1997; Mayou et al. 2002). If PTSD symptoms arise from a motor vehicle accident, the individual "at fault" for the accident would be liable not only for the distress and disability associated with pain symptoms, but for the distress and disability associated with PTSD symptoms as well (Mayou et al. 2002).

In recent years, there has been a dramatic rise in the number of claims for PTSD made to insurers following motor vehicle accidents. Part of this increase might be the result of increased sensitivity of health professionals to the potential emotional consequences of exposure to a traumatic incident involving injury. This sensitivity however might also take the form of excessively liberal diagnostic practices where symptoms associated with normal adjustment to trauma are misinterpreted as being consistent with a diagnosis of PTSD (Wakefield 1992; Bryant and Harvey 1997). It is beyond the scope of this chapter to review normal and pathologic processes of adaptation. However, recollections of trauma, intrusive thoughts and nightmares are part of the natural process of adaptation to trauma (Lazarus 1983; Horowitz, 1986; Roth and Cohen 1986). They become pathologic only when they persist intensely over time and lead to disruptions in functioning (Foa et al. 1989; McNally 1999). Unfortunately, health professionals who are not well versed in the distinguishing features of normal and pathologic adjustment to trauma may erroneously make a diagnosis of PTSD for what is essentially a normal pattern of adjustment. Once a diagnosis appears on paper, it has a tendency to take on a life of its own, and eventually the client begins to believe it as well. Careful adherence to standards of practice and respect for limits of expertise cannot be over-emphasized as they pertain to the diagnosis of PTSD.

DETERMINANTS OF PTSD ASSOCIATED WITH PAIN

At the present time, little is known about factors predictive of PTSD among chronic pain patients. The paucity of longitudinal studies and the correlational nature of the majority of studies conducted with chronic pain samples limits the nature of conclusions that can be drawn. However, as the body of literature grows, there appear to be marked similarities in the determinants of PTSD in individuals with or without pain symptoms (Asmunsdon et al. 2002).

Genetic factors have been implicated as possible determinants of PTSD. For example, True et al. (1993) reported higher concordance of PTSD in persons who had a monozygotic twin with PTSD compared with dizygotic twins. The literature further suggests that familial psychiatric history might influence the likelihood of developing PTSD. Katon et al. (1985) reported that 59.5% of patients with PTSD had first-degree relatives with chronic pain, 37.8% had first-degree relatives who abused alcohol, 29.7% had relatives with affective illness and 13.5% had families with a history of hypochondriasis. Davidson and colleagues (1985) also showed that patients with PTSD were more likely to have parents and first-degree relatives with mood, anxiety, and substance abuse disorders compared with trauma survivors who did not develop PTSD.

Cumulative lifetime stress, particularly a history of exposure to trauma, appears to be a risk factor for PTSD (Davidson et al. 1991; Breslau et al. 1991). Prior victimization, especially in childhood, has been found to be a risk factor for PTSD following rape (Resnick et al. 1992) and combat (Bremner et al. 1993; Zaidi and Foy 1994). Prior exposure to a previous traumatic event may also increase vulnerability to PTSD associated with chronic pain (Asmundson et al. 2002). In a study of motor vehicle accident victims, Blanchard et al. (1994) reported that 87% of individuals who met diagnostic criteria for PTSD reported a previous trauma. Among them, 52% reported a previous serious motor vehicle accident, and 74% reported previous trauma of another type. Hickling et al. (1992) reported that a history of depressive disorder or previous alcohol abuse was associated with a higher risk of PTSD following a motor vehicle accident. History of anxiety disorder such as phobia has also been associated with increased vulnerability to PTSD (Kuch et al. 1994).

Table 19.3 summarizes research addressing the determinants of PTSD in individuals with chronic pain. Mayou et al. (1993) examined the psychiatric consequences of road traffic accidents in a sample of 171 motor vehicle accident victims. Participants were grouped in three categories: (1) multiple injury victims who had been involved in a car accident, (2) multiple injury victims who had been involved in a motorcycle accident, and (3) whiplash injury victims who had no

Table 19.3 Determinants of PTSD among motor vehicle accident victims

Authors	Year	Sample	Variables	Measures	Results
Hickling et al.	1992	20 individuals who had been in a motor vehicle accident and had been referred to a private practice psychologist for assessment and treatment of post-traumatic headache	Prevalence of PTSD History of headache disorder History of psychiatric disorder	Detailed interview about history of headache disorders, details about the accident and assessment of previous and actual psychiatric disorder	35% of patients had a previous history of psychopathology. Among these patients, 85.7% had had previous mood disorders and 14.3% had had previous alcohol abuse
Kuch et al.	1994	55 road vehicle accident survivors with chronic pain were recruited minimum two years after injury	Previous and current psychiatric disorder	Structured clinical interview based on DSM-III-R criteria	23.8% of patients with PTSD reported a past history of other phobia
Blanchard et al.	1994	50 victims of recent motor vehicle accidents who had sought medical attention after their accidents. Participants were assessed 1 to 4 months after their accident	Psychological morbidity Previous psychiatric disorders	Structured clinical interview based on the SCID	87% of PTSD subjects reported a previous trauma. Among them, 52% reported a previous serious motor vehicle accident, and 74% reported previous trauma of another type
Mayou et al.	1993	171 consecutive road accident victims aged 18–70 with multiple injuries or whiplash neck injury	Social adjustment Nature of the accident Psychological condition Severity of injury	Semistructured interview conducted few days after the accident, at three months and one year after the accident	Psychiatric disorder at one year was associated with continuing medical and social problems. Mood disorders at one year predicted by evidence of previous psychiatric problems and initial distress. Main predictor was initial ratings of horrific intrusive memories at postaccident interview
Mayou et al.	2002	546 subjects received questionnaires at 3 months, 1 and 3 years after their motor vehicle accident	Injury severity Injury-related stresses Emotional response during trauma Physical health and emotional problems prior to accident Litigation Psychological maintaining factors	Post-traumatic Stress Symptom Scale (PSS) Self-reported scales	47% of PTSD at 1 year still suffered from PTSD at 3 years. Persistent medical and financial problems showed moderate correlations with PTSD at 3 years. Participants' initial ratings of degree of fear experienced at the time of the accident and reports of dissociation at initial assessment predicted PTSD severity at 3 years

other physical injuries. All participants were interviewed at a few days following their injury, at 3 months and one year post-injury. Results showed that emotional distress varied as a function of the type of accident. Emotional distress at 3 months was more severe in motorcycle accident victims and least severe in subjects with whiplash. Motorcycle accident victims also reported a higher level of emotional distress at one year. In subjects with multiple injuries, psychiatric symptoms were significantly related to the persistence of medical problems. High initial reports of horrific intrusive memories were associated with more severe PTSD symptoms.

Longitudinal investigations reveal that symptoms of PTSD associated with pain become chronic in a significant percentage of cases. Mayou et al. (2002) conducted a three-year prospective study examining symptom course in a sample of 546 individuals who developed PTSD following motor vehicle accidents. Results showed that 47% of individuals with PTSD at 1 year postinjury still suffered from PTSD 3 years later. Persistent medical and financial problems at 3 months and 1 year showed moderate correlations with PTSD symptoms at 3 years. Initial ratings of the intensity of fear associated with the traumatic event, as well as symptoms of dissociation, predicted severity of PTSD symptoms at 3 years. Analyses revealed that women had a higher risk of developing PTSD than men. Finally, results revealed that compensation claims at 3 months and 1 year, whether planned or initiated, were correlated with higher PTSD symptoms 3 years after the accident.

Mayou et al. (2002) also addressed the role of cognitive factors in the perpetuation of symptoms of PTSD. Analyses of cognitive measures indicated that individuals who interpreted their intrusive memories of the accident in a negative way, who presented a high level of anger, and who used rumination or thought suppression to cope with symptoms were more likely to suffer from PTSD symptoms at 3 years.

INTERVENTION APPROACHES FOR PTSD AND CHRONIC PAIN

There have been few discussions of approaches to the treatment of PTSD specific to chronic pain samples. Interventions will typically proceed by implementing a number of symptom reduction techniques that will vary as a function of the symptom profile of specific patients (McNally 1999; Rothbaum et al. 2000). There has been research to suggest that selective serotonin reuptake inhibitors (SSRIs) such as fluoxetine, sertraline and paroxetine can yield clinically meaningful reductions in debilitating symptoms of emotional distress and social impairment associated with PTSD (Shalev et al. 1996; Brady et al. 2000; Davidson et al. 2001). Cognitive behavioral interventions have also been shown to be effective in reducing PTSD symptoms

and appear particularly useful in minimizing anxiety and avoidance-related symptomatology (Hembree and Foa 2000). The use of anxiolytics in the management of PTSD symptoms has met with limited success (Braun et al. 1990). In spite of available treatments, for approximately 50% of individuals who receive a diagnosis of PTSD, symptoms are likely to follow a chronic trajectory (Kessler et al. 1995).

To illustrate, in the case of Bob presented earlier, initial goals of treatment included (1) reduction of depressive symptomatology, (2) minimization of avoidance reactions, and (3) reduction of driving fears.

One of the challenges of working with individuals with PTSD concerns the facilitation of emotional disclosure. The emotional reactions of individuals to their traumatic experience can be quite intense; so much so that some individuals might not initially be able to provide a coherent description of the traumatic incident. The intensity of this distress is often sufficient to frighten many clinicians; to the point where some clinicians will expound on the dangers of decompensation due to disclosure of trauma. However, disclosure is absolutely necessary if progress is to be made (Pennebaker 1985, 1995). If the clinician joins the client in the avoidance of emotionally distressing memories, little progress will be made.

In the initial weeks of Bob's treatment, he was encouraged to describe the details of his experience repeatedly. Since he was initially unable to master the emotional control required to describe his experience in its entirety, facilitation of disclosure proceeded in a graded fashion. At times, he was asked to describe what he was thinking when he first saw the oncoming vehicle swerve into his path; at other times he was asked to describe the sensations associated with impact, his thoughts as he approached the vehicle, the death of the young girl, the arrival of the police and ambulance, the interactions with the police, his sleepless nights, his dreams. In other words, every aspect of the trauma was revisited repeatedly.

Why the emphasis on disclosure? First and foremost, disclosure is necessary for the development of rapport and the establishment of an effective working relationship. Disclosure also forces order on the disorganized internal experience associated with trauma (Pennebaker et al. 1993). For the individual suffering from PTSD symptoms, internal experience is often characterized by tension and fear, fragmented thoughts, images related to the trauma; these different facets of internal experience will continue to intrude into consciousness and will persist in their intensity until some order is imposed (Pennebaker 1990). It is only once thoughts and images have been translated into a narrative that the individual can begin the task of gaining a sense of meaning from his or her experiences, and increasing his or her control over the management of PTSD symptoms (Greenberg and Stone 1992). Through disclosure, traumatic memories are put into words and the structure of language facilitates the process of working through the traumatic material. It is only by translating traumatic memories into a "workable" format that the client can develop effective coping strategies to deal with the trauma (Pennebaker 1993; Rothbaum et al. 2000).

Disclosure is also a form of exposure and will contribute to a deintensification of symptoms (Rachman 1980). By emphasizing disclosure as an important component of recovery, the therapist also models approach (as opposed to avoidance) strategies that will be critical to treatment success (Rothbaum et al. 2000).

Strategic use of trauma-related disclosure can lead to dramatic reductions in the intensity of symptoms within just a few sessions. Experimental research suggests that emotional disclosure leads not only to a reduction in emotional distress but may also result in a reduction in pain experience (Kelley et al. 1997; Sullivan et al. 2000). It is important to note, however, that reductions in distress subsequent to disclosure might only become apparent after an initial increase in distress immediately following disclosure (Penebaker and Beall 1986; Pennebaker et al. 1988; Pennebaker 1990; Kelley et al. 1997). Preparing the client for the possibility of an initial increase in emotional distress is important in order to prevent the possibility that the client will interpret his or her symptoms as worsening.

In the case of Bob, return to driving with a view toward returning to work was considered an important goal of intervention. Bob's time off work increased his social isolation, and contributed to mounting fears that he would not be able to return to his occupation. Making return to work a goal of treatment communicated hope and confidence in successful treatment outcome, and was considered to be necessary to achieve social re-integration, resumption of pre-injury life roles, and re-establishment of a sense of purpose in life.

Driving fears were addressed initially through imaginal exposure during treatment sessions. The most important component of the treatment of driving fears was in vivo exposure conducted with the assistance of a driving school. The clinician accompanied Bob and a driving instructor as Bob was gradually exposed to driving conditions that were progressively more and more similar to the driving situations he might encounter as part of his occupation as a truck driver.

Bob's symptoms of PTSD decreased in intensity over the course of three months of treatment. Decreased emotional distress and increased coherence of thoughts related to the trauma were the first noticeable changes. Bob was also prescribed an antidepressant (Paxil) and a sleeping aid (Imovane). These were initially provided on a weekly basis in order to minimize the possibility of suicide by overdose. Sleeping medication allowed Bob to regain the energy resources required to engage fully in the therapeutic process. Antidepressant medication appeared to "buffer" the emotional impact of distressing thoughts and images related to the trauma. The driving fears were the last symptoms to show significant improvement. Bob was able to make a successful return to work 5 months following the initiation of treatment.

When the clinician is faced with an individual who is experiencing severe mental health symptoms, there may be a tendency to take a palliative stance on treatment. Palliative strategies might include relaxation techniques and recommendation for a period of time off work. Relaxation techniques are not always effective for the client with PTSD. The quiet and stimulus reduced environment used for relaxation training often leaves the client at the mercy of a barrage of intrusive thoughts. Activity oriented interventions can often be more beneficial for calming the PTSD client since activities that are attention demanding will reduce the cognitive resources available for intrusive thoughts. The clinician must also ask the question, "what is it about staying at home that will assist in the amelioration of this condition?" While time off work might lead to a reduction of work-related stresses, it can also increase financial stresses, increase social isolation and feelings of alienation and reduce the client's ability to fulfill life roles that might be central to his or her identity. In this manner, palliative approaches to treatment can, in the long term, actually contribute to an intensification of symptoms and heightened disability.

The success of treatment for PTSD is best viewed in terms of the resumption of life roles. For Bob, this meant resumption of his roles as spouse, parent, friend and worker. The complete elimination of symptoms should never be used as either a goal of treatment or the scale on which improvement is graded. Exposure to incidents that completely overwhelm individuals' coping resources are likely to change individuals in a permanent way (Horowitz 1986). Bob will probably never be the person he was before his accident. His world view was permanently affected, his sense of the meaning of his life and life in general was altered, and the sense of "invulnerability" that characterizes the non-traumatized mind was gone forever. However, in spite of these changes, Bob was able to reintegrate himself in the world around him and find a sense of meaning and purpose in his existence.

ASSESSING THE OUTCOME OF INTERVENTIONS FOR PTSD

Structured diagnostic interviews such as the SCID (Bremmer et al. 1993), based on DSM-IV criteria are considered the most valid approach to rendering diagnoses of PTSD. Clinician ratings scales have also been developed that yield both a continuous index of PTSD symptom severity and a categorical measure of diagnostic classification (Blake et al. 1990). A number of self-report instruments have been developed to assess the severity of symptoms associated with PTSD (Falsetti et al. 1993; Davidson et al. 1997; Asmundson et al. 1998). Although these scales should not be viewed as diagnostic tools, they can be very useful as screening instruments for potential cases of PTSD, and for monitoring changes in symptom severity. Commonly used measures of PTSD symptom severity include the Impact of Events Scale (Horowitz et al. 1979), the Davidson Trauma Scale (Davidson et al. 1997), the PTSD checklist (Andrykowski et al. 1998; Weathers et al. 2001), and the Posttraumatic Stress Diagnostic Scale (Foa 1995). Changes in symptom severity can also be examined with domain-specific measures that assess the severity of depressive (e.g., BDI; Beck et al. 1996), anxious (STAI; Speilberger et al. 1970) or avoidance symptoms.

PHOBIAS AND GENERALIZED ANXIETY DISORDER

In addition to PTSD, anxiety disorders that have been discussed in relation to chronic pain include simple or social phobias, and generalized anxiety disorder (Fishbain et al. 1988; McWilliams et al. 2003). Fears are common experiences that are adaptive in many circumstances but can lead to significant life interference when they become extreme or out of keeping with the actual danger associated with a particular event or circumstance. According to the DSM-IV (APA 1994), fears are considered phobias when "the avoidance, fear, or anxious anticipation of encountering the phobic stimulus interferes significantly with the person's daily routine, occupational functioning, or social life, or if the person is markedly distressed about having the phobia."

Social phobias may be characterized by a generalized fear of most social situations, or a fear of circumscribed social situations such as speaking in public or eating in public. Specific phobias observed in pain patients might include fears of driving subsequent to a motor vehicle accident, or fears of places or activities that were associated with an occupational injury (Kuch et al. 1994; Taylor and Koch 1995; Taylor et al. 1999). Generalized anxiety disorder is characterized by excessive and uncontrollable worry about a number of life events or activities that extends over a long period of time.

Structured diagnostic interviews based on DSM-IV criteria are considered the most valid approach to diagnosing anxiety disorders associated with pain. Self report instruments can be useful tools for screening or for monitoring progress in treatment. Commonly used self-report measures of fears or phobias associated with pain include the Fear Survey Schedule (Wolpe and Lang 1964; Beck et al. 1998), the Social Phobia and Anxiety Inventory (Biedel et al. 1989), and the Fear Questionnaire (Cox et al. 1993).

In a community sample of chronic pain patients, McWilliams et al. (2003) reported prevalence rates of 7% for generalized anxiety disorder, 6% for panic disorder, 15% for social phobia, and 11% for simple phobia. In each case, the prevalence rates were found to be significantly greater than those observed in individuals without chronic pain. Although point prevalence rates of anxiety disorders in individuals with chronic pain might be higher than those of the general population, some investigators have suggested that lifetime prevalence might not differ significantly between chronic pain samples and the general population (Atkinson et al. 1991; Polatin et al. 1993; Burton et al. 1997).

Few studies have addressed the prevalence, development and time course of specific anxiety disorders in chronic pain. Clearly, there is a need for more research to document the point and lifetime prevalence rates of different anxiety disorders in individuals with chronic pain.

As a class of mental disorder, anxiety-related conditions associated with chronic pain may be as prevalent as depression (McWilliams et al. 2003). However, relative to depression, anxiety disorders associated with chronic pain have received surprisingly far less research attention. The reasons for the lack of systematic investigation of anxiety disorders in chronic pain patients are not entirely clear. It is possible that anxiety disorders might not be viewed as debilitating as depressive disorders or PTSD. Along a similar vein, anxiety might be viewed as a normal reaction to chronic pain. For example, Gatchel (1991) suggested that anxiety might be a normal reaction to the onset of persistent pain, but its expression and associated disability might become dysfunctional or pathologic as the pain condition transitions from an acute to a chronic phase. It has also been suggested that symptoms of generalized anxiety disorder observed in chronic pain patients might reflect pre-existing emotional dysfunction as opposed to a reaction to chronic pain (Polatin et al. 1993).

Although knowledge of the precise relation between pain and anxiety disorders might be limited, there is considerable research to suggest that anxiety symptoms might contribute to heightened pain experience. Numerous investigations suggest that fear of pain (or pain-related anxiety) may impact directly on pain experience. For example, it has been shown that fear of pain is associated with heightened pain reports in response to experimentally induced pain (Sullivan et al. 1995), dental pain (Sullivan and Neish 1998) and in chronic low back pain patients (McCraken et al. 1992, 1993; Vlaeyen et al. 1995).

Recently, there has been considerable discussion of the role of fear of pain in the distress and disability associated with chronic pain (Asmundson et al. 1999; Vlaeyen and Linton, 2000). The literature is not clear on whether fear of pain should be conceptualized as a specific phobia or whether it should be conceptualized as an emotional risk factor for disability (Picavet et al. 2000; Waddell et al. 2003).

The defining criteria for fear of pain are markedly similar to those of simple phobias. For example, McNeil et al. (2001) define fear of pain as a "highly specific negative emotional reaction to pain eliciting stimuli involving a high degree of mobilization for escape/avoidance behavior." Fear-avoidance is considered to be a central variable in the development of long term pain-related disability (Vlaeyen and Linton 2000).

Clinical and experimental research continues to accumulate showing that fear of pain influences the experience of pain, and pain-related disability. Individuals who score high on measures of fear of pain are less active (Bussman et al. 1998), they have reduced range of motion (McCracken et al. 1992), they are prone to discontinuing activities that are associated with pain (McCracken et al. 1993; Vlaeyen et al. 1995), and they avoid activities that they expect will be associated with pain (Waddell 1998). Fear of pain has been shown to be a better predictor of disability than medical status variables or pain itself (Waddell et al. 1993).

Escape and avoidance are two components of fear of pain that have been linked to the development of disability (Vlaeyen and Linton 2000). Escape refers to behaviors that are enacted with the goal of terminating an aversive experience. Avoidance behavior refers to behavior that postpones or averts aversive experience. Once learned, avoidance behaviors can be self-perpetuating, even in the absence of demonstrated organic pathology. Self-perpetuation of avoidance behavior occurs when individuals develop the expectation that future activities will be associated with pain (Philips 1987). Indeed, there is evidence to suggest that individuals with high levels of fear of pain actually overestimate the degree of pain that will be associated with a particular activity (McCracken et al. 1992; Crombez et al. 1996). Since avoidance behaviors occur as a result of the expectation of future pain rather than in response to pain, these behaviors can persist indefinitely because successful avoidance reduces the potential for exposure that might correct over-prediction of pain (Vlaeyen and Linton 2000).

Three of the most frequently used self-report measures of fear of pain are the Pain Anxiety Symptom Scale (PASS; McCracken et al. 1993), the Tampa Scale for Kinesiophobia (TSK; Kori et al. 1990) and the Fear-Avoidance Beliefs Questionnaire (FABQ; Waddell et al. 1993) (see also Chapter 17). The PASS assesses pain-related fear appraisals, cognitive symptoms of anxiety and physiologic symptoms of anxiety. The TSK assesses respondents' beliefs about the potential for harm associated with physical activity (Lori et al. 1990; Vlaeyen et al. 1995). The FABQ assesses fear-avoidance beliefs about physical and work-related activities. Each of these measures has been shown to predict pain-related disability better than medical status variables (Asmundson et al. 1999).

INTERVENTION IMPLICATIONS

Although there has been limited research on the specific anxiety disorders associated with chronic pain, anxiety symptoms appear to be a central target of many rehabilitation programs for chronic pain. Descriptions of intervention techniques used in pain management frequently include relaxation as well as other stress reduction strategies such as cognitive re-interpretation, problem-solving and effective communication (Turk et al. 1983; Jensen et al. 1994; Burns et al. 2003).

The recent literature on fear of pain suggests that exposure techniques might also be beneficial in the treatment of chronic pain, particularly if the goal of treatment is to minimize pain-related disability (Vlaeyen et al. 2001; George et al. 2003). The treatment approaches advocated for fear of pain are very similar to those used in the treatment of phobias. For example, Vlaeyen and his colleagues have described an exposure-based treatment program to reduce fears associated with participation in various activities (Vlaeyen et al. 2002). Reductions in fear of pain have been shown to be associated with reductions in pain-related disability. Reductions in fear of pain have also been shown to be associated with a greater probability of returning to work following occupational injury (Sullivan and Stanish 2003).

Graduated exposure interventions have been used successfully to decrease avoidance and escape behaviors associated with pain. If individuals can be encouraged to engage in activities that they fear will bring about pain, they are provided with an opportunity to correct their over-predictions (McCracken et al. 1993). Crombez et al. (1996) showed that over-predictions of pain in relation to an upcoming physical exercise were corrected prior to engaging in a second physical exercise. In other words, experience can allow individuals to alter their exaggerated predictions of threat or harm associated with potentially pain-inducing activities, and in turn, decrease the probability of avoidance behavior. Graduated exposure to activities associated with fear also leads to a reduction in the intensity of fear of pain (Lindstrom et al. 1992; Fordyce 1995; Waddell 1998).

MENTAL HEALTH INTERVENTIONS AND PAIN REHABILITATION

There has been considerable recent discussion about whether participation in pain rehabilitation interventions (e.g., physiotherapy, modified return to work) should be postponed until mental health problems have been resolved. As a general rule, waiting is a strategy that will serve to complicate even further the clinical presentation of the individual with chronic pain (Waddell 1998). Since many of the mental health conditions associated with pain are likely to persist over time, postponement of other rehabilitation interventions might be indefinite.

It should be noted that the presence of clinically significant depression or anxiety does not represent contraindications to participation in an activity-based program such as physiotherapy or modified return to work. Activity-based techniques are central components of commonly used interventions for depression and anxiety disorders (Beck et al. 1978; Beck and Emery 1985; Lewinsohn et al. 1985; Bandura 1986; D'Zurilla 1988; Mahoney 1988). As such, symptoms of depression and anxiety that accompany persistent pain are likely to respond positively to the techniques included in an activity mobilization or work reintegration program. It must be noted however that there has been a paucity of research addressing the influence of traditional rehabilitation interventions (e.g., physiotherapy, occupational therapy) on symptoms of emotional disorders. More research is needed to determine when traditional non-psychological interventions are sufficient to manage symptoms of emotional distress, and when specific mental health interventions are required.

There are two conditions, when severe, that may warrant discontinuation, postponement or consideration of immediate referral to a mental health professional: these include substance abuse and PTSD. There are unfortunate circumstances where clients attempt to self-medicate to excess with alcohol or narcotic drugs. However, excessive use can lead to health complications and may impact negatively on cognitive and behavioral functioning. Clients who are struggling to manage an alcohol or drug problem may not be able to benefit from physical rehabilitation interventions.

As noted earlier, some clients may present with post-traumatic stress symptoms associated with their pain condition. These would be most common in situations where an injury was sustained under catastrophic conditions where there was a real or apparent threat to the welfare of the client or of others in the client's milieu (e.g., motor vehicle accidents, fires, mining tragedies). The client may present with high levels of emotional distress and report disruptive and intrusive recollections (e.g., distressing thoughts and images, nightmares) of the incident. At times, emotional distress states or re-experiencing phenomena may be so severe as to compromise the individual's ability to participate fully in rehabilitation interventions.

DYNAMIC BI-DIRECTIONAL RELATIONS BETWEEN CHRONIC PAIN AND MENTAL HEALTH OUTCOMES

This present chapter has focused primarily on mental health conditions that might develop subsequent to the onset of chronic pain. There has been considerable debate about the direction of causality between chronic pain and mental health conditions. At one extreme, it has been suggested that pain symptoms that are not associated with discernible organic pathology are entirely of psychological origin (Weintraub 1988). Other researchers have emphasized the reactive nature of mental health conditions to the stresses associated with persistent pain and disability (Banks and Kerns 1996). Still others have discussed the diverse social, psychological and physical contributions to mental health outcomes associated with chronic pain (Gatchel 1991; Turk 1996).

More recent efforts have begun to emphasize the bidirectional nature of the relations between chronic pain and mental health outcomes (Banks and Kerns 1996; Asmundson et al. 2002; Sullivan et al. 2002; Burns et al. 2003). Physical symptoms, life stresses, and coping resources are in constant flux and interrelations among them can yield a very different clinical picture even in the same individual at different points in time (Gatchel 1991; Sullivan et al. 2002). Biopsychosocial models have been put forward to address the role of different determinants and outcome of chronic pain (Banks and Kerns 1996). At their current stage of development, these models might have heuristic value for research, but they remain sufficiently general and imprecise as to make their clinical utility tenuous. One of the challenges of future research will be to assess more systematically the dynamic relations among determinants of pain and mental health over time and across different contexts.

From an intervention perspective, the importance of early detection of mental health conditions associated with chronic pain is clear. (Sullivan et al. in press). Not only do mental health conditions associated with chronic pain impact negatively on quality of life, they might also play a role in prolonging or exacerbating presenting symptoms of pain and disability. Recent research showing that mental health conditions might be risk factors for chronicity following the onset of pain further highlights the importance of implementing means of detecting mental health symptoms, and providing interventions that specifically target mental health symptoms (Sullivan et al. 1992; Asmundson et al. 2002; Carroll et al. 2003).

Although the recognition of the links between chronic pain and mental health problems is paramount to effective clinical management, it is this very recognition that can also interfere with effective clinical management of the individual with chronic pain. If mental health problems are viewed as being caused by pain, there is the associated tendency to believe that mental health problems will be alleviated once pain symptoms have resolved. Such a perspective often leads to the neglect of adequate treatment of mental health problems. Clients will benefit most from treatment orientations that conceptualize mental health outcomes and chronic pain as related, but where intervention strategies are invoked to deal with pain symptoms and mental health problems as if the conditions were distinct.

The instruments in this chapter are the following:

1. For the Fear Survey Schedule, contact: langlab@nersp.nerdc.ufl.edu; or go to: http://www.edits.net/FSS.html. For a review and other versions of the FSS instrument see: http://www.measurementexperts.org/instrument/instrument_reviews.asp?detail=39.
2. The Posttraumatic Stress Diagnostic Scale can be ordered from: http://www.pearsonassessments.com
3. The Social Phobia and Anxiety Inventory can be ordered from: http://www.psychtest.com

REFERENCES

Affleck G, Tennen H, Urrows S, et al. Neuroticism and the pain-mood relation in rheumatoid arthritis: insights from a prospective daily study. J Consult Clin Psychol 1992; 60:119–126.

Aghabeigi S, Feinmann C, Harris M. Prevalence of post-traumatic stress disorder in patients with chronic idiopathic pain. Br J Oral Maxillofacial Surg 1992; 30:360–364.

American Psychiatric Association. Diagnostic and statistical manual of mental disorders: DSM-IV. American Psychiatric Association, Washington, DC, 1994.

Andrykowski MA, Cordova MJ, Studts JL, et al. PTSD after treatment for breast cancer: prevalence of diagnosis, and use of the PTSD Checklist – Civilian Version (PCL-CV) as a screening instrument. J Consult Clin Psychol 1998; 66:586–590.

Arnau RC, Meagher MW, Norris MP, et al. Psychometric properties of the Beck Depression Inventory II with primary care medical patients. Health Psychology 2001; 20:112–119.

Arnstein P, Caudill M, Mandle CL, et al. Self-efficacy as a mediator of the relationship between pain intensity, disability and depression in chronic pain patients. Pain 1999; 80:483–491.

Arnold LM, Lu, Y., Crofford LJ. et al. A double-blind, multicenter trial comparing duloxetine with placebo in the treatment of fibromyalgia patients with or without major depressive disorder. Arthritis Rheum, 2004. 50:p. 2974–2984.

Asmundson GJG, Norton GR, Allerdings MD, et al. Post-traumatic stress disorder and work related injury. J Anx Dis 1998; 12:57–69.

Asmundson GJG, Norton PJ, Norton GR. Beyond pain: The role of fear and avoidance in chronicity. Clin Psychol Rev 1999; 19:97–119.

Asmundson GJG, Coons MJ, Taylor S, et al. PTSD and the experience of pain: research and clinical implications of shares vulnerability and mutual maintenance models. Can J Psychiat 2002; 47:930–937.

Atkinson JH, Ingram RE, Kremer EF, et al. MMPI subgroups and affective disorder in chronic pain patients. J Nerv Ment Dis 1986; 174:408–413.

Atkinson JH, Slater MA, Grant I, et al. Depressed mood in chronic low back pain: relationship with stressful life events. Pain 1988; 35:47–55.

Atkinson JH, Slater MA, Patterson TL, et al. Prevalence, onset, and risk of psychiatric disorders in men with chronic low back pain: a controlled study. Pain 1991; 45:111–121.

Bandura A. Social Foundation of Thought and Action: A Social Cognitive Theory. Prentice Hall, Englewood Cliffs, NJ, 1986.

Banks SM, Kerns RD. Explaining high rates of depression in chronic pain: a diathesis-stress framework. Psychol Bull 1996; 119:95–110.

Beck AT, Rush AJ, Shaw BF, et al. Cognitive Therapy for Depression. Guilford Press, New York, 1978.

Beck AT, Emery G, Greenberg RL. Anxiety Disorders and Phobias: A Cognitive Perspective. Basic Books, New York, 1985.

Beck AT, Steer RA, Brown GK. Manual for the Beck Depression Inventory II. Psychological Corporation, San Antonio, TX, 1996.

Beck JG, Carmin CM, Henninger JA. The utility of the Fear Schedule III: an extended replication. J Anx Dis 1998; 12:177–182.

Biedel DC, Turner SM, Stanley MA, et al. The Social Phobia and Anxiety Inventory: concurrent and external validity. Behav Ther 1989; 20:417–427.

Bishop SR, Edgley K, Fisher R, et al. Screening for depression in chronic low back pain with the Beck Depression Inventory. Can J Rehab 1993; 7:143–148.

Blake D, Weathers F, Nagy L, et al. A clinician rating scale for assessing current and lifetime PTSD: the CAPS-1. Behav Therapist 1990; 13:187–188.

Blanchard EB, Hickling EJ, Taylor AE, et al. Psychological morbidity associated with motor vehicle accidents. Behav Res Ther 1994; 32:283–290.

Blumer D, Heilbronn M. Chronic pain as a variant of depressive disease: the pain-prone disorder. J Nerv Ment Dis 1982; 170:381–394.

Brady K, Pearlstein T, Asnis GM, et al. Efficacy and safety of sertraline treatment of post-traumatic stress disorder. A randomized controlled trial. JAMA 2000; 283:1837–1844.

Braun P, Greenberg D, Dasberg H, et al. Core symptoms of post traumatic stress disorder unimproved by alprazolam treatment. J Clin Psychiatry 1990; 51:236–238.

Bremner JD, Southwick SM, Johnson DR, et al. Childhood physical abuse and combat-related posttraumatic stress disorder in Vietnam veterans. Am J Psychiat 1993; 150:235–239.

Breuer J, Freud S. Studies on Hysteria. Basic Books, New York, 1957.

Bryant RA, Harvey AG. Acute stress disorder: a critical review of diagnostic issues. Clin Psychol Rev 1997; 17:757–773.

Bryant RA, Marosszeky JE, Crooks J, et al. Interaction of posttraumatic stress disorder and chronic pain following traumatic brain injury. J Head Trauma Rehabil 1999; 14:588–594.

Burns JW, Kubilus A, Bruehl S, et al. Do changes in cognitive factors influence outcome following multidisciplinary treatment for chronic pain? A cross-lagged panel analysis. J Consult Clin Psychol 2003; 71:81–91.

Bussman JBJ, van de Laar YM, Neleman MP, et al. Ambulatory accelerometry to quantify motor behavior in patients after failed back surgery. Pain 1998; 74:153–161.

Campbell, L., D. Clauw, and, F. Keefe, Persistent pain and depression: A biopsychosocial perspective. Biological Psychiatry, 2003. 54:399–409.

Cano A, Weisberg JN, Gallagher RM. Marital satisfaction and pain severity mediate the association between negative spouse responses to pain and depressive symptoms in a chronic pain patient sample. Pain Med 2000; 1:35–43.

Carroll LJ, Cassidy JD, Cote P. Factors associated with the onset of an episode of depressive symptoms in the general population. *Journal of Clinical Epidemiology*. 56(7):651–8, 2003.

. Chaves JF, Brown JM. Spontaneous cognitive strategies for the control of clinical pain and stress. J Behav Med 1987; 10:263–276.

Chibnall JT, Duckro PN. Post-traumatic stress disorder in chronic post-traumatic headache patients. Headache 1994; 34:357–361.

Ciamarella A, Grosso S, Poli P, et al. When pain is not fully explained by organic lesion: a psychiatric perspective on chronic pain patients. Eur J Pain 2004; 8:13–22.

Ciccone DS, Just N, Bandilla EB, et al. Psychological correlates of opioid use in patients with chronic non-malignant pain: a preliminary test of the downward spiral hypothesis. J Pain Symptom Manage 2000; 20:180–192.

Cohen H, Neumann L, Haiman Y, et al. Prevalence of post-traumatic stress disorder in fibromyalgia patients: overlapping syndromes or post-traumatic fibromyalgia syndrome? Semin Arthritis Rheum 2002; 32:38–50.

Cox BJ, Swinson RP, Parker JDA, et al. Confirmatory factor analysis of the Fear Questionnaire in Panic disorder with agoraphobia. Psychol Assessment 1993; 5:235–237.

Crombez G, Bijttebier P, Eccleston E, et al. The child version of the pain catastrophizing scale (PCS-C): a preliminary validation. Pain 2003; 104:639–646.

Davidson JR, Book SW, Colket JT. Assessment of a new self-rating scale for post-traumatic stress disorder. Psychol Med 1997; 27:153–160.

Davidson JR, Rothbaum BO, van der Kolk BA, et al. Multicenter, double-blind comparison of sertraline and placebo in the treatment of post traumatic stress disorder. Arch Gen Psychiatry 2001; 58:485–492.

Dersh J, Polatin PB, Gatchel RJ. Chronic pain and psychopathology: research findings and theoretical considerations. Psychom Med 2002; 64:773–786.

Dworkin RH, Gitlin MJ. Clinical aspects of depression in chronic pain patients. Clin J Pain 1991; 7:79–94.

Epping-Jordan JE, Wahlgren DR, Williams RA, et al. Transition to chronic pain in men with low back pain: predictive relationships among pain intensity, disability, and depressive symptoms. Health Psychology 1998; 17:421–427.

Falsetti SA, Resnick HS, Resnick PA, et al. The modifies PTSD Symptom Scale: a brief self-report of post-traumatic stress disorder. Behav Therapist 1993; 16:161–162.

Faucett JA. Depression in painful chronic disorders: the role of pain and conflict about pain. J Pain Sympt Manage 1994; 9:520–526.

Feinmann C. Psychogenic facial pain: presentation and treatment. J Psychosom Res 1983; 27:403–410.

Ferrari R, Russell AS. The whiplash syndrome: common sense revisited. J Rheumatol 1997; 24:618–622.

Fishbain DA, Goldberg M, Meagher BR, et al. Male and female chronic pain patients categorized by DSM-III psychiatric diagnostic criteria. Pain. 26(2):181–97, 1986.

Fishbain D, Cutler R, Rosomoff H, et al. Chronic pain-associated depression: antecedent or consequence of chronic pain? A review. Clin J Pain 1997; 13:116–137.

Fishbain D, Cutter R, Rosomoff H. Comorbid psychiatric disorders in chronic pain patients. Pain Clin 1998; 11:79–87.

Foa EB. Posttraumatic Stress Diagnostic Scale Manual. National Computer Systems, Minneapolis, MN, 1995.

Foa EB, Stekete G, Rothbaum BO. Behavioral/cognitive conceptualizations of post-traumatic stress disorder. Behav Ther 1989; 20:155–176.

Ford, CV (1995). Dimensions of somatization and hypochondriasis. In: Neurologic Clinics. Malingering and conversion reactions, ed. MI Weintraub, Philadelphia: W.B. Saunders Co. 13:241–253.

France RD, Houpt JL, Skott A, et al. Depression as a psychopathological disorder in chronic low back pain patients. J Psychosom Res 1986; 30:127–133.

France R, Krishnan K. Psychotropic drugs in chronic pain. In: France R, Krishnan K (eds). Chronic Pain. American Press, Washington, DC, 1988.

Fulop-Miller R. Triumph Over Pain. Literary Guild of America, New York, 1938.

Gatchel RJ. Early development of physical and mental deconditioning in painful spinal disorders. In: Mayer TG, Mooney V, Gatchel RJ (eds). Contemporary Conservative Care for Painful Spinal DisordersLea & Febiger, Philadelphia, PA, 1991.

Gatchel RJ, Polatin PB, Mayer TG, et al. Psychopathology and the rehabilitation of patients with chronic low back pain disability. Arch Phys Med Rehabil 1994; 75:666–670.

Geisser ME, Roth RS, Backman GE, et al. The relationship between symptoms of post-traumatic stress disorder and pain, affective disturbance and disability among patients with accident and non-accident related pain. Pain 1996; 66:207–214.

Geisser ME, Roth RS, Robinson ME. Assessing depression among persons with chronic pain using the Center for Epidemiological Studies-Depression Scale and the Beck Depression Inventory: a comparative analysis. Clin J Pain 1997; 13:163–170.

Geisser ME, Roth RS, Theisen ME, et al. Negative affect, self-report of depressive symptoms, and clinical depression: relation to the experience of chronic pain. Clin J Pain 2000; 16(2):110–120.

Gil KM, Thompson RJ, Keith BR, et al. Sickle cell disease pain in children and adolescents: change in pain frequency and coping strategies over time. J Pediatr Psychol 1993; 18:621–637.

Glynn SM, Asarnow SR, Asarnow R, et al. The development of acute post-traumatic stress disorder after orofacial injury: a prospective study in a large urban hospital. J Oral Maxillofac Surg 2003; 61:785–792.

Goldberg GM, Kerns RD, Rosenberg R. Pain-relevant support as a buffer from depression among chronic pain patients low in instrumental activity. Clin J Pain 1993; 9:34–40.

Greenberg MA, Stone AA. Emotional disclosure about traumas and its relation to health: effects of previous disclosure and trauma severity. J Pers Soc Psychol 1992; 63:75–84.

Haythornthwaite JA, Sieber WJ, Kerns RD. Depression and the chronic pain experience. Pain 1991; 46: 177–184.

Hembree EA, Foa EB. Posttraumatic stress disorder: psychological factors and psychosocial interventions. J Clin Psychiatry 2000; 61:33–39.

Hickling EJ, Blanchard EB. Post-traumatic stress disorder and motor vehicle accidents. J Anx Disor 1992; 6:285–291.

Hickling EJ, Blanchard EB, Silverman DJ, et al. Motor vehicle accidents, headaches and post-traumatic stress disorder: assessment findings in a consecutive series. Headache 1992; 32:147–151.

Hodgkiss A. Rediscovering the psychopathology of chronic pain. J Psychosom Res 1997; 42:221–224.

Horowitz MJ. Stress Response Syndromes, 2nd edn., Jason Aronson, New York, 1986.

Horowitz M, Wilner N, Alvarez W. Impact of Event Scale: a measure of subjective stress. Psychosom Med 1979; 41:209–218.

Howell S, Poulton R, Caspi A, et al. Relationship between abdominal pain subgroups in the community and psychiatric diagnosis and personality. A birth cohort. J Psychosom Res 2003; 55:179–187.

Jensen MP, Turner JA, Romano JM. Correlates of improvement in multidisciplinary treatment of chronic pain. J Consult Clin Psychol 1994; 62:172–179.

Katon W, Ries RK, Kleinmann A. A prospective study of 100 consecutive somatization patients: II. Comprehensive Psychiat 1984; 25:305–314.

Katon W, Egan K, Miller D. Chronic pain: lifetime psychiatric diagnoses and family history. Am J Psychiat 1985; 142:1156–1160.

Keefe FJ, Brown GK, Wallston KA, et al. Coping with rheumatoid arthritis pain: catastrophizing as a maladaptive strategy. Pain 1989; 37:51–56.

Kelley JE, Lumley MA, Leisen JCC. Health effects of emotional disclosure in rheumatoid arthritis patients. Health Psychol 1997; 16:331–340.

Kerns RD, Rosenberg R, Otis JD. Self-appaised problem solving and pain-relevant social support as apredictors of the experience of chronic pain. Ann Behav Med 2002; 24:100–105.

Kessler RC, Sonnega A, Bromet E, et al. Post traumatic stress disorder in the National Comorbidity Survey. Arch Gen Psychiatry 1995; 52:1048–1060.

Kinney RK, Gatchel RJ, Polatin PB, et al. Prevalence of psychopathology in acute and chronic low back pain patients. J Occup Rehabil 1993; 3:95–103.

Klinger L, Spaulding S, Polatajko H, et al. Chronic pain in the elderly: occupational adaptation as a means of coping with osteoarthritis of the hip and/or knee. Clin J Pain 1999; 15:275–283.

Kramlinger KG, Swanson DW, Maruta T. Are patients with chronic pain depressed? Am J Psychiatry 1983; 140:747–749.

Krishnan KRR, France RD, Pelton S, et al. Chronic pain and depression: II.Symptoms of anxiety in chronic low back pain patients and their relationship to subtypes of depression. Pain 1985; 22:289–294.

Kuch K, Swinson RP, Kirby M. Post-traumatic stress disorder after car accidents. Can J Psychiat 1985; 30:426–427.

Kuch K, Cox BJ, Evans RJ, et al. To what extent do anxiety and depression interact with chronic pain? Can J Psychiat 1993; 38:36–38.

Kuch K, Cox BJ, Evans R, et al. Phobias, panic, and pain in survivors of road vehicle accidents. J Anx Disor 1994; 8:181–187.

Lazarus RS. The cost and benefits of denial. In: Breznitz S (ed). The Denial of Stress. International Universities Press, New York, 1983.

Lewinsohn PM, Hoberman PM, Teri L, et al. An integrative theory of depression. In: Reiss S, Bootzin RR (eds). Theoretical Issues in Behavior TherapyAcademic Press, New York, 1985.

Lindsay PG, Wyckoff M. The depression pain syndrome and its response to antidepressants. Psychosomatics 1981; 22:571–577.

Lindstrom I, Ohlund C, Eek C, et al. The effect of graded activity on patients with subacute low back pain: a randomized prospective clinical study with an operant-conditioning behavioral approach. Phys Ther 1992; 72:279–290.

Kori SH, Miller RP, Todd DD. Kinesophobia: a new view of chronic pain behavior. Pain Manage 1990:Jan35–43.

Love AW. Depression in chronic low back pain patients: diagnostic efficiency of three self-report questionnaires. J Clin Psychol 1987; 43:84–89.

Madland G, Feinmann C, Newman S. Factors associated with anxiety and depression in facial arthromyalgia. Pain 2000; 84:225–232.

Magni G, Moreshi C, Rigatti-Luchini S, et al. Prospective study on the relationship between depressive symptoms and chronic musculoskeletal pain. Pain 1994; 56:289–298.

Maxwell D, Gatchel RJ, Mayer TG. Cognitive predictors of depression in chronic low back pain: toward an inclusive model. J Behav Med 1998; 21:131–143.

Mayou R, Bryant B. Outcome of "whiplash" neck injury. Injury 1996; 27:617–623.

Mayou R, Bryant B, Duthie R. Psychiatric consequences of road traffic accidents. Br Med J 1993; 307:647–651.

Mayou RA, Ehlers A, Bryant B. Posttraumatic stress disorder after motor vehicle accidents: 3-year follow-up of a prospective longitudinal study. Behav Res Ther 2002; 40:665–675.

McCracken LM. Learning to live with the pain: acceptance of pain predicts adjustment in persons with chronic pain. Pain 1998; 74:21–27.

McCracken LM, Zayfert C, Gross RT. The Pain Anxiety Scale: development and validation of a scale to measure fear of pain. Pain 1992; 50:67–73.

McCracken LM, Gross RT, Sorg PJ, et al. Prediction of pain in patients with chronic low back pain: effects of inaccurate prediction and pain-related anxiety. Behav Ther 1993; 31:647–652.

McNally R. Post-traumatic stress disorder. In: Millon T, Blaney PH, Davis RD (eds). Oxford Textbook of Psychopathology: Oxford University Press, Oxford, 1999:341–351.

McWilliams LA, Cox B.J, Enns MW. Mood and anxiety disorders associated with chronic pain: an examination in a nationally representative sample. Pain 2003; 106:127–133.

Morley S, Williams AC, de C, Black S. A confirmatory factor analysis of the Beck Depression Inventory in chronic pain. Pain 2002; 99:157–165.

Nicassio PM, Radojevic V, Schoenfeld-Smith K, et al. The contribution of family cohesion and the pain-coping process to depressive symptoms in fibromyalgia. Ann Behav Med 1995; 17:349–356.

Pennebaker JC. Emotion, disclosure, and health: an overview. In: Pennebaker JC (ed). Emotion, Disclosure, and Health. American Psychological Association, Washington, DC, 1995.

Pennebaker JW. Traumatic experience and psychosomatic disease: exploring the roles of behavioural inhibition, obsession, and confiding. Can Psychol 1985; 26: 82–95.

Pennebaker JW. Opening Up: The Healing Power of Confiding in Others. William Morrow, New York, 1990.

Pennebaker JW. Putting stress into words: health, linguistic, and therapeutic implications. Behav Res Ther 1993; 31:539–548.

Pennebaker JW, Beall SK. Confronting a traumatic event: toward an understanding of inhibition and disease. J Abnorm Psychol 1986; 95:274–281.

Pennebaker JW, Kiecolt-Glaser JK, Glaser R. Disclosure of traumas and immune function: health implications for psychotherapy. J Consulting Clin Psychol 1988; 56:238–245.

Polatin PB. Integration of pharmacotherapy and psychological treatment of chronic pain. In: Gatchel RJ, Turk DC (eds). Psychological Approaches to Pain ManagementGuilford Press, New York, 1996.

Polatin PB, Kinney RK, Gatchel RJ, et al. Psychiatric illness and chronic low-back pain: the mind and the spine – which goes first? Spine 1993; 18:66–71.

Rabin C, O'Leary A, Neighbors C, et al. Pain and depression experienced by women with interstitial cystitis. Women Health 2000; 31:67–81.

Rachman S. Emotional processing. Behav Res Ther 1980; 18:51–61.

Radloff LS. The CES-D Scale: a self-reported depression scale for research in the general population. Appl Psychol Meas 1977; 1:385–401.

Rainville J, Sobel JB, Hartigan C, et al. The effect of compensation involvement on the reporting of pain and disability by patients referred for rehabilitation of chronic low back pain. Spine 1997; 26:2016–2024.

Reid GJ, Gilbert CA, McGrath PJ. The Pain Coping Questionnaire: preliminary validation. Pain 1998; 76:83–96.

Remick RA, Blasberg B, Campos PE, et al. Psychiatric disorders associated with atypical facial pain. Can J Psychiat 1983; 28:178–181.

Resnick HS, Kilpatrick DG, Best CL. Vulnerability stress factors in development of posttraumatic stress disorder. J Nerv Ment Dis 1992; 180:424–430.

Rodin G, Craven J, Littlefield C. Depression in the Medically Ill: An Integrated Approach. Bruner/Mazel, New York, 1991.

Romano JM, Turner JA. Chronic pain and depression: does the evidence support a relationship? Psychol Bull 1985; 97:18–34.

Rosenstiel AK, Keefe FJ. The use of coping strategies in chronic low back pain patients: relationship to patient characteristics and current adjustment. Pain 1983; 17:33–44.

Roth S, Cohen LJ. Approach avoidance and coping with stress. Am Psychologist 1986; 41:813–819.

Rothbaum BO, Meadows EA, Resick P, et al. Cognitive-bahavioral therapy. In: Foa FB, Keane TM, Friedman MJ (eds). Effective Treatments for PTSD: Practice Guidelines from the International Society for Traumatic Stress StudiesGuilford Press, New York, 2000.

Rush AJ, Polatin P, Gatchel RJ. Depression and chronic low back pain. Spine 2000; 25:2566–2571.

Sharp TJ, Harvey AG. Chronic pain and post-traumatic stress disorder: mutual maintenance? Clin Psychol Rev 2001; 21:857–877.

Sist TC, Florio GA, Miner MF, et al. The relationship between depression and pain language in cancer and chronic non-cancer pain patients. J Pain Sympt Manage 1998; 15:350–358.

Smith, Timothy W; O'Keeffe, Jennifer L; Christensen, Alan J. Cognitive distortion and depression in chronic pain: Association with diagnosed disorders. *Journal of Consulting and Clinical Psychology*. Vol 62(1) 1994, 195-198.

Spanos NP, Radtke-Bodorik HL, Ferguson JD, et al. The effects of hypnotic susceptibility, suggestions for analgesia, and utilization of cognitive strategies on the reduction of pain. J Abnorm Psychol 1979; 88:282–292.

Spielberger CD, Gorsuch RL, Lushen RE. Manual for the State Trait Anxiety Inventory. Counselling Psychologists Press, Palo Alto, CA, 1970.

Spiegel K, Kalb R, Pasternak GW: Analgesic activity of tricyclic antidepressants. Ann Neurol 1983; 13:462–465.

Sternbach RA. Pain Patients: Traits and Treatment. Academic Press, New York, 1974.

Sullivan MJL, D'Eon JL. Relation between catastrophizing and depression in chronic pain patients. J Abnorm Psychol 1990; 99:260–263.

Sullivan MJL, Neish N. Catastrophizing, anxiety and pain during dental hygiene treatment. Community Dent Oral Epidemiol 1998; 37:243–250.

Sullivan MJL, Stanish WD. Psychologically based occupational rehabilitation: the Pain-Disability Prevention Program. Clin J Pain 2003; 19:97–104.

Sullivan MJL, Reesor K, Mikail S, Fisher R. The treatment of depression in chronic low back pain: review and recommendations. Pain 1992; 50:5–13.

Sullivan MJL, Bishop S, Pivik J. The Pain Catastrophizing Scale: development and validation. Psychol Assess 1995; 7:524–532.

Sullivan MJL, Tripp D, Rodgers W, et al. Catastrophizing and pain perception in sports participants. J Appl Sport Psychol 2000; 12:151–167.

Sullivan MJL, Thorn B, Haythornthwaite JA, et al. Theoretical perspectives on the relation between catastrophizing and pain. Clin J Pain 2001; 17:52–64.

Sullivan MJL, Rodgers WM, Wilson PM, et al. An experimental investigation of the relation between catastrophizing and activity intolerance. Pain 2002; 100:47–53.

Sullivan MJL, Stanish W, Sullivan ME, et al. Differential predictors of pain and disability in patients with whiplash injuries. Pain Res Manage 2002; 7:68–74.

Sullivan MJL, Adams H., Thibault, P, et al. (2006) Initial depression severity and the trajectory of recovery following cognitive-behavioural intervention for chronic pain. Journal of Occupational Rehabilitation; 16:63–74.

Sullivan MJL, Ward, LC, Tripp, D., et al. Secondary prevention of work disability: community-based psychosocial intervention for musculoskeletal disorders. Journal of Occupational Rehabilitation 2005; 15:377–392.

Sullivan MJL, Thibault, P., Savard A, et al. Psychological risk factors for prolonged pain and disability following recovery from cancer. In M. Feuerstein (Ed.), Handbook of Cancer Survivorship. New York, Springer, 2006.

Sullivan MJL, Adams H., Tripp, D., et al. Stage of chronicity and treatment response in depressed patients with musculoskeletal injuries. Pain, in press.

Szasz T.S. Pain and pleasure: A study of bodily-feelings. New York: Basics Books,1957.

Taylor S, Koch WJ. Anxiety disorders due to motor vehicle accidents: nature and treatment. Clin Psychol Rev 1995; 15:721–738.

Taylor SE, Deane FP, Podd JV. Stability of driving fear acquisition pathways over one year. Behav Res Ther 1999; 37:927–939.

Thorn BE, Boothy J, Sullivan MJL. Targeted treatment of catastrophizing in the management of chronic pain. Cogn Behav Prac 2002; 9:127–138.

Trief PM, Carnrike CLM Jr, Drudge O. Chronic pain and depression is social support relevant? Psychol Rep 1995; 76:227–236.

True WR, Rise J, Eisen S, et al. A twin study of genetic and environmental contributions to liability for posttraumatic stress symptoms. Arch Gen Psychiat 1993; 50:257–264.

Turk DC, Salovey P. Chronic pain as a variant of depressive disease: a critical reappraisal. J Nerv Ment Dis 1984; 172:398–404.

Turk DC, Okifuji A, Scharff L. Chronic pain and depression: role of perceived impact and perceived control in different age cohorts. Pain 1995; 61:93–101.

Turner JA, Aaron LA. Pain-related catastrophizing: What is it? Pain 2001; 17:65–71.

Turner JA, Clancy S. Strategies for coping with chronic low back pain: relationships to pain and disability. Pain 1986; 24:355–364.

Turner JA, Romano JM. Self-report screening measures for depression in chronic pain patients. J Clin Psychol 1984; 40:909–913.

Turner JA, Jensen MP, Warms CA, et al. Catastrophizing is associated with pain intensity, psychological distress, and pain-related disability among individuals with chronic pain after spinal cord injury. Pain. 98(1–2): 127–34, 2002.

Turner JA, Mancl L, Aaron LA. Pain-related catastrophizing: a daily process study. Pain 2004; 110:103–111.

Vlaeyen JWS, Linton SJ. Fear-avoidance and its consequences in chronic musculoskeletal pain: a state of the art. Pain 2000; 85:317–332.

Vlaeyen JW, De Jong JR, Onghena P, et al. Can pain-related fear be reduced? The application of cognitive-behavioral exposure in vivo. Pain Res Manage 2002; 7:144–153.

Vowles KE, Gross RT, Sorrell JT. Predicting work status following interdisciplinary treatment for chronic pain. Eur J Pain 2004; 8:351–358.

Waddell G, Newton M, Henderson I, et al. A Fear-Avoidance Beliefs Questionnaire (FABQ) and the role of fear-avoidance beliefs in chronic low back pain and disability. Pain 1993; 52:157–168.

Waddell G, Burton AK, Main CJ. Screening to Identify People at Risk of Long-Term Incapacity for Work. Royal Society of Medicine Press, London, 2003.

Wakefield JC. Disorder as harmful dysfunction: a conceptual critique of DSM-III-Rs definition of mental disorder. Psychol Rev 1992; 99:232–247.

Wasan AD, Davar G, Jamison R. The association between negative affect and opioid analgesia in patients with discogenic low back pain. Pain 2005; 117(3):450–461.

Weathers FW, Keane TM, Davidson JR. Clinician-administered PTSD scale: a review of the first ten years of research. Depress Anx 2001; 13:132–156.

Weintraub MI. Regional pain is usually hysterical. Arch Neurol 1988; 44:914–915.

Wesley, A. LaVonne; Gatchel, Robert J; Gorofalo, John Paul, et al. Toward more accurate use of the Beck Depression Inventory with chronic back pain patients. Clinical Journal of Pain. Vol 15(2) 1999, 117-121.

White AD. A History of the Warfare of Science with Theology in Christendom. Appleton and Company, New York, 1896.

Wijeratne, Chanaka; Shome, Sushmita; Hickie, Ian, et al. An age-based comparison of chronic pain clinic patients. International Journal of Geriatric Psychiatry. Vol 16(5) 2001, 477-483.

Wilson, Keith G; Mikail, Samuel F; D'Eon, Joyce L, et al. Alternative diagnostic criteria for major depressive disorder in patients with chronic pain. Pain. Vol 91(3) 2001, 227-234.

Wilson, Keith G; Eriksson, Mariane Y; D'Eon, Joyce L, et al. Major depression and insomnia in chronic pain. Clinical Journal of Pain. Vol 18(2) 2002, 77-83.

Wolpe J, Lang PJ. A fear schedule for use in behaviour therapy. Behav Res Ther 1964; 2:27–30.

Zaidi LY, Foy DW. Childhood abuse and combat-related PTSD. J Trauma Stress 1994; 7:33–42.

Zung WW. A self-rating depression scale. Arch Gen Psychiat. 1965; 12:63–70.

FURTHER READING

Asmundson GJG, Bonin MF, Frombach IK, et al. Evidence of a disposition toward fearfulness and vulnerability to post-traumatic stress in dysfunctional pain patients. Behav Res Ther 2000; 38:801–812.

Breslau N, Davis GC, Andreski P, et al. 1991 Traumatic events and posttraumatic stress disorder in an urban population of young adults. Arch Gen Psychiat 1993; 48:216–222.

Brown GK. A causal analysis of chronic pain and depression. J Abnorm Psychol 1990; 99:127–137.

Burns JW. Repression predicts outcome of multidisciplinary treatment of chronic pain. Health Psychol 2000; 19:75–84.

Burton AK, Tillotson KM, Main CJ, et al. Psychosocial predictors of outcome in acute and subchronic low back trouble. Spine 1995; 20:722–728.

Crombez G, Vlaeyen JWS, Heuts PH TG, et al. Fear of pain is more disabling than fear itself. Evidence for the role of pain-related fear in chronic back pain disability. Pain 1999; 80:329–340.

D'Zurilla T. Problem-Solving Therapy: A Social Competence Approach to Clinical Intervention. Springer, New York, 1986.

Engel GL. "Psychogenic" pain and the pain-prone patient. Am J Med 1959; 26:899–918.

Hadjistavropoulos HD, Asmundson GJG, Kowalyk KM. Measures of anxiety: is there a difference in their ability to predict functioning at three-month follow-up among pain patients? Eur J Pain 2004; 8:1–11.

Hamilton MA. A rating scale for depression. J Neurol Neurosurg Psychiatry 1960; 23:56–62.

Ingram RE. Toward an information processing analysis of depression. Cog Ther Res 1984; 8:443–478.

Jacobsen PB, Butler RW. Relation of cognitive coping and catastrophizing to acute pain and analgesic use following breast cancer surgery. J Behav Med 1996; 19:17–29.

Kerns RD, Haythornthwaite J. Depression among chronic pain patients: cognitive-behavioral analysis and effects on rehabilitation outcome. J Consult Clin Psychol 1988; 56:870–876.

Klenerman L, Slade PD, Stanley M, et al. The prediction of chronicity in patients with an acute attack of low back pain in a general practice setting. Spine 1995; 20:478–484.

Mahoney MJ. Human Change Processes: The Scientific Foundations of Psychotherapy. Basic Books, New York, 1991.

Maupassant G. Sur l'eau [originally published 1875]. M Walter Dunne, New York, 1903.

McNeil DW, Au AR, Zvolensky MJ, et al. Fear of pain in orofacial pain patients. Pain 2000; 89:245–252.

Osman A, Barrios FX, Kopper BA, et al. Factor structure, reliability, and validity of the Pain Catastrophizing Scale. J Behav Med 1997; 20:589–605.

Picavet HS, Vlaeyen JW, Schouten JS. Pain catastrophizing and kinesiophobia: predictors of chronic low back pain. Am J Epidemiol 2002; 156:1028–1034.

Scholten-Peeters GMG, Verhagen AP, Bekkering GE, et al. Prognostic factors of whiplash-associated disorders: a systematic review of prospective cohort studies. Pain 2003; 104:303–322.

Selling LS. Men Against Madness. Greenberg, New York, 1948.

Smith TW, O'Keeffe JL, Christensen A.J. Cognitive distortion and depression in chronic pain: association with diagnosed disorders. J Consult Clin Psychol 1984; 62:195–198.

Speigel K, Kalb R, Pasternak G. Analgesic activity of tricyclic antidepressants. Ann Neurol 1983; 13:462–465.

Szasz TS. Pain and Pleasure: A Study of Bodily Feelings. Tavistock, London, 1969.

Trief PM, Grant W, Fredrickson B. A prospective study of psychological predictors of lumbar surgery outcome. Spine 2000; 25:2616–2621.

Vlaeyen JWS, Kole-Snijders AMJ, Rotteveel A, et al. The role of fear of movement/(re)injury in pain disability. J Occup Rehabil 1995a; 5:235–252.

Vlaeyen JWS, Kole-Snijders AMJ, Boeren RBG, et al. Fear of movement/(re) injury in chronic low back pain and its relation to behavioral performance. Pain 1995b; 62:363–372.

Whitwell JR. Historical Notes on Psychiatry. Lewis and Co., London, 1936.

Measuring work outcomes with a focus on health-related work productivity loss

Benjamin C. Amick III • David Gimeno

INTRODUCTION

Measuring work outcomes in pain research is not uncommon. Recent pain research indicates that traditional outcome measures focusing on absenteeism substantially underestimate the lost productivity associated with pain and pain conditions. We contend pain researchers should measure the productivity losses associated with on-the-job decrements on work role performance, which are referred to as "presenteeism." Recommendations for pain researchers when assessing work outcomes are for them to consider labor force status, the time loss and time until return to work as well as health-related work role performance while at work. In this chapter, we review a range of presenteeism measures pain researchers can choose from. While no measure has extensive research supporting its use, several measures are based on a broad conceptualization of work, have good reliability and validity, have been shown to be related to independent economic data and are responsive to change.

Adapting a list from our earlier review, there are six reasons for measuring work outcomes in pain research (Amick et al. 2000):

- To assess productivity loss in clinical trials testing new pain medications or treatment protocols.
- To evaluate the effectiveness of health services targeting pain management and new treatment protocols for managing pain.
- To target injury and re-injury prevention programs reducing common pain conditions.
- To evaluate the effectiveness of work re-organization projects such as ergonomic changes to reduce musculoskeletal pain.
- To improve provider–worker and provider–safety engineer interaction to improve clinical and worksite management of persons with pain conditions.
- To inform policy discussions on the role of health and healthcare in business and global competitiveness.

In the most comprehensive US study, common pain conditions including headache, back pain, arthritis pain and musculoskeletal pain resulted in about 5 hours per week of lost productive time (Stewart et al. 2003a). Health-related lost productivity cost US employers US$61 billion per year. Over 75% of the loss was related to reduced performance while working and not work absence

(Stewart et al. 2003a). Blyth and colleagues (2003) found one-third of the full or part time workers in their community study reported one or more days absent due to chronic pain in the past six months. To their surprise, 97% reported working in pain and 60% of those working in pain reported pain reduced their work effectiveness. Even among those reporting no lost workdays, 50% reported reduced work effectiveness. Accordingly, the authors instructed pain researchers interested in capturing productivity loss and economic impact to assess health-related work role performance. Pain researchers interested in measuring work outcomes are confronted with a new intellectual landscape.

Work outcomes assessment has recently been subsumed within the new health and productivity movement (Mayne et al. 2004). Health and productivity has emerged as a new field of inquiry in public health integrating health and labor economics, health services research and occupational medicine (Edington and Burton 2003; Loeppke et al. 2003; Lofland et al. 2004; Ozminkowski et al. 2004; Prasad et al. 2004). Consequently, work outcomes researchers have shifted their measurement focus. Typically work outcomes measures would include days absent from work or days until return to work, job accommodation or light duty and/or lost productivity measured by workers' compensation, sick leave (sickness absence) and disability. As illustrated (Blyth et al. 2003), to capture the full work impact requires a broader approach that considers not only lost productivity associated with health-related absence from work, but also lost productivity at work ("presenteeism"). In this chapter, we present a review of the extent of health-related work performance measures and build on prior work (Amick et al. 2000) to suggest a series of work outcomes to measure in pain research.

Figure 20.1 guides our work outcomes perspective. Work role functioning (WRF) occupies a central place in the model. Business productivity is a direct result of work role functioning. WRF represents the latent concept typically of interest in work outcomes research, but often measured with a variety of indicators. WRF can be seen as a continuum that varies from working successfully (i.e., the ability to meet all work demands for a given state of health) to work absence (i.e., the inability to meet any work demand for a given health state). Examples of this part of the continuum are sickness absence and short-term and long-term sick leave (disability). Time until return to work is the flip side of being absent. Work role functioning is not independently determined by work demands and health, but rather by their joint influence. Practically, improving WRF requires changes in health and work as indicated by intersecting lines leading to WRF. Healthcare directly affects health status through pills and other medical treatments; directly affects work role functioning through prescribing absence or work modifications (e.g., light duty); and moderates the impact of demands and health on WRF by specifying health-related job accommodations (i.e., primarily changing work demands). Healthcare is determined by the societal

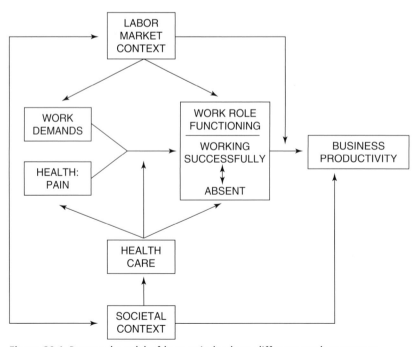

Figure 20.1 Proposed model of how pain leads to different work outcomes.

context through healthcare policy. Also, societal industrial and economic policy/regulations affect business productivity. Finally, the local labor market context (e.g., the industrial/occupational mix and economic development of the region) directly affects work demands; directly affects work role functioning (e.g., through sickness absence and workers' compensation regulations); and moderates the relationship between WRF and business productivity (e.g., through the relationship of the local economy to the global economy). Situating pain research in this broader model demonstrates the salience of the topic to society.

WHY FOCUS ON THE WORK ROLE?

Numerous quality of life measures have role functioning scales that capture a range of roles. For example, the SF-36 examines work and other usual activities. However, it is unclear when a person responds if the person is focused on the work or non-work (leisure time and household) roles or both. It is easy to imagine a worker with arthritis going to work and working with diminished effectiveness due to pain, but when returning home to not engage in leisure time or household activities because these activities don't contribute to the family income. Furthermore, the economic evaluation of these scales is less intuitive conceptually and practically. How do we value leisure time roles? Alternatively, work is a role intrinsically valued economically. Thus numerous instruments have emerged to capture the combined effects of not being at work – absenteeism – and being at work but not successfully meeting all work role demands – "presenteeism." These are often summed into a lost productivity estimate. The ability to provide an economic interpretation to pain research is a core reason for using work role-specific measures.

A second, more practical reason to focus on the work role is the limited utility of accumulating absences. As reported above (Stewart et al. 2003a,c), studies have found lost productivity related to pain or pain-related conditions mainly occurs when a person is working, not as a result of absences. In our earlier paper we reported similar findings from a clinical trial of sumatriptan (Adelman et al. 1996). Given the known validity and reliability issues associated with counting health-related absences (Johns 1994) and the above evidence, work outcomes research should emerge as a major element in pain research.

A third reason for considering health-related work role performance has to do with the translation of knowledge to practice. What if by using absenteeism measures instead of presenteeism measures different prevention targets are identified? In our research we have examined predictors of work absence (Katz et al. 2005) and health-related work role functioning (Amick et al. 2004) in a cohort of workers undergoing carpal tunnel surgery. At six month follow-up, baseline health-related work role functioning, improved self-efficacy and working in a supportive organization predicted successful health-related work role functioning. In contrast, having multiple pain sites, stable or declining self-efficacy, having an attorney involved in work injury and having low income predicted work absence at six months. Clearly, using work role functioning identifies healthcare (self-efficacy improvement) and the worksite (supportive organization) as points of intervention. These are identified in Figure 20.1. Work absence predictors were individual (pain sites and income), healthcare (self-efficacy) and the legal system (attorney). We are only beginning to learn about what predicts health-related work role performance, but the choice of focusing on the work role over nonparticipation in the work role leads to different prevention strategies.

GENERIC ROLE-SPECIFIC MEASUREMENT AS A NEW PARADIGM

Generic quality of life role functioning measures are useful for capturing total role burden, but not useful for specifically assessing pain's impact on work role performance. Consequently, we argued for a new class of measures, generic role-specific measures (Amick et al. 2000). What makes the measure generic is that it captures the meaningful diversity in the role, thus making the measure applicable to all individuals participating in the role. It implies a different development process where the role itself is conceptually described and measured rather than assembling a series of clinically relevant items and empirically identifying those that "hang together." There is a finite set of roles individuals participate in during their life. We have developed measures for four roles: work, college student, household and leisure time (Schmidt et al. 2002; Vidrine et al. 2004). To accomplish this for the work role requires development of a set of work demand questions representative of demands in the labor market. How a worker's health status affects the ability to meet these demands would then measure health-related work role performance.

There is no broad consensus on how to conceptualize the work role. In our own work (Amick et al. 2000; Lerner et al. 2001), we have considered five broad work dimensions:

- Physical demands: the range of dynamic and physical loads required to accomplish work.
- Social demands: the interaction demands of engaging both people in the workplace and clients.
- Psychological/cognitive demands: the cognitive demands associated with doing the work.

- Work scheduling/time management demands: the required demands to manage the workday from beginning to end.
- Output/production demands: the demands of completing work on time and with high quality to the satisfaction of supervisors and the respondent.

Without a clear conception of the work role, pain researchers run the risk of overestimating or underestimating pain's impact on work role performance. A unique challenge in work role measurement emerges: the need for short measures that captures the diversity of demands in the work role. For those seeking short measures, summary or overall estimates may be the best and simplest solution, but little evidence exists in support of simple measures and their use depends primarily on the research questions being answered.

HEALTH-RELATED WORK ROLE PERFORMANCE MEASURES

Numerous instruments have emerged measuring health-related work role performance and lost productivity. Pain researchers are challenged by the choices. We briefly review these measures (summarized in Table 20.1) and then discuss current issues in measuring work outcomes. We do not consider the scientific literature sufficiently populated with well-designed studies to recommend one instrument over another. Rather, we consider the measurement of health-related work role performance and lost productivity an advance in work outcomes measurement. The order of instrument description was chosen randomly and does not indicate any preference on the authors' part. Unlike prior reviews (Loeppke et al. 2003), we describe only instruments/measures published in peer-review journals.

Occupational Role Questionnaire (ORQ) (Kopec and Esdaile 1998). The ORQ assesses limitations in an individual's ability to perform the occupational role. The ORQ measures two aspects of working life: *job productivity* (works more slowly, cuts down on extra work, takes more frequent and longer rest breaks, is less able to concentrate) and *job satisfaction* (has less opportunity to upgrade skills, is more likely to lose job, is less satisfied, needs more help from co-workers). The 8 items are aggregated into a single summary measure with high internal consistency (alpha = 0.88), test–retest reliability (0.91), and predictive validity [correlates with the TyPE Low Back Pain Form ($r = -0.37$) and the Roland–Morris Disability Scale ($r = -0.51$)]. The ORQ was developed in 137 ambulatory subjects seeking professional help for back pain in Canada and is available in French. The questionnaire is in the public domain (Kopec and Esdaile 1998).

The ORQ presents five potential problems. First, whether the items reflect a robust conception of the work role required in generic work role-specific instruments is unclear. The scale captures job conditions, job attitudes, organizational practices (i.e., upgrade skills), and company performance (i.e., lose job). Second, using a population with back injuries for item selection could produce a measure of limited generalizability. Third, the respondent is asked to perform a complicated cognitive task requiring extensive recall and cognitive comparisons. The individual must translate the question into their work situation, assess the degree health interferes with the job, compare their current situation to past situations and endorse either "a lot," "somewhat," "a little," or "not at all." The recall period is not specified. Fourth, there exist no economic data supporting the ORQ as a measure of lost productivity. Fifth, there is no information on responsiveness to change.

Work Limitations Questionnaire (WLQ) (Lerner et al. 2001). The WLQ measures the on-the-job performance impact of chronic conditions and their treatment. The WLQ was developed from focus groups, cognitive interview and comparison of different versions in 277 employed patients with different chronic conditions. 25 items measure 4 dimensions: time management, physical demands, output demands and psychosocial demands, which combines mental demands and social demands. The response categories are the percentage of time a person has difficulty meeting the specific demand (all, most, some, a slight bit, none) over two weeks. In addition, a sixth category, "does not apply to my job," allows workers to answer each item faithfully. For ease of response, 100% is placed under "all the time," 50% under "some of the time" and 0% under "none of the time." An advantage of the percentage time response is that it provides an immediate economic translation.

The four WLQ scales have high reliability (alpha between 0.80 and 0.92) and were significantly related to the Short Form-36 Health Survey (SF-36) role limitations scales indicating high validity (Lerner et al. 2003). The WLQ has been used in samples with osteoarthritis (Lerner et al. 2002), depression (Lerner et al. 2004) and rheumatoid arthritis (Burton et al. 2004). Several WLQ scales (time management, physical job demands, and output demands) predict objectively measured productivity (measured as the log of units produced per hour) in call centre operators and material handlers (Lerner et al. 2003). Shorter versions of the WLQ have been used in the literature (Allen and Bunn 2003a,b; Allen et al. 2003; Bunn et al. 2003; Burton et al. 2004; Beaton and Kennedy 2005; Walker et al. 2005), but little research has been done supporting a short form. WLQ versions exist in English for USA and Canada, French for Canada, and Spanish for the USA. The WLQ questionnaire is available upon request to the authors (at www.benamick.com).

The WLQ has the advantage of being based on a robust conceptual model of work better ensuring its

Table 20.1 Characteristics of health and productivity measurement instruments

Title	Items	Response scale type	Recall period	Pain-related conditions studied	Summary score	Internal consistency/ reliability	Test-retest reliability	Construct validity*
ORQ	8	4-point scale (a lot, somewhat, a little, not at all)	Not specified	Back pain	Yes	0.82–0.88	0.80–0.91	Yes
WLQ	25	5-point frequency scale (all, most, some, slight/ bit, none, not part of job)	2 weeks	Osteoarthritis, arthritis, low back pain	Yes	0.88–0.91	NA	Yes
WL-26	26	5-point frequency scale (all, most, half, some, none, not part of job)	4 weeks	Musculoskeletal disorders	Yes	0.80–0.92	NA	Yes
WPAI	6–9[†]	Asking for the no. of hours or days and how much did health problems affect your regular daily activities or work (in an 11-point Likert scale)	1 week	Adaptable (see text for details)	Yes	0.69–0.95	NA	Yes (partial)
MWPLQ	29	Asking for the no. of hours or days and 7-point difficulty degree scale from "no difficulty" to "so much difficulty, couldn't do at all," not part of job	The most recent migraine headache	Migraine headache Angina pectoris	Yes	0.86–0.95	NA	Yes
MBQ	9	Varies with question (see text)	4 weeks/1 year	Migraine	Yes	NA	NA	NA
HRPQ-D	9	Asking for the no. of hours and percent effectiveness	1 day	None	Yes	NA	NA	Yes
WPSI	22	No. of hours/days experiencing the health problem, unproductive and missed	2 weeks/3 and 12 months	Arthritis, rheumatism, migraine	No	NA	0.66–0.74 (split sample)	Yes (partial)
SPS	6	5-point Likert scale	4 weeks	None, but adaptable	Yes	0.80	NA	Yes

(Continued)

Table 20.1 Characteristics of health and productivity measurement instruments—Cont'd

Title	Items	Response scale type	Recall period	Pain-related conditions studied	Summary score	Internal consistency/ reliability	Test–retest reliability	Construct validity*
EWPS	25	5-point frequency scale (from never to almost always)	1 week	None	Yes	0.80–0.93	0.92	Yes
HLQ	23	Varies with module	2 weeks	Migraine	Yes	NA	NA	Yes(partial)
HPQ	24	11-point Likert scale (from "worst" to "top" performance)	Present state, 4 weeks, 1 year	Arthritis, rheumatism, migraine, chronic pain, stomach ulcer	Yes	NA	NA	Yes
WHI	‡	Varies with item	2 weeks	Headache, arthritis, back pain, menstrual pain	Yes	NA	NA	Yes (partial)

*We used a dichotomous label (Yes/No) due to the great variability on the methods used to establish construct validity.

†Six items for the general questionnaire and up to 9 for the different specific health problem questionnaires.

‡The WHI is a 15-minute computer-assisted interview with skip patterns which may change the total number of items that are finally asked.

NA = not available.

relevance to the range of jobs in the economy, has data on economic interpretation, but has been used in a small number of chronic conditions and only data based on a very small sample (n=42) exists on responsiveness to change using a 16-item WLQ version (Beaton and Kennedy).

WL-26 (Amick et al. 2000). The WL-26 is grounded in the same conceptual framework and drew items from the same item pool as the WLQ. The WL-26 was originally designed for use in populations with occupational illnesses and injuries, but has been used in population and clinic samples with a particular emphasis on clinics managing a variety of musculoskeletal disorders (Amick et al. 2000). The WL-26 differs from the WLQ. The WL-26 uses a 4-week recall period rather than a 2-week recall period. A 4-week recall period was chosen since the range of work demands will typically be experienced over a monthly production cycle. The WL-26 conceptualizes the work role in five work demand categories disaggregating psychological and social demands. The WL-26 uses a single response set for all questions (i.e., difficulty meeting work demands compared to the WLQ which uses ability to meet demands for the physical demand questions). The WL-26 uses "half the time" as the middle category (50%) rather than "some of the time." Given the different response values and the inclusion of additional items there may be differences in scale performance, although no research has compared the two questionnaires. The WL-26 has been used to discriminate upper extremity functioning and hand-wrist severity in 298 workers. Preliminary data on its clinical utility has been obtained from 78 workers following a 2- to 3-month physical therapy course. The WL-26 questionnaire is available in the public domain (Amick et al. 2000) and recently a Canadian French version has been developed (Durand et al. 2005). A shorter 15-item version designed as a summary measure (alpha = 0.91) has been used in several recent studies to predict return to work and work role functioning in a sample of workers undergoing carpal tunnel release surgery (Amick et al. 2004; Gimeno et al. 2005; Katz et al. 2005). These data showed that the WL-26 is responsive to change, but the short version only intended to create a summary score. Therefore, further research should be done to corroborate this finding.

Like the WLQ, the WL-26 is based on a broad work model of work. The instrument has been used in populations with musculoskeletal injuries, workers' compensation claimants and for other occupational illnesses. Small amounts of data exist on responsiveness to change, but no data exist on economic interpretation of scale scores.

Work Productivity and Activity Impairment Instrument (WPAI) (Reilly et al. 1993, 1996). The WPAI questionnaire was developed to measure general health and symptom severity effects on work productivity and regular activities. The WPAI asks 6 questions about time worked, lost work time, reduced performance while at work and the extent work impairment limited individual work and reduced performance while doing regular daily activities (housework, schoolwork, and leisure) during the previous 7 days. An overall work productivity score can be computed by multiplying time worked in the past week by effectiveness while working.

There is a generic version of the WPAI (WPAI-GH) to measure the impact of general health status on productivity and four different versions for specific health problems. Specific WPAI questionnaires exist for: patients with gastro-esophageal reflux disease symptoms (WPAI-GERD) (Wahlqvist et al. 2002), patients with allergies (WPAI-AS) (Murray et al. 2002), subjects with chronic obstructive pulmonary disease (WPAI-COPD) (Stahl et al. 2003), and chronic hand dermatitis (WPAI-ChHD) (Reilly et al. 2003) and irritable bowel syndrome (Dean et al. 2005), as well as many other health problems (see: http://www.reillyassociates.net). The generic WPAI could be adapted by pain researchers substituting the term "pain" or "chronic pain condition" for the term "problem." Recently, the recall period was changed to 4 weeks to assess productivity losses related to the common cold (Bramley et al. 2002). Such changes limit comparability across studies. The authors advise against using the WPAI for systemic diseases and complicated conditions. More details can be obtained at http://www.reillyassociates.net (accessed June 12, 2007).

Two WPAI-GH versions, self-administered and interviewer administered, were fielded in 106 subjects who reported a symptom or health problem during the past 7 days. The interview versions performed better on most psychometric tests. While WPAI scores correlated positively with SF-36 role functioning and symptom severity measures, the strength and variability in correlations suggest further psychometric testing. Again, the lack of sample representativeness raises questions of generalizability. US Spanish and Brazilian Portuguese versions have been published (Gawlicki et al. 2006; Ciconnelli et al. 2006).

The WPAI is based on a limited conceptualization of work and has multiple versions for use in different populations. There is limited data on economic interpretation or responsiveness to change (Wahlqvist et al. 2007).

Migraine Work and Productivity Loss Questionnaire (MWPLQ) (Davies et al. 1999; Lerner et al. 1999; Dasbach et al. 2000). The MWPLQ is an early version of the WLQ developed specifically for migraines. Like the WLQ, the MWPLQ development was initiated with a thorough work role conceptualization with specific content areas refined through focus groups ($n = 18$) and telephone interviews ($n = 144$). All work was done in migraineurs assessing the impact of an acute migraine attack and its treatment on a person's ability to perform paid work.

The MWPLQ captures both absenteeism and presenteeism regarding the most recent migraine headache. Three items ask about the name of the job and the main things to do, hours worked per week in the main job and, if it is the case, hours worked per week in a second job. A skip question asks people not working for pay during the migraine headache or its treatment. Five questions ask about work time (in hours) loss because of migraine or migraine treatment, before and after initial dose, and time worked while having symptoms during the entire migraine episode. On-the-job difficulty performing work (presenteeism) is assessed with 18 items covering seven domains: time management, work quality, work quantity, bodily effort, interpersonal demands, mental effort, and environmental factors. In addition, to capture the difficulty experienced on all work-related tasks a global question is asked. Difficulty items use a 6-point degree of difficulty scale from "no difficulty" to "so much difficulty couldn't do it at all." A "does not apply to my work" option is provided to allow subjects to opt out of items not relevant to their jobs. In addition, subjects are asked to rate their on-the-job percent effectiveness during the entire time period the migraine lasted. A total on-the-job work loss score can be computed by adding the worked paid hours missed and $(100 - \%$ effectiveness$/100) \times$ hours worked with migraine.

The MWPLQ has been shown to be valid to capture work loss and difficulty in 164 migraineurs patients of a triple-blind placebo-controlled randomized clinical trial (Davies et al. 1999). The difficulty domains had high reliability (alpha between 0.86 and 0.95). The correlations between these domains and the 24-h Migraine Quality of Life Questionnaire (MQoLQ) were between -0.31 and -0.65 and with the SF-36 were between -0.11 and -0.29. The global work difficulty question is highly correlated with the difficulty domains (all $r > 0.70$), with the MQoLQ domains (-0.41 to -0.58) and correlates low with the SF-36 (-0.13). The authors suggested this global question might be sufficient to capture the overall effect, although the specific domains give a more complete view of the migraine's impact on work difficulty. A similar questionnaire has been developed for chronic stable angina pectoris (Lerner et al. 1998). The questionnaire is in the public domain (Davies et al. 1999).

The MWPLQ is based on a broad conceptualization of work, but has only been used among migraineurs and has no data on economic interpretation or responsiveness to change.

Migraine Background Questionnaire (MBQ) (Gerth et al. 2001). The MBQ was developed to assess the economic burden of migraine-associated illness. The MBQ follows the Osterhaus method (Osterhaus et al. 1992) to capture information on migraine presence (migraine frequency, days worked with migraine, hours worked negatively affected by migraine, percent effectiveness of working with migraine, missed work days (paid and unpaid) because of migraine) and healthcare resource utilization (emergency treatment, medical visits, and hospitalizations). Some questions have a recall period of 4 weeks, while for others it is 12 months. A score

on the total hours of work loss is computed similarly to the WPAI and the MWPLQ.

The development process included a test within 25 countries over Europe, Latin and North America, and other regions, comprising more than 2600 clinic-based patients. Only one other study used the MBQ, a clinical trial of a migraine therapy drug in 134 patients in Canada (Lambert et al. 2002). However, in both studies psychometric data regarding reliability or validity is not provided, and results have to be taken with caution. Study sample selection methods may cause the sample not to be representative of all migraineur patients.

The MBQ is not based on a broad conceptualization of work and has only been used among migraineurs. There is not data available on economic interpretation or responsiveness to change.

Health-Related Productivity Questionnaire Diary (HRPQ-D) (Kumar et al. 2003). The HRPQ-D was designed to capture data on premature retirement or reduction from full to part-time, planned and missed paid and unpaid work hours and classes (for students), and the health-related impact on effectiveness. Presenteeism is calculated using the number of planned and missed hours.

Three main concerns apply to this instrument regarding its generalizability: first, it was developed in Parkinson's disease patients using focus groups; second, it has been used only in one study with 43 young school-going patients with mononucleosis within the USA; third, the HRPQ-D overall productivity measure showed a moderate correlation with symptoms scores ($r = 0.58$), but high variability when considering individual productivity scores. Therefore, much work needs to be done to provide users with reliability and validity information. The diary version questionnaire is in the public domain (Kumar et al. 2003).

The HRPQ-D is not based on a broad conceptualization of work and has only been used in several disease groups. There are no data available on economic interpretation or responsiveness to change.

Work Productivity Short Inventory (WPSI) (Goetzel et al. 2003a; Ozminkowski et al. 2003). The WPSI was developed to assess the economic impact of health-related on-the-job and off-the-job productivity losses. It assesses productivity loss associated with 15 common medical conditions identified through literature review, contacting employers and physicians. Eleven of the 15 health problems refer to respondents' health conditions while 4 request data on the impact of providing care to relatives, both children and elders. Thus, the WPSI targets specific medical conditions where interventions potentially yield the greatest overall cost saving opportunities.

Three versions varying in recall period (2 weeks, 3 and 12 months) were tested in 212 subjects reporting whether they experienced the health problem and whether the health problem has impacted absenteeism and presenteeism. Financial (or "dollar") metrics for each health problem (summing costs related to absenteeism and presenteeism) were created taking into account the estimated average hourly employee compensation (Goetzel et al. 2001). Reliability analyses did not indicate whether one recall period performed better. The WPSI evidence for construct and predictive validity is inconclusive. Correlation between self-reported general health status and absenteeism and presenteeism were unclear and evidence for construct validity was mixed. The WPSI is also referred to as the Wellness Inventory Survey and it is in the public domain (Goetzel et al. 2003a).

The WPSI is not based on a broad conceptualization of work, but is designed to examine a range of health conditions (Lamb et al. 2006). Data exist on economic interpretation, but no data exist in responsiveness to change.

Stanford Presenteeism Scale (SPS) (Koopman et al. 2002). The SPS instrument was developed to measure the impact of health problems on workers' performance and productivity at work. Presenteeism is conceptualized as a health-related decrease in functioning while at work during the last month. The SPS captures two domains of presenteeism: *work focus* or process outcome and *psychological focus* or the cognitive, emotional and behavioral engagement.

The first version of the SPS included 32 items (SPS-32) (Lynch and Riedel 2001), and after an item-reduction strategy a six-item scale remained (SPS-6). A total presenteeism score can be computed by summing the six items. Respondents are asked to express their agreement with each statement on a 5-point Likert scale. The SPS-6 psychometric properties were tested in 175 municipal employees. Reliability was high (alpha = 0.80) and validity analyses showed a high correlation with other self-reported work productivity measures ($r = 0.47$ and $r = 0.53$), job satisfaction ($r = 0.15$) and job stress ($r = -0.22$). The SPS-6 is in the public domain (Koopman et al. 2002). A Japanese version has been developed (Wada et al. 2007).

The SPS-6 shortness is an advantage in studies where lost productivity is a secondary objective. But it has not been used in studies of pain conditions and therefore it is unclear whether it could be widely applicable in pain research. Testing in a white-collar population may not make the instrument generalizable to blue-collar populations. Moreover, some relevant information such as the number of worked hours or hours absent are not asked, making it difficult to estimate total lost productive time. The SPS-6 is not based on a broad conceptualization of work, but is designed for use in general populations. Data do not exist on economic interpretation or responsiveness to change.

Endicott Work Productivity Scale (EWPS) (Endicott and Nee 1997). The EWPS assesses the degree a medical condition affects the individual's work functioning. Only sample items of the English version can be found in the public domain (Endicott and Nee

1997) although a full version in Turkish language has been published (Uguz et al. 2004). The EWPS includes 25 items assessing the work impact of a range of mental and medical disorders. Respondents are asked to rate on a 5-point frequency scale (from never to almost always) the presence of a behavior, feeling or attitude during the last week. In addition, questions regarding the number of planned work hours, the number of worked hours and the reasons for working less than planned are asked. The EWPS was developed in 110 outpatients seeking major depression treatment and community subjects. Reliability was very good (ICC = 0.92, and alpha = 0.93 for the patient sample and alpha = 0.80 for the nonpatient sample). Correlations with several illness severity measures (HAM-D, SCL-90 and Global Clinical Index of Severity) were between 0.27 and 0.61 demonstrating predictive validity. Since development, the instrument has been used only in one more study to evaluate the economic impact of premenstrual syndrome (Borenstein et al. 2003). Consequently, much work is needed to assess the instrument's properties and relevance for pain researchers.

The EWPS is not based on a broad conceptualization of work. It has been used in a small number of populations, but no studies with pain populations. Data do not exist on economic interpretation or responsiveness to change.

Health and Labor Questionnaire (HLQ) (van Roijen et al. 1996). The HLQ was developed to collect quantitative data on the relationship between illness, treatment and work performance over the past two weeks and to estimate economic production losses. The HLQ has 23 items divided in 4 modules: (1) absence from paid work, (2) productivity reduced at paid work, (3) unpaid production, and (4) impediments to paid and unpaid work. Summed scores for each module are obtained. In module 2, the respondent estimates the number of additional hours they should work to compensate for production losses due to sickness absence on seven items (concentration, working, work pace, need to be alone, decision making, work postponement, and taking over work by other workers) with a 4-point frequency response scale (from never to always).

The HLQ has been applied in several studies, some of them unpublished (van Roijen et al. 1995), involving: a representative general population sample ($n = 667$), a migraineur sample ($n = 846$), a spinal cord injury sample ($n = 44$), a sample of patients waiting for hip or knee surgery ($n = 107$) and a diabetes mellitus sample (Lavigne et al. 2003). The reliability (response rates ranging from 58% to 81%, missing values from 5% to 11%, 10 minutes for completion, and respondents' remarks on the questionnaire) and validity (for modules 1 and 3 results were consistent with available national data; for module 2 a comparison with lost productivity estimates) results have limited utility for psychometric interpretation. Recent research has shown moderate construct validity in relation to general physical and mental health measures

(Meerding et al. 2005). The same study based on a sample of industrial and construction workers found the HLQ not to be applicable to low educated population or jobs that do not allow catching up on backlogs. The HLQ is available in Dutch and English upon request (van Roijen et al. 1996).

The HLQ is not based on a broad conceptualization of work, but covers a range of work tasks and activities. The HLQ has been used in a range of clinical populations. There is no information on the correspondence of the role performance measure with economic data and no information on responsiveness to change.

Health and Work Performance Questionnaire (HPQ) (Kessler et al. 2003). The HPQ was developed by the World Health Organization (WHO) as part of the WHO Composite International Diagnostic Interview. The HPQ focuses on the global impact of health on different aspects of the work role: work performance, work absence, and critical incidents (i.e., work-related accidents, special work successes and failures). The HPQ has three sections on health, work and demographics. In the health section subjects are asked to rate their overall and mental health, and the experience of several common health-related conditions (and if they are being treated), health professional visits, and hospitalizations. The work section includes questions on occupation, supervisory tasks, work quantity (expected work hours, missed days according to different reasons), work quality (subjects have to make a complex cognitive task by rating their own and their co-workers' overall work performance, a frequency assessment of various situations implying reduced performance and to rate their usual performance with their past performance, and with co-workers) and critical incidents. Different recall periods are used ranging from present state, past 4 weeks (most commonly used) and past year. An international data consortium and coordination center has been created to facilitate the collection, analysis and comparison of studies using the HPQ. The WHO is carrying out nationally representative surveys in over 30 countries covering around 250,000 interviews.

The HPQ self-reported work performance and work absence measures have been tested against administrative records in four different occupation samples ($N = 2350$). Results show good concordance between self-reported and company absence records (Wang et al. 2003). Response rates varied between 30% and 57% but the researchers argue the large samples mitigate bias. The HPQ has been shown to correlate with a range of independent economic performance outcomes (Kessler et al. 2004). The HPQ has very good reliability, validity and sensitivity to change. However, indicators used were uncommon for questionnaire development, which limits psychometric interpretation (Kessler et al. 2004). Different versions of the HPQ, including two clinical trial versions and an internet-based version, are available at http://www.hcp.med.harvard.edu/hpq (accessed June 21, 2007).

The HPQ is not based on a broad conceptualization of work. It has been used in a wide range of populations and disorders (see Kessler et al. 2005), and has been shown to correspond to economic information. Responsive to change data is presented, but further studies on responsiveness are needed.

Work and Health Interview (WHI) (Stewart et al. 2003a, 2004). The WHI is a computer-assisted telephone interview developed to measure lost productive work time during the last two weeks related to 22 specific health conditions. Among six different versions, a version with a two-week recall period was selected based on the optimal balance between over and under-reporting bias. The WHI consists of 8 modules: informed consent, occupational status, maternity/disability leave, health assessment, job tasks, lost productive work time, lifestyle and demographics. The lost productive work time module measures both absenteeism, as the sum of missed workdays and reduced work hours on workdays (i.e., late start, early departure, or missed time while at work), and presenteeism, as reduced work performance. Presenteeism scales included five questions on how often, on average, the worker lost concentration, has repeated a job, worked more slowly than usual, felt fatigued at work, and did nothing at work on days not feeling well. A sixth question asked to rate the average time it took to start working on days not feeling well. A presenteeism score is computed as the average percentage of lost productive time (Stewart et al. 2004).

The WHI lost productive time scores have been compared with real-time electronic data for 196 customer-service employees. Pearson's correlations were 0.54 for total productive time and 0.86 for total missed hours indicating the WHI is a valid estimator of lost productive time. In addition, the correlation with independent productivity measures was high ($r = 0.46$).

The WHI has been used in the American Productivity Audit (APA), which captures a large nationally representative US workforce sample of almost 29,000 workers. Initial findings about depression (Stewart et al. 2003b) and common pain conditions (Stewart et al. 2003c) and pain exacerbation (Ricci et al. 2005; 2006) have been published. The WHI is available by request from the authors (Stewart et al. 2003c).

The WHI was not based on a broad conceptualization of work, but has been used in a wide range of populations. While correspondence with independent economic data is available, no data is presented on responsiveness to change.

SELECTED ISSUES IN HEALTH-RELATED WORK ROLE PERFORMANCE MEASUREMENT

Overall, many of the reviewed instruments have proved to be applicable across many health problems as well as across many occupations. A few are applicable across different countries. Pain researchers reading the above descriptions recognize the measurement of health-related work performance research is at an early stage. Instruments differ in the occupational populations and health conditions sampled, scale length and content, and recall periods. In many cases, small samples have been used to test the questionnaire's psychometric properties. Several instruments focus on specific health conditions or a list of common health disorders, but they seem to be adaptable to other health conditions. Studies considering the performance of multiple instruments would advance the field. Moreover, for prevention more knowledge about whether the measures can detect changes over time is needed.

The issue of responsiveness to change is critical for pain researchers. Few interventions have been done using these health-related work role performance measures. Figure 20.2 shows data from our prospective study of workers undergoing carpal tunnel surgery (Amick et al. 2004; Gimeno et al. 2005; Katz et al. 2005). In this figure we compare baseline work role functioning to functioning at 6 months post carpal tunnel surgery. Work role functioning in this sample is measured with a reduced WL-26 and varies from 0 (absent from work) to 100 (able to meet all job demands given the worker's health). The population is divided into three groups. In the "working well" group workers had to report a baseline work role functioning (WRF) score greater than or equal to 90. For the "working hurt" group, baseline WRF scores varied from 75 to 89. Finally the "working injured" group had baseline WRF scores less than 75. To understand how to interpret the WRF values let's consider the working injured group average baseline score of

58. A score of 58 means that almost 50% of the time (one half a work week) a worker cannot meet the demands of his or her job because of health.

There are several observations to make about Figure 20.2. First, not all workers respond equally to carpal tunnel surgery. Workers who were "working well" before surgery do not change with surgery. However, the "working injured" improved by 20 points or the equivalent of one working day. Simply, carpal tunnel surgery improved work role performance one full day. Given where you start affects where you end up, pain researchers should take care when presenting cross-sectional or retrospective data on change. Additionally, even in prospective designs baseline levels need to be considered. The second obvious point is that WRF identifies groups that may benefit more from either healthcare or worksite prevention activities. An open question is whether this is true of other pain conditions or among chronic pain patients.

All the measures presented use self-report data on work performance. Reliability and validity of some of the reviewed measures are unclear and more research is strongly needed (Mattke et al. 2007). The generalized perception among health professionals and many researchers and managers that individuals cannot give a reliable evaluation of their own health status is a common myth. Rather, we consider it important to continue to do research examining the construct validity of self-reported measures. A more fundamental question is, does the measure capture the information it is hypothesized to have measured?

Another approach is to capture productivity and health data from unobtrusive measures (e.g., electronic performance measurement systems and health claims

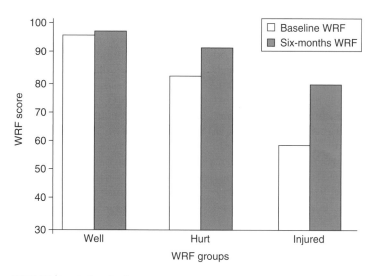

WRF: Work role functioning

Figure 20.2 Work outcomes following carpal tunnel surgery: a comparison of baseline and six-month postsurgery work role functioning.

systems) and then look at the correspondence between health claims and productivity to develop estimates of health-related lost productivity. An example is the Worker Productivity Index (WPI). The WPI consists of two lost productivity measures: time away from the job because of illness, including scattered illness and short-term disability absences; and time lost because of a failure to maintain the department's productivity standard, a measure of presenteeism (see Burton et al. 2001). The WPI was developed in "First Card," a major US credit card company where the data used to calculate the WPI is collected via the information system for customer service employees. Employee productivity and quality are measured in two ways: (1) supervisors monitor randomly selected calls for the correctness of the information provided by the employees, as well as their interpersonal skills, and (2) a computer-based system that automatically registers task-related time variables. Since the employee "logs off" the system when leaving the workstation, work time is directly measured. Generalization of the WPI approach to other workplaces and jobs seems difficult. Nevertheless, research should include studies of the relationship of self-reports to unobtrusive performance and productivity measures and to using the self-reported measures in intervention studies observing predicted changes.

While Figure 20.1 shows a direct relationship between work role functioning and business productivity, the relationship is not perfect. Pain researchers need to prevent work outcome measures from being used to "blame the worker" as a poor performer. Business productivity is more than simply the sum of work role functioning measures for all individuals. For example, teams and teamwork create production buffers against performance decrements. Work role functioning is just one indicator among a range of indicators that inform decision makers on business productivity.

Instead, we see work role functioning measures as tools to help in the management of health and work organization. As Figure 20.1 shows, healthcare research can affect work role functioning through three pathways. Similarly, work demands can be modified through an occupational safety and health intervention. DeRango et al. (2003) have shown that one-third of the impact of an ergonomic intervention on health is through pain reductions. Therefore, investing in health improvement is more than simply an investment in healthcare for employers (Shamansky 2002; Goetzel et al. 2003b).

Furthermore, not all work-role functioning measurement will lead to the same prevention strategies. In our presentation of data from the worker cohort undergoing carpal tunnel surgery we showed that the type of prevention activities identified changes if a researcher uses work absence versus a health-related work role performance measure. Work role performance measurement focuses prevention on both the worksite and the healthcare system. This creates intellectual challenges in synthesizing

research and in making recommendations on how to translate knowledge into practice.

Perhaps the most important observation to make about the instruments described above is that the majority were developed in the USA. Only a few instruments are in languages other than English. As Figure 20.1 shows, societal context affects work role functioning through healthcare and the labor market context. Given the unique nature of the US healthcare system and labor market, we caution pain researchers in assuming instruments are generalizable to other international labor markets. Translational research by pain researchers is an important intermediate step.

While presenteeism is being discussed in the European Union (EU) (Aronsson et al. 2005), the majority of the EU research community has used sickness absence as a major economic indicator of disease burden (Kristensen 1991; Marmot et al. 1995; Kivimaki et al. 2003). Presenteeism is used particularly in relation to job insecurity, to explain why workers with temporary contracts had less sickness absence than their counterparts in permanent contracts (Virtanen et al. 2003; Gimeno et al. 2004), but studies of productivity consequences are lacking. A central theme of this chapter is the need to capture the productivity consequences of working while ill. The simple number of days away from work gives only a partial lost productivity estimate. Most health-related productivity reductions appear to occur while workers are at work, not absent from work.

Finally, we return to Figure 20.1 and remind pain researchers that the determinants of work role functioning are multifactorial. Companies vary according to the prevalence of specific health conditions in their workplace and the product they produce or the services they provide. The sickness benefits a worker receives, supervisor or co-worker pressure to attend work, the amount of job responsibility, organizational policies and practices, or labor market regulations may affect the presence and extent of absenteeism and presenteeism in an organization.

CONCLUSION

Following our earlier consensus work (Amick et al. 2000), we recommend that pain researchers consider the following measures when trying to assess work outcomes. First, labor force status (i.e., employed in usual job, does light duty or placed on restricted work assignment, on paid, sick or unpaid leave, is unemployed because of a health problem, a student, a homemaker, or receiving disability). Labor force status should be assessed at least at two meaningful points such as first clinic visit and last clinic visit. Second, the time loss (e.g., sickness absence) and time until return to work are important to capture. Such data can often be collected from the worker, employer, insurer or social security agency. However, many workers in pain experience no time loss and thus we strongly recommend capturing health-related work role performance. The completeness of any work outcomes assessment depends on the research questions and other competing demands placed on the respondent.

REFERENCES

Adelman JU, Sharfman M, Johnson R, et al. Impact of oral sumatriptan on workplace productivity, health-related quality of life, health care use, and patient satisfaction with medication in nurses with migraine. Am J Managed Care 1996; 10:1407–1416.

Allen HM, Bunn WB. Using self-report and adverse event measures to track health's impact on productivity in known groups. J Occup Environ Med 2003a; 45:973–983.

Allen HM, Bunn WB. Validating self-reported measures of productivity at work: a case for their credibility in a heavy manufacturing setting. J Occup Environ Med 2003b; 45:926–940.

Allen HM, Borden SIV, Pikelny DB, et al. An intervention to promote appropriate management of allergies in a heavy manufacturing workforce: evaluating health and productivity outcomes. J Occup Environ Med 2003; 45:956–972.

Amick BC III, Lerner D, Rogers WH, et al. A review of health-related work outcome measures and their uses, and recommended measures. Spine 2000; 25:3152–3160.

Amick BC III, Habeck RV, Ossmann J, et al. Predictors of successful work role functioning after carpal tunnel release surgery. J Occup Environ Med 2004; 46:490–500.

Aronsson G, Gustafsson K. Sickness presenteeism: prevalence, attendance-pressure factors, and an outline of a model for research. J Occup Environ Med 2005; 47:958–966.

Beaton DE, Kennedy CA. Beyond return to work: testing a measure of at-work disability in workers with musculoskeletal pain. Qual Life Res 2005; 14:1869–1879.

Blyth FM, March LM, Cousins MJ. Chronic pain-related disability and use of analgesia and health services in a Sydney community. Med J Australia 2003; 179:84–87.

Borenstein JE, Dean BB, Endicott J, et al. Health and economic impact of the premenstrual syndrome. J Reprod Med 2003; 48:515–524.

Bramley TJ, Lerner D, Sarnes M. Productivity losses related to the common cold. J Occup Environ Med 2002; 44:822–829.

Burton WN, Conti DJ, Chen CY, et al. The impact of allergies and allergy treatment on worker productivity. J Occup Environ Med 2001; 43:64–71.

Burton WN, Chen CY, Conti DJ, et al. Caregiving for ill dependents and its association with employee health risks and productivity. J Occup Environ Med 2004; 46:1048–1056.

Bunn WB, Pikelny DB, Paralkar S, et al. The burden of allergies – and the capacity of medications to reduce this burden – in a heavy manufacturing environment. J Occup Environ Med 2003; 45:941–955.

Burton WN, Pransky G, Conti DJ, et al. The association of medical conditions and presenteeism. J Occup Environ Med 2004; 46:S38–S45.

Ciconelli RM, Soarez PC, Kowalski CC, et al. The Brazilian Portuguese version of the Work Productivity and Activity Impairment: General Health (WPAI-GH) Questionnaire. Sao Paulo Med J 2006; 124(6):325–332.

Dasbach EJ, Carides GW, Gerth WC, et al. Work and productivity loss in the rizatriptan multiple attack study. Cephalalgia 2000; 20:830–834.

Davies GM, Santanello N, Gerth W, et al. Validation of a migraine work and productivity loss questionnaire for use in migraine studies. Cephalalgia 1999; 19:497–502.

Dean BB, Aguilar D, Barghout V, et al. Impairment in work productivity and health-related quality of life in patients with IBS. Am J Manag Care 2005(1 Suppl):S17–S26.

DeRango K, Amick BC III, Robertson M, et al. The Productivity Consequences of Two Ergonomic Interventions. Rep. No. Working Paper 286. Toronto, Canada, 2003.

Edington DW, Burton WN. Health and productivity. In McCunney RJ (ed). A Practical Approach to Occupational and Environmental Medicine, 3rd edn. Lippincott Williams and Wilkins, Philadelphia, PA, 2003.

Endicott J, Nee J. Endicott Work Productivity Scale (EWPS): a new measure to assess treatment effects. Psychopharmacol Bull 1997; 33:13–16.

Gawlicki MC, Reilly MC, Popielnicki A, et al. Linguistic validation of the US Spanish work productivity and activity impairment questionnaire, general health version. Value Health 2006; 9(3):199–204.

Gerth WC, Carides GW, Dasbach EJ, et al. The multinational impact of migraine symptoms on healthcare utilisation and work loss. Pharmacoeconomics 2001; 19:197–206.

Gimeno D, Benavides FG, Amick BC III, et al. Psychosocial factors and work related sickness absence among permanent and non-permanent employees. J Epidemiol Community Health 2004; 58:870–876.

Gimeno D, Amick BC III, Habeck RV, et al. The role of job strain on return to work after carpal tunnel surgery. J Occup Environ Med 2005; 62:778–785.

Goetzel RZ, Guindon AM, Turshen IJ, et al. Health and productivity management: establishing key performance measures, benchmarks, and best practices. J Occup Environ Med 2001; 43:10–17.

Goetzel RZ, Ozminkowski RJ, Long SR. Development and reliability analysis of the Work Productivity Short Inventory (WPSI) instrument measuring employee health and productivity. J Occup Environ Med 2003a; 45:743–762.

Goetzel RZ, Hawkins K, Ozminkowski RJ, et al. The health and productivity cost burden of the "top 10" physical and mental health conditions affecting six large US employers in 1999. J Occup Environ Med 2003b; 45:5–14.

Johns G. Absenteeism estimates by employees and managers: divergent perspectives and self-serving perceptions. J Appl Psychol 1994; 79:229–239.

Katz JN, Amick BC III, Keller R, et al. Determinants of work absence following surgery for carpal tunnel syndrome. Am J Ind Med 2005; 47(2):120–130.

Kessler RC, Adler L, Ames M, et al. The prevalence and effects of adult attention deficit/hyperactivity disorder on work performance in a nationally representative sample of workers. J Occup Environ Med 2005; 47:565–572.

Kessler RC, Barber C, Beck A, et al. The world health organization health and work performance questionnaire (HPQ). J Occup Environ Med 2003; 45:156–174.

Kessler RC, Ames M, Hymel PA, et al. Using the World Health Organization Health and Work Performance Questionnaire (HPQ) to evaluate the indirect workplace costs of illness. J Occup Environ Med 2004; 46:S23–S37.

Kivimaki M, Head J, Ferrie JE, et al. Sickness absence as a global measure of health: evidence from mortality in the Whitehall II prospective cohort study. Br Med J 2003; 327:364–368.

Koopman C, Pelletier KR, Murray JF, et al. Stanford presenteeism scale: health status and employee productivity. J Occup Environ Med 2002; 44:14–20.

Kopec JA, Esdaile JM. Occupational role performance in persons with back pain. Disability Rehabil 1998; 20:373–379.

Kristensen TS. Sickness absence and work strain among Danish slaughterhouse workers: an analysis of absence from work regarded as coping behavior. Social Sci Med 1991; 32:15–27.

Kumar RN, Hass SL, Li JZM, et al. Validation of the Health-Related Productivity Questionnaire Diary (HRPQ-D) on a sample of patients with infectious mononucleosis: results from a phase 1 multicenter clinical trial. J Occup Environ Med 2003; 45:899–907.

Lamb CE, Ratner PH, Johnson CE, et al. Economic impact of workplace productivity losses due to allergic rhinitis compared with select medical conditions in the United States from an employer perspective. Curr Med Res Opin 2006; 22:1203–1210.

Lambert J, Carides GW, Meloche JP, et al. Impact of migraine symptoms on health care use and work loss in Canada in patients randomly assigned in a phase III clinical trial. Canad J Clin Pharmacol 2002; 9:158–164.

Lavigne JE, Phelps CE, Mushlin A, et al. Reductions in individual work productivity associated with type 2 diabetes mellitus. Pharmacoeconomics 2003; 21:1123–1134.

Lerner DJ, Amick BC III, Malspeis S, et al. The Angina-related Limitations at Work Questionnaire. Quality Life Res 1998; 7:23–32.

Lerner DJ, Amick BC III, Malspeis S, et al. The migraine work and productivity loss questionnaire: concepts and design. Quality Life Res 1999; 8:699–710.

Lerner D, Amick BC III, Rogers WH, et al. The Work Limitations Questionnaire. Med Care 2001; 39:72–85.

Lerner D, Reed JI, Massarotti E, et al. The Work Limitations Questionnaire's validity and reliability among patients with osteoarthritis. J Clin Epidemiol 2002; 55:197–208.

Lerner D, Amick BC III, Lee JC, et al. Relationship of employee-reported work limitations to work productivity. Med Care 2003; 41:649–659.

Lerner D, Adler DA, Chang H, et al. The clinical and occupational correlates of work productivity loss among employed patients with depression. J Occup Environ Med 2004; 46:S46–S55.

Loeppke R, Hymel PA, Lofland JH, et al. Health-related workplace productivity measurement: general and migraine-specific recommendations from the ACOEM expert panel. J Occup Environ Med 2003; 45:349–359.

Lofland JH, Pizzi L, Frick KD. A review of health-related workplace productivity loss instruments. Pharmacoeconomics 2004; 22:165–184.

Lynch W, Riedel J. Measuring Employee Productivity. A Guide to Self-Assessment Tools. William M Mercer and Institute for Health and Productivity Management, Phoenix and Scottdale, AZ, 2001.

Marmot M, Feeney A, Shipley M, et al. Sickness absence as a measure of health-status and functioning: from the UK Whitehall-Study. J Epidemiol Community Health 1995; 49:124–130.

Mattke S, Balakrishnan A, Bergamo G, et al. A review of methods to measure health-related productivity loss. Am J Manag Care 2007; 13:211–217.

Mayne TJ, Howard K, Brandt-Rauf PW. Measuring and evaluating the effects of disease on workplace productivity [supplement introduction]. J Occup Environ Med 2004; 46:S1–S2.

Meerding WJ, IJzelenberg W, Koopmanschap MA, et al. Health problems lead to considerable productivity loss at work among workers with high physical load jobs. J Clin Epidemiol 2005; 58(5):517–523.

Murray JJ, Nathan RA, Bronsky EA, et al. Comprehensive evaluation of cetirizine in the management of seasonal allergic rhinitis: impact on symptoms, quality of life, productivity, and activity impairment. Allergy Asthma Proc 2002; 23:391–398.

Osterhaus JT, Gutterman DL, Plachetka JR. Healthcare resource and lost labour costs of migraine headache in the US. Pharmacoeconomics 1992; 2:67–76.

Ozminkowski RJ, Goetzel RZ, Long SR. A validity analysis of the work productivity short inventory (WPSI) instrument measuring employee health and productivity. J Occup Environ Med 2003; 45:1183–1195.

Ozminkowski RJ, Goetzel RZ, Chang S, et al. The application of two health and productivity instruments at a large employer. J Occup Environ Med 2004; 46:635–648.

Prasad M, Wahlqvist P, Shikiar R, et al. A review of self-report instruments measuring health-related work productivity: a patient-reported outcomes perspective. Pharmacoeconomics 2004; 22:225–244.

Reilly MC, Zbrozek AS, Dukes EM. The validity and reproducibility of a work productivity and activity impairment instrument. Pharmacoeconomics 1993; 4:353–365.

Reilly MC, Tanner A, Meltzer EO. Work, classroom and activity impairment instruments: validation studies in allergic rhinitis. Clin Drug Invest 1996; 11:278–288.

Reilly MC, Lavin PT, Kahler KH, et al. Validation of the Dermatology Life Quality Index and the work productivity and activity impairment-chronic hand dermatitis, questionnaire in chronic hand dermatitis. J Am Acad Dermatol 2003; 48:128–130.

Ricci JA, Stewart WF, Chee E, et al. Pain exacerbation as a major source of lost productive time in US workers with arthritis. Arthritis Rheum 2005; 53:673–681.

Ricci JA, Stewart WF, Chee E, et al. Back pain exacerbations and lost productive time costs in United States workers. Spine 2006; 31:3052–3060.

Schmidt L, Amick BC III, Katz JNEB. Evaluation of Upper Extremity Student-Role Functioning Scale using item response theory. Work 2002; 19:105–116.

Shamansky SL. Presenteeism…or when being there is not being there. Public Health Nurs 2002; 19:79–80.

Stahl E, Jansson SA, Jonsson AC, et al. Health-related quality of life, utility, and productivity outcomes instruments:

ease of completion by subjects with COPD. Health Quality Life Outcomes 2003; 1:18.

Stewart WF, Ricci JA, Chee E, et al. Lost productive work time costs from health conditions in the United States: results from the American productivity audit. J Occup Environ Med 2003a; 45:1234–1246.

Stewart WF, Ricci JA, Chee E, et al. Cost of lost productive work time among US workers with depression. JAMA 2003b; 289:3135–3144.

Stewart WF, Ricci JA, Chee E, et al. Lost productive time and cost due to common pain conditions in the US workforce. JAMA 2003c; 290:2443–2454.

Stewart WF, Ricci JA, Leotta C. Health-related lost productive time (LPT): recall interval and bias in LPT estimates. J Occup Environ Med 2004; 46:S12–S22.

Uguz S, Inanc BY, Yerlikaya EE, et al Reliability and validity of Turkish form of Endicott Work Productivity Scale. Turk Psikiyatri Derg 2004; 15:209–214.

van Roijen L, Essink-Bot ML, Koopmanschap MA, et al. Societal perspective on the burden of migraine in the Netherlands. Pharmacoeconomics 1995; 7:170–179.

van Roijen L, Essink-Bot ML, Koopmanschap MA, et al. Labor and health status in economic evaluation of health care: the health and labor questionnaire. Int J Technol Assessment Health Care 1996; 12:405–415.

Vidrine DJ, Amick BC III, Gritz ER, et al. Validity of the Household and Leisure Time Activities questionnaire (HLTA) in a multiethnic HIV-positive population. AIDS Care 2004; 16:187–197.

Virtanen M, Kivimaki M, Elovainio M, et al. From insecure to secure employment: changes in work, health, health related behaviours, and sickness absence. J Occup Environ Med 2003; 60:948–953.

Wada K, Moriyama M, Narai R, et al. The effect of chronic health conditions on work performance in Japanese companies. Sangyo Eiseigaku Zasshi 2007; 49(3): 103–109.

Wahlqvist P, Carlsson J, Stalhammar NO, et al. Validity of a Work Productivity and Activity Impairment questionnaire for patients with symptoms of gastro-esophageal reflux disease (WPAI-GERD): results from a cross-sectional study. Value Health 2002; 5:106–113.

Wahlqvist P, Guyatt GH, Armstrong D, et al. The Work Productivity and Activity Impairment Questionnaire for Patients with Gastroesophageal Reflux Disease (WPAI-GERD): Responsiveness to Change and English Language Validation. Pharmacoeconomics 2007; 25:385–396.

Walker N, Michaud K, Wolfe F. Work limitations among working persons with rheumatoid arthritis: results, reliability, and validity of the work limitations questionnaire in 836 patients. J Rheumatol 2005; 32:1006–1012.

Wang PS, Beck A, Berglund P, et al. Chronic medical conditions and work performance in the health and work performance questionnaire calibration surveys. J Occup Environ Med 2003; 45:1303–1311.

FURTHER READING

Durand MJ, Vachon B, Hing QN, et al. The cross-cultural adpadation of the work role functioning questionnaire. Int J Rehabil Res 2004; 27(4):261–268.

Sullivan S. Making the business case for health and productivity management. J Occup Environ Med 2004; 46:S56–S61.

21

Outcomes research in older adults with pain: status and future

Rollin M. Gallagher • Jana Mossey

INTRODUCTION

THE PUBLIC HEALTH PROBLEM OF PAIN IN THE ELDERLY

The increased incidence of falls, chronic diseases, and other health problems associated with aging places older adults at higher risk for experiencing both acute and chronic pain. As the evidence mounts that pain in older adults is common, morbid, inadequately treated, and costly, the management of pain in the elderly has become a growing burden on our health care system and a challenging problem on the public health agenda (Weiner et al. 2003; Mossey and Gallagher 2004a). In this older adult population, we lack definitive epidemiologic data regarding the prevalence of pain and pain disorders, the experience of pain as it impacts quality of life, and the societal costs for its care (Gallagher et al. 2000a). As well, there is a paucity of clinical data pertinent to the treatment and management of pain in older populations, and there are few definitive guidelines concerning the measurement of pain or the tools to be used to evaluate the benefits of promising interventions. This chapter begins with a brief summary of current findings regarding the epidemiology of pain in elderly populations and addresses problems that affect epidemiologic studies of pain in such individuals, including the definition and identification of pain and painful disorders, sampling bias related to institutionalization and mortality, and the effects of gender, and psychiatric comorbidity. With this as background, the remainder of the chapter is focused on issues related to the requirements for the rigorous measurement of pain and the specification and measurement of pain treatment outcomes.

The current state of pain measurement and outcomes assessment in treatment studies of older persons is reviewed, current and future challenges to researchers in developing adequate measures of pain and related outcomes are addressed, and an agenda for further work to increase the scientific basis for conducting outcomes research with older pain patients is proposed.

DEFINITION AND IDENTIFICATION OF PAIN AND PAINFUL DISORDERS

Appreciating the methodologic challenges of studying outcomes in chronic pain requires an understanding of how cases for study are defined and identified. Consider the well-known IASP definition of pain: "Pain is an unpleasant sensory and emotional experience associated with actual and potential tissue damage, or described in terms of such damage." According to this definition chronic pain is pain which persists beyond normal tissue healing (suggested as three months). However, this definition presents with a number of difficulties that complicate the study of epidemiology of pain in older adults and the measurement of treatment outcomes. Initial difficulties are with *case definition* and *case ascertainment* (Harkins et al. 1994). Whereas *case definition* of acute pain is usually determined by its cause (e.g., injury or disease), in chronic pain, *case definition* is often determined by both its cause and its effects (e.g., pain levels, persistence and recurrence, or interference with function) which largely determine a patient's perception of pain, its clinical management and the use of resources. The other issue is that of *case ascertainment* or *identification*. Many common pain problems may seriously afflict the person but are short lived because of rapid resolution (e.g., fractures) or increased mortality (e.g., cancer unresponsive to treatment) and so are not reflected in cross-sectional prevalence studies. Chronic pain conditions known to increase in prevalence with age, such as neuropathic pain caused by injury or disease (e.g., neuralgias, post-cancer treatment, central poststroke pain, post-herpetic neuralgias, diabetic neuropathy), are less likely to be featured because of their low incidence compared to the high frequency and chronicity of degenerative joint disease. Also direct approaches at *case ascertainment* (or identification) are hampered by a number of factors including a focus on specific diseases or conditions rather than pain as a case-defining entity itself, the use of pain clinic or institutionalized populations as a sampling frame leading to results which cannot be generalized to the community from which they arise, the use of unvalidated measurement instruments, and direct patient questioning. This last point is important to note because of the frequently weak relationship between the pain reported on specific questioning and pain considered severe enough by the patient to warrant treatment or to affect functioning (Williams 1995), reflecting the multidimensional influences on pain perception and pain behavior. Most prevalence studies are unable to incorporate the large number of questions needed to adequately describe the pain experience: where is the site of pain; is it continuous or intermittent; what has been its duration; what is its quality and severity at different times; how is it aggravated and relieved; how has it been treated; what is its effect on quality of life; how does it affect mood; and what is its effect on care givers? Usually the reason these questions remain unanswered is because most epidemiologic studies of pain in the elderly are not conducted with the primary object of examining the problem of pain. Pain is either an afterthought, a minor aspect of

the study in hand or the results were derived later from a general data source by a second group of researchers (Herr and Mobily 1997). Only recently has the concept of chronic pain as a group of diseases (e.g., painful peripheral neuropathies, post-herpetic neuralgia, CRPS, etc.), with evolving understanding of distinct causes, pathophysiology, and course, been deemed worthy of specific research focus.

PREVALENCE OF PAIN IN ELDERLY POPULATIONS

In their lifetime, an estimated 80–85% of persons aged 65 and older will experience a clinically significant health problem that will predispose them to pain (Roy and Thomas 1987). Of this population, 25–50% will experience pain that interferes with quality of life, and the percentage will increase to 45–80% amongst those living in nursing homes (Roy and Thomas 1986). Institutional samples report higher rates than community samples. The previously discussed methodologic challenges in case identification and ascertainment demonstrate considerable variation in the prevalence rates depending upon the methodology used. The limited data available suggest that approximately 36–83% of the elderly population report some degree of pain that may interfere with life's activities and quality of life (Brody and Kleban 1983). Age-specific morbidity rates for persistent pain generally increase with age for most, though not all, conditions.

In the most methodologically sound cross-sectional population-based study thus far, the Iowa 65+ Study (Wright et al. 1995), data on pain complaints were obtained as a part of an ongoing project specifically designed to explore a broad range of physical, mental, and social characteristics in all non-institutionalized persons 65 years and older living in two rural Midwestern counties ($N = 3693$). Eight-six percent reported some type of pain in the last year, and 59% of those with pain reported multiple pain complaints. A significant relationship was found between pain and age, with those over 85 years or older less likely to report pain. The review by Gibson and Helme (2001) of 11 pain prevalence studies that contained sufficient detail to allow comparison of overall pain rates across a wide age range collectively suggests a peak or a plateau in the prevalence of pain by age 65 and a decline in reported pain in the "old" old (75–84 years old) and the "oldest" old (85+).

There may be several reasons for the apparent decrease in the prevalence of pain with age. First, it is important to note that there is no laboratory or clinical evidence for a change in pain sensitivity with age, which makes pain unique amongst the senses, which otherwise have well-documented age-related deterioration (Harkins 2003, p. 8). The elderly may be more reluctant to report painful symptoms than younger individuals (Ferrell et al. 1990). The decrease in pain in community dwelling adults may be an artifact of higher mortality rates or an increased likelihood of institutionalization for those more ill (Parmelee 1996). Kareholdt and Brattberg (1998) analyzed the mortality risk of pain complaints in ages 53–98 for the period 1968–1991 using a proportional hazard regression. Headache, chest pain, abdominal pain, rectal pain and pain in the extremities showed increased risk with age whereas there was no incremental risk for back pain or pain in the hips/shoulder.

GENDER EFFECTS ON PAIN IN THE ELDERLY

The issue of sex difference in the prevalence of pain in the elderly has not been investigated specifically. Almost 60% of persons more than 65 years old are women, and by the year 2020, 73% of those aged 85 and above will be women. Given this disproportionate representation, any gender differences in pain complaints could greatly affect age-specific pain prevalence estimates. Most, though not all, studies report an increased prevalence of pain in females, with females tending to report pain in multiple sites. However, the Iowa 65+ Study (Wright et al. 1995) found no gender difference in the overall prevalence of pain, and, although finding a higher prevalence of multiple pain complaints in females, the differences were not statistically significant. The magnitude of gender differences in pain prevalence may depend upon the type of disease. Rheumatoid arthritis, osteoarthritis, headache, and fibromyalgia are more common in women, whereas gout, ankylosing spondylitis and coronary heart disease are more common in men. Sex-related biologic factors, differential lifetime exposures to factors causing injuries or diseases and sociocultural factors in illness behavior probably contribute to some of these differences; but further research is needed to clarify this issue.

PREVALENCE OF PAINFUL CONDITIONS AND SITES OF PAIN IN THE ELDERLY

Clinical syndromes in the elderly causing pain include cancer, osteoarthritis, rheumatoid arthritis, temporal arteritis, polymyalgia rheumatica, osteoporosis, osteomalacia, cervical spondylosis, angina, herpes zoster, post-herpetic neuralgia, trigeminal neuralgia, sympathetic dystrophies, spinal stenosis and neuropathies (idiopathic, postsurgical, radiation, toxic, diabetic, alcohol, malnutrition), (Skevington 1998). The site of reported pain is a source of major variation in prevalence figures between different studies. The most common sites of pain in residents of a long term care facility in descending order of frequency were backaches, joint pains, hand and foot pain, muscle pain, neck pain, headaches, stomach pains, bone pains and

chest pain (Parmelee et al. 1991). In reviewing different studies in which the site and cause of pain vary, certain trends emerge. The prevalence of articular pain and hand and foot pain more than doubles in adults over 65 years old when compared to young adults. Conversely, the prevalence of headache shows a progressive decrease after its peak prevalence at 45–50 years of age. Chest pain also peaks in middle age but declines thereafter in spite of the high mortality from ischemic heart disease. The trend for abdominal pain is similar whereas back pain does not co-vary with age. A summary would be that head, abdominal and chest pain frequency are reduced in older people and that joint pain is increased (Herr and Mobily 1997).

TREATMENT OF PAIN IN THE ELDERLY

Review of the literature concerning the effectiveness of different pain treatment and management approaches for the elderly reveals a plethora of articles and commentaries and a dearth of useful, valid and reproducible clinical findings regarding the efficacy and effectiveness of specific treatments. This reflects:

1. The fact that the elderly are not a homogeneous group. In addition to idiosyncratic life histories, co-morbid disease states, and sociodemographic characteristics, older individuals who are cognitively intact are different, in fundamental ways, from those who are cognitively impaired. Those residing in a residential or nursing home setting differ from those who are community dwelling.
2. The subjective experience of pain reflects characteristics of the individual, the source or causes and the locations of the pain (often which are multiple), and the pathophysiologic and/or functional processes involved (often which are multiple).
3. Few treatment studies have focused on the elderly. Rather, many randomized and nonrandomized studies to evaluate the efficacy and effectiveness of pharmacologic and nonpharmacologic interventions for pain have included older individuals but only as part of the "adult population" studied. Consequently, there is little available data on sufficiently large older populations to provide evidence based treatment protocols for this age group.
4. Many pain treatment studies are specific to a particular treatment approach and/or type or location of pain syndrome and cannot readily be generalized to the larger older adult population.

Despite the relative absence of "hard" data from which to formulate pain condition specific, evidence based treatment approaches, there is some consensus regarding the general management of pain in older individuals. Guidelines for the management of pain in the elderly have been published by the American Geriatrics Society (American Geriatrics Society 2002).

In summary the following general management approaches are recommended:

1. Initial multidisciplinary evaluation of pain using reliable, valid, and responsive instruments. These should be designed to obtain information on the characteristics of the current and previous episodes of pain as well as the individual's physical, social, and emotional functioning, his or her knowledge and beliefs regarding pain and possible treatment approaches, especially pharmacologic ones, and the impact of the pain condition on the individual's significant others.
2. Frequent reassessment of pain using the same baseline instruments validated to reflect accurately clinically important changes in health status.
3. Rational use of pharmacologic agents, such as anti-inflammatory analgesics, adjuvant analgesics and opioid analgesics. Use must be governed by the principles of adequate clinical trials, and, when necessary, treatments must be designed to control pain and improve functioning, while reflecting rational polypharmacy, and balancing effectiveness against side effect burden and toxicity risk. Measures of effectiveness, in addition to efficacy, should include adherence, pain relief, and functional improvement.
4. Treatment of comorbid depression and/or anxiety using both antidepressant and anti-anxiety medications and psychosocial therapies.
5. Development of more effective strategies for coping with pain using cognitive-behavioral approaches and education.
6. Whenever possible, inclusion of physical therapy and exercises.

In their reporting, the AGS Panel provided an assessment of the "evidence base" for each recommendation. While some recommendations reflected the findings from at least one randomized clinical trial, treatment protocols applicable to specific patient categories that can be implemented by treating physicians were not identified. Rather, the recommendations that reflected randomized clinical trial data were general in nature, e.g., the need for careful evaluation of pain, the value of pharmacologic agents. The recurring emphasis in the AGS Panel report was the need for thorough and continuous patient evaluation monitoring, consideration of the multiple and interacting effects of each treatment component, and attentiveness to the unique medical, physical, and psychosocial deficits and resources of the individual elderly patient.

While the AGS Panel recommended initial and follow-up multidimensional evaluations of pain and its impact on the functioning and life quality of the individual, no measurement instruments for pain, individual functioning, or quality of life were identified. If evidence based treatments for pain in the elderly are to be developed, however, appropriate measurement of these variables is essential. Despite the importance of assessing pain, medical, physical functioning, and psychosocial variables that are meaningful at the level of the individual, there is a surprising absence of well documented reliable, valid, and precise measurement instruments that are appropriate for use with older individuals and that are sufficiently responsive to detect change in the person's status over time when it does occur and to accurately document the status-quo when no change has taken place. The paucity of appropriate measurement instruments does not imply the absence of scales. Indeed, many different measures are available. For the most part, however, their appropriateness for outcome evaluation of pain related interventions has not been well demonstrated. The following separately addresses issues related to the measurement of pain in the elderly and to the identification and measurement of "outcomes" relevant to pain treatments.

MEASUREMENT OF PAIN IN THE ELDERLY

There is an extensive research related to measurement of pain in the elderly. However, while there is some consensus regarding the aspects of pain that should be measured and several instruments that are commonly used, there is little consensus regarding the best measure to use to monitor the effectiveness of interventions directed towards either cognitively intact older individuals or those who have varying degrees of cognitive impairment. As noted by others (McDowell and Newell 1996; Fitzpatrick et al. 1998; Haywood et al. 2004), longitudinal assessment of pain for the purposes of evaluating treatment success requires assessment tools that: (1) comprehensively tap relevant pain dimensions; (2) meet established standards of reliability and validity; (3) are responsive over time to "clinically significant" changes and for which the "minimum important difference" is known and can be detected; (4) have appropriate levels of precision; (5) are acceptable to the clinician and the respondent; and (6) are feasible to administer. Development of quality measurement tools is a tall order especially when dealing with a subjective phenomenon like pain that not only reflects an individual's comfort and accuracy in reporting but also reflects idiosyncratic ways in which pain may be perceived and interpreted.

FACTORS THAT INFLUENCE PAIN PERCEPTION AND/OR REPORTING

While the literature regarding the importance of cognitive functioning for pain perception is unclear (Gagliesi 2001), the level of cognitive functioning and ability to communicate are important factors affecting the ability to report pain. Individuals who are not verbal or who are not reliable verbal informants due to short-term memory deficits cannot easily report pain levels. The instrument development for this group of individuals is reported in a separate section below. The following refers to individuals who have sufficient cognitive integrity to communicate, either verbally or in writing, information regarding the pain they currently experience. Since the early studies reported by Zola (1966), the importance of cultural background for both pain perception and reporting has been understood and documented. With respect to the older individual, many factors other than cultural background and idiosyncratic or disease-related neurologic processing appear to affect how pain is perceived and reported. Several studies have noted an apparent decrease in either the perception or reporting of pain with age (Gaston-Johansson et al. 1999; Goth 2000; Gibson and Helme 2001; Pickering et al. 2002). This does not appear to be due to age related changes in nociception as there is an absence of firm evidence that such changes occur (Gloth 2000; Herr 2002). Investigators have observed several factors that appear to reduce pain reporting such as: (1) acceptance of pain as a normative accompaniment of aging (Gaston-Johansson et al. 1999); (2) stoicism, especially among males (Cook and Chastain 2001); (3) the desire not to be viewed as a "complainer." In contrast, associations with non-specific anxiety (Bishop et al. 2001), pain related fear and anxiety (Keefe et al. 1987), poor coping strategies regarding pain management, and depression and pain reporting have been observed. The consistency of these associations, however, remains unclear. For example, in one of our studies of Caucasian independently living elders, individuals with high depressive symptoms as indicated by the Geriatric Depression Scale (GDS) (Yesavage et al. 1983) were not more likely than those with low symptoms to report any pain but were considerably more likely to report pain with activity limitations (Mossey and Gallagher 2004a). In a second unpublished study, similar individuals with high depressive symptoms (as indicated by the Center for Epidemiologic Depression Scale (CES-D), (Radloff 1977) were much more likely than others to report any pain but only as likely as those with low depressive symptoms to report activity limiting pain. These findings were based on analyses of cross-sectional data. The absence of data regarding the presence of conditions that might be expected to result in pain, however, precludes causal interpretations of the direction of the association. In a study reported by Creamer et al. (1999), anxiety but not depressive symptoms were related to reporting pain among individuals with osteoarthritis of the knee but only among women who had no obvious clinically relevant evidence from standing anteroposterior radiographs of the knee. Some studies have suggested that women are more likely to report pain than men. Again, consistency is lacking for this

finding. In our studies, once the effects of depressive symptom levels and number of health conditions were taken into account, no gender effects for pain reporting were observed.

Although the above suggests that there is incomplete evidence regarding a number of different psychological and social factors that should be taken into account when interpreting the pain reports given by older individuals, several different approaches to measuring pain in the elderly are being used by researchers and clinicians. While no one ideal pain measure for use with the elderly (Bird 2003; Herr et al. 2004) has been identified that meets the criteria for an adequate measurement tool (reliability, validity, comprehensiveness, responsiveness to change, feasibility and acceptability), they can be classified into unidimensional or multidimensional scales.

UNIDIMENSIONAL SCALES

Unidimensional rating scales typically measure pain intensity with one of the extreme poles reserved for those who report "no pain." Included are:

1. The 10cm visual analog scale (VAS) in which the tester asks the patient to pick a point that represents their pain on a 10cm line anchored on the left end by the verbal descriptor "No pain" and, on the right end, "Pain as bad as it could be." The VAS is validated in adult populations, not specifically in older adults, and has been widely used in research studies of pain. The literature reports failure rates of the VAS in up to 30% of elderly subjects (Gagliese and Melzack 1997; Herr and Mobily 1993).
2. Numerical scales range from 0 "no pain" to 10 or to 100 "pain as bad as it could be" or "worst possible pain." The numeric rating scale (NRS) (an 11-point scale ranging from 0 to 10 with verbal descriptors associated with most or all of the numbers) has been validated in treatment studies demonstrating that a 2-point change is clinically meaningful (Farrar et al. 2001, 2003).
3. Horizontal or vertical "Box Scales" (these scales follow either a VAS or a NRS format but are displayed as a series of boxes rather than lines) also have been used with older individuals. Box scales have 21 discrete levels (Doctor et al. 1995; Jensen et al. 1998).
4. The verbal rating scale (VRS). Often a scale with 5 pain descriptors that represent increasing pain intensity such as "mild...horrible...excruciating" (Chibnall and Tait 2001).
5. Behavioral rating scales (BRS). These are observational scales designed to measure pain behavior as an indicator of pain intensity.
6. Two pictorial scales: the Pain Thermometer (gradations are indicated by verbal descriptors) and the Faces of Pain Scale (different facial expressions purportedly indicating different levels of pain).

The above types of scales differ in the degree of abstract thinking required for a rating to be made and in the ease of quantification. The VAS and the NRS scale formats are both more abstract than the others but inherently more quantifiable. The VAS can be administered verbally. Moreover, by changing the objective of the rating, the VAS, the NRS, and the Box Scales can be expanded to include more pain dimensions than simply pain intensity. However, these approaches require the individual to be able to conceptualize his or her pain along a numeric continuum. Our experience with the use of the VAS and the NRS suggests that a sizeable minority of patients in a chronic pain clinic, over 30%, had some difficulty with this requirement (Mossey et al. 2005). Depending on the number of ordered categories, the reading ability and cognitive integrity of the individual, verbal rating scales tend to be more user friendly. In a comparison of a VAS and a 5 point VRS measure administered to osteoarthritis patients who had been involved in a randomized, double blind study, Averbuch and Katzper (2004) observed that the scales were equally effective in determining the average osteoarthritic pain reported by the 2 treatment groups. For each level of the VRS, however, the VAS scores ranged widely, indicating what others have concluded about the lack of concurrent validity (agreement with other measures of pain in the same individual) of the VAS in the elderly (Gagliese 2001, p. 120). The authors recommended the development of a measurement scale that combined features of both VAS and VRS ratings.

In contrast to the VAS, NRS, and VRS measures, the Pain Thermometer and the Faces of Pain Scale (FPS) do not require reading ability. However, their use is limited to individuals who have adequate visual acuity. The FPS may be difficult to interpret clinically because the faces indicate emotional distress, as well as pain (Herr et al. 1998). As well, the FPS is particularly limited for research purposes because it cannot readily be quantified; therefore, change over time is difficult to evaluate.

In the only study we have identified in which more than 2 pain scales were compared, Chibnall and Tait (2001) administered 4 scales to 90 individuals 55 or older who were patients in a subacute care facility. The battery included: (1) the VRS (Melzack 1975); (2) the FPS adapted for elderly populations by Herr et al. (1998); (3) a 21-point, horizontal Box Scale (BS-21) developed by Jensen et al. (1998) in which 0 was labeled "no pain" and 100 was labeled "pain as bad as it could be"; and (4) 2 vertical 21 level Box Scales (GBS-1 and GBS-U) (Doctor et al. 1995), measuring intensity and pain unpleasantness, in which verbal descriptors were associated with 13 boxes. In analyses limited to 33 cognitively intact (Mini Mental State Exam (MMSE) $\geq$ 22) (Folstein et al. 1975) and 42 cognitively impaired (MMSE < 22) who completed 1 week of data collection, the BS-21 as a measure of pain intensity demonstrated greater reliability and validity than the other scales and performed remarkably well even with those individuals who had mild-to-moderate cognitive integrity.

MULTIDIMENSIONAL PAIN SCALES

Pain intensity is but one indicator of the overall pain experience and its impact on a person. Clinicians and researchers seek ways of obtaining information about other factors that influence both the impairment associated with the pain and the outcome of treatment. A number of scales have been developed that reflect the multidimensionality of pain including measures of: intensity, severity, duration, persistence, and degree to which the pain limits physical, social, and psychological functioning. Multidimensional scales such as the McGill Pain Questionnaire (MPQ; see also Chapter 5) (Melzack 1975) often include some questions that follow a VRS format that yield ordered responses as well as others that provide categorical data. The MPQ may be the most widely used and evaluated (McDowell and Newell 1996) multidimensional scale. Although there is some controversy, it appears to tap sensory, affective and evaluative dimensions (McDowell and Newell 1996). While the MPQ has been used with older individuals, Ferrell et al. (1995) observed individuals with visual or hearing problems had difficulty completing it. Its complexity also makes it inappropriate for use with cognitively impaired older individuals. An adaptation of the MPQ, the 5 item Philadelphia Geriatric Center Pain Scale (PGC Pain Scale) (Parmelee et al. 1991), has successfully been used with several older community dwelling and institutional samples (Mossey and Gallagher 2004a,b). This scale taps pain intensity, duration, severity, and extent of pain related physical limitation. Psychometric evaluations of the PGC Pain Scale for use with older individuals indicate it to have high internal consistency (standardized alpha of 0.91) (Parmelee et al. 1991) and test–retest reliability of 0.84 (Parmelee et al. 1993).

The Brief Pain Inventory (BPI) (Cleeland 1985; see also Chapter 22), initially developed to measure the severity and impact of cancer pain, reflects some of the same dimensions as the MPQ but is shorter. The BPI also includes questions on pain history and contains a diagram of a human figure where the patient can locate current pain sites. Although it appears to have been used with older individuals (Bird 2003), its psychometric properties with this group have not been evaluated.

Greater information yield is an advantage of multidimensional pain scales. This is particularly salient during initial evaluations when it is important to develop a comprehensive understanding of an individual's pain conditions; however, the number of questions and heavy reliance on verbal skills make such scales problematic for cognitively impaired individuals (Bird 2003). While the multidimensionality of a scale makes it attractive in the clinical and research setting, it also creates dilemmas in terms of both cross-sectional and longitudinal interpretation. Specifically, the composite scores that are frequently computed for such measures may yield identical scores for quite different pain profiles; more problematic, in assessing longitudinal change, composite multidimensional scale scores do not identify the dimensions within which change has occurred.

Also, many multidimensional scales exist to assess specific outcomes of interest to those who are conducting pain treatment programs. The outcomes that are most often considered include: physical function measured in several ways, such as ability to perform discrete physical activities (i.e., walking, lifting, and pushing) or ability to improve performance on designated physical challenges (i.e., walking endurance on treadmill, lifting strength, repetitive lifting, climbing a ladder, etc.), usually measured by a combination of time and task intensity; instrumental activities of daily living and self-care activities of daily living; and quality and valuation of life. Little has been done, however, to evaluate the ability for most of the measures to detect real clinically relevant longitudinal change.

In addition to the above general multidimensional pain scales, there are numerous disease specific pain scales (e.g., for arthritis, cancer, neuropathic pain), which, with the exception of age-related diseases such as arthritis, have not been developed and validated for use with older individuals. Presumably they function well in cognitively intact older adults and can be clinically useful. While some disease specific information may be useful and relevant, outcomes research with the objective of generating the evidence with which to develop evidence based pain treatment and management protocols requires at least a core pain assessment tool that can be embedded in all outcome studies.

PAIN DOMAIN-SPECIFIC SUBSCALES OF LARGER HEALTH QUALITY OF LIFE SCALES

A large number of multidimensional general health and/or health quality of life scales have been developed and some, such as the Medical Outcomes Study (MOS), Short Form 36-item Health Survey (SF-36) (Ware and Sherbourne 1992; see Chapter 1), and the European Quality of Life Instrument (EuroQol) EQ-5D (Brooks 1996; see Chapter 1), have included a "Bodily Pain" domain. Typically such scales include 1–3 questions on pain. The SF-36, for example, contains 2 ordinal scaled items that tap pain intensity and pain interference in normal work. Although the health quality of life scales have been used extensively and have

undergone cross-national and cross-cultural evaluations, the use of the pain subscales as the primary indicator of pain during clinical evaluations has not been advocated. However, there has been extensive interest in using the pain subscale to describe population pain levels, to compare two populations, and to assess population or treatment group changes over time. By far, the SF-36 was the most widely used and tested. Although the results have been mixed, adequate reliability and validity for most or all SF-36 domain scales has been observed and the data support the use of the SF-36 with older individuals at the group level (Haywood et al. 2004). The responsiveness of the health quality of life scales to detect individual level change over time, however, has not been clearly demonstrated. There is some evidence that the quality of life dimensions of the SF-36 and the EuroQol are responsive to change in morbidity levels in older community dwelling individuals who have lower levels of morbidity (Tidermark et al. 2003). Studies of the responsiveness of the SF-36 pain items when used with older individuals are limited and the few results not promising. In one study, Bombardier et al. (1995) compared the utility of the SF-36 with the Western Ontario and McMaster Universities Osteoarthritis Index (WOMAC; Chapter 16) for measurement of outcomes following knee replacement surgery in a sample of over 1000 Medicare beneficiaries. They concluded that the SF-36 was better than the WOMAC in measuring differences in general health status but that the WOMAC was superior in discriminating differences in factors relevant to knee pain and functioning.

In response to the inability of the SF-36 Bodily Pain subscale to adequately document over-time change in pain, Rogers et al. have developed an instrument to track such changes in adult populations (Rogers et al. 2000a,b; Chapter 17). Their Treatment Outcomes in Pain Survey, TOPS, has augmented the SF-36 instrument with additional questions to tap specific dimensions of pain intensity, severity, and pain related limitations in physical and emotional functioning. Described as a multidimensional measure of pain, Rogers et al. (2000b) have reported excellent reliability and validity and good responsiveness to over-time change. Their comparisons with the SF-36 bodily pain items indicate the TOPS to be more efficient in documenting subtle change in pain symptoms as well as other pain related dimensions. The TOPS represents an exceedingly promising instrument for use in monitoring outcomes of pain treatment and management studies. While it is evident from their published work that older individuals have been studied (over 200 individuals aged 60 and older were included in their second evaluation study (Rogers et al. 2000b) and over 100 in their evaluation of pain management programs (Wittink et al. 2007)), the TOPS continues to be fully evaluated with older individuals.

LONGITUDINAL PAIN ASSESSMENT FOR OUTCOME STUDIES

Many different approaches to assessing the pain experienced by older individuals have been identified. Although no one scale or approach has been singled out as "the one to be used," it is likely that, among individuals with relatively good cognitive capacity, several will perform well enough to reliably and validly distinguish older persons according to low, medium, and high levels of pain. While this level of distinction may suffice for many purposes, it is not adequate for the outcome evaluation of pain management or treatment protocols. As noted previously, to merit such use, a scale must be reliable and valid, but it also must be responsive to change, have high levels of precision, be feasible to administer over repeated assessments and acceptable to the respondent and the assessor. A measurement tool to conduct longitudinal assessment of pain in older individuals, even if it did meet all these requirements, must take into account several additional issues:

Pain, particularly in older individuals, is often not limited to only one site or to one etiologic problem. In our studies of older individuals, for example, respondents were asked to indicate whether they were bothered by a health problem such as arthritis, heart disease, lung disease, and, if so, whether the condition caused them pain. Of the 600 community dwelling individuals 70 years or older in one study, 52.5% reported that they experienced pain related to two or more health problems. A measurement instrument to assess pain longitudinally, especially if a particular treatment is being evaluated, will need the capacity to distinguish site and/or disease-specific change. Without providing for this, investigators will likely find, as we have, that older individuals express confusion and frustration because they do not know how to describe two different changes on one VAS scale or how to "correctly" pick the pain location or type that should be recording on the scale.

Meaningful, clinically significant change in pain among older individuals that demonstrates treatment or management success has not been determined. Stated differently, short of the obliteration of pain, no consensus exists regarding the reduction in a pain level, measured by virtually any of the above scales, that can be classified as definitely "of importance" to patients (Guyatt et al. 1992; Fitzpatrick et al. 1998). In older individuals where there are multiple etiologies for their pain, where pain may be experienced at several different locations, and where physical, social, and emotional well-being may be influenced by many factors unrelated to pain, this problem is magnified many times.

HEALTH QUALITY OF LIFE AND OTHER OUTCOMES OF IMPORTANCE FOR PAIN-RELATED OUTCOMES RESEARCH WITH OLDER INDIVIDUALS

The inappropriateness of limiting outcomes of clinical care and research to a cure or a significant reduction in core symptoms has been widely recognized. This is especially true when considering older individuals whose main pain condition(s) and comorbid medical conditions are likely to be chronic in nature and interrelated. In addition to diminished pain, relevant outcome categories particularly for older individuals include those at the following levels:

1. The patient level (e.g., mental health, especially in terms of depressed mood, clinical depression, anxiety, fear, and/or rage); level of physical functioning; performance of self-care and other activities associated with independent functioning; engagement in physical exercise; involvement in personally meaningful or necessary activities (e.g., leisure past-times, employment, community service); involvement in satisfying relationships with "significant others" and members of personal community; sense of self-efficacy; degree of adherence to treatment regimens and recommendations; competence in identifying and using effective strategies to cope with physical, emotional, environmental stresses.
2. The "family" level (e.g., mental health (especially in terms of depressed mood, clinical depression, anxiety, or rage) of closest family members or other important others); involvement in personally meaningful activities; involvement in "role appropriate" activities such as employment, parenting, etc.; competence in identifying and using effective strategies to cope with physical, emotional, and environmental stresses.
3. The community level (e.g., healthcare resources consumed by the patient and his/her family; healthcare service costs).

Quality of life represents the most often suggested patient specific "outcome" proposed as an evaluation indicator for clinical studies. Health-related quality of life indices of those with chronic nonmalignant pain are among the lowest observed for any medical condition. Multiple factors determine quality of life. In a study of pain epidemiology and health-related quality of life in 150 chronic nonmalignant pain patients consecutively referred to a Danish multidisciplinary pain center, Becker et al. (1997) showed that, as compared with the normal population, pain patients had significantly reduced physical, psychological and social well being as assessed by Medical Outcome Study-Short Form (SF-36), Hospital Depression and Anxiety Scale

(HAD) and Psychological General Well Being Scale (PGWB). Skevington (1998) examined the impact of pain on quality of life and its components in a representative sample of 320 well people and patients selected from all major categories of illness. Quality of life was assessed using a new, multidimensional, multilingual generic profile designed for cross-cultural use in healthcare, developed by the World Health Organization Quality of Life (WHOQOL) Group. Pain and discomfort made a significant impact on perceptions of general quality of life related to health. Furthermore, the presence of pain affected perceptions of five of the six domains of quality of life. Gallagher et al. (2000b) examined the quality of life, as measured by the SF-36, in a consecutive sample of 4056 patients admitted to a pain clinic in rural Georgia. Patients over 75 years old (mean 80.6 [sd 4.5]) with pain ($N = 530$) differed little from patients under 75 (mean 51.9 [sd 12.9]) with pain ($N = 2724$) on all dimensions of the SF-36, but differed considerably from healthy norms for the same age groups. Their results suggest that cognitively intact older adults (those who are capable of completing the SF-36) do not differ from younger adults in the multiple dimensions of quality of life measured by the SF-36. Thus quality of life is one of the most important contemporary measures in health care. When quality of life has been studied in pain research, it has been observed that scales measuring quality of life are often more responsive to changes in clinical condition than pain measures themselves. This fact underscores the importance for systematic inclusion of these measures in investigating pain.

While a large number of important dimensions have been identified above, with few exceptions, "quality of life" has been conceptualized and operationally defined in terms of "health-related quality of life." The National Centre for Health Outcomes Development, Department of Public Health, University of Oxford, has published a thorough evaluation of health status and quality of life outcome measures for use with older individuals (Haywood et al. 2004). In summary, the authors have reviewed two of the three types of measurement tools that are currently available to measure patient assessed health related quality of life: (1) generic instruments developed for use with the general population, and (2) instruments developed for use with older populations. With the exception of one instrument, these are all multidimensional, although the number and nature of the dimensions vary across instruments.

GENERIC PATIENT-ASSESSED HEALTH QUALITY OF LIFE MEASURES

Fifteen different measures were reviewed including such instruments as the SF-36, the Sickness Impact Profile (Bergner et al. 1976), the European Quality of Life Instrument (EuroQol), and the Nottingham Health Profile (Hunt et al. 1985) (see also Chapter 1). Of these, only the SF-36 had been used with older individuals with sufficient frequency (over 90 published studies) to warrant mention here. Haywood et al. suggested that, overall, the studies provided evidence for scale reliability and validity. However, the reviewers suggest that the SF-36 performs better when used with older populations with lower morbidity levels. Moreover, Rogers et al. (2000b) convincingly argue and provide supporting data that demonstrate the inadequacies of the SF-36 as an instrument to document change in pain or the physical, social, or emotional outcomes pertinent to its treatment. Their observation is even more salient with respect to older patients where serious comorbidity commonly occurs. With respect to the elderly, comorbid depression, at subthreshold, minor, and major depression levels, represents a critically important factor that affects the relationship between pain and physical function as well as the longitudinal course of pain. Our studies, for example, show individuals with any level of elevated depressive symptoms to be at substantial increased risk of limitations in physical function over and above their self-reported pain (Mossey et al. 2000; Mossey and Gallagher 2004a). An important implication of this research is that treatment of comorbid depression is an essential component of pain treatment and measurement of depression a requirement for outcome studies of pain management approaches. Neither the SF-36 nor any of the other generic health quality of life measures reviewed by Haywood et al. (2004) included adequate assessment of depressive symptoms.

MULTIDIMENSIONAL INSTRUMENTS DEVELOPED SPECIFICALLY FOR OLDER INDIVIDUALS

Haywood et al. (2004) have reviewed 18 multidimensional self report instruments that have been developed for use with older individuals. Included are such assessment batteries as: the Comprehensive Assessment and Referral Evaluation (CARE) (Gurland et al. 1977), the Older American Resource Study (OARS) Multidimensional Functional Assessment Questionnaire (OMFAQ) (Fillenbaum and Smyer 1981), the Philadelphia Geriatric Center Multilevel Assessment Instrument (MAI) (Lawton et al. 1982) and the Wellness Index (WI) (Slivinske et al. 1996). While the majority of these were not developed as health quality of life instruments, the dimensions tapped were sufficiently congruent with those thought to be quality of life domains that they have begun to be used to assess quality of life. The Philadelphia Geriatric MAI, for example, was initially developed for use in research studies. The several domains included – activities of daily living, cognition, perceived environment, personal adjustment, physical health, social interaction, and time use – have made it attractive as a tool for assessing quality of life. As Haywood et al. (2004, p. 13) report, with few exceptions, evaluation of most instruments is limited to one study. Moreover, while several instruments have evidence of internal consistency or test – retest reliability to justify their use to document group level change, the Philadelphia Geriatric MAI (Lawton et al. 1982) and the Wellness Index (Slivinske et al. 1996) are the only two that appear able to document change at an individual level.

Instruments developed specifically for use with older individuals have several advantages over generic measures. Dimensions most salient to older individuals are more likely to be included. For example, cognitive functioning is measured in 6 of the 18 geriatric specific instruments and in none of the 15 generic measures Haywood et al. have reviewed. Moreover, by developing the instruments specifically for use with older individuals, issues related to item wording, instrument length, and respondent burden that might affect the response rates and reliability are more likely to have been successfully addressed. Despite this, however, such instruments share with the generic instruments the inability to adequately measure an individual's level of depression.

Generic health quality of life instruments and those developed specifically for use with older individuals, for the most part, have the advantage of relative brevity. Studies conducted in clinical settings or structured measurement of patient outcomes as part of routine clinical practice are restricted in the extent of respondent and assessor burden that can be tolerated. When data collection expectations are too high, patient refusal and/or assessor distractions result in missed assessments and missing data. It is partly for these reasons that a measurement battery that includes reliable and sensitive indices of important quality of life domains as well as permits reliable and valid assessment of clinically relevant conditions such as depression or anxiety or performance based measures of physical function does not currently exist. In the context of assessment of older individuals, brevity is particularly salient because response rates, respondent comprehension and instrument completion, and data quality are substantially improved when interviews are conducted than when self administered questionnaires are used.

LONGITUDINAL ASSESSMENT OF HEALTH QUALITY OF LIFE AND OTHER PAIN OUTCOME MEASURES

Both the limited responsiveness to change of many pain related indicators and the absence of a clear understanding of what constitutes change in pain that is meaningful to the patient have been noted above. Responsiveness to change and quantification of clinically significant change are also problems for health quality of life and other pain outcome measures. As Goodman (2003) notes, the problems associated with measurement of over-time change is exacerbated because, even if a measure is responsive and change is detected, the absence of a "gold standard" makes interpretation and evaluation of results difficult.

PAIN ASSESSMENT IN THE COGNITIVELY IMPAIRED

Since pain is inherently a subjective experience, clinicians and family members caring for a person with pain generally rely on patient self-report about the intensity of pain and the effectiveness of treatment. However, when patients cannot communicate because of physical or mental impairments, the burden is on others to decide, by a combination of intuition, deduction and observation, whether a person is suffering in pain and whether relief is provided. Thus the "subjectivity" of pain is transferred from the suffering person to the observing and treating clinician or care-giver, leading to a situation in which observer bias, not patient suffering, may determine treatment. Reports of widespread under-treatment of pain in such circumstances have confirmed this scenario. Thus considerable efforts have been made to lessen the "guesswork" inherent to observer judgments by developing reliable observational methods for assessing pain and the outcomes of treatment. Since older adults comprise the large majority of persons with cognitive and physical impairments preventing communication about pain and suffering, the focus of most studies has been on this population.

The rating of facial expressions and verbal and non-verbal vocalizations have undergone the most study. Cognitively intact persons have been used to understand the nature and accuracy of observer ratings. In general, raters of facial expressions judged the pain of older adults as more severe than younger adults, despite equivalent subjective ratings of pain. It is not clear whether this is due to observer bias or to age-related differences in facial expression or a combination of these (Matheson 1997). In fact, studies of younger patients in clinical settings show that healthcare workers generally underestimate pain (Allcock 1996). Weiner et al. (1999) studied cognitively intact older adults and showed concordance between self-report and observer ratings, that musculoskeletal disease and medications predicted pain ratings, that relatives tended to overestimate pain and that patient self-reports were influenced by depression co-morbidity unobserved by raters. Generally, nurses both underestimate and overestimate pain in these samples (Weiner et al. 1998, 1999). Studies of cognitively impaired elderly generally show relatively high failure rates for most self-report measures (Gagliesi 2001). In a study of behavioral indicators of pain in verbal but confused older adults with acute pain, Miller et al. (1996) found generally good inter-rater reliability but that facial expressions were difficult to judge. Some work has been done in correlating facial expressions and physiologic reactions to an acute pain stimulus in cognitively impaired elderly, but it is generally inconclusive. In summary, much work needs to be done in developing valid measures for assessing outcomes of older persons with dementia and other cognitive impairments. Clinicians must base their judgment upon a combination of their knowledge of probable level of nociception, patient expression and verbalizations when activating probable nociception (e.g., moving, ambulating, procedures), and patient responses behaviorally and physiologically to treatment (Weiner and Herr 2003).

SUMMARY: WHERE WE ARE NOW

It is evident from the preceding that, with respect to the measurement of pain and quality of life, we cannot specify the optimum measurement tools appropriate for use in rigorous outcomes research of pain treatment and management programs targeted to older individuals. Either such tools have yet to be developed or, like the TOPS, have not yet been adequately evaluated in samples of older persons. We do not, however, suggest a moratorium on outcomes research with older individuals pending the identification of the "best tools." Rather we recommend that current evaluations of pain treatment and management approaches use the tools that the evidence indicates to be closest to meeting the requirements identified in the preceding for outcomes research.

NEXT STEPS: WHERE DO WE GO FROM HERE?

The authors recommend a multi-step process to developing a battery that could be used with cognitively intact older adults. It should be structured in such a way that comprehensive baseline data could be obtained and a subset of the battery would be appropriate for collecting follow-up treatment and outcomes data. Such a battery would yield information useful to both the clinician and the researcher.

First, for patient samples, obtain a standard baseline health background database that includes a detailed pain history and treatment history. The authors have developed the Health Background Questionnaire for Pain (HBQ-P), that incorporates the TOPS, for entry into web-based data registry, either by scanning (the paper and pencil questionnaire has been formatted for that purpose) or online (Herr et al. 2002). Although

the performance of this tool has been tested in one pain clinic (Mossey et al. 2005), it has yet to be validated in larger samples of elderly patients with pain.

Second, develop a variant of the NRS such as the box scales in which different levels are highlighted with descriptive adjectives and the poles are anchored at the extremes. This instrument could be self-administered or administered by an interviewer for the visually impaired.

Third, using this same format, develop several different scales to tap pain intensity, pain duration, and pain-associated limitation of function. A standard format will make interpretation easier for clinicians who will be using these data to help them make clinical decisions. As an example, the simplicity and ease of administration of the Brief Pain Inventory (BPI), an NRS that evaluates patients in five different domains, has led to its widespread clinical use in cancer pain management.

Fourth, using these instruments, make provision to separately assess the contributions of different sites of pain, since the older adult often has more than one site. In pain management, each site may be treated differently, depending on pathology and function, so that following each separately will yield more specificity to the evaluation of the outcome of treatment.

Fifth, further evaluate the adequacy of the TOPS as a measure of quality of life for older individuals. Modifying the SF-36 for pain, as does the TOPS, has the advantage of enabling investigators to compare the relative illness burden of pain diseases and disorders with other chronic disease groups.

Sixth, measure comorbid depression because of both its high prevalence in elderly pain samples and its negative impact on outcomes (Lebowitz et al. 1991; Mossey and Gallagher 2004a). Short of a clinical evaluation by a trained interviewer, a brief version of the Center for Epidemiology Studies – Depression Scale (CES-D) (Radloff 1977) may be useful. The Beck Depression Inventory (BDI) is widely used in pain clinics. However, the CES-D has been shown to have better sensitivity and almost equal specificity as the BDI (Geisser et al. 1997), and is more sensitive to changes in depression severity. This may be because it has fewer somatic items than the BDI (Bradley et al. 2000), which is an advantage particularly in the elderly who tend to have potentially confounding physical symptoms of somatic disease. In unpublished analyses of data from a study of community dwelling elderly women, one of the authors (JM) observed Pearson correlation coefficients of .97 between the full CES-D and the version in which dichotomized item response categories were used. As well, Andresen et al. (1994) have evaluated a 10 item CES-D version for use with older individuals. This showed close agreement with the full version and acceptable test – retest reliability.

Seventh, consider expansion of the quality of life dimensions assessed in many quality of life scales such as the SF-36. Research with community dwelling and institutional based older individuals, for example, suggests that quality of time use is an important dimension of overall quality of life (Lawton et al. 1999a). A 7 item quality of time use scale developed by Lawton has been used extensively with older individuals; Cronbach alpha calculated from a sample of 600 community dwelling elders greater than 70 years of age was 0.74. The scale is easy to administer and is well tolerated. As well, it is strongly correlated with other dimensions of quality of life and with a global measure of "valuation of life" comprised of 13 items measuring hope, futurity, purpose, and meaning (Lawton et al. 1999b).

In designing new measurement components, it will be particularly important to address the issue of what constitutes a meaningful level of change in pain level or quality of life indicators. There is a growing body of literature that considers several promising approaches to defining the parameters of "meaningful change" and/or the "minimum important difference." (See Fitzpatrick et al. (1998), Haywood (2004), Beaton et al. (2001), and Liang et al. (2002) for review and discussion of this literature and Rogers et al. (2000b) for a discussion on the use of "effect size statistic" to quantify meaningful change in the TOPS subscales.) In brief, Haywood et al. (2004) identify two common methods to determine meaningful change, distribution-based and anchor-based approaches. The "effect size statistic" presented in the work of Rogers et al. (2000b) is an example of the distribution-based approach in which change over time in a measure is considered in relation to a measure of the scale's variability. Anchor-based approaches consider change in a measure relative to an external criterion. While the development of these methodologies for outcomes research is very important, neither of these approaches queries patients to ascertain if they have experienced a meaningful change. Cepeda et al. (2003) have reported some encouraging work in this area. They compared the agreement between "patient-reported percentage pain reduction" and computed changes in their pre and post treatment NRS scores indicating pain intensity. Using data from over 700 patients (of whom 25% were age 60 or greater) they concluded that change in the NRS scores and "patient-reported percentage pain reduction" could be used interchangeably. This work provides the basis for further methodologic development and extension to older pain patient populations.

The above recommendations are generally consistent with those made by the Initiative on Methods, Measurement, and Pain Assessment in Clinical Trials (IMPACT III) working group (Turk et al. 2006) and the panel that developed a consensus statement on pain assessments for older individuals (Hadjistavropoulos et al. 2007) While both working groups advocate the development

of multi-dimensional pain assessment tools and the latter provided an encyclopedic compendium of instruments to tap the pain dimensions relevant to older persons, the realization of widely applicable, psychometrically appropriate and acceptable battery remains the immediate challenge.

CONCLUSION

Pain and its effects on health status and quality of life are rapidly growing clinical and public health problems as our population ages and accrues risk for pain-causing diseases and injuries and their morbidities. Although considerable progress has been made in developing reliable and valid methods of evaluating pain and its effects in individuals and in populations, benefiting the work of both clinician and investigator, considerable work remains to be done. The pain field is challenged to develop a standard evaluation procedure using validated outcome measures. This procedure should accomplish several goals: it should provide discriminating data for the epidemiologist and clinical investigator; it should generate clinically meaningful information related to the characteristics of pain and quality of life that will be useful to health care providers making clinical decisions, such as outcome measures that are sensitive to meaningful clinical change in the individual patient; and it should provide information useful to health planners and policy makers by using widely used measures of health status and quality of life. The TOPS (Rogers 2000a,b) is such a promising instrument, which, if imbedded into a general, standardized health background database and used widely, can generate the large data registry needed to advance our development of evidence-based pain practice in pain care for the elderly. The obstacles to achieving these goals reside primarily in the organizational structures and economics of our health care system and the research enterprise, which presently cannot foster the large-scale cooperative networks needed for success. Policy makers and health planners need to help. We are particularly challenged in developing reliable and valid outcome measures to assess and treat pain in the rapidly growing population of cognitively impaired older adults. Overall, the parallel development and intersection of organized clinical and research enterprises in both geriatrics and pain medicine promises important new discoveries about the nature of pain in the older adult. This intersection also anticipates the development of new evidence-based treatments that will reduce suffering and improve the quality of life for older patients and their families.

REFERENCES

Allcock N. Factors affecting the assessment of postoperative pain: a literature review. J Adv Nurs 1996; 24:1144–1151.

American Geriatrics Society. The management of persistent pain in older persons: AGS Panel on persistent pain in older persons: JAGS 2002; 50:S205–S224.

Andresen EM, Malmgren JA, Carter WB, et al. Screening for depression in well older adults: evaluation of a short form of the CES-D (Center for Epidemiologic Studies Depression Scale). Am J Preventive Med 1994; 10(2): 77–78.

Averbuch M, Katzper M. Assessment of visual analog versus categorical scale for measurement of osteoarthritis pain. J Clin Pharmacol 2004; 44:368–372.

Beaton DE, Bombardier C, Katz JN, et al. A taxonomy for responsiveness. J Clin Epidemiol 2001; 54:1204–1217.

Becker N, Bondifaard TA, Oslen AL, et al. Pain epidemiology and health related quality of life in chronic malignant pain patients referred to a Danish multidisciplinary pain center. Pain 1997; 73:393–400.

Bergner M, Bobbitt RA, Pollard WE, et al. The Sickness Impact Profile: validation of a health status measure. Med Care 1976; 14:57–67.

Bird J. Selection of pain measurement tools. Nurs Standard 2003; 18:33–39.

Bishop KL, Ferraro FR, Borowiak DM. Pain management in older adults: role of fear and avoidance. Clin Geronto 2001; 23:33–42.

Bombardier C, Melfi CA, Paul J, et al. Comparison of a generic and a disease-specific measure of pain and physical function after knee replacement surgery. Med Care 1995; 33:AS131–AS144.

Bradley LA, McKendree-Smith NL, Alarcon GS. Pain complaints in patients with fibromyalgia versus chronic fatigue syndrome. Curr Rev Pain 2000; 4(2):148–157.

Brody EM, Kleban MH. Day to day mental and physical health symptoms of older people: a report on health logs. Gerontologist 1983; 23:75–85.

Brooks R. EuroQol: the current status of play. Health Policy 1996; 37:53–72.

Cepeda MS, Africano JM, Polo R, et al. Agreement between percentage pain reductions calculated from numeric rating scores of pain intensity and those reported by patients with acute or cancer pain. Pain 2003; 106:439–442.

Chibnall JT, Tait RC. Pain assessment in cognitively impaired and unimpaired older adults: a comparison of four scales. Pain 2001; 92:173–186.

Cleeland CS. Measurement and prevalence of pain in cancer. Semin Onco Nurs 1985; 1:87–92.

Cook AJ, Chastain DC. The classification of patients with chronic pain: age and sex differences. Pain Res Manage 2001; 6:142–151.

Creamer P, Lethbridge-Cejuka M, Costa P, et al. The relationship of anxiety and depression with self-reported knee pain in the community: data from the Baltimore Longitudinal Study of Aging. Arthritis Care Res 1999; 12:3–7.

Doctor JN, Slater MA, Atkinson JH. The descriptor differential scale of pain intensity: an evaluation of item and scale properties. Pain 1995; 61:251–260.

Farrar JT, Young JP Jr., LaMoreaux L, et al. Clinical importance of changes in chronic pain intensity measured on an 11-point numerical pain rating scale. Pain 2001; 94(2):149–158.

Farrar JT, Berlin JA, Strom BL. Clinically important changes in acute pain outcome measures: a validation study. J Pain Sympt Manage 2003; 25(5):406–411.

Ferrell BA, Ferrell BR, Osterweil D. Pain in the nursing home. J Am Geriat Soc 1990; 38:409–414.

Ferrell BA, Ferrell BR, Rivera L. Pain in cognitively impaired nursing home patients. J Pain Sympt Manage 1995; 10(8):591–598.

Fillenbaum GG, Smyer MA. The development, validity and reliability of the OARS Multidimensional Functional Assessment Questionnaire. J Am Geriat Soc 1981; 33:698–706.

Fitzpatrick R, Davey C, Buxton MJ, et al. Evaluating patient-based outcome measures for use in clinical trials. Health Technol Assessment 1998; 2(14) (National Coordinating Centre for Health Technology Assessment, Southampton, UK; available at www.ncchta.org/htacd. htm).

Folstein MF, Folstein SE, McHugh PR. "Mini-Mental State": a practical method for grading the cognitive status of patients for the clinician. J Psychiatr Res 1975; 12:189–198.

Gagliesi L. Assessment of pain in elderly people. In: Turk D, Melzack R (eds). Handbook of Pain Assessment, 2nd edn. Guilford Press, New York, 2001:119–133.

Gallagher RM, Mossey JM, Mody SH, et al. Quality of Life (SF-36®) in chronic pain sufferers 75 years of age and older: the impact of age and chronic pain in a clinical setting. Pain Med 2000b; 1:205–206.

Gallagher RM, Verma S, Mossey JM. Sources of late-life pain and risk factors for disability. Geriatrics 2000a; 55:40–48.

Gaston-Johansson F, Johansson F, Johansson N. Undertreatment of pain in the elderly: causes and prevention. Ann Long-Term Care 1999; 7:190–196.

Geisser ME, Roth RS, Robinson ME. Assessing depression among persons with chronic pain using the Center for Epidemiological Studies – Depression Scale and the Beck Depression Inventory: a comparative analysis. Clin J Pain 1997; 13(2):163–171.

Gibson SJ, Helme RD. Age-related differences in pain perception and report. Clinics Geriatric Med 2001; 17:433–456.

Goodman GR. Outcome measurement in pain management: issues of disease complexity and uncertain outcomes. J Nurs Care Qual 2003; 18:105–111.

Gloth FM. Geriatric pain. Factors that limit pain relief Gloth and increase complications. Geriatrics 2000; 55:46–4851–54.

Gurland B, Kuriansky J, Sharpe L, et al. The comprehensive assessment and referral evaluation (CARE) rationale, development and reliability. Int J Aging Human Devel 1977; 8:9–42.

Guyatt GH, Kirshner B, Jaeschke R. Measuring health status: what are the necessary measurement properties? J Clin Epidemiol 1992; 45:1341–1345.

Hadjistavropoulos T, Herr K, et al. An interdisciplinary expert consensus statement on assessment of pain in older persons. Clin J Pain 2007; 23 (I); Supplement S1 – S43.

Harkins SW. What is unique about the older adult's pain experience? In: Weiner DK, Herr K, Rudy TE (eds). Persistent Pain in Older Adults. Springer, New York, 2003.

Harkins SW, Price D, Bush FM. Geriatric pain. In: Wall PD, Melzack R (eds). Textbook of Pain. Churchill Livingstone, London, 1994.

Haywood KL, Garratt AM, Schmidt LJ, et al. Health status and quality of life in older people: a structured review of patient-assessed health instruments. Report from the Patient-assessed Health Instruments Group to the Department of Health, April 2004 (website: www.phi. uhce.ox.as.uk).

Herr K. Chronic pain: challenges and assessment strategies. J Gerontol Nurs 2002; 28:20–30.

Herr K, Mobily P. Comparison of selected pain assessment tools for use with the elderly. Appl Nurs Res 1993; 6:39–46.

Herr KA, Mobily PR. Chronic pain in the elderly. In: Smithson E, Tripp-Reiner T (eds). Advances in Gerontological Nursing: Chronic Illness and the Older Adult. Springer, New York, 1997:82–111.

Herr KA, Mobily PR, Kohout FJ, et al. Evaluation of the Faces Pain Scale for use with the elderly. Clin J Pain 1998; 14:29–35.

Herr KA, Spratt K, Mobily PB, et al. Pain intensity assessment in older adults. Use of experimental pain to compare psychometric properties and usability of selected pain scales with younger adults. Clin J Pain 2004; 20:207–219.

Hunt SM, McEwen J, McKenna SP. Measuring health status: a new tool for clinicians and epidemiologists. J R Coll Gen Pract 1985; 35:185–188.

Jensen MP, Miller L, Fisher LD. Assessment of pain during medical procedures: a comparison of three scales. Clin J Pain 1998; 14:343–349.

Kareholt I, Brattberg G. Pain and mortality risk among elderly persons in Sweden. Pain 1998; 77(3):271–278.

Keefe FJ, Caldwell DS, Queen KT. Pain coping strategies in osteoarthritis patients. J Consult Clin Psychol 1987; 55:208–212.

Lawton MP, Moss M, Fulcomer M, et al. A research and service oriented multilevel assessment instrument. J Gerontol 1982; 37:91–99.

Lawton MP, Winter L, Kleban MH, et al. Affect and quality of life: objective and subjective. J Aging Health 1999a; 11:169–198.

Lawton MP, Moss M, Hoffman C, et al. Health, valuation of life, and the wish to live. Gerontologist 1999b; 39:406–416.

Liang MH, Lew RA, Stuck G, et al. Measuring clinically important changes with patient-oriented questionnaires. Med Care 2002; 40(suppl):II45–II53.

Matheson DH. The painful truth. Interpretation of facial expressions of pain in older adults. J Non-verbal Behav 1997; 21:223–238.

McDowell I, Newell C. Measuring Health. A Guide to Rating Scales and Questionnaires. Oxford University Press, New York, 1996:346–352.

Melzack R. The McGill Pain Questionnaire: major properties and scoring methods. Pain 1975; 1:277–299.

Miller J, Neelson V, Dalton J, et al. The assessment of discomfort in elderly confused patients: a preliminary study. J Neurosci Nurs 1996; 28:175–183.

Mossey J, Gallagher RM. The longitudinal occurrence and impact of comorbid chronic pain and chronic depression over two years in continuing care retirement community residents. Pain Med 2004a; 5(4):335–348.

Mossey JM, Gallagher RM. The impact of co-morbid activity limiting pain and sub-threshold or major depression on socio-economically and racially diverse elderly residents of urban neighborhoods. Pain Med 2004b.

Mossey JM, Gallagher RM, Tirumalasetti F. The effects of pain and depression on the physical functioning of a continuing care retirement community. Pain Med 2000; 1:340–350.

Mossey JM, Kerr ND, Gallagher RM. Evaluation of the Health Background Questionnaire (HBQ-P): a clinical tool for use with pain management patients and the TOPS-Uniform Outcomes Measures-Xeris (TUX) protocols. Pain Med 2005; 6(6):443–451.

Parmelee PA. Pain in cognitively impaired older persons. Clin Geriat Med 1996; 12:473–487.

Parmelee PA, Katz IR, Lawton MP. The relation of pain to depression in the institutionalized aged. J Gerontol Psychol Sci 1991; 46:15–21.

Parmelee PA, Smith B, Katz IR. Pain complaints and cognitive status among elderly institutional residents. J Am Geriatr Soc 1993; 41:517–522.

Pickering G, Jourdan D, Eschalier A, et al. Impact of age, gender and cognitive functioning on pain perception. Gerontology 2002; 48:112–118.

Radloff LS. The CES-D Score: a self-report depression scale for research in the general population. Appl Psychol Meas 1977; 1:385–401.

Rogers WH, Wittink H, Wagner A, et al. Assessing individual outcomes during outpatient multidisciplinary chronic pain treatment by means of an augmented SF-36. Pain Med 2000a; 1:44–54.

Rogers WH, Wittink H, Ashburn MA, et al. Using the "TOPS," an outcomes instrument for multidisciplinary outpatient pain treatment. Pain Med 2000b; 1:55–67.

Roy R, Thomas MR. Survey of chronic pain in an elderly population. Can Fam Physician 1986; 32:513–516.

Roy R, Thomas MR. Elderly persons with and without pain: a comparative study. Clin J Pain 1987; 3:102–106.

Skevington SM. Investigating the relationship between pain and discomfort and quality of life using the WHOQOL. Pain 1998; 76:395–406.

Slivinske LR, Fitch VL, Morawski DP. The Wellness Index: developing an instrument to assess elders' well-being. J Gerontol Social Work 1996; 25:185–204.

Tidermark J, Zethraeus N, Svensson O, et al. Responsiveness of the EuroQol (EQ-5D) and the SF-36 in elderly patients with displaced femoral neck fractures. Quality Life Res 2003; 12:1069–1079.

Turk DC, et al. Developing patient-oriented outcome measures for pain clinical trials: IMPACT recommendations. Pain 2006; 125:208–215.

Ware J, Sherbourne CD. The MOS 36-item short form health survey (SF-36): I. Conceptual framework and item selection. Med Care 1992; 30:473–483.

Weiner DK, Herr K. Comprehensive interdisciplinary assessment and treatment planning: an integrative overview. In: Weiner DK, Rudy TE, Herr K (eds). Persistent Pain in Older Adults. Springer, New York, 2003:18–57.

Weiner DK, Peterson B, Keefe FJ. Evaluating persistent pain in long-term care residents: what role for pain maps? Pain 1998; 76:249–257.

Weiner DK, Peterson B, Ladd K, et al. Pain in nursing home residents: an exploration of prevalence, staff perspectives, and practical aspects of measurement. Clin J Pain 1999; 15:92–101.

Weiner DK, Haggerty CL, Kritchevsky SB, et al. Health, Aging and Body Composition Research Group. How does low back pain impact physical function in independent, well-functioning older adults? Evidence from the Health ABC Cohort and implications for the future. Pain Med 2003; 4(4):311–320.

Williams ME. The American Geriatric Society's Complete Guide to Aging and Health. Harmony Books, New York, 1995:453–460.

Wittink HM, Rogers WH, Lipman AG, et al. Older and younger adults in pain management programs in the United States: Differences and similarities. Pain Medicine 2006; 7(2):151–163.

Wright D, Barrows S, Fisher AD, et al. Influence of physical, psychological and behavioral factors on consultation for low back pain. Br J Rheumatol 1995; 34:156–161.

Yesavage JA, Brink TL, Rose TL, et al. Development and validation of a geriatric depression screening scale: a preliminary report. J Psychiatric Res 1983; 17:37–49.

Zola IK. Culture and symptoms: an analysis of patients' presenting complaints. Am Sociological Rev 1966; 31:615–630.

CHAPTER
22

Outcomes measurement in cancer pain

Xin Shelley Wang • Charles S. Cleeland

INTRODUCTION: WHY MEASURE CANCER PAIN OUTCOMES?

Despite nearly three decades of multidisciplinary and multinational efforts toward managing cancer pain, undertreated pain remains an issue in oncology care across the globe. Even in developed countries like the USA, where there are fewer restrictions on opioid use and greater availability of analgesics, inadequate pain control continues to be a major complaint within the cancer population (Cleeland et al. 2003). Chronic cancer pain impacts not only the individual, in terms of physical, cognitive, and affective functioning, but also the community, in terms of social issues like family impact and reduction of work productivity. Outcome measures that evaluate cancer pain management are necessary and very important for routine pain management practice, pain epidemiology studies, pain intervention clinical trials, and for quality assurance in cancer care.

Outcome measures typically quantify either economic or patient health outcomes. There are three types of efficiency analyses for economic pain outcome measures: cost-effectiveness, cost-utility, and cost-benefit, which are not the concern of this chapter. In this chapter, we review common features of available patient health outcome measures of the efficacy of cancer pain management. These can include measures of differences in pain severity, perceptions of pain relief and daily functioning, adequacy of pain management, satisfaction with treatment, symptom burden, and health-related quality of life. We also discuss pertinent methodologic issues and the application of outcome measure in cancer pain research.

THE APPROACH AND CONSTRUCT OF CANCER PAIN OUTCOME MEASURES

FEATURES OF CANCER PAIN OUTCOME MEASURES

The ideal outcome measure should be sensitive, reproducible, and widely applicable. It may be either a subjective or objective measure. To evaluate the effectiveness of cancer pain management, an outcome measure must be useful and meaningful to both health care professionals and patients. From a methodologic standpoint, the ideal outcome measurement tool should be reliable, validated, and responsive to changes within particular study populations. From a practice standpoint, it must be feasible for use with different types of practice settings or research projects. Patient outcome measures, especially repeated measures, must be easy to use and intuitive for patients. Among the commonly used patient outcome measures, pain intensity scales easily meet these requirements.

Patient-reported outcome (PRO) is widely accepted by cancer pain researchers and regulatory agencies, such as the Food and Drug Administration, as the gold standard for measuring pain to make practical judgments about how treatment should progress or whether treatments work. Quantitative research into the impact of cancer pain across cultures has found meaningful cutoff points for mild, moderate, and severe pain (Cleeland et al. 1996; Serlin et al. 1995). These patient outcome variables become important relative to "hard" endpoints such as survival or time to recurrence. In addition, the qualitative pain literature, such as reports on patient preference studies, has contributed to the description of pain quality, pattern, history, expectation of pain relief, and potential causes.

Outcome tools for professional use also include so-called objective measure components, such as analgesic use and other pain management factors that could be important within particular projects. For example, a measurement of pain sensitivity may be helpful in pediatric oncology settings for effectively targeting pain-vulnerable children for psychological intervention. Preliminary analyses indicate that an empirically supported intervention for procedural distress is efficacious for those children who are most pain-sensitive (Chen and Craske 2000).

MAJOR TYPES OF OUTCOME MEASURE FOR CANCER PAIN

Although validated and standardized pain assessment tools are widely used, there is limited consensus about which measures are the most appropriate for evaluating the adequacy of cancer pain treatment. It may be unreasonable to expect a single gold-standard outcome measure for cancer pain to be fitted for multidimensional needs, which vary by type of research and practice situation. Healthcare professionals and policy makers will need to make choices about which patient outcome measures to use and how to interpret them to patients.

Cancer pain literature suggests that the outcome measures commonly used for evaluating pain and its treatment effects can be classified into five types. The first type, patient self-report of pain intensity (i.e., severity), uses a simple and straightforward scale (Ventafridda et al. 1987; Walker et al. 1988; Grond et al.

1991, 1993; Jamison and Brown 1991; Zech et al. 1995; Jensen et al. 1996). This is the tool most frequently used for monitoring pain. The second type, also a patient's self-report outcome measure, includes pain relief and patient satisfaction scales. The third group consists of scales with pain assessment as a component of the construct, such as pain interference scales, and measures of functional status such as health-related quality-of-life scales. The fourth type is the measures of symptom burden. The fifth comprises is the treatment outcome measures of adequacy of cancer pain management, namely the pain management indexes, which relate the level of analgesics to the patient's reported level of pain (Cleeland et al. 1994).

Pain intensity assessment tools

Pain is a complex subjective experience that includes multiple dimensions. Melzack and Casey (1970) suggested that pain consists of three dimensions based on the underlying neurophysiology of pain mechanisms: sensory-discriminative, motivational-affective, and cognitive-evaluative. More commonly, researchers have found that two dimensions adequately describe patient's self-reports of pain, variously described as "pain" and "reaction to pain" (Beecher 1959), "sensory-discriminative" and "attitudinal" (Clark and Yang 1983), or "sensory" and "reactive" (Cleeland 1989). The sensory dimension is often assessed by pain severity or intensity ratings. The reactive dimension has been equated with the distress and interference caused by pain (Cleeland 1989).

Pain severity is the dominant factor determining the effects of pain on the patient and the urgency of the treatment process. Many adults with mild pain function quite effectively, and their pain does not seriously impair their daily activities. As pain severity increases, however, it typically disrupts many areas of the patient's life (Serlin et al. 1995). Current guidelines for pain treatment from the Agency for Health Care Policy and Research, the American Pain Society, the National Comprehensive Cancer Network, and the World Health Organization (WHO) all use a determination of pain severity as the primary item of information in specifying treatment (Jacox et al. 1994; WHO 1996; American Pain Society 1999; Grossman et al. 1999).

Many standardized quantitative pain questionnaires assess pain severity and also other factors related to pain. Using pain assessment instruments minimizes many patient-reporting biases and assists health care professionals in obtaining complete information. Using pain scales that assign a metric to pain intensity and interference makes pain an "objective" symptom, similar to other signs and symptoms such as blood pressure and heart rate. By making pain "objective," standard questions allow patients to feel free to report its presence and severity, and also to report treatment efficacy. Patients are often less concerned about acknowledging the failure of a treatment on a questionnaire than in response to questions put to them by their health care providers.

Types of pain assessment scales

Several reliable and valid methods for scaling the severity or intensity of pain have been developed in the past twenty years of pain research, including visual analog scales (VAS), numeric rating scales (NRS), and verbal descriptor scales (VDS) (Jensen et al. 1986; De Conno et al. 1994; Price et al. 1994). Efforts have been made to determine the clinical meaning of a rating decrease for each type of scale, in both children (Powell et al. 2001) and adults (Farrar et al. 2000). Jensen details these efforts in Chapter 5.

Verbal descriptor scales have long been used in pain research (Lasagna 1980). Patients are asked to pick a category, such as "none," "mild," "moderate," "severe," or "excruciating," that best describes their pain intensity. Although VDS have proven useful in research and clinical settings, these scales assume that patients comprehend the meaning of the descriptors and define them in the same way. This assumption is questionable when patients have diverse educational, cultural, or linguistic backgrounds (Cleeland 1991a).

Visual analogue scales (VAS) are frequently used in clinical and research settings (Wallenstein 1984). The patient is asked to determine how much of the VAS, usually a straight line, is equivalent to or analogous with the severity of the pain. The VAS has proven useful in studies comparing the effectiveness of analgesic drugs and other pain treatments. However, the VAS concept may be difficult for some patients to comprehend (Ferraz et al. 1990).

Numerical rating scales (NRS) are often more easily understood by patients than VAS or VDS. NRS are becoming increasingly popular and have made their way into mainstream medicine (Rowbotham 2001). NRS measure pain intensity by asking the patient to select a number to represent their pain severity. The most commonly used NRS uses an 11-point scale of 0 to 10. The numbers are typically arrayed along a horizontal line, with 0 on the left labeled as "no pain," and 10 on the right labeled with a phrase such as "pain as bad as you can imagine." As the intensity of cancer-related pain is often variable, patients can be asked to rate their pain at the time of responding to the scale, and also at its "worst," "least" and "average" over the last 24 hours. The use of numbers may remove some sources of cultural and linguistic variation (Cleeland 1989). Using NRS is recommended in many pain treatment guidelines (Grossman et al. 1999). The validity and reliability of NRS are well established (Kremer and Atkinson 1981; Syrjala 1987; McGuire 1988; de Wit et al. 2001).

Ratings of pain intensity obtained using the NRS, VDS, and VAS are highly intercorrelated, with the NRS and VAS most highly correlated with one another (Jensen et al. 1986; Syrjala 1987; De Conno et al. 1994). The NRS has been found to be more reliable than the VAS in clinical trials, especially with less-educated patients (Ferraz et al. 1990). Oral versions of the NRS are easily administered to very sick patients who are unable to write.

Commonly used pain questionnaires

Among the most commonly used outcome measures for monitoring pain and estimating treatment effects based on patient self-report of pain intensity (Ventafridda et al. 1987; Walker et al. 1988; Grond et al. 1991, 1993; Jamison and Brown 1991; Zech et al. 1995; Jensen et al. 1996), three have been validated in the cancer population and are short enough to be considered for repeated clinical or research administration to cancer patients.

The Brief Pain Inventory (BPI; Cleeland 1989) is designed specifically for the assessment of cancer-related pain. The BPI provides information on pain severity and the degree to which pain interferes with patients' functioning. The BPI uses 0–10 numeric rating scales. Since cancer-related pain can be quite variable over the course of a day, the BPI asks patients to rate their pain intensity at the time of responding ("pain now"), and also at its worst, least, and average over the last 24 hours. In the long version of the BPI, severity ratings are made for the previous week. BPI ratings have been shown to be a valid measure of pain due to their strong association with other measures of pain severity, sensitivity to change, and strong association with daily pain diary ratings (Jensen and Karoly 2001). All severity items have shown good responsiveness to change over time (Mendoza et al. 2004a,b).

The BPI also asks patients to rate how much pain interferes with seven aspects of life, including general activity, walking, normal work, relations with other people, mood, sleep, and enjoyment of life. The mean of patient ratings on the pain interference items can be used to determine a pain interference score. As "pain worst" becomes more severe, an increasing number of pain interference items are rated as impaired. The BPI also asks patients to rate the amount of relief that they feel their current pain treatment provides. This item can be considered an indication of patients' satisfaction with their current pain treatment. In addition, the BPI long form asks patients to provide a graphic representation of the location of their pain along with characteristics of the pain.

The development of the BPI may serve as a model for the construction of further instruments to assess the effects of cancer and other diseases. The initial version of the BPI was the Wisconsin Brief Pain Questionnaire (WBPQ; Daut and Cleeland 1982). To develop this tool, we gathered and administered existing pain scales to samples of cancer patients with pain. Patients were also interviewed to determine if important aspects of pain were missing in the questionnaires. Most existing scales were (a) too long, (b) had several items not relevant to cancer patients, or (c) required responses that patients felt were ambiguous. The WBPQ was designed as a new instrument that allowed patients to give several ratings of the severity of their pain and to rate the degree to which their pain had a negative influence on several aspects of their lives (e.g., activity, mood, sleep, relations with others, and work). The questionnaire was brief, taking less than 10 minutes to complete, and was designed to be self-administered without extensive instruction. Tests of the WBPQ (Daut et al. 1982, 1983) demonstrated that it had satisfactory reliability, sensitivity, and validity.

Based on these studies, items with little information yield (little variation) were dropped, and the scaling of responses was made uniform (0–10 scales for pain at its worst, least, average and now, and 0–10 scales for how much pain interferes with walking, work, activity, mood, enjoyment of life, and relations with others). The new instrument became the BPI (Cleeland 1989; Cleeland and Ryan 1994). Comparable information is obtained by self-administration and by interviewer administration. The BPI has demonstrated content, construct, concurrent and discriminative validity (Cleeland and Ryan 1994).

The BPI has been used by the Eastern Cooperative Oncology Group to determine the prevalence and severity of pain, its impact on patient function, and how it was treated. A group-wide study enrolled consecutive outpatients with recurrent or metastatic cancer from 80 centers. BPI data from 1261 patients were available (Cleeland et al. 1994). Factor analysis verified the separate pain severity and interference factors found in prior research. Alphas for the four pain severity items (0.80 to 0.87) and the seven pain interference items (0.89 to 0.92) demonstrated the internal consistency of these two scales. Consistent with other studies, patients who rated their worst pain as 5 or more on 11-point severity scales reported significantly more functional impairment due to pain. Of the 1,061 patients who had not had recent surgery (to exclude postoperative pain), 65% reported pain during the past week other than that which they had experienced before being ill, and 41% reported their worst pain at a level of 5 or greater.

As a measure of cancer pain, the BPI demonstrates a number of advantages over other questionnaires. It is short and can be completed by most patients in two or three minutes. Depending on the patient, it can be self-administered, given in a clinical interview, or administered over the telephone. The BPI has demonstrated good test–retest reliability over short intervals. Evidence for the validity of the BPI comes from multiple studies

of cancer patients (Cleeland 1989, 1991a). For example, patients with metastatic disease reported more severe pain and greater interference in daily activities due to pain than did patients without metastatic disease.

Another advantage of the BPI is its availability in multiple languages. The BPI has been administered to cancer patients in numerous countries in Europe, Central and South America, Asia, and the Middle East. Validation studies from these countries suggest that cancer patients from very different cultural and linguistic groups rate pain severity and pain interference in a similar fashion (Serlin et al. 1995; Cleeland et al. 1996; 1997a). Factor analyses of patients' BPI responses reveal two similar factors, pain severity and pain interference, that are remarkably consistent across cultures and languages.

The Memorial Pain Assessment Card (MPAC) consists of three VAS that assess pain intensity, pain relief, and mood, and one 8-point VDS that provides another measure of pain intensity (Fishman et al. 1987). This instrument is short and can be administered in the hospital or clinic setting. Some patients may have difficulty comprehending the VAS and VDS.

The McGill Pain Questionnaire short form (SF-MPQ; see also Chapter 5) consists of 11 sensory (e.g., sharp, shooting) and 4 affective (e.g., sickening, fearful) verbal descriptors (Melzack 1987). The patient is asked to rate each descriptor on an intensity scale of 0 (none) to 3 (severe). Three pain scores are calculated from the SF-MPQ: the sensory, affective, and total pain-rating index. In addition, patients rate their present pain intensity on a 0–5 scale and a VAS. The SF-MPQ provides important information about the affective component of pain that is not included in many pain questionnaires. However, some of the verbal descriptors and VAS scales may be difficult for patients to comprehend and may be interpreted differently by patients of various educational, linguistic, or cultural backgrounds.

Pain relief and patient satisfaction scales

The second type of commonly used patient outcome measures for evaluating pain treatment are pain relief and patient satisfaction scales.

Pain relief scales. Pain relief scales measure change in pain intensity over time, rather than adequacy (De Conno et al. 1994), with a weighted judgment about the effect of the pain treatment (Wallenstein 1984; Cleeland 1991b). Patients are asked to compare themselves on a scale that starts for everyone at the same level of "no change" or "worsening pain" and ends at "complete relief" (Syrjala and Chapman 1984; Takeda 1986; Walker et al. 1988; Goisis et al. 1989). Various studies have shown partial or complete pain relief in up to 93% of patients (Goisis et al. 1989; de Wit et al. 1999).

Pain relief scales can be used to indicate whether pain remained the same, was relieved, or worsened. Combining a pain relief scale with a pain severity scale, this might be helpful to test the response shift in certain patients, because one of the assumptions in longitudinal pain assessment is that a certain pain rating level has the same meaning for all patients so that there is no other expected interpretation for the same level over time.

Patient satisfaction scales. The Patient Satisfaction Scale (Ware et al. 1983) rates how satisfied patients are with their pain treatment on a 5-point scale, from "very satisfied" (1), to "very dissatisfied" (5). The scores are then classified into "adequate" (1–3) or "inadequate" (4–5) treatment. An evaluation of patient satisfaction with pain management becomes one component of a total quality assurance program on pain management recommended by the American Pain Society (APS) (Miaskowski et al. 1994; Ward and Gordon 1996). The Agency for Health Care Policy and Research (AHCPR) proposed the Patient Satisfaction Scale as one of the criteria by which the success of pain guidelines should be investigated (Jacox et al. 1994). Studies measuring patient satisfaction showed modest to extremely high proportions of patients (59% to 93%) who were satisfied with pain relief or cancer pain treatment or with the responsiveness of the staff (Miaskowski et al. 1994; Ward et al. 1994; Zhukovsky et al. 1995).

Despite a growing consensus that global measures of treatment satisfaction should be included in clinical trials (Wright 1999; Wu et al. 2001; Turk et al. 2003), little research has been performed that clarifies the meaning or validity of such measures. Jensen et al. (2004) reported the validity of global satisfaction ratings as assessing something other than pain intensity or change in pain intensity, and therefore support the use of such measures, as recommended by experts in the field of pain assessment in clinical trials (Turk et al. 2003). The predictors of satisfaction in the context of an analgesia clinical trial, including treatment regimen, age, worst pain experienced, pain interference with functioning, morphine equivalent dose taken, and number of opioid-related symptoms (e.g., nausea, fatigue), were all associated with satisfaction with the overall performance of the study medications at day 1. These findings indicate that the study participants considered more than one factor when estimating their satisfaction with the study medications, and that the changes produced by the treatment (e.g., decreased pain, opioid-related symptoms) mediated, in part, the effects of treatment on treatment satisfaction.

However, research on the correlates of satisfaction with general pain treatment indicates that patients tend to report high levels of treatment satisfaction, even when pain severity remains relatively high (e.g., Jamison et al. 1997; Miaskowski et al. 1994; Dawson et al. 2002). Data from de Wit's study (1999) shows satisfaction ratings that are skewed toward the high end of the scale. A majority of patients (68%) who were somewhat or very satisfied reported moderate to severe pain at baseline. These results are in concurrence with other studies of patient satisfaction with pain treatment, underscoring a critical concern about the appropriateness of patient satisfaction as an outcome measure (Ward and Gordon 1996; Hester et al. 1997). Factors that are associated with pain treatment satisfaction include higher levels of perceived support and lower levels of depression, higher levels of internal locus of control, and various aspects of the patient–health care provider relationship, such as perceptions that the provider appears caring or is making efforts to provide pain relief, perceived quality of caregiver communication, and confidence and trust in the treatment provider (Jensen et al. 2004). When patients do not know what quality of pain treatment to expect, they will not necessarily be dissatisfied when their pain is severe. This suggests the role of patients' preferences and their expectation of pain relief cannot be ignored. Without checking the quality of pain treatment in the specific sample, researchers should be careful about drawing conclusions from satisfaction results.

Other outcome measures used for cancer pain

In addition to severity, self report of how pain affects the patient's function is of paramount importance (Turk et al. 2003). Measures of the impact of pain may be included in pain scales or may be measured independently using health-related quality of life measures.

Pain interference. The BPI measures both pain severity and pain interference. The interference items of the BPI are sensitive to variables such as severity of disease and dose changes in drug trials. Results from other and our own studies indicate that the Interference subscale is both valid and reliable across disease type. In a placebo-controlled trial of sustained-release oxycodone, Roth et al. (2000) reported that patients receiving oxycodone showed significant improvement in their functioning from baseline. Of interest is the sensitivity to dose treatment response of the Interference subscale, i.e., a larger effect is associated with a higher dose of drug.

The sensitivity of the Interference subscale is demonstrated by reduction in mean interference rating of at least one point or half a standard deviation in most phase II trials and randomized controlled trials, such as postherpetic neuralgia (Katz et al. 2002; White et al. 2003), low back pain (Gammaitoni et al. 2003; White et al. 2003), bone metastases (Goetz et al. 2004), cancer-related neuropathy (Hardy et al. 2001) and diabetic neuropathy (White et al. 2003).

Health-related quality of life measures. Common symptoms of cancer and cancer treatment adversely affect patients' daily functioning, and have become a major health problem in their own right. The adverse impact of pain, for example, on health outcomes such as function (Cleeland et al. 1994; Serlin et al. 1995;

Given et al. 2000), affective status (Given et al. 1994; Turk et al. 1995; Rudy et al. 1998), and quality of life (Ahmedzai 1995; Wang et al. 1999) among patient populations is well documented.

Improving a patient's quality of life (QOL) is a goal of all medical treatment. QOL is best viewed as a subjective evaluation of life as a whole (de Haes 1988). Based on the WHO definition of health (WHO 1948), QOL includes psychological and social functioning as well as physical functioning, and incorporates positive aspects of well-being as well as negative aspects of disease and infirmity. In 1996 the American Society of Clinical Oncology (ASCO) stated that QOL was an endpoint secondary only to survival (ASCO 1996). The US Food and Drug Administration (FDA) has recommended that QOL is a more important measure for treatment efficacy than most other traditional endpoints for drugs that do not have an impact on survival (Bietz et al. 1996). Health-related QOL measures, such as the SF-36 (Ware and Sherbourne 1992), EORTC–30 (Aaronson et al. 1993), and FACT (Cella et al. 1993), always include pain as an item or subscale and have been used in many pain intervention trials to evaluate the effectiveness of therapy as it affects QOL.

Among health researchers, a common consensus is that QOL is a multidimensional construct composed of at least four dimensions: physical function (i.e., daily activities, self care, etc.), psychological function (i.e., emotional/mental, mood), social role function (i.e., social interactions, family dynamics), and disease/ treatment symptoms (i.e., pain, nausea, fatigue). The comprehensive nature of quality of life, however, is both one of its attractions and its difficulties as an outcome measure. Using QOL measures in practice may assist in gaining insight into the effects of pain on their patients' QOL. This information may be useful in developing treatment programs that minimize pain and its associated side effects while maximizing patients' well-being (Bonomi et al. 2000).

The impact of cancer pain on health-related QOL has been studied (Wang et al. 1999). Increasing severity of pain was associated with worsening health-related functioning, even when an estimate of disease severity was taken into account. The correlation between pain severity and impairment was nonlinear. Functional health and well-being were significantly less impaired for cancer patients with no or mild pain than for patients with moderate or severe pain. The impairment of patients with moderate and severe pain did not differ. Providing pain relief should significantly improve the functional status of cancer patients.

Measures of symptom burden

In cancer patients undergoing aggressive treatment or with advanced-stage disease, severe pain is almost always accompanied by other cancer-related symptoms, such as fatigue, sleep disturbance, distress, poor appetite, and others. The concept of "symptom burden" may be operationally defined as a summative indicator of: (1) the severity of the symptoms most associated with a disease or treatment, and (2) a summary of the patient's perception of the impact of these symptoms on daily living, including activity, mood, ability to work, and ability to relate to others. Symptom burden is another outcome measure for following the impact of the disease and multiple treatment-related symptoms, and is a meaningful way to justify treatment for pain.

Several symptom scales have been developed for use with cancer patients. Any of these scales, if the salient symptoms and the degree to which these symptoms interfere with patient functioning are represented, could serve as the basis for measuring symptom burden. Such scales include the Symptom Distress Scale (McCorkle and Young 1978), the Memorial Symptom Assessment Scale (Portenoy et al. 1994), the Rotterdam Symptom Checklist (de Haes et al. 1990), and the M. D. Anderson Symptom Inventory (MDASI; Cleeland et al. 2000).

We developed the MDASI as a brief measure of the severity and impact of cancer-related symptoms. It is based on tools we developed to assess the severity and interference of single symptoms, including the BPI and the Brief Fatigue Inventory (BFI) (Mendoza et al. 1999). The "core" MDASI is a 19-item scale consisting of 13 symptoms frequently reported by cancer patients: pain, fatigue, nausea, disturbed sleep, emotional distress, shortness of breath, lack of appetite, drowsiness, dry mouth, sadness, vomiting, difficulty remembering, and numbness or tingling. It also contains six items that describe how much the symptoms have interfered with different aspects of the patient's life during the past 24 hours: general activity, mood, walking ability, normal work (including both work outside the home and housework), relations with other people, and enjoyment of life. Both the symptom and the interference items are rated on an 11-point scale, with 0 being "does not interfere" and 10 being "completely interferes." The validation process for the MDASI has been reported elsewhere (Cleeland et al. 2000).

Based on our experience with pain, we believe that the relationship between symptom severity and the degree of the symptom's interference in functions such as activity and mood may help determine the level of symptom severity, which may in turn direct treatment. In particular, we have found that pain intensity ratings have a corresponding degree of interference with function. Mild, moderate, and severe pain differentially affect the functioning of cancer patients (Serlin et al. 1995). This classification is now incorporated into several guidelines for the management of pain. Recent studies also indicate that the severity of cancer-related fatigue can be classified in the same fashion, suggesting that a patient's report of fatigue severity might directly contribute to treatment recommendations (Mendoza et al. 1999). A similar methodology might be applied to other cancer-related symptoms (i.e., sleep disturbance, negative affect, cognitive impairment) to help determine levels of severity that may help guide treatment decisions.

Symptom burden as a construct differs from QOL and moves in an inverse direction. With increased pain severity, QOL would be decreased and symptom burden would be increased. Symptom burden may have advantages over QOL measures for interpreting potential outcomes to patients. In clinical practice, it may be difficult to make sense of a finding of improvement in QOL scores. For example, the finding that a treatment is associated with a 10-point improvement in QOL as opposed to a 15-point improvement is not intuitive to a clinician or patient. Because of this, physicians discussing treatment options with their patients must find a way to interpret and then to explain findings presented as improvements in QOL. In contrast, both patient and clinician should have an easier choice to make when given the information that, although two treatments have similar survival benefit, one of the treatments was associated with significantly less pain, fatigue, and sleep disturbance. As a multidimensional construct, a measure of QOL may include aspects that go beyond the impact of cancer or its treatment. Measuring symptom burden, with particular emphasis on pain, would be a more direct way to address the impact of pain management.

Treatment outcome measures

Pain treatment outcome measures attempt to reflect the appropriateness of pain management in studies of quality of care. An example of a pain treatment outcome measure is the Pain Management Index (PMI) (Cleeland et al. 1994), which takes into consideration not only self-reported pain intensity levels, but also pain management as indicated by the strength of the analgesic prescribed . There are several types of PMI.

Cleeland's PMI (Cleeland et al. 1994) is based upon the patient's BPI "pain worst" rating, scored as 0 (no pain), 1 (1–3, mild pain), 2 (4–7, moderate pain), or 3 (8–10, severe pain). The most potent level of analgesic drug prescribed by the clinician is similarly categorized, scored as 0 (no analgesic drug), 1 (nonopioid), 2 (weak opioid), or 3 (strong opioid). The pain level score is subtracted from the analgesic level score. Cleeland's PMI can thus range from −3 (a patient receiving no analgesic drugs [score 0] who is in severe pain [score 3]) to +3 (a patient receiving strong opioids [score 3] who is pain-free [score 0]). These scores are then dichotomized: negative scores indicate inadequate orders for analgesic drugs, and scores of 0 or higher are considered to be conservative indicators of

acceptable treatment. Cleeland's PMI has been used in pain studies to rate the adequacy of pain management in the study setting over time, or to facilitate comparisons among study settings, such as in the USA, France, Netherlands, Greece, China, India and Japan (Cleeland et al. 1993, 1994; Larue 1995; Wang et al. 1996; de Wit et al. 1997, 1999; Uki et al. 1998; Saxena et al. 1999; Wang et al. 2002; Okuyama et al. 2004).

A variation on Cleeland's PMI was developed by Ward and colleagues (Ward et al. 1993; Ward and Hernandez 1994). Ward's PMI also uses the BPI "pain worst" rating and scores pain and analgesic strength in the same way, but it incorporates analgesics as used by a patient instead of analgesics as prescribed by the physician. In the hospital, some patients had difficulty reporting what pain medication was prescribed; in contrast, patients at home were better informed. Evidence of the validity of this PMI has been demonstrated by Ward et al.

The Amsterdam Pain Management Index, also based on Cleeland's PMI, compares patients' present pain intensity, average pain intensity, and worst pain intensity with a composite score of all opioid and nonopioid analgesics used (nonadherence is incorporated), while correcting for what a patient considers as a tolerable level of pain on the Tolerable Pain Intensity scale (de Wit et al. 2001). The categorized pain scores are subtracted from the categorized level of analgesic drugs used. Results range from −4 to +4, and are further dichotomized into "inadequate use of analgesics" (score −4 to −1), and "adequate use of analgesics" (score 0–4). The impact of Tolerable Pain Intensity on the adequacy of pain treatment has not been established, so the value of including patients' Tolerable Pain Intensity is unclear.

The aforementioned PMI treatment outcome measures correlate a patient's self-report of pain to the pain treatment itself. They are crude measures of the adequacy of pain treatment. Although using a PMI to evaluate pain treatment has shown satisfactory results in some studies, all PMIs are based on the World Health Organization's analgesic ladder, which does not take into account such pain-related issues as diagnosis, tumor extension, cancer treatment, potency of the pain drug, dosage, number of pain drugs used, duration of treatment, adverse reactions, and clarity of instruction. Ideally, when evaluating pain treatment for an individual patient, clinicians and researchers should consider these various pain-related aspects, especially dose, schedule, route of administration, and the best drug for the patient's particular type of pain. Although the PMI is thus not ideal for assessing individual treatment, it is nonetheless a robust and attractive measure for comparing pain management by practice setting and progress over time, and for providing basic information about and feedback from pain epidemiology studies to policymakers, consumer groups, and the media.

APPLICATION OF OUTCOME RESEARCH TO CANCER PAIN

CHOOSING PAIN OUTCOME MEASURES

Outcome measures are important for describing the effectiveness of a treatment. However, no single outcome measure has received widespread acceptance for evaluating cancer pain treatment. In a randomized clinical trial, de Wit et al. (1999) examined by factor analysis the underlying constructs – pain severity, pain management index, and satisfaction – of several outcome measures. The factor structures of the outcome measures did not overlap, loading in three areas. Three factors clearly emerged, explaining most of the variability in the different scales. The results provide support for the conclusion that the different types of outcome measures do not measure a single underlying construct.

The Amsterdam, Cleeland, and Ward PMIs appear to show satisfactory results in distinguishing between subgroups of patients reported to be nonadherent and patients reported to be adherent. In contrast, the pain intensity assessment tools, pain relief scales, and patient satisfaction scales do not clearly differentiate between groups known to be different.

CATEGORIZING PAIN SEVERITY: THE USE OF CUT POINTS

Categorizing a pain severity rating as "mild," "moderate," or "severe" is a crucial step in the assessment process and determines the urgency of the treatment process. For example, the three-step analgesic ladder in the WHO guidelines for cancer pain management recommends a family of analgesic drugs based on the three categories of pain intensity (WHO, 1986, 1996). Thus, the implementation of pain treatment guidelines necessitates the categorization of pain intensity.

In data sets from several countries' BPI validation studies, there appeared to be natural breaks in the amount of functional interference that patients reported, dependent upon the severity of their pain. These breaks or cut points suggested that we might define "mild," "moderate," and "severe" pain in terms of the interference burden produced. In a subsequent study (Serlin et al. 1995) we addressed the question of defining categories of pain severity and determining whether cross-cultural differences existed. The subjects were patients with metastatic cancer and pain who participated in collaborative projects in the Philippines, France, China, and the USA. Our goals were: (1) to determine at what level we can best distinguish "mild" pain from "moderate" pain, (2) to determine at what level we can best distinguish "moderate" pain from "severe" pain and (3) to evaluate whether the national origin of the sample makes a difference in these separations.

Within the context of an NRS, "mild," "moderate," and "severe" pain can be defined as ranges of patient responses to a numerical rating of pain at its worst. In the literature, a pain intensity of either 3 or 4 on a 0–10 scale has been the upper boundary for mild pain, while pain severity of 4 or 5 has been the lower boundary for moderate pain. Similarly, a pain intensity of either 6 or 7 has been the upper boundary for moderate pain, while pain severity of 7 or 8 has been the lower boundary for severe pain. The ranges for each category of pain severity are based on the degree of interference with function associated with each category (Serlin et al. 1995). Since clinically important differences in pain severity levels are expected to be associated with large differences in self-reported interference, in the Serlin et al. study (1995) we evaluated which one of these four possible pairings of category boundaries could distinguish the three levels of pain severity. Multivariate analyses of variance revealed that the optimal boundaries along the pain intensity scale for cancer patients could be set at 1–4 for "mild," 5–6 for "moderate," and 7–10 for "severe" pain.

Mild pain (1–4 worst pain) will most often call for a mild analgesic (acetaminophen or a nonsteroidal anti-inflammatory) or a moderate analgesic such as oxycodone or hydrocodone (Grossman et al. 1999). Mild pain typically causes the least interference with function. However, patients with mild pain can benefit from education about the need to report pain when it occurs, when it gets worse, or if it is not relieved by current treatment. *Moderate pain* (5–6 worst pain) calls for a more aggressive analgesic program and thorough assessment of the impact of the pain on the patient's life. Since pain at this level is impairing multiple areas of a patient's functioning, a follow-up contact should be made within 24 to 72 hours of the clinic visit to assess the efficacy of the pain treatment provided. *Severe pain* (7–10 worst pain) mandates very aggressive analgesic treatment with a strong opioid such as morphine. Follow-up contact should occur within 24 hours after the initial assessment. A comprehensive evaluation of the impact of the pain is necessary to determine if the patient needs psychosocial support or other behavioral treatments.

DETERMINING CLINICALLY MEANINGFUL PAIN REDUCTION

Although pain studies often include serial measures of pain intensity and pain relief assessment, the precise relationship between the two has been an interesting research question in longitudinal trials for chronic cancer pain (Rowbotham 2001). Practically speaking, what do changes in pain intensity mean to patients, and what does a clinically important difference mean to clinicians? Variability in patients' expressions and physicians' interpretations may contribute to disagreement on pain severity (Todd 1994). In fact, there is no method to objectively measure the complex internal process of pain perception; patient self-reports remain the "gold standard" (Melzack 1983).

Methodologic challenges arise from the fact that rating scale descriptors, such as the "mild," "moderate," and "severe" categories of NRS scales, may mean different things to different people, because the 0–10 NRS is not linear (Cleeland 1989; Max and Laska 1991; Serlin et al. 1995). In children, a one-unit decrement in NRS has been reported to be the threshold for clinical significance (Powell et al. 2001). Cepeda's study of adult cancer patients supports this conclusion, finding that a change of 1.3 units was the threshold for minimal pain relief if the baseline pain intensity was moderate, while 1.8 units was the threshold if the baseline pain intensity was severe (Cepeda et al. 2003a). Further, the clinical meaning of changes in the NRS for patients with cancer or chronic noncancer pain may differ from that for patients with acute pain, because cancer pain affects coping abilities and mood (Jacox et al. 1994).

In another study of cancer pain relief, "adequate relief" was defined not by asking patients what degree of relief they perceived as acceptable, but by their no longer requiring additional opioid doses as rescue medication (Farrar et al. 2000). Simply asking patients whether they require further analgesia seems a logical alternative, making pain measurement and the definition of the minimum clinically important difference unnecessary. However, a patient's decision to refuse analgesia may be based on concerns other than pain severity.

The proportion of subjects with a specific percentage reduction in pain intensity is increasingly used by researchers to evaluate treatment efficacy. A cutoff of 50% to dichotomize pain intensity outcomes is commonly used to calculate number-needed-to-treat (NNT) (Moore et al. 1996, 1997a,b). Although a 50% decline in pain intensity correlates well with other measures of pain intensity and pain relief, the clinical meaning to patients with acute pain of specific percentage reductions in pain intensity is unknown. Cepeda et al. (2003b) found that, regardless of baseline pain severity, the minimal change in the NRS that is noticeable to patients (i.e., identified with minimal improvement) is 20%. The American College of Rheumatologists (ACR) has defined improvement as a 20% decrease in pain (Felson et al. 1995, 1998). For achieving higher degrees of pain relief, the percent reduction has to be 35% if baseline pain is of moderate intensity, or 44% if baseline pain is severe. Therefore, using a cutoff of 50% to dichotomize pain intensity outcomes for calculation of NNT may be too stringent.

In studies of patients with chronic and cancer pain, Farrar et al. found that the meaning of a percent reduction did not vary with the intensity of the pain (Farrar et al. 2001), and that a 30–33% decline in VAS was judged to be clinically important relief by patients (Farrar et al. 2000, 2001).

Sensitivity and specificity analyses of patients with complex regional pain syndrome type 1 showed that a relative pain reduction cut-off point of 50% and an absolute pain reduction of 3-cm on the VAS were most likely to result in patients reporting their treatment as "successful" on the Global Perceived Effect for their pain relief over the same time periods (Forouzanfar et al. 2003).

Understanding the meaning of changes in the NRS and how percentage pain reductions correlate with patients' perceptions of adequate pain control is indispensable for assessing the effectiveness of pain treatment. It may allow physicians to better interpret patient refusal of analgesia (Lee et al. 2003).

INTERPRETING CROSS-CULTURAL CHANGES IN CANCER PAIN MANAGEMENT

How do sociocultural, attitudinal, and economic variables influence pain experience? Given the multidimensional nature of pain, these factors confound the interpretation of "good pain management." Although research suggests that culture does not affect pain thresholds or pain intensity ratings (Cleeland et al. 1997a), culture probably does impact people's behavioral responses to pain and their interpretations of the meaning of pain. Similarly, people's attitudes and beliefs regarding pain and pain treatment undoubtedly influence their responses to pain and pain interventions. Patients' understanding and knowledge of pain also impact their reactions to the pain experience and pain treatments. Beyond individual pain data, economic factors, such as a patient's ability to pay for pain medications, also have a powerful impact on the success of pain treatments in large-scale pain epidemiology studies.

Our first evidence that cancer patients from two widely different cultural and linguistic backgrounds might rate their pain in a similar fashion was the study of Vietnamese cancer patients and cancer patients in Wisconsin. We made cross-cultural comparisons by examining BPI responses on pain severity and interference (Cleeland et al. 1988). A common factor analysis with oblimin rotation was applied to the matrix of intercorrelations for each patient sample. Two factors with an eigenvalue greater than one emerged in both analyses. These two factors accounted for 67% of the variance in the responses of the Wisconsin sample and 65% of the variance in the Vietnamese sample. One factor consisted of the four pain intensity items, and the second factor was composed of the seven interference items. For both cancer groups, the severity of pain was rated somewhat independently from ratings of the interference that pain caused in important dimensions of the patients' lives.

A study of four cultural groups (Cleeland et al. 1997a) demonstrated that cancer pain patients from diverse populations show fairly consistent patterns in relating pain intensity to pain interference. The relative effects of pain severity on interference were comparable across the three severity levels (mild, moderate, and severe) for each nation. While there are slight differences in the specific interference items affected by pain across cultures, the overall impact of pain severity on interference appears to be the same.

Comparisons of pain intervention trials across different countries and cultures require psychometrically sound, culturally adapted outcome measures. Several foreign language versions of the BPI have been developed using well-established methods (e.g., forward and backward translations) by firms such as MAPI in France and Oxford Outcomes in the United Kingdom. We have used the resultant translations in our epidemiologic studies. The psychometric properties and the utility of the BPI have been examined in the traditional character structure of Chinese characters used in Taiwan and Hong Kong (Ger et al. 1999), the simplified Chinese character structures used in mainland China (Wang et al. 1996), Spanish (Badia et al. 2003), Cebuano (Laudico et al. 2002), French (Larue et al. 1995), German (Radbruch et al. 1999), Greek (Mystakidou et al. 2001), Hebrew (Shvartzman et al. 2003), Hindi (Saxena et al. 1999), Italian (Caraceni et al. 1996), Japanese (Uki et al. 1998), Korean (Yun et al. 2004), Norwegian (Klepstad et al. 2002), and Vietnamese (Cleeland et al. 1988). Data collection for additional language versions has been completed for Arabic, Czech, Croatian, Dutch, Russian, Swedish, Slovak, and Slovenian. Versions of the BPI in Afrikaans, Danish, Estonian, Polish, and several African languages such as Sepedi, Xhosa, and Zulu were also linguistically validated.

USING OUTCOME MEASURES IN PAIN RESEARCH DESIGN

As treatments that depend on subjective outcomes emerge, how such treatments will be valued becomes a major issue. Will patients, given subjective outcome information about treatments, opt to complete them? Will physicians use this outcome information to recommend and prescribe treatments? When such treatments are being developed, will approval agencies decide they are beneficial? Will agencies (public and private health funders) decide that such treatments are worth paying for? Thus, when a treatment offers little or no survival advantage, yet seems to improve how patients feel, judgments about the worth of the treatment will be made by several audiences who will ultimately determine whether or not the treatment is effective, should be approved, and will be used.

It is evident that different outcome measures generate different results, making it difficult to compare multiple cancer pain management intervention trials when various outcome measures have been used. Pain intensity assessment tools, pain relief scales, patient satisfaction scales, and pain management indexes are used interchangeably for the evaluation of pain treatment (Jadad and Browman 1995), which results in substantial differences in reported adequacy of cancer pain treatment. When a pain relief scale or a patient satisfaction scale is used, cancer pain treatment is most frequently evaluated as adequate. However, when pain intensity scales or pain management indexes are used, most studies show high percentages of inadequate cancer pain treatment. On the basis of the diversity of results, it seems that each of the different measures has its own advantages and disadvantages for the evaluation of pain treatment, and that commonly used groups of outcome measures cover different aspects of patients' pain experience.

The AHCPR (Jacox et al. 1994) and the APS (Max 1991) recommend using pain intensity scales and patient satisfaction scales as outcome measures. Pain treatment is primarily evaluated unidimensionally. However, because pain is a multidimensional concept, the physiologic, sensory, affective, cognitive, behavioral, and sociocultural dimensions should be integrated to evaluate pain treatment. Further psychometric analyses are needed to identify instruments for evaluating pain treatment in patients with cancer in a variety of situations. As long as the various outcomes are not consistent within one dimension, a unidimensional instrument must first be identified.

The PMI has good potential for beneficial use in pain epidemiology studies, such as using the PMI to advocate cancer pain management for minority populations. The two largest ethnic minority groups with cancer in the USA are African Americans and Hispanics. Among the more than one million cancer patients newly diagnosed each year in the United States, minority patients, particularly economically disadvantaged and underserved patients, tend to present with later stages of disease than nonminority patients. Thus, they are at risk for the development of pain that is often associated with metastatic or recurrent disease. Patients treated in minority settings were three times more likely to be undermedicated than patients seen in nonminority settings (Cleeland et al. 1994). A follow-up study showed that 65% of the minority patients with pain did not receive the WHO recommended analgesics for their pain, as compared with 38% of patients from nonminority settings in the previous study (Cleeland et al. 1997b). The minority patients reported less pain relief and were less likely to be adequately assessed for their pain than nonminority patients.

CLINICAL APPLICATION

Factors to consider in selecting measures of outcomes include feasibility, sensitivity to treatment effects, clinical utility, and clinical vs. statistical significance. Pain intensity markers, based on pain intensity scores, are most frequently used in pain research and allow for the establishment of descriptive and treatment-action cut points. For example, the APS Quality of Care Committee (1995) has advocated the use of a value of 5 or greater on a 0–10 NRS as a starting point for eliciting an immediate assessment of pain treatment.

Much of the research done with the BPI has been with cancer patients in epidemiologic studies (Cleeland et al. 1994; Beck and Falkson 2001) or in clinical trials (DuPen et al. 1999; Ward et al. 2000). However, the BPI is also widely used as an outcome measure in clinical trials to assess pain in other chronic conditions, including HIV/AIDS (Smith et al. 2002; Evans et al. 2003), phantom limb pain (Jensen et al. 2002), critical limb ischemia (Mitchell and Fallon 2002), Fabry disease (Schiffmann et al. 2001), osteoarthritis (Roth et al. 2000; Thie et al. 2001), and painful neuropathy (Semenchuk et al. 2001). The BPI has also been useful for patients undergoing coronary artery bypass grafting (Mendoza et al. 2004a, b). Novel uses of the BPI included measuring pain at the injection site associated with the administration of vaccine (Su et al. 2000). Nonrandomized studies using the BPI in other chronic conditions include low back pain (Gammaitoni et al. 2003), chronic hemiplegia (Yu et al. 2001), osteoarthritis (Keller et al. 2004), AIDS (Breitbart et al. 1996), and painful diabetic neuropathy (Galer et al. 2000). A recent consensus panel recommended that the two domains measured by the BPI – pain severity and its impact on functioning (pain interference) – be included in the conduct of all chronic pain clinical trials (IMMPACT; Turk et al. 2003; see Chapter 18). This panel specifically identified the interference items of the BPI, measured using ratings of 0–10, as one of the two scales to assess pain-related function. Since we began systematically tracking requests for the BPI in 2006, 157 requests came from pharmaceutical companies intending to use the BPI as a primary or secondary outcome measure in their clinical trials.

Longitudinal assessment is another application for the BPI. The BPI or a modified version has been successfully used over 2-week periods for patients who have undergone coronary artery bypass grafting (Mendoza et al. 2004a). With its brevity and simplicity, patients were able to respond to the BPI with minimal burden, as attested by few missing data over the 14-day study period. As described above, the use of mild, moderate, and severe classifications is a simple and useful means of describing patients' pain based on pain-related interference with function. The pain severity level cut points developed for chronic pain by Serlin et al. (1995) applied equally well to postoperative pain; according to that classification scheme, 18% of patients reported moderate pain and 14% reported severe pain after day 3. Only 9% of patients reported experiencing moderate-to-severe pain approximately 2 weeks later, at the end of the study. Because most patients experience only mild pain 6 days after surgery, long-term clinical trials of postoperative pain control may be more efficient and cost-effective if they focus on the subset of patients with persistent moderate or severe pain (Mendoza et al. 2004b). This categorization could also be a meaningful outcome measure in clinical trials and is well suited for an emerging analysis scheme called "responder analysis."

BPI-based computerized adaptive testing of pain is a promising new application. Clinical trials where pain is the primary or secondary outcome usually require additional dimensions of patient-reported outcomes besides those covered by the BPI, such as questions that assess the quality of the pain, its location, its temporal pattern, the treatment history of the patients, their functional and affective status, and satisfaction with past treatment. Beginning with BPI assessment, the computerized model is designed as a decision tree with branches that will be followed if appropriate screening indicates a treatment need. The model divides the pain assessment procedure into three steps: (1) assessing pain severity, (2) assessing pain characteristics, and (3) assessing pain impact. A comprehensive assessment includes screening at all steps, with step 1 having the highest priority. Use of item response theory (IRT) would be extremely helpful in streamlining the gathering of information for steps in the decision tree. Assessing pain severity in the first step of the decision tree makes it possible to define, based on the BPI, "mild," "moderate," and "severe" pain. These categories of pain severity are based on the degree of interference with function associated with each category (Serlin et al. 1995).

Studies of symptoms and their measurement have almost exclusively examined a single symptom at a time (e.g., studies of pain, studies of nausea and vomiting, studies of fatigue). However, anyone who has a cancer or who treats cancer knows that symptoms often occur as a cluster and that symptoms can exacerbate one another. For example, pain is often linked with affective disturbance, sleep problems, difficulties with concentration, and fatigue in many advanced cancers. The need to assess multiple symptoms simultaneously is clear. However, the acceptance of symptom burden as a patient outcome measure for clinical trials, clinical treatment, and policy decisions will require further conceptual elaboration and clinical research (Cleeland and Reyes-Gibby 2002). The evolution of cancer pain research suggests how symptom burden research might evolve. With further development, symptom burden has many potential benefits as a patient outcome summary measure: it is more sensitive to differences in treatment toxicities, and it is easy for patients, health care professionals, and policy makers to understand and use as the basis for treatment choices and priorities.

Pain outcome measures could also be used for quality assurance (Cleeland et al. 2003). Cancer patients should be guaranteed the best possible pain management; therefore, poorly treated pain is a quality assurance issue. Pain assessment tools provide a method for routine monitoring and charting of pain in the hospital or clinic setting. Numerical scales seem best suited for easy tracking of pain. The Joint Committee on Accreditation of Healthcare Organizations has developed standards for the assessment and management of pain in health care organizations. Hospitals and other health care facilities will be expected to demonstrate compliance with these standards when they are reviewed for accreditation. The standards include the regular assessment and recording of patients' pain levels in dynamic patient care. The success of using simple pain outcome measures in the Veterans' Administration Hospital System proved their role in developing standardized cancer care (Cleeland et al. 2003).

Caution should be exercised when comparing and making judgments regarding "adequate" pain management in a practice, because it is not always known whether the high variance of patients receiving inadequate pain treatment is due to differences in defining adequate pain medication, heterogeneity of patient groups, or differences in the quality of the pain treatment itself.

CONCLUSION

Although improvements in the treatment of cancer-related pain have been significant over the last 20 years, undertreatment continues to exist. The most important issue for promoting widespread, adequate pain management has been the impact of valid pain measurement (Carr and Goudas 1999). Armed with a better understanding of the different types of pain outcome measurements, investigators will be able to select the most appropriate measures for epidemiologic studies of cancer pain, etiology studies, pain intervention trials, and clinical practice. The findings from extensive research on the BPI have provided strong support for its use as a standardized cancer pain assessment tool. The measurement and management of cancer-related pain presents a model for how to think of the evolution and acceptance of the measurement and management of other symptoms and other diseases.

INSTRUMENTS

For permission to use the Symptom Distress Scale, please contact Professor McCorkle at ruth.mccorkle @yale.edu. For the Rotterdam Symptom Checklist the manual and the questionnaire can be found at: http://www.med.rug.nl/nch/rscl.pdf.

REFERENCES

Aaronson NK, Ahmedzai S, Bergman B, et al. The European Organization for Research and Treatment of Cancer QLQ-C30: a quality-of-life instrument for use in international clinical trials in oncology. J Natl Cancer Inst 1993; 85:365–376.

American Pain Society. Principles of Analgesic Use in the Treatment of Acute Pain and Cancer Pain. APS, Glenview, IL, 1999.

American Society of Clinical Oncology. Outcomes of cancer treatment for technology assessment and cancer treatment guidelines. J Clin Oncol 1996; 14:671–679.

Badia X, Muriel C, Gracia A, et al. Validation of the Spanish version of the Brief Pain Inventory in patients with oncological pain [Spanish]. Med Clin Barc 2003; 120:52–59.

Beck SL, Falkson G. Prevalence and management of cancer pain in South Africa. Pain 2001; 94:75–84.

Beecher HK. Measurement of Subjective Responses: Quantitative Effects of Drugs. Oxford University Press, New York, 1959.

Bietz J, Gnecco C, Justice R. Quality of life endpoints in cancer clinical trials: the US Food and Drug Administration perspective. JNCI Monogr 1996; 20:7–9.

Bonomi AE, Shikiar R, Legro MW. Quality-of-life assessment in acute, chronic, and cancer pain: a pharmacist's guide. J Am Pharm Assoc Wash 2000; 40:352.

Breitbart W, McDonald MV, Rosenfeld B, et al. Pain in ambulatory AIDS patients: I. Pain characteristics and medical correlates. Pain 1996; 68:315–321.

Caraceni A, Mendoza TR, Mencaglia E, et al. A validation study of an Italian version of the Brief Pain Inventory (Breve Questionario per la Valutazione del Dolore). Pain 1996; 65:87–92.

Carr DB, Goudas LC. Acute pain. Lancet 1999; 353:2051–2058.

Cella DF, Tulsky DS, Gray G, et al. The Functional Assessment of Cancer Therapy scale: development and validation of the general measure. J Clin Oncol 1993; 11:570–579.

Cepeda MS, Africano JM, Polo R, et al. What decline in pain intensity is meaningful to patients with acute pain? Pain 2003a; 105:151–157.

Cepeda MS, Africano JM, Polo R, et al. Agreement between percentage pain reductions calculated from numeric rating scores of pain intensity and those reported by patients with acute or cancer pain. Pain 2003b; 106: 439–442.

Chen E, Craske MG, Katz ER, et al. Pain-sensitive temperament: does it predict procedural distress and response to psychological treatment among children with cancer? J Pediatr Psychol 2000; 25:269–278.

Cleeland CS. Measurement of pain by subjective report. In: Chapman CR, Loeser JD (eds). Issues in Pain Measurement. Raven Press, New York, 1989:391–403.

Cleeland CS. Research in cancer pain: what we know and what we need to know. Cancer 1991a; 67:823–827.

Cleeland CS. Pain assessment in cancer. In: Osoba D (ed). Effect of Cancer on Quality of Life. CRC Press, Boca Raton, FL, 1991b:294–305.

Cleeland CS. Cancer-related symptoms. Semin Radiat Oncol 2000; 10:175–190.

Cleeland CS, Reyes-Gibby CC. When is it justified to treat symptoms? Measuring symptom burden. Oncology (Huntingt) 2002; 16:64–70.

Cleeland CS, Ladinsky JL, Serlin RC, et al. Multidimensional measurement of cancer pain: comparisons of US and Vietnamese patients. J Pain Sympt Manage 1988; 3:23–27.

Cleeland CS, Gonin R, Baez L, et al. Pain and treatment of pain in minority patients with cancer. The Eastern Cooperative Oncology Group Minority Outpatient Pain Study. Ann Intern Med 1993; 127:813–816.

Cleeland CS, Gonin R, Hatfield AK, et al. Pain and its treatment in outpatients with metastatic cancer. N Engl J Med 1994; 330:592–594.

Cleeland CS, Nakamura Y, Mendoza TR, et al. Dimensions of the impact of cancer pain in a four country sample: new information from multidimensional scaling. Pain 1996; 67:267–273.

Cleeland CS, Serlin RC, Nakamura Y, et al. Effects of culture and language on ratings of cancer pain and patterns of functional interference. In: Jensen TS, Turner JA, Wiesenfeld-Hallin Z (eds). Progress in Pain Research and Management, Proceedings of the 8th World Congress on Pain. IASP Press, Seattle, WA, 1997a:35–51.

Cleeland CS, Gonin R, Baez L, et al. Pain and treatment of pain in minority outpatients with cancer. The Eastern Cooperative Oncology Group minority outpatient pain study. Ann Int Med 1997b; 127:813–816.

Cleeland CS, Mendoza TR, Wang XS, et al. Assessing symptom distress in cancer patients: the M. D. Anderson Symptom Inventory. Cancer 2000; 89:1634–1646.

Cleeland CS, Reyes-Gibby CC, Schall M, et al. Rapid improvement in pain management: the Veterans Health Administration and the institute for healthcare improvement collaborative. Clin J Pain 2003; 19:298–305.

Daut RL, Cleeland CS. The prevalence and severity of pain in cancer. Cancer 1982; 50:1913–1918.

Daut RL, Cleeland CS, Flanery RC. Development of the Wisconsin Brief Pain Questionnaire to assess pain in cancer and other diseases. Pain 1983; 17:197–210.

Dawson R, Spross JA, Jablonski ES, et al. Probing the paradox of patients' satisfaction with inadequate pain management. J Pain Sympt Manage 2002; 23: 211–220.

De Conno F, Caraceni A, Gamba A, et al. Pain measurement in cancer patients: a comparison of six methods. Pain 1994; 57:161–166.

de Haes JC, van Knippenberg FC, Neijt JP. Measuring psychological and physical distress in cancer patients: structure and application of the Rotterdam Symptom Checklist. Br J Cancer 1990; 62:1034–1038.

de Wit R, van Dam F, Abu-Saad HH, et al. Empirical comparison of commonly used measures to evaluate pain treatment in cancer patients with chronic pain. J Clin Oncol 1999; 17:1280.

de Wit R, van Dam F, Loonstra S, et al. The Amsterdam Pain Management Index compared to eight frequently used outcome measures to evaluate the adequacy of pain treatment in cancer patients with chronic pain. Pain 2001; 91:339–349.

DuPen SL, DuPen AR, Polissar N, et al. Implementing guidelines for cancer pain management: results of a randomized controlled clinical trial. J Clin Oncol 1999; 17:361–370.

Evans S, Fishman B, Spielman L, et al. Randomized trial of cognitive behavior therapy versus supportive psychotherapy for HIV-related peripheral neuropathic pain. Psychosomatics 2003; 44:44–50.

Farrar JT. What is clinically meaningful: outcome measures in pain clinical trials. Clin J Pain 2000; 16:S106–S112.

Farrar JT, Portenoy RK, Berlin JA, et al. Defining the clinically important difference in pain outcome measures. Pain 2000; 88:287–294.

Farrar JT, Young JP, LaMoreaux L, et al. Clinical importance of changes in chronic pain intensity measured on an 11-point numerical pain rating scale. Pain 2001; 94:149–158.

Felson DT, Anderson JJ, Boers M, et al. American College of Rheumatology. Preliminary definition of improvement in rheumatoid arthritis. Arthritis Rheum 1995; 38:727–735.

Felson DT, Anderson JJ, Lange ML, et al. Should improvement in rheumatoid arthritis clinical trials be defined as fifty percent or seventy percent improvement in core set measures, rather than twenty percent? Arthritis Rheum 1998; 41:1564–1570.

Ferraz MB, Quaresma MR, Aquino LR, et al. Reliability of pain scales in the assessment of literate and illiterate patients with rheumatoid arthritis. J Rheumatol 1990; 17:1022–1024.

Fishman B, Pasternak S, Wallenstein SL, et al. The Memorial Pain Assessment Card. A valid instrument for the evaluation of cancer pain. Cancer 1987; 60:1151–1158.

Forouzanfar T, Weber WE, Kemler M, et al. What is a meaningful pain reduction in patients with complex regional pain syndrome type 1? Clin J Pain 2003; 19: 281–285.

Galer BS, Gianas A, Jensen MP. Painful diabetic polyneuropathy: epidemiology, pain description, and quality of life. Diabetes Res Clin Pract 2000; 47:123–128.

Gammaitoni AR, Galer BS, Lacouture P, et al. Effectiveness and safety of new oxycodone/acetaminophen formulations with reduced acetaminophen for the treatment of low back pain. Pain Med 2003; 4:21–30.

Ger LP, Ho ST, Sun WZ, et al. Validation of the Brief Pain Inventory in a Taiwanese population. J Pain Sympt Manage 1999; 18:316–322.

Given CW, Given B, Azzouz F, et al. Comparison of changes in physical functioning of elderly patients with new diagnoses of cancer. Med Care 2000; 38:482–493.

Goetz MP, Callstrom MR, Charboneau JW, et al. Percutaneous image-guided radiofrequency ablation of painful metastases involving bone: a multicenter study. J Clin Oncol 2004; 22:300–306.

Goisis A, Gorini M, Ratti R, et al. Application of a WHO protocol on medical therapy for oncologic pain in an internal medicine hospital. Tumori 1989; 75:470–472.

Grond S, Zech D, Schug SA, et al. Validation of World Health Organization guidelines for cancer pain relief during the last days and hours of life. J Pain Sympt Manage 1991; 6:411–422.

Grond S, Zech D, Lynch J, et al. Validation of World Health Organization guidelines for pain relief in head and neck cancer. A prospective study. Ann Otol Rhinol Laryngol 1993; 102:342–348.

Grossman SA, Benedetti C, Payne R, et al. NCCN practice guidelines for cancer pain. Oncology 1999; 13:33–44.

Hardy JR, Rees EA, Gwilliam B, et al. A phase II study to establish the efficacy and toxicity of sodium valproate in patients with cancer-related neuropathic pain. J Pain Sympt Manage 2001; 21:204–209.

Hester NO, Miller KL, Foster RL, et al. Symptom management outcomes. Do they reflect variations in care delivery systems? Med Care 1997; 35:NS69–NS83.

Jacox A, Carr DB, Payne R, et al. Management of cancer pain. Clinical practice guideline No. 9. AHCPR Publication no. 94-0592. Agency for Health Care Policy and Research, US Department of Health and Human Services, Public Health Service, Rockville, MD, 1994.

Jadad AR, Browman GP. The WHO analgesic ladder for cancer pain management: stepping up the quality of its evaluation. JAMA 1995; 274:1870–1873.

Jamison RN, Brown GK. Validation of hourly pain intensity profiles with chronic pain patients. Pain 1991; 45:123–128.

Jensen MP, Karoly P. Self-report scales and procedures for assessing pain in adults. In: Turk DC, Melzack R (eds). Handbook of Pain Assessment, 2nd edn. Guilford Press, New York, 2001:15–34.

Jensen MP, Karoly P, Braver S. The measurement of clinical pain intensity: a comparison of six methods. Pain 1986; 27:117–126.

Jensen MP, Turner LR, Turner JA, et al. The use of multiple-item scales for pain intensity measurement in chronic pain patients. Pain 1996; 67:35–40.

Jensen MP, Ehde DM, Hoffman AJ, et al. Cognitions, coping and social environment predict adjustment to phantom limb pain. Pain 2002; 95:133–142.

Jensen MP, Mendoza T, Hanna DB, et al. The analgesic effects that underlie patient satisfaction with treatment. Pain 2004; 110(1–2):480–487.

Katz NP, Gammaitoni AR, Davis MW, et al. Lidocaine patch 5% reduces pain intensity and interference with quality of life in patients with postherpetic neuralgia: an effectiveness trial. Pain Med 2002; 3:324–332.

Keller S, Bann CM, Dodd SL, et al. Validity of the Brief Pain Inventory for use in documenting the outcomes of patients with noncancer pain. Clin J Pain 2004; 20:309–318.

Klepstad P, Loge JH, Borchgrevink PC, et al. The Norwegian Brief Pain Inventory questionnaire: translation and validation in cancer pain patients. J Pain Sympt Manage 2002; 24:517–525.

Kremer E, Atkinson JH Jr. Pain measurement: construct validity of the affective dimension of the McGill Pain Questionnaire with chronic benign pain patients. Pain 1981; 11:93–100.

Larue F, Colleau SM, Brasseur L, et al. Multicentre study of cancer pain and its treatment in France. Br Med J 1995; 310:1034–1037.

Laudico AV, Mendoza TR, Siguan SS, et al. Measuring cancer pain intensity and its effect on daily functioning: validation of the Cebuano version of the Brief Pain Inventory (BPI-Ce). Philipp J Surg Spec 2002; 57:94–99.

Lee JS, Hobden E, Stiell IG, et al. Clinically important change in the visual analog scale after adequate pain control. Acad Emerg Med 2003; 10:1128–1130.

Max M. American Pain Society quality assurance standards for relief of acute pain and cancer pain. In: Bond M, Charlton J, Woolf C (eds). Proceedings of the 6th World Congress on Pain. Elsevier, Amsterdam, 1991:186–189.

Max MB, Laska EM. Single-dose analgesic comparisons. In: Max MB, Portenoy RK, Laska EM (eds). The Design of Analgesic Clinical Trials. Raven Press, New York, 1991:55–96.

McCorkle R, Young K. Development of a symptom distress scale. Cancer Nurs 1978; 1:373–378.

McGuire DB. Measuring pain. In: Frank-Stromborg M (ed). Instruments for Clinical Nursing Research. Appleton & Lange, Norwalk, CT, 1988:333–356.

Melzack R. Concepts of pain measurement. In: Melzack R (ed). Pain Measurement and Assessment. Raven Press, New York, 1983:1–50.

Melzack R. The short-form McGill Pain Questionnaire. Pain 1987; 30:191–197.

Melzack R, Casey KL. The affective dimension of pain. In: Arnold MB (ed). Loyola University of Chicago. Feelings and Emotions: The Loyola Symposium. Academic Press, New York, 1970.

Mendoza TR, Wang XS, Cleeland CS, et al. The rapid assessment of fatigue severity in cancer patients: use of the Brief Fatigue Inventory. Cancer 1999; 85:1186–1196.

Mendoza TR, Chen C, Brugger A, et al. The utility and validity of the modified brief pain inventory in a multiple-dose postoperative analgesic trial. Clin J Pain 2004a; 20:357–362.

Mendoza TR, Chen C, Brugger A, et al. Lessons learned from a multiple-dose post-operative analgesic trial. Pain 2004b; 109(1–2):103–109.

Miaskowski C, Nichols R, Brody R, et al. Assessment of patient satisfaction utilizing the American Pain Society's quality assurance standards on acute and cancer-related pain. Clin J Pain 1994; 9:5–11.

Mitchell AC, Fallon MT. A single infusion of intravenous ketamine improves pain relief in patients with critical limb ischaemia: results of a double blind randomised controlled trial. Pain 2002; 97:275–281.

Moore A, McQuay H, Gavaghan D. Deriving dichotomous outcome measures from continuous data in randomised controlled trials of analgesics. Pain 1996; 66:229–237.

Moore A, Moore O, McQuay H, et al. Deriving dichotomous outcome measures from continuous data in randomised controlled trials of analgesics: use of pain intensity and visual analogue scales. Pain 1997a; 69:311–315.

Moore A, McQuay H, Gavaghan D. Deriving dichotomous outcome measures from continuous data in randomised controlled trials of analgesics: verification from independent data. Pain 1997b; 69:127–130.

Mystakidou K, Mendoza T, Tsilika E, et al. Greek Brief Pain Inventory: validation and utility in cancer pain. Oncology 2001; 60:35–42.

Okuyama T, Wang XS, Akechi T, et al. Adequacy of cancer pain management in a Japanese cancer hospital. Jpn J Clin Oncol 2004; 34:37–42.

Portenoy RK, Thaler HT, Kornblith AB, et al. The Memorial Symptom Assessment Scale: an instrument for the evaluation of symptom prevalence, characteristics and distress. Eur J Cancer 1994; 30A:1326–1336.

Powell CV, Kelly AM, Williams A. Determining the minimum clinically significant difference in visual analog pain score for children. Ann Emerg Med 2001; 37:28–31.

Price DD, Bush FM, Long S, et al. A comparison of pain measurement characteristics of mechanical visual analogue and simple numerical rating scales. Pain 1994; 56:217–226.

Radbruch L, Loick G, Kiencke P, et al. Validation of the German version of the Brief Pain Inventory. J Pain Sympt Manage 1999; 18:180–187.

Roth SH, Fleischmann RM, Burch FX, et al. Around-the-clock, controlled-release oxycodone therapy for osteoarthritis-related pain: placebo-controlled trial and long-term evaluation. Arch Int Med 2000; 160:853–860.

Rowbotham MC. What is a "clinically meaningful" reduction in pain? Pain 2001; 94:131–132.

Rudy TE, Kerns RD, Turk DC. Chronic pain and depression: toward a cognitive-behavioral mediation model. Pain 1988; 35:129–140.

Saxena A, Mendoza T, Cleeland CS. The assessment of cancer pain in north India: the validation of the Hindi Brief Pain Inventory – BPI-H. J Pain Sympt Manage 1999; 17:27–41.

Schiffmann R, Kopp JB, Austin HA III, et al. Enzyme replacement therapy in Fabry disease: a randomized controlled trial. JAMA 2001; 285:2743–2749.

Semenchuk MR, Sherman S, Davis B. Double-blind, randomized trial of bupropion SR for the treatment of neuropathic pain. Neurology 2001; 57:1583–1588.

Serlin RC, Mendoza TR, Nakamura Y, et al. When is cancer pain mild, moderate or severe? Grading pain severity by its interference with function. Pain 1995; 61:277–284.

Shvartzman P, Friger M, Shani A, et al. Pain control in ambulatory cancer patients: can we do better? J Pain Sympt Manage 2003; 26:716–722.

Smith MY, Egert J, Winkel G, et al. The impact of PTSD on pain experience in persons with HIV/AIDS. Pain 2002; 98:9–17.

Su L, Tucker R, Frey SE, et al. Measuring injection-site pain associated with vaccine administration in adults: a randomised, double-blind, placebo-controlled clinical trial. J Epidemiol Biostat 2000; 5:359–365.

Syrjala KL. The measurement of pain. In: McGuire DB, Yarbro CH (eds). Cancer Pain Management. WB Saunders, Philadelphia, PA, 1987:133–150.

Syrjala KL, Chapman CR. Measurement of clinical pain: a review and integration of research findings. In: Benedetti C (ed). Advances in Pain Research and Therapy. Raven Press, New York, 1984.

Takeda F. Results of field-testing in Japan of the WHO draft interim guidelines on relief of cancer pain. The Pain Clinic 1986; 1:83–89.

Thie NM, Prasad NG, Major PW. Evaluation of glucosamine sulfate compared to ibuprofen for the treatment of temporomandibular joint osteoarthritis: a randomized double blind controlled 3 month clinical trial. J Rheumatol 2001; 28:1347–1355.

Todd K. Standardized pain control research. JAMA 1994; 271:925–928.

Turk DC, Okifuji A, Scharff L. Chronic pain and depression: role of perceived impact and perceived control in different age cohorts. Pain 1995; 61:93–101.

Turk DC, Dworkin RH, Allen RR, et al. Core outcome domains for chronic pain clinical trials: IMMPACT recommendations. Pain 2003; 106:337–345.

Uki J, Mendoza T, Cleeland CS, et al. A brief cancer pain assessment tool in Japanese: the utility of the Japanese Brief Pain Inventory – BPI-J. J Pain Sympt Manage 1998; 16:364–373.

Ventafridda V, Tamburini M, Caraceni A, et al. A validation study of the WHO method for cancer pain relief. Cancer 1987; 59:850–856.

Walker VA, Hoskin PJ, Hanks GW, et al. Evaluation of WHO analgesic guidelines for cancer pain in a hospital-based palliative care unit. J Pain Sympt Manage 1988; 3:145–149.

Wallenstein S. Measurement of pain and analgesia in cancer patients. Cancer 1984; 53(suppl 10):2260–2264.

Wang XS, Mendoza TR, Gao SZ, et al. The Chinese version of the Brief Pain Inventory (BPI-C): its development and use in a study of cancer pain. Pain 1996; 67:407–416.

Wang XS, Cleeland CS, Mendoza TR, et al. The effects of pain severity on health-related quality of life. Cancer 1999; 86:1848–1855.

Wang XS, Li TD, Yu SY, et al. Brief report on the status of pain and palliative care in China. J Pain Sympt Manage 2002; 24:177–179.

Ward SE, Gordon D. Application of the American Pain Society quality assurance standards. Pain 1994; 56:299–306.

Ward SE, Gordon DB. Patient satisfaction and pain severity as outcomes in pain management: a longitudinal view of one setting's experience. J Pain Sympt Manage 1996; 11:242–251.

Ward SE, Hernandez L. Patient-related barriers to management of cancer pain in Puerto Rico. Pain 1994; 58:233–238.

Ward SE, Goldberg N, Miller-McCauley V, et al. Patient-related barriers to management of cancer pain. Pain 1993; 52:319–324.

Ward S, Donovan HS, Owen B, et al. An individualized intervention to overcome patient-related barriers to pain management in women with gynecologic cancers. Res Nurs Health 2000; 23:393–405.

Ware JE, Sherbourne CS. The MOS 36-item Short-form Health Survey (SF-36): I. Conceptual framework and item selection. Med Care 1992; 30:473–483.

Ware JE, Snyder MK, Wright WR, et al. Defining and measuring patient satisfaction with care. Eval Prog Plan 1983; 6:247–263.

White WT, Patel N, Drass M, et al. Lidocaine patch 5% with systemic analgesics such as gabapentin: a rational polypharmacy approach for the treatment of chronic pain. Pain Med 2003; 4:321–330.

Wright JG. Outcomes research: what to measure. World J Surg 1999; 23:1224–1226.

Wu CL, Naqibuddin M, Fleisher LA. Measurement of patient satisfaction as an outcome of regional anesthesia and analgesia: a systematic review. Reg Anesth Pain Med 2001; 26:196–208.

Yu DT, Chae J, Walker ME, et al. Percutaneous intramuscular neuromuscular electric stimulation for the treatment of shoulder subluxation and pain in patients with chronic hemiplegia: a pilot study. Arch Phys Med Rehabil 2001; 82:20–25.

Zech DF, Grond S, Lynch J, et al. Validation of World Health Organization guidelines for cancer pain relief: a 10-year prospective study. Pain 1995; 63:65–76.

Zhukovsky DS, Gorowski E, Hausdorff J, et al. Unmet analgesic needs in cancer patients. J Pain Sympt Manage 1995; 10:113–119.

FURTHER READING

Ahmedzai S. Recent clinical trials of pain control: impact on quality of life. Eur J Cancer 1995; 31A(suppl 6):S2–S7.

American Pain Society. Principles of Analgesic Use in the Treatment of Acute Pain and Chronic Cancer Pain: A Concise Guide to Medical Practice. APS, Skokie, IL, 1992.

American Pain Society Quality of Care Committee. Quality improvement guidelines for the treatment of acute pain and cancer pain [abstract]. JAMA 1995; 274:1874–1880.

Anderson KO, Mendoza TR, Valero V, et al. Minority cancer patients and their providers: pain management attitudes and practice. Cancer 2000; 88:1929–1938.

Burris HA 3rd, Moore MJ, Andersen J, et al. Improvements in survival and clinical benefit with gemcitabine as first-line therapy for patients with advanced pancreas cancer: a randomized trial. J Clin Oncol 1997; 15:2403–2413.

Cleeland CS. Pain control: public and physicians' attitudes. In: Hill CS Jr, Fields WS (eds). Advances in Pain Research and Therapy, vol 11. Raven Press, New York, 1989b:81–89.

Cleeland CS, Ryan KM. Pain assessment: global use of the Brief Pain Inventory. Ann Acad Med Singapore 1994b; 23:129–138.

Dietrick-Gallagher M, Polomano R, Carrick L. Pain as a quality management initiative. J Nurs Care Qual 1994; 9:30–42.

Jamison RN, Ross MJ, Hoopman P, et al. Assessment of postoperative pain management: patient satisfaction and perceived helpfulness. Clin J Pain 1997; 13:229–236.

Lasagna L. Analgesic methodology: a brief history and commentary. J Clin Pharmacol 1980; 20:373–376.

Steer CB, Marx GM, Harper PG. Is there quality in clinical benefit? Ann Oncol 2001; 12:1191–1193.

World Health Organization. Constitution of the World Health Organization. Handbook of Basic Documents. WHO, Geneva, 1948.

World Health Organization. Cancer Pain Relief. WHO, Geneva, 1986.

World Health Organization. Cancer Pain Relief and Palliative Care. WHO, Geneva, 1996.

Yun YH, Mendoza T, Heo DS, et al. Development of a cancer pain assessment tool in Korea: a validation study of a Korean version of the Brief Pain Inventory. Oncology 2004; 66:439–444.

CHAPTER
23

Palliative care outcome measures: translating research into practice

Gwenyth R. Wallen • Harriët M. Wittink • Ann Berger • Daniel B. Carr

INTRODUCTION

The first modern hospice was founded in the United Kingdom in 1967 by Dr. Cicely Saunders in response to the unmet needs of terminally ill patients and their families. At the beginning of the modern hospice movement, emphasis was placed on the last days or weeks of a patient's life. In the past few decades the scope of palliative care has expanded to include earlier and earlier stages in the trajectory of incurable disease (Kaasa and De Conno 2001). There is an increasing expectation that the control of pain and other symptoms and the relief of suffering throughout the spectrum of the disease should be included in the best of what health care has to offer (Cleeland 2001).

Since the founding of the first modern hospice, palliative care services have grown explosively, albeit unevenly, and are likely to multiply even more in the decades to come. As attention to and resources allocated for palliative care have increased, so has the need to evaluate the quality and impact of such treatment. The World Health Organization defines palliative care as "an approach which improves the quality of life of patients and their families facing the problem [sic] associated with life-threatening illness, through the prevention and relief of suffering by means of early identification and impeccable assessment and treatment of pain and other problems, physical, psychosocial and spiritual" (http://www.who.int/cancer/palliative/definition/en/) (2003). This definition reflects a recent evolution in the goals of medical care, particularly towards the end of life, from cure towards better symptom control, improved functioning and enhanced HRQOL. Palliative care is an interdisciplinary, collaborative, individual-centered approach concerned with physical, psychosocial, and spiritual care in progressive disease. It focuses on both the quality of life remaining to patients and on supporting their families and those close to them (Higginson 1999). Patients with advanced malignancies and incurable diseases require individualized complements of palliative care, where the emphasis extends beyond pain and symptom management to include the resolution of emotional, social, psychological and spiritual problems, the provision of information, improved communication, and support for the family (Higginson et al. 2002; Standing Medical Advisory Committee 1992).

Driving this evolution is the recognition that the disease burden for patients with advanced cancer often includes a large variety of severe physical and psychological symptoms (Berger et al. 1998). Pain, fatigue and depression are prominent contributors to the suffering of patients who have cancer (Goudas et al. 2001). The prevalence of cancer-related pain according to epidemiologic studies ranges from 14 to 100%, depending on the setting. While the prevalence rates for major depressive disorders or clinically significant depressive symptoms in patients with cancer range from 10 to 25% (Carr et al. 2002), wide variations in the prevalence of fatigue (4–91%) have been described in patients undergoing chemotherapy, radiation therapy or other treatments. The prevalence of fatigue in patients receiving palliative care has been reported as being from 48 to 75% and in cancer survivors as being from 17 to 56%. Hospitalized patients with cancer or non-cancer diagnoses, judged to be near the end of life, experience many symptoms that are frequent, moderately severe and moderately distressing (Tranmer et al. 2003). A number of authors have found pain to be the most frequent symptom (Walsh et al. 2000; Stromgren et al. 2002; Goodwin et al. 2003) but others have reported fatigue or weakness to be more common (Sarna 1993; Guo et al. 2001; Tranmer et al. 2003), while still others have reported breathlessness (Higginson and McCarthy 1989) or poor appetite (Brescia et al. 1990; Lichter and Hunt 1990) as most prevalent. Results from epidemiologic studies such as these vary by the target population examined and the methods used to establish the presence of each outcome, both of which are quite heterogeneous in studies of pain control and palliative care (Stromgren et al. 2002).

In the Institute of Medicine (IOM) report *Improving Palliative Care for Cancer*, Cleeland (2001) describes three broad categories in which research is needed to improve overall care and reduce distress at the end of life:

1. descriptive and epidemiologic studies that operationalize the individual needs of both patients and their caregivers, determine the prevalence and severity of the symptom distress they experience, and lay the foundation for additional research into the causes and treatment for this distress;
2. biomedical and behavioral studies of specific symptoms experienced by patients and the treatments for these symptoms; and
3. investigations that focus on patient care delivery and methods to improve this care through the optimal use of available treatments.

A major criticism of the evaluation research conducted in the field of palliative care has been the lack of standardization, or consensus, in outcome measures. One study by Hearn and Higginson (1999) found that

41 different outcome measures had been used to evaluate palliative care for advanced cancer patients. Similarly, a recent evidence report (Carr et al. 2002) on management of cancer-related symptoms issued by the US Agency for Healthcare Research and Quality (AHRQ) calculated the number of different tools employed in randomized controlled trials (RCTs) of treatments for pain, depression and fatigue. This report found that 125 distinct tools to assess pain were employed in the 218 RCTs of pain control retrieved from the literature between 1966 and 2001. Equally problematic, only a small fraction (5%) of papers concerned with cancer symptoms assessed pain, depression and fatigue concurrently despite prevalence studies and consensus reports suggesting the importance of investigating these three cancer-related symptoms simultaneously.

Although the uniformity, comprehensiveness and validity of outcome measures for the treatment of all types of pain lag behind those of equally high-impact conditions that affect the public's health (e.g., in cardiology, psychiatry or oncology) these lags are even more pronounced for cancer-related pain than for non-cancer pain (Goudas et al. 2001). From 1990 to 1999 the annual number of publications on the development and evaluation of patient-assessed measures rose from 144 to 650, of which 30% were in oncology. Reports of disease-specific measures rose exponentially, although there is little standardization in the use of such measures within clinical trials (Garratt et al. 2002). Much more research has addressed functional assessment, and how pain management influences function, in patients with acute or chronic non-cancer pain than in those whose pain results from malignancy (McQuay and Moore 1998). The more limited progress in outcomes research related to cancer symptoms may reflect the increased complexity and multidimensional nature of this field.

Adequate management of physical and psychosocial distress of patients and their families is the main objective of palliative care. The WHO model of care (World Health Organization 1990) proposed for cancer suggests that there is a complex interplay between treatments aimed at prolonging life, or curing the patient, and those palliative treatments aimed at controlling physical and psychosocial symptoms. Unrelieved symptoms are a major detriment to patients' HRQOL, including their ability to function. In surveys on factors considered important at the end of life, pain and symptom control is overwhelmingly ranked as most important by patients with advanced chronic illnesses. Pain, however, continues to be frequently inadequately controlled in cancer patients (Cleeland 1998; Goudas et al. 2001; Carr et al. 2002). Measuring symptoms in conjunction with HRQOL should therefore be at the heart of palliative care. Yet despite the distress that symptoms can cause, and the importance of their control, comprehensive symptom assessment is not yet a part of routine cancer care. Symptom measurement scales are the basis for adequate symptom assessment and control. Problems with symptom assessment are recognized as major barriers to good symptom control, and in part result from communication gaps between patients and their healthcare providers. Routine application of standard outcome assessment tools can help improve communication and facilitate the detection of symptoms, documentation of their severity, and assessment of the effectiveness of treatment (Cleeland et al. 2000).

In 2002 Higginson and colleagues published a systematic review of the literature utilizing both a qualitative meta-synthesis and a quantitative meta-analysis to determine whether hospital-based palliative care teams improve the process or outcomes for patients and their families at the end of life. Findings regarding the efficacy of hospital palliative care teams reveal a lack of well designed clinical research (Higginson et al. 2002). Nine studies were found which specifically explored the intervention of hospital-based palliative care teams (Bruera 1989; Wenk 1991; Zwahlen 1991; Bennett and Corcoran 1994; Ellershaw 1995; McQuillan 1996; Axelsson and Christensen 1998; Axelsson and Sjoden 1998; Edmonds et al. 1998). In addition, four studies were found which examined broader interventions but included a component of hospital palliative care or the use of a support team (Higginson and McCarthy 1989; Ventafridda et al. 1990; Addinton-Hall et al. 1992; Higginson et al. 1992). The nature of the interventions varied widely, ranging from individual nurses with unspecified training to multi-professional teams. Outcomes of interest included pain, quality of life, patient satisfaction, varied symptoms including nausea and fatigue, and service related outcomes. Only one of these studies was a randomized controlled trial where a hospital team was examined as part of other services. Furthermore, comparison groups were subject to bias and the analyses were not adjusted for confounding variables. Despite small sample sizes and relatively high attrition rates, most studies indicated a small positive effect for the hospital-based team. Higginson and colleagues (2002) concluded that, although hospital-based palliative care teams appear to offer some benefits, the study designs need to be improved and different models for providing pain and palliative support in the hospital need to be compared. Mazzocato and colleagues (2001) have identified many of the same outcome variables as those described by other researchers and those that will be included in the current review, including pain, symptoms, depression, coping, family structure and communication with health care professionals. They have further suggested a move towards more rigorous prospective, controlled, randomized trials in an effort to reduce potential biases.

The present review provides an introduction to basic concepts of outcomes assessment relevant to pain control and palliative care. Although many of the outcome measures presented in this chapter focus on palliative care evaluation trials in advanced cancer, the measurement of palliative care outcomes is equally important in other incurable diseases including but not limited to neurodegenerative diseases, end-stage renal, hepatic, cardiac and pulmonary diseases, and terminal HIV/AIDS. We also present some widely applied tools for the measurement of symptoms and HRQOL used in clinical outcomes research and bedside palliative care. Such measurement is the foundation of evidence-based practice, including continuous quality improvement and clinical practice guidelines. Due to the individualized, multidimensional, and evolving nature of palliative care outcomes, we will also briefly examine the use of mixed methods approaches where data generated from the quantitative tools described in this review are combined with in-depth qualitative inquiry.

This review is systematic in that the identification of the instruments presented, and the descriptions (when the data permitted) of their reliability and validity, are based upon results of Medline spanning 1966 to early 2004, Embase, and Cochrane Library searches. Additionally, the authors manually searched reference lists of articles published by experts in the field of palliative care (Wiffen 2003). Unfortunately, meta-analyses and systematic reviews in most areas of health care have been more concerned with the types of interventions examined and the quality of the relevant studies rather than with the heterogeneity of the outcomes used (McQuay and Moore 1998; Kahn et al. 2002). In the field of palliative care, there is a paucity of evidence-based practice guidelines, and comparative data to determine the most effective models of care are lacking (Lipscomb and Snyder 2002; Max 2003). Few systematic reviews exist on palliative care services and the reviews that do exist concluded that there is a lack of good quality evidence on which to base conclusions due to heterogeneous interventions and outcomes (Lipman et al. 2000; Goodwin et al. 2002; Higginson et al. 2002).

OUTCOME TOOLS FOR SYMPTOM ASSESSMENT

The patient's physical symptoms, as well as psychological, social and spiritual problems, may be described as "the palliative needs." In a recent study of cancer symptoms in patients receiving palliative care, pain was recorded most frequently (92%), followed by fatigue, anorexia, nausea, depression/sadness, poor physical function and impaired concentration or memory (Stromgren et al. 2002). Symptoms can be assessed by unidimensional scales that measure only one symptom at a time such as pain or fatigue, or by multidimensional scales that measure a range of symptoms. In controlled cancer trials the most frequently used instruments were the 0–10 visual analogue scales (VAS) of pain intensity (54%), the EORTC-QLQ C-30 (8%), the Hospital Anxiety and Depression Scale (HADS; 8%) and the Profile of Mood States (POMS; 8%). All other instruments were used in fewer than 3% of the reporting on controlled trials (Carr et al. 2002).

PAIN ASSESSMENT IN PALLIATIVE CARE

Pain in general is a unique challenge to outcomes research due to the importance of subjective information, not least when the pain is due to cancer. "Cancer pain" comprises acute pain, chronic pain, tumor specific pain and treatment- (including procedure-) related pain and is a major cause of impaired quality of life (Jacox et al. 1994). The majority of patients with cancer experience pain at some point during their course of treatment and the likelihood of pain increases, as does its average severity, with advancing cancer stage. Physical functioning, work, family and social relationships are usually impaired by pain. Many approaches to the measurement of pain attributes have evolved, but the selection and application of these approaches in palliative care has often been capricious and idiosyncratic (Caraceni et al. 2002). By far the most frequently employed pain measures in cancer clinical trials have been unidimensional scales of pain intensity, followed by scales of pain relief, then measures of peak and summed pain intensity differences between experimental and control groups (Carr et al. 2002).

An Expert Working Group of the European Association of Palliative Care (EAPC) has issued recommendations for pain measurement tools and methods in clinical research in palliative care (Caraceni et al. 2002). The group recommends that standardized pain assessment measures be applied. Visual analogue scales (VAS), verbal rating scales (VRS) and numerical rating scales (NRS) are considered valid to assess pain intensity in clinical trials and in other types of palliative care studies (see Chapters 5 and 22).

Among the multidimensional questionnaires designed to assess pain, the McGill Pain Questionnaire and Brief Pain Inventory have been recommended by the Expert Working Group of the EAPC because they have been validated in many languages. The group withheld recommending the Memorial Pain Assessment Card (MPAC) because it had not been validated in languages other than English at the time (Caraceni et al. 2002).

Von Korff (2000) cautions that multiple factors influence patients' pain reports, including time of day. Aggregated pain measures have therefore been shown to be more reliable and more sensitive to treatment effects than single item measures (Jensen and McFarland 1993). Aggregated pain measures are scores derived from multiple measures. For instance, the average of three concurrent responses to a 100 mm Visual Analogue Scale or of pain intensity ratings of current, average and best pain can be taken (Dworkin et al. 1990). A composite measure shown in cancer pain patients to have high internal consistency (Cronbach alpha > 0.8) consists of an average of ratings on a 0–10 scale of current, least and average pain (Serlin et al. 1995). Jensen et al. (1999) report that individual 0–10 pain intensity ratings have sufficient psychometric strength to be used in chronic pain research, especially in studies with large sample sizes, but composites of 0–10 ratings may be more useful when maximal reliability is necessary such as in studies with small sample sizes or in the monitoring of an individual patient.

The McGill Pain Questionnaire (MPQ)

The McGill Pain Questionnaire (MPQ) provides estimates of the sensory, affective, and evaluative dimensions of pain (Melzack 1975; see also Chapter 5). It is one of the most frequently used instruments for pain measurement and is considered useful for evaluating the efficacy and effectiveness of pain treatments, and as a diagnostic aid (Graham et al. 1980; Melzack 1985). It takes 5–10 minutes to administer. A short form has been developed (SF-MPQ) that takes 2–5 minutes to complete (Melzack 1987). In addition to collecting information about diagnosis, drug therapy, pain and medical history, and other symptoms and modifying features, the MPQ also contains a list of words that describe pain, divided into groups pertaining to the sensory, affective, and evaluative dimensions of the pain experience. It has been validated in cancer pain (Graham et al. 1980). The MPQ is widely used, including in numerous studies of terminally ill patients (Melzack et al. 1976, 1979; Kane et al. 1985). Dobratz (2001) used the MPQ in patients with advanced cancer in home hospice care in a qualitative study. The patients chose words that described four main pain patterns: "tiring and exhausting" (11.5%), "troublesome and annoying" (8.8%), "dull and aching" (7.7%), and "nauseating and sickening" (6.8%), supporting content validity in terminal patients. Repeated administrations of the MPQ to cancer patients revealed a consistency index ranging from 66 to 80% (Melzack 1975; Graham et al. 1980). The instrument has discriminative validity in types of pain, with cancer patients scoring higher than non-cancer patients (Majani et al. 2003). The MPQ is available in Spanish, Danish, Dutch, Arabic, Chinese, French, German, Italian, Japanese, Norwegian, Polish, and Slovak.

Brief Pain Inventory (BPI)

The Brief Pain Inventory (BPI) is a 56 item pain assessment tool for cancer patients developed by the Pain Research Group of the WHO Collaborating Center for

Symptom Evaluation and Cancer Care of the University of Wisconsin. It requires approximately 10 minutes to complete (Daut et al. 1983; Cleeland and Ryan 1994; see also Chapter 22). The purpose of the BPI is to assess the severity of pain and the impact of pain on daily functions. Pain intensity is scored on a 0–10 NRS on which 0 represents "no pain at all" and 10 represents "the worst possible pain" a patient may have. Patients rate their worst, least, average and immediate pain severity, pain relief ranging from 0 to 100%. Additionally seven numerical scales for functional interference factors caused by pain are measured in the areas of daily activity, mood, walking, sleeping, movement, enjoyment of life and relationships with others. Assessment areas include severity of pain, impact of pain on daily function, location of pain, pain medications and the amount of pain relief in the past 24 hours or the past week. The BPI is also available in a shortened form, the BPI-SF, a 15 item tool that takes 5 minutes to fill out (Cleeland and Ryan 1994). The internal consistency ranges from a Cronbach's alpha of 0.77 to 0.91. The level of pain assessed by the BPI can be divided into categories of "mild" (1–4), "moderate" (5–6) and "severe" (7–10) pain based on the amount of pain-related interference with function (Serlin et al. 1995). The BPI has been used as an outcome measure in advanced cancer patients, but in one study it was concluded that for routine clinical use with repeated assessments the BPI is not brief enough, and that the short form of the BPI (BPI-SF) is too short (Twycross et al. 1996). It has been validated for use in multiple languages including Cebuano, Chinese, Dutch/Flemish, English, Filipino, French, German, Greek, Hindi, Italian, Japanese, Korean, Norwegian, Spanish, Swedish, Taiwanese, Thai, Vietnamese, and others ongoing. In validating a Taiwanese version of the BPI-SF, Ger et al. (1999) demonstrated significant positive correlations between pain severity, advancing stage of disease and declining performance status. BPI questions about functioning are subject to both floor and ceiling effects.

To use the BPI in a publication or clinical or research trial, one must obtain permission and must agree not to alter its format. Permission is granted free of charge. Please see http://www.mdanderson.org/departments/PRG/ (accessed June 31, 2005).

Memorial Pain Assessment Card (MPAC)

The Memorial Pain Assessment Card (MPAC) is a self-administered 4-item, 8.5 by 11 inch card with eight pain intensity descriptors and three visual analogue scales that measure pain intensity, pain relief, and mood that is brief enough to use in the clinical setting (Fishman et al. 1987). It is composed of a visual analogue scale (MPAC1), a verbal descriptor scale that measures pain intensity (MPAC2), and visual analogue scales that measure pain relief (MPAC3) and mood (MPAC4). The verbal rating scale of pain severity is scored from 1 (no

pain) to 8 (excruciating pain). Shannon et al. (1995) found that cognitively unimpaired terminal patients were able to use the categorical scale, but a large percentage (25%) were unable to complete the visual analogue scales for pain intensity and mood. In another (medication) study on terminally ill patients, 85% of the sample were too ill to complete the MPAC repeatedly (Miller et al. 1999). Elderly hospice patients' choice of words to describe their pain had little overlap with the words used in the MPAC (Duggleby 2002).

Gracely Pain Scale (GPS)

The Gracely Pain Scale (GPS) is a ratio scale originally designed to measure both the intensity and unpleasantness of the individual's experimental pain sensation with the aid of verbal pain descriptors (Gracely et al. 1978, 1982). Most measures of clinical pain magnitude use a single measurement derived from a numerical, visual-analogue, or verbal scale of pain intensity. However, with the GPS individuals are asked to select along a continuum of 13 verbal descriptors that are arranged according to the amount of pain intensity they describe. First the patient is asked to select one of the word descriptors along the graphic continuum and then they are asked to select a corresponding number. The intensity scale is administered followed by the unpleasantness scale. It is important to administer both scales because the intensity of a pain sensation and the unpleasantness of this sensation are different. Gracely provides an example of this by describing sometimes weak or mild pains (like an earache in the middle of the night) as more unpleasant than the more intense pains (like getting an injection). The multiple verbal descriptors cover the entire pain range, minimizing floor and ceiling effects (Gracely and Kwilosz 1988). Based on ratio-scaling techniques, the magnitudes assigned to the descriptors demonstrate good internal consistency, reliability and objectivity (Max et al. 1992; McArthur et al. 2000). Although the GPS has not been widely adopted in the clinical palliative care arena, it has been used in clinical trials examining neuropathic pain in HIV (McArthur et al. 2000) and diabetic (Max et al. 1992) patients.

FATIGUE ASSESSMENT

Fatigue is one of the most commonly reported symptoms in patients in palliative care. Fatigue in cancer patients is associated with psychological disturbance, symptom distress and decreases in functional status and consequently has a profound impact on HRQOL. Until very recently, fatigue has not been measured routinely despite its effect on HRQOL. Most commonly, fatigue is found as one item on a scale measuring functional status or mood (Mendoza et al. 1999). Several HRQOL instruments contain items that measure vitality, but fatigue in the terminally ill population may not be the same as the lack of vitality in other populations. The concurrent validity of three fatigue measures, the Brief Fatigue Inventory (BFI) (Mendoza et al. 1999), the Functional Assessment of Cancer Therapy Fatigue Subscale (FACT-F) (Yellen et al. 1997), and the lack of energy item from the Memorial Symptom Assessment Scale Short Form (MSAS-SF) (Portenoy et al. 1994), has been established in a cancer population (Hwang et al. 2003).

The National Comprehensive Cancer Network (NCCN) has published practice guidelines for cancer-related fatigue in which frequent assessment of fatigue is recommended (Mock et al. 2000). The use of a simple 0–10 numerical self-report scale or verbal scale is recommended to assess the severity of fatigue in clinical settings. This recommendation is based on a study by Piper et al. (1999) correlating self-report scores on a 0–10 scale of fatigue with the physical functioning (PF) scale from the SF-36. They found a significant reduction in SF-36 PF scores when fatigue scores were ≥ 7. If moderate or severe fatigue is reported, the NCCN panel recommends a focused history and physical examination and evaluation of the pattern of fatigue, associated symptoms, and its interference with normal functioning. Five potential causes should be addressed because they are common and potentially reversible: pain, emotional distress, sleep disturbance, anemia and hypothyroidism (Mock et al. 2000; Barnes and Bruera 2002). Cancer-related fatigue criteria have been proposed for the International Classification of Disease 10th revision – Clinical Modification (Cella et al. 1998). For an overview of fatigue outcome tools, see Table 23.1.

Brief Fatigue Inventory (BFI)

The Brief Fatigue Inventory (BFI) (Mendoza et al. 1999) is a self-report instrument based on the Brief Pain Inventory (BPI). It consists of 9 items that are measured on a 0–10 numeric rating scale. Three items ask patients to rate the severity of their fatigue ranging from 0 (no fatigue) to 10 (fatigue as bad as you can imagine) at its "worst," "usual" and "now" during normal waking hours. Six items assess the degree that fatigue has interfered with different aspects of the patient's life during the past 24 hours (this can be changed to last week). The interference items include general activity, mood, walking ability, normal work (including housework and work outside the home), relationships with others, and enjoyment of life. The interference items are scaled from 0 (no interference) to 10 (complete interference). The tool was validated on 305 inpatients and outpatients with cancer and a comparison group of 290 community dwelling adults. Factor analysis showed that the BFI measures a single construct. The arithmetic mean of the nine BFI scores can be used as a global BFI score. Discriminant validity was supported by significantly different BFI scores across different

performance status ratings based on the ECOG scale. Good internal consistency was demonstrated in the initial psychometric testing of the BFI, with a Cronbach's alpha coefficient of 0.94 (Mendoza et al. 1999). The BFI has been validated in numerous languages. Most recently, the Chinese translation of the BFI (BFI-C) was tested in 249 Chinese cancer patients with multiple diagnoses. Internal consistency of the fatigue severity (alpha = 0.92) and fatigue interference (alpha = 0.90) scales in this Chinese sample was high (Wang et al. 2004).

Functional Assessment of Cancer Therapy-Fatigue (FACT-F)

The Functional Assessment of Cancer Therapy-Fatigue (FACT-F) was designed to measure the fatigue symptoms of cancer patients with anemia (Yellen et al. 1997). It consists of 28 items of the widely translated Functional Assessment of Cancer Therapy-General (FACT-G; Cella et al. 1993) to assess HRQOL and an additional 13 items to address fatigue. Each item is rated on a 5 point Likert scale ranging from 0 (not at all) to 4 (very much so). The FACT-F is a unidimensional measure of fatigue that demonstrates good test–retest and internal reliability and has concurrent validity. High scores reflect fewer problems, i.e., better HRQOL. Fatigue subscale scores have a significant inverse relationship with ECOG scores, meaning that high FACT-F scores are associated with better functional status. The entire questionnaire may be too long to be given to cancer patients in a clinical setting. The 13-item fatigue subscale, however, does meet the requirement of a rapidly administered scale (Mendoza et al. 1999).

To obtain the instrument see: http://www.facit.org/qview/qlist.aspx (accessed July 31, 2005).

Piper Fatigue Scale (PFS)

The original scale assesses subjective fatigue using responses to a 46 item visual analogue scale (Piper et al. 1987). The original instrument has shown good internal consistency with a Cronbach's alpha of 0.85, and has been validated in multiple studies. The revised PFS (Piper et al. 1998) consists of 22 items which are rated on 0–10 scales, with word anchors that vary from generic ("none" to "a great deal") to specific ("able to concentrate" to "unable to concentrate"). The scale measures four dimensions of subjective fatigue: behavior/severity; affective; meaning/sensory; and cognitive/mood. The 22 items are used to calculate the four subscale scores and the total fatigue score. The total fatigue score is divided by 22 to normalize it on a numeric 0–10 scale. Severity of the fatigue is coded from none (0), mild (1–3), moderate (4–6) to severe (7–10). Standardized alpha for the entire 22 item scale was alpha = 0.97.

Table 23.1 Outcome tools for the measurement of fatigue

Instrument (time to complete)	Items/domains	Publication	Reliability	Validity	Language other than English
BFI Brief Fatigue Inventory	9 items, 1 domain	Mendoza et al. (1999)	Internal consistency: alpha = 0.96	Construct validity through factor analysis. Concurrent validity with the fatigue subscale of the FACT and the vigor and fatigue subscales of the POMS	German, Japanese, Arabic, Chinese, Korean, Russian, Taiwanese
FACT-F Functional Assessment of Cancer Therapy-Fatigue	28 items from the Fact-General + 13 items to assess fatigue (the 13 items form one domain)	Yellen et al. (1997)	FACT-G: test–retest reliability = 0.82–0.92 FACT-F: test–retest reliability = 0.87 Internal consistency: alpha = 0.93–0.95	Discriminant validity with ECOG scores, convergent validity with POMS fatigue and Piper fatigue scales. Discriminant validity for hemoglobin and physical performance levels	FACT-G: Afrikaans, Arabic, Bulgarian, Chinese-Simplified, Chinese-Traditional, Chinese for Hong Kong, Chinese for Malaysia, Chinese for Singapore, Chinese for Taiwan, Croatian, Czech, Danish, Dutch, Estonian, Finnish, French, Georgian, German, Greek, Hebrew, Hindi, Hungarian, Indonesian, Italian, Japanese, Korean, Latvian, Lithuanian, Malay, Marathi, Norwegian, Pedi, Polish, Portuguese, Romanian, Russian, Russian for Israel, Russian for USA, Serbian, Slovak, Slovene, Spanish, Swedish, Tagalog, Telugu, Thai, Tswana, Turkish, Zulu
Piper Fatigue Self-Report Scale – revised (PFS)	22 items, four subscales: behavioral/severity (6 items), affective meaning (5 items), sensory (5 items) and cognitive/mood 6 items)	Piper et al. (1987, 1998)	Internal consistency: alpha = 0.97	Construct validity through factor analysis	No

FUNCTIONAL ABILITY ASSESSMENT

Functional status can be measured using the Karnofsky Performance Status Scale (Karnofsky et al. 1948), the Zubrod Scale (Zubrod 1960) or the Eastern Cooperative Oncology Group (ECOG) Scale (Oken et al. 1982). The recently developed Edmonton Functional Assessment Tool (EFAT) attempts to measure some activities of daily living and a number of impairments common in palliative care patients that may interfere with ability to carry out activities of daily living (Kaasa et al. 1997). Functional status scales have previously been used as proxy measures of HRQOL. Because they only measure one domain of the construct, they are not considered HRQOL measures by current standards. Performance status is widely used to select adult patients for entry into clinical trials. For this purpose broad assessment tools are used as described below and in Table 23.2. Although these performance status instruments can provide a quick and useful description of a population of patients, they are less successful in conveying the specific needs and challenges of an individual patient (Gillis and Donovan 2001). An ECOG level of 2 for instance ("Ambulatory and capable of all self care but unable to carry out any work activities." "Up and about more than 50% of waking hours") specifies very little about the quality and quantity of a person's physical functioning. For example: "ambulatory" with the aid of a rolling walker is a different level of physical functioning than being "ambulatory" without any assistive devices. What is not readily apparent is how marginal a patient's hold on independence may be, and the extent that further minor losses may impair his or her ability to function. A brief period of bed rest or limited mobility may lead to functional loss sufficient to result in dependence in gait and transfers (Gillis and Donovan 2001). The ability to function independently allows a patient to remain at home and has a significant impact on the family members' burden of care. Functional ability is a major consideration in discharge and advanced care planning and is

an important outcome in the evaluation of the adequacy of symptom control. Despite the importance that the level of functional ability has to patients, family and care providers in daily life, clinical care and research, there is a relative lack of instruments to assess functional ability in palliative care. For an overview of functional assessment tools, see Table 23.2.

Edmonton Functional Assessment Test (EFAT)

The Edmonton Functional Assessment Test (EFAT) is based on the perspective of functional status within the domains of impairment and disability as defined by the WHO (1980) in a sample of terminal cancer patients (Kaasa et al. 1997). A clinician-rated tool, the EFAT consists of Part I, which includes 10 items of functional status, and Part II, which contains a single item that summarizes overall performance status. Each item is scored on a 4-point numerical rating scale. A 0 rating represents independent functional status and a 3 rating represents complete loss of functional status. The item scores are summed and expressed as a proportion of the total number of items evaluated. Higher scores indicate more functional dependence. The instrument has good inter-rater reliability, although agreement for the sensation, pain and mental alertness items was lower than acceptable. The EFAT has good content, concurrent, and construct validity. The next generation of the EFAT, known as EFAT-2, was

Table 23.2 Outcome tools for the measurement of physical functioning

Instrument (time to complete)	Items/domains	Publication	Reliability	Validity	Language other than English
ECOG Eastern Cooperative Oncology Group (<1 minute)	1 domain: physical functioning	Oken et al. (1982)	Inter-rater reliability ICC = 0.81	KPS	No
EFAT Edmonton Functional Assessment Tool (not reported)	10 items + global performance status: communication, mental alert, pain, sensation, respiratory function, balance, mobility, activity level, wheelchair mobility, ADL	Kaasa et al. (1997)	Inter-rater reliability ICC = 0.88	Concurrent validity with ECOG and Karnofsky Discriminant validity functional status hospital and home patients	No
KPS Karnofsky Performance Scale (<1 minute)	1 domain: physical functioning	Karnofsky et al. (1948)	Inter-rater reliability ICC = 0.71	Concurrent validity with ECOG, predictive validity survival	Numerous
Zubrod Scale (<1 minute)	1 domain: physical functioning	Zubrod (1960)	Unknown	Unknown	Unknown

developed and tested on 275 patients in an acute palliative care unit (Kaasa and Wessel 2001). Factor analysis revealed two main factors: physical and non-physical (cognitive/affective). Pain was identified as an independent item and did not correlate with any other item. Cronbach's alpha was 0.86. Inter-rater reliability for the EFAT-2 is good with an intraclass correlation (ICC) of 0.95–0.97 (Kaasa et al. 2000).

Eastern Cooperative Oncology Group (ECOG)

The Eastern Cooperative Oncology Group (ECOG) measure (Zubrod 1960; Oken et al. 1982) is a clinician-rated instrument with 6 statements ranging from 0 (fully active, able to maintain all pre-disease performance without restriction) to 5 (dead). The instrument is used to assess disease severity, how a patient's disease is progressing, how the disease affects the daily living abilities of the patient, and to determine appropriate treatment and prognosis. Inter-rater reliability between physicians was reported as Kendall's correlation 0.75, and between patients and physicians as 0.59 (Conill et al. 1990). The WHO has developed a performance status classification for patients similar to the ECOG scale (Wester et al. 1996).

Karnofsky Performance Scale (KPS)

The Karnofsky Performance Scale (KPS) is considered the "gold standard" for assessment of functional status in patients with cancer (Karnofsky et al. 1948). The KPS measures one dimension using a 101-point scale that ranges from normal functioning (100) to dead (0). Subjects are grouped into one of three categories: no special care needed (80–100), varying amounts of assistance needed (50–70) and unable to care for self–requires equivalent of institutional or hospital care; disease may be progressing rapidly (0–40). Inter-rater reliability between physicians resulted in a Kendall's correlation of 0.76, while the Kendall's correlation between patients and physicians equaled 0.65 (Conill et al. 1990). In another study the inter-rater reliability of 47 National Health Service interviewers was found to be 0.97 (Mor et al. 1984). The KPS has strong correlations with physical capacities such as balance and stair climbing. It has shown predictive validity for survival in terminal cancer patients (Mor et al. 1984). The KPS has been criticized for having a floor effect (Verger et al. 1992; Kaasa et al. 1997). The Modified Karnofsky Performance Scale (MKPS) is a nine category scale which addresses both physical performance and level of pain (Jones et al. 1984).

Zubrod scale

The Zubrod scale is a clinician-rated list with 5 categories: 0 – normal activity, asymptomatic; 1 – symptomatic, fully ambulatory; 2 – symptomatic, in bed less than 50% of the time; 3 – symptomatic, in bed more than 50% of the time; and 4 – fully bedridden (Zubrod 1960). The Zubrod scale should be rated according to patient ability; i.e., if the patient stays in bed even though capable of normal activity, the rating should be "0." No information on the reliability and validity of the Zubrod scale could be found.

DEPRESSION ASSESSMENT

In addition to the assessment of pain, symptoms and functional status, it is important to explore psychosocial issues in palliative care patients and their families. The prevalence rates of major depressive disorders and depressive symptoms appear to be between 10–25% in patients with cancer. This prevalence is about four times that for the general population (Carr et al. 2002). The instruments that have been most often used to assess depression in cancer patients are the Hospital Anxiety and Depression Scale (HADS) and the Profile of Mood States (POMS) (Carr et al. 2002). In a review regarding depression in patients with advanced cancer and among mixed hospice populations Hotopf et al. (2002) report that the most widely used assessment of depression was the HADS, which gave a median prevalence of "definite depression" (i.e., a score on the depression subscale of > 10) of 29%. Studies that used psychiatric interviews indicated a prevalence of major depressive disorder ranging from 5% to 26%, with a median of 15%. Studies were generally small, had high numbers of non-responders, and rarely gave confidence intervals for estimates of prevalence. Ita et al. (2003) report that almost two-thirds of the palliative care population in their study had comorbid psychiatric illness. One-third of these disorders had not been identified or treated appropriately prior to admission.

Because depression may go undetected and untreated in medical care, the importance of screening tools and rapid assessment has been emphasized. The National Comprehensive Cancer Network (NCCN) practice guidelines for the management of psychosocial distress recommend the use of the Distress Thermometer, a modified visual analogue scale (National Comprehensive Cancer Network 1999). Single-item Interview Screening, the Visual Analogue Scale (VAS) and the Distress Thermometer have all been used in patients with advanced stages of cancer (Chochinov et al. 1997; Roth et al. 1998). The VAS has shown poor screening performance (sensitivity 0.72; specificity 0.50) (Chochinov et al. 1997). Many of the patients in palliative care present with vegetative symptoms of depression, such as changes in appetite and loss of energy, because of their illness. Therefore, in screening patients for depression and depressive symptoms, screening items should not include somatic symptoms. An overview of outcome tools to screen for depression and depressive symptoms in palliative care is presented in Table 23.3.

Table 23.3 Outcome tools for screening for depression and depressive symptoms

Instrument (time to complete)	Items/domains	Publication	Reliability	Validity	Language other than English
Distress Thermometer (<1 minute)	1 item	Roth et al. (1998); Ransom et al. (2006) and Jacobsen et al. (2005)		Convergent validity with HADS, BSI-18 and CESD	Japanese
HADS Hospital Anxiety and Depression Scale	14 items, 2 domains: anxiety and depression	Zigmond and Snaith (1983)	Test–retest reliability > 0.80 (2 weeks) Internal consistency: depression, alpha = 0.81–0.90; anxiety, alpha = 0.80–0.93	Content validity by factor analysis, convergent validity with distress thermometer Discriminant validity	The HADS is available in all languages of Western Europe and many of Eastern Europe, Scandinavia, along with some African and Far East languages
POMS-SF Profile of Mood States (3–5 minutes)	37 items, 6 domains: tension/anxiety, depression/dejection, anger/hostility, fatigue/inertia, vigor/activity, confusion/bewilderment	McNair et al. (1971); Shacham (1983)	Internal consistency: alpha = 0.78–0.91	Content validity by factor analysis Convergent and discriminant validity CES-D, MOS SF-20, KPS	Czech, Danish, Dutch, Finnish, French, German, Greek, Italian, Japanese, Norwegian, Polish, Russian, Spanish, Swedish

The Distress Thermometer

The Distress Thermometer is a self-report screening tool for psychological distress in patients with cancer (Roth et al. 1998). It reports distress on a thermometer configured as an 11-point Likert scale, labeled from 0 (no distress) to 10 (extreme distress). A score of 5 (labeled as moderate distress) is defined as the cut-off point. Optimal cut-off points were between 4 and 5 in a Japanese study with a sensitivity of 0.84 and a specificity of 0.61 (Akizuki et al. 2003). The Distress Thermometer was found to be valid in assessing distress in informal caregivers of patients with advanced stages of cancer (Ingham et al. 2003).

Hospital Anxiety and Depression Scale (HADS)

The Hospital Anxiety and Depression Scale (HADS) is a 14-item self-report scale that has been validated for use in cancer patients (Zigmond and Snaith 1983). It has two subscales, each comprised of seven items regarding depression and anxiety. Patients rate how they felt during the previous week on a 4-point Likert scale. Total scores range from 0 to 42 and a higher score indicates greater depression and anxiety. Ibbotson et al. (1994) found that an overall cutoff score of ≥ 15 resulted in

80% sensitivity, 76% specificity, and a positive predictive value of 41%. It is particularly useful because of the absence of questions regarding physical symptoms, which may be confused with psychological symptoms in medically ill patients. The HADS has been used in more than 200 studies worldwide. The reliability and validity of the instrument in international studies has been reviewed by Herrmann (1997). The HADS is generally found acceptable by (sick) patients and to have good to excellent reliability (alpha = 0.85) and validity (Lloyd-Williams et al. 2001). Akizuki et al. (2003) found the HADS to be the most sensitive screening tool in a sample of Japanese cancer patients with a sensitivity of 0.89 and a specificity of 0.65. A study of 100 patients with a prognosis of 6 months or less suggests that the HADS scale performs differently, with a less sensitive threshold, in individuals with advanced metastatic cancer with respect to the subscales and factor structure (Lloyd-Williams et al. 2001).

Profile of Mood States (POMS)

The Profile of Mood States (POMS) is a 65 item self-report instrument of subjective mood states that attempts to measure emotional state "now"

(McNair et al. 1971). Adjectives are rated on a five-point rating scale ranging from 0 (not at all) to 4 (extremely). Responses are summed to yield both sub-scale scores and a total mood disturbance score. In an effort to facilitate the use of the POMS with patients under stress or having pain, a shorter version of the POMS was developed in a sample of cancer patients (Shacham 1983). Each of the original POMS scales was reduced by 2 to 7 items without losing internal consistency. The shortened version consists of 37 items, each rated on the same 5-point scale (from not at all to extremely) as in the 65 item instrument. Baker et al. (2002) examined the POMS Short Form (POMS-SF) for its psychometric quality in cancer patients and found the instrument to be reliable and valid. Two sub-scales of the POMS have been used to assess fatigue in cancer patients: the POMS fatigue and the POMS vigor subscales (McNair et al. 1971).

Beck Depression Inventory (BDI)

The Beck Depression Inventory (BDI) was developed to screen for the presence and severity of depression in adults (Beck et al. 1961). The BDI contains 21 items. Each item is concerned with a particular aspect of the experience and symptomatology of depression that are rated on a four-point intensity scale rather than on a frequency dimension. A rating of three indicates the most severe, while zero indicates the absence of a problem in that area. Thus, the greater the score, the more depressed the individual. There is evidence that the BDI is reliable and valid with adults, including the elderly, with internal consistency (alpha = 0.91) and predictive validity (0.85) reported to be high (Gallagher et al. 1983).

Zung Self-Rating Depression Scale

The Zung Self-Rating Depression Scale (ZSDS) is a 20-item measure of the symptoms of depression (Passik et al. 2000). Patients are asked to rate each item according to how they have been feeling during the preceding week. Item responses are ranked by symptom frequency from 1 to 4, with some of the items being reverse scored. A raw score is calculated from the sum of the 20 items. This raw score is then converted to the "SDS Index" which is a percentage of the depression that is measured by the scale. It is important to note that scores on the Zung do not yield a clinical diagnosis of depression, but indicate a level of depressive symptoms that may have clinical significance. The ZSDS has been established as a valid and reliable measure of depressive symptoms (Gabrys and Peters 1985; Agrell and Dehlin 1989; Biggs et al. 1978).

Center for Epidemiologic Studies Depression Scale (CES-D)

The Center for Epidemiologic Studies Depression Scale (CES-D) is designed to assess current frequency of depressive symptoms, with emphasis on depressed affect or mood. The CES-D was originally intended for use with cross-sectional samples in survey research. In contrast to other commonly used measures of depression such as the Beck Depression Inventory (BDI), the CES-D was not designed for use as a clinical intake measure for the evaluation of illness severity over the course of psychiatric treatment. The CES-D has 20 items and 6 domains: depressed mood, feelings of guilt and worthlessness, feelings of helplessness and hopelessness, psychomotor retardation, loss of appetite, and sleep disturbance. Patients are asked how frequently they experienced a given symptom in the past week. Responses include: "rarely or none of the time (less than 1 day)," "some or a little of the time (1–2 days)," "occasionally or a moderate amount of time (3–4 days)," "most of the time (5–7 days)." Each of the frequency levels is assigned a numerical score from 0 (rarely or none of the time) to 3 (most or all of the time). Four of the items (numbers 4, 8, 12, and 16) are worded in a positive (non-depressed) direction to help avoid response set and to assess positive affect (or its absence). Scores range from 0 to 60, with higher scores indicating a higher degree of symptomatology. Because this scale includes symptoms that are common in terminally ill patients such as loss of appetite and sleeplessness, the results may be skewed toward a higher degree of depressive symptoms regardless of mood. The CES-D was validated in both household surveys and in psychiatric settings. Test–retest reliabilities have been reported ranging from 0.32 for 12 months to 0.67 for 4 weeks. Internal consistency of the measure has been good. Split-half correlations were reported as 0.85 for patient groups and 0.77 for normal groups. Coefficient alpha and Spearman-Brown coefficients were 0.90 or above for both the normal volunteers as well as the patients (Radloff 1977; Shaver and Brennan 1991).

MULTIDIMENSIONAL SYMPTOM ASSESSMENT

A variety of multidimensional outcome measures exist that can assess physical, psychological and emotional symptoms simultaneously in individuals receiving palliative care. These are presented in Table 23.4.

Edmonton Symptom Assessment Scale (ESAS)

The Edmonton Symptom Assessment Scale (ESAS) was developed for use in symptom assessment of palliative care patients. The ESAS is designed to be completed on admission and then twice-a-day thereafter (Bruera et al. 1991). It consists of nine 100 mm visual analogue scales for pain, activity, nausea, depression, anxiety, drowsiness, appetite, shortness of breath and sensation of well-being. An optional tenth item may be added by the patient. The patient is asked to make a mark along the 100 mm line with the far left indicating the least

Table 23.4 Outcome tools for the measurement of multiple symptoms

Instrument (time to complete)	Items/domains	Publication	Reliability	Validity	Language other than English
ESAS Edmonton Symptom Assessment System (few minutes)	10 items; pain, activity, nausea, depression, anxiety, drowsiness, appetite, well-being, shortness of breath	Bruera et al. (1991)	Inter-rater 0.5–0.9 Overall Cronbach alpha = 0.79 Test–retest summary distress measure = Rs 0.86 at 2 days and 0.45 at 1 week	Concurrent validity with STAS, MSAS KPS, BPI, RSCL Discriminant validity in/ outpatients	Chinese, French, German, Italian, Polish, Spanish
MPAC Memorial Pain Assessment Card (1 minute)	8 pain intensity descriptors and three visual analogue scales that measure pain intensity, pain relief, and mood	Fishman et al. (1987)	NR*	Construct validity with MPQ, the POMS, the Zung Anxiety Scale and HRSD, FACES, COOP pain subscale and a numeric rating scale	German
MSAS Memorial Symptom Assessment Scale	32 items, 3 domains that measure psychological symptoms, physical symptoms and global distress	Portenoy et al. (1994)	Internal reliability: PSYCH alpha = 0.88, PHYS-H alpha = 0.83, PHYS-L alpha = 0.53	Convergent validity with the FLIC, Karnofsky, Symptom Distress Scale	No
MSAS-SF Memorial Symptom Assessment Scale Short Form	3 domains that measure psychological symptoms, physical symptoms and global distress	Chang et al. (2000)	Cronbach alpha = 0.76–0.87 Test–retest 1 day 0.86–0.94; 1 week 0.4–0.84	Convergent validity with FACT-G Discriminant validity in/ outpatients	No
MDASI M.D. Anderson Symptom Inventory (less than 5 minutes)	19 items, 2 domains: symptoms (13 items) and interference (6 items)	Cleeland et al. (2000)	Internal consistency: symptoms alpha = 0.82–0.91; interference alpha = 0.87–0.94	Content validity by factor analysis Construct validity with disease and treatment severity	Arabic, Chinese, French, Japanese, Korean, Russian, Spanish, Tagalog, Taiwanese, Vietnamese
RSCL Rotterdam Symptom Checklist (8 minutes)	38 items, 3 domains: physical symptom distress (23 items), psychological symptom distress (7 items), activities	de Haes et al. (1990)	Internal consistency: alpha = 0.82–0.88	Convergent validity with ESAS and BPI, HADS	English, Finnish, French, German, Hungarian, IsiZulu, Italian, Portuguese (2 versions),

Table 23.4 Outcome tools for the measurement of multiple symptoms—Cont'd

Instrument (time to complete)	Items/domains	Publication	Reliability	Validity	Language other than English
	level scale (8 items)				Servic, Spanish, Tjecho-Slovene
SDS Symptom Distress Scale (5–10 minutes)	13 items; nausea, mood, loss of appetite, insomnia, pain, mobility, fatigue, appearance, bowel pattern, concentration	McCorkle and Young (1978)	Internal consistency: alpha = 0.97	Convergent validity	Dutch, French Canadian, Italian, Spanish, Swedish, Taiwanese

*(HRSD), Hamilton Rating Scale for Depression.

degree of symptoms they are experiencing and the far right the "worst" degree of symptoms. The sum of patient responses to the nine standard symptoms is the ESAS distress score. A numeric rating scale can be substituted for the VAS. A newer version of the ESAS includes an additional VAS for shortness of breath. In non-hospice patients with a diagnosis of cancer the ESAS satisfied criteria for test–retest reliability and internal consistency, criterion and concurrent validity (Chang et al. 2000).

For the instrument see: http://www.palliative.org/PC/ClinicalInfo/AssessmentTools/AssessmentToolsIDX.html (accessed July 31, 2005).

Memorial Symptom Assessment Scale (MSAS)

The Memorial Symptom Assessment Scale (MSAS) is a self-administered 32-item questionnaire (Portenoy et al. 1994). Factor analysis revealed various subscales: psychological state, which can be divided into an emotional symptom subgroup and a concentration subgroup; high frequency physical symptoms, which can be divided into a subgroup related to pain and pain treatment, and a subgroup related to gastrointestinal distress; and low frequency symptoms. The authors also sought to identify a brief subscale that could be used as a measure of global symptom distress. The combination of ten items including frequency of emotional symptoms and distress items from pain and treatment revealed the highest correlations, and was termed the MSAS Global Distress Index (MSAS-GDI). The MSAS-GDI is the average of the frequency of four prevalent psychological symptoms (feeling sad, worrying, feeling irritable and feeling nervous) and the distress associated with six prevalent physical symptoms (lack of appetite, lack of energy, pain, feeling drowsy, constipation and dry mouth). A short version (MSAS-SF) has been developed and validated in AIDS, cancer and

non-cancer patients (Chang et al. 2000). It has been validated for use in children aged 10–18 (MSAS 10–18), and recently for children aged 7–12 (MSAS 7–12) (Collins et al. 2000, 2002). It has been tested in terminal patients with end-stage congestive heart disease, chronic obstructive pulmonary disease, cirrhosis and metastatic cancer (Kutner et al. 2001; Tranmer et al. 2003). There was a significant difference in the prevalence of selected physical symptoms, but no significant difference in psychological symptoms, between cancer and non-cancer patients. Even participants who were seriously ill were able to complete the measure with little difficulty. Internal consistencies for the psychological subscale and for the physical subscale groupings were good, with Cronbach's alpha coefficients ranging from 0.77 to 0.85 and 0.78 to 0.87 respectively (Tranmer et al. 2003). Tranmer and colleagues report that while the strength of MSAS lies in its comprehensiveness and the detailed assessment of the frequency, severity and distress of each symptom, its weakness is its length, which may limit its utility in the clinic.

M. D. Anderson Symptom Inventory (MDASI)

The M. D. Anderson Symptom Inventory (MDASI) (Cleeland et al. 2000; see Chapter 22) is based on instruments previously developed by this group, the BPI (Cleeland et al. 1994) and the BFI (Mendoza et al. 1999). Each symptom is rated on a 10-point Likert scale to indicate the presence and severity of each symptom, with 0 meaning "not present" and 10 meaning "as bad as you can imagine." Patients are asked to rate each symptom at its worst in the past 24 hours. The instrument also includes ratings of how much symptoms interfered with different aspects of a patient's life in the past 24 hours. These interference items include general activity, mood, work (both outside the home and housework), relations with other people, walking and enjoyment of life. The interference items were also rated from 0 to 10 with 0 meaning "no interference" and 10 "interfered completely." An original item pool of 26 symptom items was tested for validity and reliability. Hierarchical cluster analysis followed by principal axis factor analysis and the best subset regression model technique yielded a 13-item model with two underlying constructs to predict symptom distress: (1) a general symptom severity factor including pain, fatigue, disturbed sleep, emotional distress, shortness of breath, drowsy, dry mouth, sad, remembering and numbness or tingling; and (2) a gastrointestinal factor including nausea and emesis (Cleeland et al. 2000). Cronbach's alpha for the two sets of symptoms and the interference scales have shown a high degree of internal consistency with alpha values of 0.85–0.87; 0.82–0.87; and 0.91–0.94 respectively in validation and cross-validation samples. The instrument has been validated on inpatients and outpatients with various types of cancer. The MDASI was shown to be sensitive to disease severity with higher scores being associated with higher ECOG scores (poorer performance). MDASI modules for specific types of cancer are being developed.

Rotterdam Symptom Check List (RSCL)

The Rotterdam Symptom Check List (RSCL) is a 38-item questionnaire widely accepted for use in patients with cancer (de Haes et al. 1990). The questionnaire can be completed by the patient and interviewer or a proxy. Patients are asked to rate the extent to which a particular symptom bothered them during either the past 3 days or the past week, using a 4-point Likert scale. Possible answers include "not at all," "a little," "quite a bit" and "very much." A manual in PDF format that includes instructions, for instance, on dealing with missing data, transforming scores and translations is available on the internet (see: http://coo.med.rug.nl/nch/rscl.pdf, accessed July 31, 2005). Philip et al. (1998) report face validity, construct and criterion validity, as well as repeatability of the RSCL in a sample of palliative care patients. The RSCL was found to perform well as a screening tool for anxiety and depression and to perform better than the HADS in those with progressive disease (Ibbotson et al. 1994). The instrument has been criticized for being too lengthy and for using verbal descriptors that may be difficult for some patients to understand.

Symptom Distress Scale (SDS)

The Symptom Distress Scale (SDS) is a self-report instrument that measures the level of distress with respect to 13 symptoms: pain (frequency and intensity), nausea (frequency and intensity), appetite, bowel pattern, breathing, cough, fatigue, insomnia, concentration, appearance and mood (McCorkle and Young 1978). Responses are rated on a 5-point Likert scale

ranging from 1 (no distress) to 5 (extreme distress). The total score ranges from 13 to 65 with higher scores reflecting greater distress. Items rated 3 or higher are considered to indicate serious distress. A total summed score of 25 or above indicates moderate distress; scores of 33 or above indicate severe distress that requires immediate intervention (McCorkle et al. 1999). Sarna (1993) found that symptom distress was strongly correlated to QOL ($r = 0.72$, $P < 0.001$) and functional status ($r = 0.71$, $P < 0.001$) in a sample of female patients with lung cancer. The SDS is responsive to change (McCorkle et al. 1989). Construct validity was supported when the SDS was compared to specific patient characteristics (McCorkle et al. 1994). Concurrent validity has been documented in various studies where the SDS has been compared to a variety of other tools with correlations ranging from 0.40 to 0.81 (McCorkle et al. 1999). Internal consistency has been reported in numerous studies and ranges from 0.70 to 0.92. The scale is short enough for sick patients to complete, but may not adequately capture the intensity of symptom distress felt by patients and may not include symptoms important for the care of some patients (Cleeland et al. 2000).

DESCRIPTIONS OF HEALTH-RELATED QUALITY OF LIFE (HRQOL) MEASURES

Broadly speaking, quality of life (QOL) includes not only health, but also other dimensions of life that reflect the aggregate impact of food, shelter, safety, living standards, and social and physical environmental factors (Greenfield and Nelson 1992). Outcomes related to QOL are of particular importance in trials comparing treatments that yield similar (or no) impact on disease progression and survival (Sanders et al. 1998). The use of quality of life measures in clinical practice can serve to shift the focus of treatment plans and evaluations from the disease to the patient (Higginson and Carr 2001). In palliative care, many authors have emphasized the importance of outcomes related to existential, spiritual and family domains as well. The definition of health by the WHO as "a state of complete *physical*, *mental* and *social* well being and not merely the absence of disease or infirmity" (WHO 1948) emphasizes that health, while a single dimension of QOL, itself comprises multiple dimensions. According to the WHO definition, health encompasses not only function at a biologic level, but also an individual's ability to perform physically, psychologically and socially in the everyday environment. The multidimensional concept of health-related quality of life (HRQOL) follows from this definition. Symptoms and HRQOL are related because pain and fatigue are associated with psychological disturbances, distress, and decreases in functional status (Guo et al. 2001). To date, however, most of the instruments applied to monitor and report the health status of patients with incurable diseases (both cancer and non-cancer) do not address components of HRQOL distinct from symptoms per se. Although reporting on HRQOL in RCTs has increased over the past decade, the proportion is below 10% for cancer pain trials, and there is a lack of a consensus standard for HRQOL measurement and reporting in this context (Sanders et al. 1998; Garratt et al. 2002). For instance, one review on HRQOL in patients with lung cancer identified 151 relevant reports (Montazeri et al. 1998). In aggregate, over 50 instruments were used to measure HRQOL or one of its dimensions. Garratt et al. (2002) examined the growth of HRQOL measures and their availability across healthcare specialties. From 1990 to 1999 reports of new instrument development and evaluation rose from 144 to 650 per year. Forty-six percent of these new instruments were disease- or population-specific, 22% were generic, and 18% were dimension-specific. A consistent issue with many of the palliative care studies is the use of outcome measures that are not responsive to change, and not validated or not appropriate for the palliative care population (Osoba 2002). As the choice of HRQOL instruments employed for a particular trial can affect both the results and conclusions, it is important to consider carefully which instrument is most likely to detect important differences relevant to the patients' lives in the specific setting of each planned trial (King et al. 1996).

HRQOL and health status are terms that are often used interchangeably, although they originally referred to different concepts. HRQOL encompasses the dimensions of health and well-being that have consequences for the daily lives of individual patients. HRQOL may include biologic markers, but it emphasizes indicators of physical functioning, mental health, social functioning and other health-related concepts, such as pain, fatigue and perceived well-being (Greenfield and Nelson 1992). Most measures operationalize HRQOL according to the WHO (1948) definition of health, with at least a physical, an emotional and a social dimension. A growing body of work discusses the use of generic versus condition-specific instruments and the number of instruments that aim to measure HRQOL is continually expanding. Historically, few instruments have been developed with careful attention to the principles of test construction and evaluation.

Quantifying HRQOL measures involves either scoring each domain separately, or combining the results from all domains to an index score. In the context of palliative care, the use of standardized HRQOL measures has been criticized for not taking into account each individual patient's view on what he or she considers important, or "quality," in life. Thus, HRQOL measures should be used as an adjunct to measuring disease specific outcomes rather than a substitute for them (Higginson and Carr 2001). Different groups of

patients attach a range of weights to the same domains (between-patient variation), and the weight that individual patients assign to the same domain at different points in their life may also change (within-patient variation) (Carr and Higginson 2001). Several authors (O'Boyle and Waldron 1997; Carr and Higginson 2001) argue that if an instrument does not truly capture the individual quality of life of a particular patient, it is not likely that it is valid for that individual nor responsive to change after treatment, because the instrument does not measure what is important to the patient. Based on these arguments, individualized measures are being developed and are receiving increasing attention (e.g., SEIQoL – see below), although more work needs to be done. An overview of HRQOL and QOL instruments is presented in Table 23.5 (see also Chapter 1).

Nottingham Health Profile

The Nottingham Health Profile (NHP; see also Chapter 1) is a self-report generic HRQOL instrument. The instrument is reliable and valid, but not used extensively in palliative care due to its length (Hunt and McEwen 1980; Hunt et al. 1981).

Short-Form 36 (SF-36)

The Short-Form 36 (SF-36; see also Chapter 1) is the most widely used generic HRQOL instrument with more than 3500 publications worldwide (Ware and Sherbourne 1992). One study (Kuenstner et al. 2002) comparing the EORTC QLQ-C30 with the SF-36 and the FLIC found good convergent validity of physical dimensions and emotional functioning between the three questionnaires, consistent with other studies. All three instruments were able to discriminate between patients with varying HRQOL status, supporting discriminant validity. Convergent validity was poor for the social subscales and the overall health ratings. The authors warned that comparison of overall health scores across studies that use different HRQOL instruments may lead to erroneous conclusions as the different overall health questions may actually tap into dissimilar concepts.

Sickness Impact Profile (SIP)

The Sickness Impact Profile (SIP; see Chapter 1) is a 136 item self-report. Although often used for outcomes assessment in chronic non-cancer pain, it is used much less in palliative care (Bergner et al. 1981). Witteveen et al. (1999) used the RSCL and the SIP in a sample of cancer and non-cancer patients. The RSCL and the SIP correlated well in psychological and physical dimensions in patients with advanced cancer, but this correlation was not observed in end stage cancer patients. The authors concluded that their data indicated that the HRQOL of end stage cancer patients cannot be reliably assessed with a symptom-based

Table 23.5 Outcome tools for the measurement of HRQOL

Instrument (time to complete)	Items/domains	Publication	Reliability	Validity	Language other than English
Generic					
NHP Nottingham Health Profile (10–15 minutes)	45 items: 38 in part I and 7 in part II. Physical abilities, pain, sleep, social isolation, emotional reactions, and energy level (6 +) A second section includes optional questions about work, social and sex life, interests and hobbies, and holidays	Hunt and McEwen (1980); Hunt et al. (1981)	Internal consistency: alpha = 0.77–0.85 for the first section and alpha = 0.44–0.86 for the second section in a sample of patients with osteoarthritis	Concurrent validity SIP, SF-36, RSCL	Arabic, Danish, Dutch, English US, Finnish, French, German, Hungarian, Italian, Japanese, Norwegian, Spanish, Swedish
SF-36 (10–15 minutes)	36 items, 8 domains: physical functioning, role-physical, bodily pain, general health, vitality, social functioning, role-emotional and mental health	Ware and Sherbourne (1992)	Cronbach alphas in both general and chronic disease populations range from 0.78 to 0.93	EORTC QLQ-C30	Afrikaans, Armenian, Bulgarian, Chinese for Hong Kong, Chinese for Singapore, Chinese for Taiwan, Chinese for USA, Croatian, Czech, Danish, Dutch, Finnish, French, German, Greek, Hebrew, Hungarian, Italian, Japanese, Kiswahili, Korean, Latvian, Lithuanian, Norwegian, Polish, Portuguese, Romanian, Russian, Serbian, Slovak, Slovenian, Spanish, Swedish, Turkish
SIP Sickness Impact Profile	136 items, 12 domains: sleep and rest, emotional	Bergner et al. (1981)	Test–retest reliability $r = 0.92$ Internal	NHP SF-36	Arabic, Chinese for Hong Kong, Danish, English

Table 23.5 Outcome tools for the measurement of HRQOL—Cont'd

Instrument (time to complete)	Items/domains	Publication	Reliability	Validity	Language other than English
(20–30 minutes)	behavior, body care and movement, home management, mobility, social interaction, ambulation, alertness behavior, communication, work, recreation and pastimes, eating		consistency: alpha = 0.94	EQ-5D MMPI	for UK, Finnish, French, French for Belgium, Dutch, Dutch for Belgium, German, Italian, Norwegian, Portuguese, Russian, Spanish, Spanish for USA (Chicano Spanish for Southwest USA), Swedish, Tamil, Thai
Disease specific					
BHI Brief Hospice Inventory (a few minutes)	17 items, 2 domains: physical/ psychological symptoms and quality of life/ satisfaction	Guo et al. (2001)	Test–retest 0.58–0.63 Internal consistency: symptoms, alpha = 0.88; QOL/ satisfaction, alpha = 0.94 (patient); symptoms, alpha = 0.89; QOL/ satisfaction, alpha = 0.94 (care giver)	Construct (factor analysis)	No
EORTC QLQ-C30 European Organization for Research and Treatment of Cancer Quality of Life Questionnaire (11–12 minutes)	30 items, 9 multi-item scales: 5 functional, 3 symptom and a global quality of life scale	Aaronson et al. (1993)	Test–retest reliability ranges from 0.59 for quality of life to 0.72 for physical functioning Internal consistency: alpha = 0.54–0.86	Construct validity with POS Convergent validity with SF-36 and FLIC	Afrikaans, Arabic, Bulgarian, Chinese, Croatian, Czech, Danish, Dutch, English, Finnish, French, German, Greek, Gujarati, Hebrew, Hungarian, Hindi, Iranian, Italian, Japanese, Korean, Lithuanian, Malaysian, Marathi, Norwegian, Persian, Polish, Portuguese ×2, Romanian, Russian, Serbian, Slovakian, Slovenian,

(Continued)

Table 23.5 Outcome tools for the measurement of HRQOL—Cont'd

Instrument (time to complete)	Items/domains	Publication	Reliability	Validity	Language other than English
					Sesotho, Spanish, Swedish, Taiwanese, Thai, Turkish, Xhosa
FLIC Functional Living Index Cancer (<10 minutes)	22 items, 5 domains: physical well-being and ability, emotional state, sociability, family situation, nausea	Schipper et al. (1984)	Internal consistency: alpha = 0.90	Construct validity by factor analysis Convergent-discriminant validity was shown with independent measures of symptoms and anxiety	Afrikaans, German for Austria, Chinese (Mandarin), Danish, Dutch, Dutch for Belgium, Finnish, French, French for Canada, German, Greek, Italian, Japanese, Luganda, Malay, Nobele, Portuguese, Shona, Spanish, Swedish
HRCA-QL Hebrew Rehabilitation Centre for Aged Quality of Life Index (1–2 minutes)	5 items; mobility, daily living, health attitude, support	Morris et al. (1986)	Internal consistency: alpha = 0.70–0.78 Test–retest = 0.89 Inter-rater reliability = 0.67	Concurrent validity with Karnofsky, and IADL index, STAS	Spanish
MQOL McGill Quality of Life Questionnaire (10–30 minutes)	17 items; physical symptoms, psychological symptoms, outlook on life and meaningful existence	Cohen et al. (1995)	Internal consistency: alpha = 0.89	Concurrent validity with Spitzer Quality of Life	Spanish, Taiwanese
MQLS McMaster Quality of Life Scale	32 items; physical symptoms, functional status, social functioning, emotional status, cognition, sleep and rest, energy and vitality, general life satisfaction, meaning of life	Sterkenburg et al. (1996)	Inter-rater reliability 0.83–0.95 Internal consistency: alpha = 0.62–0.79	Concurrent validity with Spitzer Quality of Life	No
POS Palliative Care Outcome	12 items; pain, other symptoms, patient anxiety,	Hearn and Higginson (1999);	Test–retest reliability 0.74–1.00	Construct validity with EORTC QLQ-C30 and STAS	No

Table 23.5 Outcome tools for the measurement of HRQOL—Cont'd

Instrument (time to complete)	Items/domains	Publication	Reliability	Validity	Language other than English
Scale (10 minutes)	family anxiety, information, support, life worthwhile, self-worth, wasted time and personal affairs	Goodwin et al. (2003)	Internal consistency: alpha = 0.65 (patients), alpha = 0.70 (staff)		
Spitzer QLI Spitzer Quality of Life Index (5 minutes)	5 items	Spitzer et al. (1981); Addington-Hall et al. (1990)	Internal consistency: alpha = 0.66–0.80	Convergent validity with POMS and HADS	Dutch, French, German, Italian, Spanish
SEIQoL Schedule for the Evaluation of Individual Quality of Life	30 items, 5 domains nominated by the individual	McGee et al. (1991)	Internal consistency: alpha = 0.48–0.74	Construct validity, concurrent validity with McMaster Quality of Life and HADS	No official translations

instrument alone, but must be supplemented by other instruments such as the SIP.

Brief Hospice Inventory (BHI)

The Brief Hospice Inventory (BHI) is a 17-item, self-administered questionnaire, using 0–10 numeric ratings which allow for the symptoms to be classified as severe or non-severe (Guo et al. 2001). This method of classification was based on the BPI. The instrument was validated in hospice patients, of whom 47% had cancer. A two factor fit was established; one for 8 physical and psychological symptoms (pain, tiredness, nausea, loss of appetite and shortness of breath; depression, anxiety and distress related to self-care ability) and the other for QOL outcomes and satisfaction (perceptions of hospice care: overall symptom management, sense of being cared for and helpfulness of hospice care; quality of life issues: comfort, feeling of life as a gift versus a burden, sense of quality of life and fulfillment of previously identified goals for the preceding week). Symptom scores were significantly correlated with QOL scores for patients and caregivers.

European Organization for Research and Treatment of Cancer Quality of Life Questionnaire (EORTC QLQ-C30)

The European Organization for Research and Treatment of Cancer Quality of Life Questionnaire (EORTC QLQ-C30) is a 30-item self-report designed for use in a wide range of cancer patient populations, and is intended to be supplemented by more specific questionnaire modules (Aaronson et al. 1993). It is the most frequently used tool in cancer care and palliative care studies (Montazeri et al. 1998; Kuenstner et al. 2002). The EORTC QLQ-C30 contains five functional scales (physical, role, cognitive, emotional and social) and three symptom scales (fatigue, pain and nausea/vomiting), as well as several single item symptom measures and a global health/QOL scale. Twenty-eight of the 30 questions are constructed as 4-point Likert scales with verbal anchors for each category. The remaining two questions are 7-point Likert scales with verbal anchors for the end-point. All subscales and individual items are transformed to 0–100 scales. Higher scores on the functional scales indicate a higher level of functioning while higher scores on the symptom scales indicate an increased presence of the symptom (Klee et al. 1999). Eleven disease specific modules have been developed. Strömgren et al. (2002), in their study of symptomatology of cancer patients in palliative care, found that the EORTC QOL-C30 covered the most frequent symptoms, but not drowsiness. This deficiency can be solved by adding the ESAS. The Greek translation of the EORTC QLQ-C30 was validated on a palliative care sample. The instrument was found to be useful in detecting the effectiveness of palliative treatment over time. Reliability was good (pretreatment from 0.57 to 0.79, during treatment from 0.56 to 0.75), especially for the functioning scale. In addition, very good validity was found in all the approaches used (Kyriaki et al. 2001).

To obtain the instrument please see: http://www.eortc.be/home/qol/ (accessed July 31, 2005).

Functional Living Index Cancer (FLIC)

The Functional Living Index Cancer (FLIC) is a 22-item self-completed questionnaire with 7-point Likert/linear analogue scales with verbal anchors on both sides (Schipper et al. 1984). The FLIC items are summed to provide an index score. Higher scores indicate better HRQOL. Several studies have demonstrated the multidimensional nature of the FLIC (Morrow et al. 1992; King et al. 1996). The instrument is reliable and valid and has been used as a standard against which to validate other HRQOL instruments.

To use the instrument, contact Dr. H. Schipper for permission at: Harvey Schipper, M.D., World Health Organization, Collaborating Centre for Quality of Life in Cancer Care, St. Boniface General Hospital Research Centre, 351 Tache Avenue, Winnipeg, Manitoba, Canada R2H 2A6.

Hebrew Rehabilitation Centre for the Aged Quality of Life (HRCA-QL)

The Hebrew Rehabilitation Centre for the Aged Quality of Life (HRCA-QL) is a version of the Quality of Life Index by Spitzer et al. (1981), specifically adapted for patients with advanced cancer (Morris et al. 1986). It is a multidimensional index with scores ranging from 0 (worst) to 10 (best). This index represents the summation of the scores for 5 items (mobility, daily living, health, attitude and outlook). The instrument was recently found to be reliable and valid in a sample of 200 patients with terminal cancer (Llobera et al. 2003). Criterion validity was established by significant correlations with the Karnofsky Performance Scale and the IADL index. This instrument is sensitive to change: when the clinical situation of a patient changed, important differences were seen in the index scores. When clinical conditions deteriorated the index score decreased dramatically. Predictive validity was supported by high correlations with survival (Llobera et al. 2003).

McGill Quality of Life Questionnaire (MQOL)

The McGill Quality of Life Questionnaire (MQOL) has been validated in patients with cancer receiving palliative care at home (Cohen et al. 1995). The MQOL is a 17-item questionnaire with each item rated on a 0–10 scale. It asks patients at all phases of illness, including those receiving treatment and those who have been treated, to list the physical symptoms that are most problematic. The first three symptom items are open-ended, thereby allowing patients to report only a few severe symptoms. Previous studies have found that a difference of 2.6 in the MQOL total score corresponded to changing a "bad day" into a "good day." The support domain was excluded from one study as it results in data that has a skewed distribution, is not sensitive to change, and its omission does not influence previously reported MQOL total score results (Cohen et al. 2001). Goodwin and colleagues (2003) report that the MQOL has limited utility in palliative day care patients as the measure does not identify items that are important to this patient group, such as that meeting people improved their QOL.

To use this tool, contact the author at robin.cohen@mcgill.ca to obtain a copy of this tool. You will be asked to sign a user form. There is no charge if it is not being used for profit.

McMaster Quality of Life Scale (MQLS)

The McMaster Quality of Life Scale (MQLS) assesses quality of life from the palliative patient's perspective (Sterkenburg et al. 1996). Sterkenburg et al. investigated the psychometric properties of the MQLS in a palliative care population and found that although ratings by different people (patient, family, staff) were correlated, systematic differences were found according to source of rating, which suggests that proxy rating (substituting family or staff ratings for a patient rating) should be avoided. The MQLS was sensitive to changes in the patient's QOL.

Support Team Assessment Schedule (STAS)

The Support Team Assessment Schedule (STAS) was designed to test the effectiveness of palliative care with multidisciplinary cancer support teams (Higginson and McCarthy 1993). The STAS has 17 items, each scaled from 0 (best) to 4 (worst). Ten of the items assess the status of the patient and family while the remaining seven items assess the services delivered. The tool was found to be valid, reliable, and practical in individuals in late stages of terminal illnesses living in community settings in the United Kingdom (Higginson and McCarthy 1993). Carson and colleagues (2000) found the STAS to be less valid and reliable in their Canadian study; however, they state that the STAS continues to offer a frame of reference for areas of patient need that should be monitored and assessed.

Palliative Care Outcome Scale (POS)

The Palliative Care Outcome Scale (POS) was developed using data from a review of other outcome measures that had been used, or were proposed for use, in evaluating the palliative care of patients with advanced cancer (Hearn and Higginson 1997, 1999). Ten questions were selected for inclusion based upon reliable and valid questions used in other measures that covered the physical, psychological and spiritual domains of life within the scope of palliative care. Eight of the questions are scored on a 5-point scale ranging from zero to 4; question 9 is scored on a 3-point scale and question 10 on a 4-point scale. There are staff- and patient-completed versions of the form. The form was found to have good test–retest reliability and internal consistency as well as face and content validity. Construct validity was supported by significant correlations of the subscales of the EORTC QLQ-C30 with the patient-completed POS, and significant correlations of the STAS with the staff-completed POS. Responsiveness to change was established for patient- and staff-rated pain and family anxiety; however, in a recent study a floor effect was noted for the items "time wasted on appointments," "given enough information" and "practical matters addressed" (Goodwin et al. 2003). Furthermore, these items did not show any change over time. The level of agreement between patient and staff completed forms as measured by Cohen's kappa was acceptable for all items except family anxiety and support, but improved to acceptable agreement for all items by the second assessment.

For more information and to order the instrument and its User Guide see: http://www.kcl.ac.uk/depsta/pallia tive/pos/pospub.html (accessed July 31, 2005).

Palliative Care Assessment (PACA)

The Palliative Care Assessment (PACA) symptom assessment tool was specifically developed to evaluate the effectiveness of a hospital palliative care team intervention (Ellershaw et al. 1995; Jack et al. 2003). The PACA tool measures level of symptom control for pain, anorexia, nausea, insomnia and constipation using 4-point scales ranging from 0 to 3 as follows: 0 represents absence of symptom; 1, symptom present, not affecting daily life; 2, present, moderate effect on daily life; and 3, present, daily life dominated by the symptom. The PACA has been shown to correlate with the McCorkle SDS and has an inter-rater reliability of 0.44–1.0. Reliability was assessed by cross-observer analysis (Ellershaw et al. 1995; Hearn and Higginson 1997).

The Spitzer QL-Index

The Spitzer QL-Index is one of the earliest QOL instruments to measure activity level, social support, and mental well being (Spitzer et al. 1981). The scale is intended to be completed by a healthcare professional and consists of five items.

Schedule for the Evaluation of Individual Quality of Life (SEIQoL)

The Schedule for the Evaluation of Individual Quality of Life (SEIQoL) includes two components to assess individual quality of life (McGee et al. 1991). First, it asks patients to choose and describe five domains they believe are the most important to their QOL at that moment. Then they are asked to rate how good or bad life is in each of those domains. One hundred mm vertical bars, where 0 mm = "worst possible," and 100 mm = "best possible," are used to rate the domains. The SEI-QoL-DW, which has been employed in a study to measure quality of life in cancer patients, uses visual analogue scales in place of the 30 hypothetical profiles used in the original longer SEIQoL (Montgomery et al. 2002).

MIXED METHODS IN PALLIATIVE CARE OUTCOMES RESEARCH

Although standard quantitative measures may provide a general picture of where an individual falls as compared to the population being studied, each patient *is* in reality so unique that qualitative methods are imperative if we are to gain a true picture of each individual's pain and symptom experience (Wallen and Berger 2004). For example, suffering is often mentioned in conjunction with pain and symptoms, yet the experience is so personal that it has been difficult to quantify despite the fact that the relief from suffering is a central goal for palliative care.

Investigations and evaluation of pain and palliative care outcomes have historically taken an "either–or" approach when it comes to the use of quantitative or qualitative methods despite recommendations of experts in our field. It is time to combine the best of what randomized clinical trials offer with in-depth qualitative inquiry (Wallen and Berger 2004). Mixed methods, also known as methodologic triangulation, allows the investigator to utilize multiple methods to collect and interpret data about a given phenomenon. The combination of qualitative and quantitative measures followed by simultaneous and complementary data analysis is known as a parallel/simultaneous mixed methods design (Tashakori and Teddlie 1998, 2003). Results of the multivariate analyses of the quantitative data are juxtaposed with thematic results of the qualitative analyses. This combination of methods ascribes to Patton's view that "qualitative data can put flesh on the bones of quantitative results, bringing the results to life through in-depth case elaborations" (Patton 2002, p. 193).

IMPLICATIONS FOR PALLIATIVE CARE PRACTICE

Outcomes assessment in palliative care is in transition. Instruments exist that measure one or more dimensions of one symptom or a number of symptoms. The terms HRQOL and QOL have been used interchangeably and are defined and measured in a wide variety of manners. Instruments exist that measure:

1. the need for care by patients and their families (Osse et al. 2000);
2. the objectives of palliative care such as the Support Team Assessment Schedule, the Palliative Core Standards and the Palliative Care Assessment (Hearn and Higginson 1997);
3. satisfaction with care (Kristjanson 1993); and
4. the quality of dying and death (Patrick et al. 2003).

Despite the abundance of instruments, insufficient attention has been given to the assessment of physical functioning in all types of palliative care patients and to the assessment of symptoms in patients with cognitive impairments, such as the elderly with dementia. Prior to selecting or developing instruments to assess QOL and quality of care, it is useful to have a comprehensive conceptual framework that specifies and defines all relevant domains that are appropriate for describing and evaluating end-of-life care and how it affects patients and families (Stewart et al. 1999). Stewart et al. have proposed a conceptual model that considers the patient, family and loved ones as important. Another conceptual model to consider is the International Classification of Functioning, Disability and Health (WHO 2001).

Outcome instruments are used in hospitals, hospice, day care, and in the community. Various instruments are also used at the various stages of terminal disease, although it is often unclear how "sick" the patients are that are included in each study. A prognostic or life expectancy rating scale of where patients are in the palliative care process is urgently needed.

A number of the instruments correlate with each other on subscales or domains, but the correlations are moderate. This diversity suggests that while different instruments attempt to measure the same concept, they may tap into different dimensions of the same concept and may therefore not be comparable. The results of investigations should thus not be interpreted independently from the instruments used and an interpretation of results must be based on the content of the items of the respective questionnaires (Holzner et al. 2001). Furthermore, most of the outcome instrument validation studies focus on patients with cancer rather than a broad spectrum of life-threatening illnesses.

Palliative care comprises care for patients who cannot be cured. Predictions for the year 2025 show an aging population, with more people dying worldwide from chronic or progressive diseases than acute conditions (Higginson 1999). Non-cancer patients with active, progressive, far-advanced diseases have traditionally not been fully integrated into the palliative care movement. For instance, in an annual series of surveys covering England, Wales, Scotland and Northern Ireland on the activity of palliative care inpatient services

in 1997/1998, only 2.4% of patients had a non-cancer diagnosis (Eve and Higginson 2000). Most of the outcome tools discussed in this paper have not been validated in a non-cancer, terminally ill population, yet they should be.

Despite the plethora of outcomes assessment studies, few papers explicitly discuss the relationship between symptom management and HRQOL. Symptom management is at the core of palliative care and HRQOL is central to the desired outcomes of that care. The use of patient-centered outcome measures allows patients to introduce and discuss concerns they might not otherwise voice. No tool will be used if it is too burdensome (too long or too difficult to understand). Instruments must be easily understood, administered, and interpreted by both clinicians and patients. No instrument is ideal for all intended uses; questionnaires are available in a variety of forms and many of these can be readily incorporated into clinical care and research. The dying experience differs not only by individual, but across health care systems, and across social and cultural groups (Patrick et al. 2001). The goal of preventing suffering and improving quality of life in patients with life threatening diseases could become a reality by accurately quantifying the variability in individuals, by replicating palliative care systems, providers and processes that provide the highest quality dying experience for different individuals.

CONCLUSION

Outcomes assessment is a dynamic area, particularly as it stands at the interface between routine practice and new standards for pain assessment and treatment applied by the Joint Commission for the Assessment of Healthcare Organizations. Systematic measurement and documentation of HRQOL is a useful, clinically relevant approach to incorporate patient preferences into front-line medical decision making. Doing so is expected to improve overall patient satisfaction with care (Marvel et al. 1999). It is clear that a comprehensive assessment of palliative care outcomes is unlikely to occur with the use of any single measure (Mazzocato et al. 2001). It is only through the combination of valid and reliable tools and appropriate methods that a full picture of the individual's overall health and well-being will be achieved.

The dissemination of ever-simpler and more powerful means to capture data electronically in everyday health care (Jadad 2000) opens new opportunities for understanding which treatments are effective, and for whom, and may provide irrefutable evidence that we who provide palliative care do add patient-centered value to the health care enterprise.

The following are websites to visit for measurement tools:

http://www.chcr.brown.edu/PCOC/toolkit.htm (overview of palliative care outcomes instruments)

http://www.eortc.be/home/qol/ (for information on the EORTC group)

http://www.qolid.org/ (for general information and listing of existing translations)

http://www.jr2.ox.ac.uk/bandolier/ (pain research at Bandolier EBM)

http://www.ahcpr.gov/ (Agency for Healthcare Research and Quality).

REFERENCES

Aaronson NK, Ahmedzai S, Bergman B, et al. The European Organization for Research and Treatment of Cancer QLQ-C30: a quality-of-life instrument for use in international clinical trials in oncology. J Natl Cancer Inst 1993; 85:365–376.

Addinton-Hall J, MacDonald, Anderson HR, Chambelain, Freeling P, Bland JM, Raftery JP. Randomised controlled trial of effects of coordinating care for terminally ill patients. British Medical Journal 1992; 305:1317–1322.

Addington-Hall JM, MacDonald LD, Anderson HR (1990) Can the Spitzer Quality of Life Index help to reduce prognostic uncertainty in terminal care? Br J Cancer 62:695–699.

Agrell B, Dehlin O. Comparison of six depression scales in geriatric stroke patients. Stroke 1989; 20:1190–1194.

Akizuki N, Akechi T, Nakanishi T, Yoshikawa E, Okamura M, Nakano T, Murakami Y, Uchitomi Y (2003) Development of a brief screening interview for adjustment disorders and major depression in patients with cancer. Cancer 2003; 97:2605–2613.

Axelsson B, Christensen SB. Evaluation of a hospital-based care support service with particular regard to financial outcome measures. Palliative Medicine 1998; 12:41–49.

Axelsson B, Sjoden PO. Quality of life of cancer patients and their spouses in palliative home care. Palliative Medicine 1998; 12:29–39.

Baker F, Denniston M, Zabora J, Polland A, Dudley WN. A POMS short form for cancer patients: psychometric and structural evaluation. Psychooncology 2002; 11:273–81.

Barnes EA, Bruera E. Fatigue in patients with advanced cancer: a review. Int J Gynecol. Cancer 2002; 12:424–8.

Beck AT, Ward CH, Mendelson M, et al. An inventory for measuring depression. Archives of General Psychiatry 1961; 4:561.

Bennett M, Corcoran G. The impact on community palliative care services of a hospital palliative care team. Palliative Medicine 1994; 8:237–244.

Berger AM, Portenoy RK, Weissman DE. Principles and Practice of Supportive Oncology. Lippincott-Raven, Philadelphia, 1998.

Bergner M, Bobbitt RA, Carter WB, Gilson BS. The Sickness Impact Profile: development and final revision of a health status measure. Medical Care 1981; 19:787–805.

Biggs JT, Wilie LT, Ziegler VE. Validity of the Zung Self-Rating Depression Scale. Br J Psychiatry 1978; 132:381–385.

Brescia FJ, Adler D, Gray G, Ryan MA, Cimino J, Mamtani R. Hospitalized advanced cancer patients: a profile. J Pain Symptom Manage 1990; 5:221–227.

Bruera E. Influence of the pain and symptom control team on the patterns of treatment of pain and other symptoms in a cancer centre. J Pain Symptom Manage 1989; 4:112–116.

Bruera E, Kuehn N, Miller MJ, Selmser P, Macmillan K. The Edmonton Symptom Assessment System (ESAS): a simple method for the assessment of palliative care patients. J Palliat Care 1991; 7:6–9.

Caraceni A, Cherny N, Fainsinger R, Kaasa S, Poulain P, Radbruch L, De Conno F, and the Steering Committeee of the EAPC Research Network. Pain measurement tools and methods in clinical research in palliative care: recommendations of an Expert Working Group of the European Association of Palliative Care. J Pain Symptom Manage 2002; 23:239–55.

Carr AJ, Higginson IJ. Are quality of life measures patient centred. BMJ 2001; 322:1357–1360.

Carr D, Goudas L, Lawrence D, Pirl W, Lau J, DeVine D, Kupelnick B, Miller K (2002) Management of Cancer Symptoms: Pain, Depression, and Fatigue. Evidence report/Technology Assessment no.61 and Prepared by the New England Medical Center Evidence Based Practice under contract No.290-97-0019. 02-E032. Agency for Healthcare Research and Quality, U.S. Department of Health and Human Services, Rockville, MD. Ref Type: Report.

Carr DB, Wiffen P, Fairman F, LeMaitre M. The Cochrane collaboration and its Pain, Palliative and Supportive Care review group. In: Max M. (ed.). Pain 1999 - an updated review. Refresher course syllabus IASP press, Seattle, 1999:399–410.

Carson MG, Fitch MI, Vachon ML. Measuring outcomes in palliative care: a reliability and validity study of the Support Team Assessment Schedule. Palliat Med 2000; 14:25–36.

Cella D, Peterman A, Passik S, Jacobsen P, Breitbart W. Progress toward guidelines for the management of fatigue. Oncology (Huntingt) 1998; 12:369–377.

Chang VT, Hwang SS, Feuerman M. Validation of the Edmonton Symptom Assessment Scale. Cancer 2000; 88:2164–2171.

Chang VT, Hwang SS, Feuerman M, Kasimis BS, Thaler HT. The memorial symptom assessment scale short form (MSAS-SF). Cancer 2000; 89:1162–71.

Chochinov HM, Wilson KG, Enns M, Lander S. "Are you depressed?" Screening for depression in the terminally ill. Am.J Psychiatry 1997; 154:674–676.

Cleeland CS. Undertreatment of cancer pain in elderly patients. JAMA 1998; 279:1914–1915.

Cleeland CS. Cross-cutting research issues: a research agenda for reducing distress of patients with cancer. In: Foley KM, Gelband H (eds). Improving Palliative Care for Cancer (Chapter 8). National Academy Press, Washington, D.C, 2001:233–274.

Cleeland CS, Mendoza TR, Wang XS, Chou C, Harle MT, Morrissey M, Engstrom MC (2000) Assessing symptom distress in cancer patients: the M.D. Anderson Symptom Inventory. Cancer 2000; 89:1634–1646.

Cleeland CS, Ryan KM. Pain assessment: global use of the Brief Pain Inventory. Ann Acad. Med Singapore 1994; 23:129–138.

Cohen SR, Boston P, Mount BM, Porterfield P. Changes in quality of life following admission to palliative care units. Palliat.Med 2001; 15:363–371.

Cohen SR, Mount BM, Strobel MG, Bui F. The McGill Quality of Life Questionnaire: a measure of quality of life appropriate for people with advanced disease. A preliminary study of validity and acceptability. Palliat Med 1995; 9:207–219.

Collins JJ, Byrnes ME, Dunkel IJ, Lapin J, Nadel T, Thaler HT, Polyak T, Rapkin B, Portenoy RK (2000) The measurement of symptoms in children with cancer. J Pain Symptom Manage 2000; 19:363–377.

Collins JJ, Devine TD, Dick GS, Johnson EA, Kilham HA, Pinkerton CR, Stevens MM, Thaler HT, Portenoy RK (2002) The measurement of symptoms in young children with cancer: the validation of the Memorial Symptom Assessment Scale in children aged 7-12. J Pain Symptom Manage 2002; 23:10–16.

Conill C, Verger E, Salamero M. Performance status assessment in cancer patients. Cancer 1990; 65:1864–1866.

Curt GA, Breitbart W, Cella D, Groopman JE, et al. Impact of cancer-related fatigue on the lives of patients: new findings from the Fatigue Coalition. Oncologist 2000; 5:353–360.

Curtis EB, Krech R, Walsh TD. Common symptoms in patients with advanced cancer. J Palliat Care 1991; 7:25–29.

Daut RL, Cleeland CS, Flanery RC. Development of the Wisconsin Brief Pain Questionnaire to assess pain in cancer and other diseases. Pain 1983; 17:197–210.

de Haes JC, van Knippenberg FC, Neijt JP. Measuring psychological and physical distress in cancer patients: structure and application of the Rotterdam Symptom Checklist. Br J Cancer 1990; 62:1034–1038.

Dobratz MC. Patterns of advanced cancer pain in home hospice patients. Cancer Nurs 2001; 24:294–299.

Donaldson GW, Moinpour CM. Individual differences in quality-of-life treatment response. Med Care 2002; 40: III39–III53.

Duggleby W. The language of pain at the end of life. Pain Manag Nurs 2002; 3:154–60.

Dworkin SF, Von Korff M, Whitney CW, LeResche L, Dicker BG, Barlow W. Measurement of characteristic pain intensity in field pain research. Pain Supplement 1990; 5:S290.

Echeverri TA, Acosta OV. Palliative care: the hospice concept. Pain Clinical Updates 1996; 4:1–4.

Edmonds PM, Stuttaford JM, Penny J, Lynch, A.M. Chamberlain J. Do hospital palliative care teams improve symptom control? Use of modified STAS as an evaluative tool. Palliative Medicine 1998; 12:345–351.

Ellershaw JE, Peat SJ, Boys LC. Assessing the effectiveness of a hospital palliative care team. Palliat Med 1995; 9:145–152.

Epstein RS, Sherwood LM. From outcomes research to disease management: A guide for the perplexed. Ann Intern Med 1996; 124:832–837.

Eve A, Higginson IJ. Minimum dataset activity for hospice and hospital palliative care services in the UK 1997/98. Palliat Med 2000; 14:395–404.

Fainsinger R, Miller MJ, Bruera E, Hanson J, MacEachern T. Symptom control during the last week of life on a palliative care unit. J Palliat Care 1991; 7:5–11.

Field MJ, Cassell CK. Approaching Death: Improving Care at the End of Life. Institute of Medicine. National Academy Press, Washington, D.C, 1997.

Fischer D, Stewart AL, Bloch DA, Lorig K, Laurent D, Holman H. Capturing the patient's view of change as a clinical outcome measure. JAMA 1999; 282:1157–1162.

Fishman B, Pasternak S, Wallenstein SL, Houde RW, Holland JC, Foley KM. The Memorial Pain Assessment Card. A valid instrument for the evaluation of cancer pain. Cancer 1987; 60:1151–1158.

Foreman MD. Measuring cognitive status. In: Frank-Stromborg M, Olsen SJ (eds). Instruments for Clinical Health-Care Research, 2nd, Jones and Bartlett Publishers, Sudbury,Massachusetts, 1997:86–113.

Gabrys JB, Peters K. Reliability, discriminant and predictive validity of the Zung Self-Rating Depression Scale. Psych Rep 1985; 57:1091–1096.

Gallagher D, Breckenridge J, Steinmetz J, Thompson L. The Beck Depression Inventory and research diagnostic criteria: Congruence in an older population. J Consult Clin Psychol 1983; 51:945–946.

Gandek B, Ware JE, Aaronson NK, Apolone G, Bjorner JB, Brazier JE, Bullinger M, Kaasa S, Leplege A, Prieto L, Sullivan M (1998) Cross-validation of item selection and scoring for the SF-12 Health Survey in nine countries: results from the IQOLA Project. International Quality of Life Assessment. J Clin.Epidemiol 1998; 51:1171–1178.

Garratt A, Schmidt L, Mackintosh A, Fitzpatrick R. Quality of life measurement: bibliographic study of patient assessed health outcome measures. BMJ 2002; 324:1417.

Ger LP, Ho ST, Sun WZ, Wang MS, Cleeland CS. Validation of the Brief Pain Inventory in a Taiwanese population. J Pain Symptom Manage 1999; 18:316–322.

Gerteis M, Edgman-Levitan S, Daley J, Delbanco T. Through the patient's eyes: understanding and promoting patient-centered care. Jossey-Bass, San Francisco, 1993.

Gillis TA, Donovan ES. Rehabilitation following bone marrow transplantation. Cancer 2001; 92:998–1007.

Given B, Given C, Azzouz F, Stommel M. Physical functioning of elderly cancer patients prior to diagnosis and following initial treatment. Nurs Res 2001; 50:222–232.

Given CW, Given B, Azzouz F, Kozachik S, Stommel M. Predictors of pain and fatigue in the year following diagnosis among elderly cancer patients. J Pain Symptom Manage 2001; 21:456–466.

Goodwin DM, Higginson IJ, Edwards AG, Finlay IG, Cook AM, Hood K, Douglas HR, Normand CE (2002) An evaluation of systematic reviews of palliative care services. J Palliat Care 2002; 18:77–83.

Goodwin DM, Higginson IJ, Myers K, Douglas HR, Normand CE. Effectiveness of palliative day care in improving pain, symptom control, and quality of life. J Pain Symptom Manage 2003; 25:202–12.

Goudas LC, Carr DB, Balk E, Ioannidis JP, Terrin N, Bloch R, Chew P, Goudas M, Lau J (2001) Management of cancer pain. www.ahrq.gov/clinic/canpainsum Evidence Report/ Technology Assessment: Number 35. Agency for Healthcare Research and Quality, Public Health Service,

US Department of Health and Human Services, Rockville, MD, 2001.

Gracely RH, Dubner R, McGrath P. Fentanyl reduces the intensity of painful tooth pulp sensations: Controlling for detection of active drugs. Anesthesia and Analgesia 1982; 9:751–755.

Gracely RH, Kwilosz DM. The Descriptor Differential Scale: Applying psychophysical principles to clinical assessment. Pain 1988; 35:279–288.

Gracely RH, McGrath P, Dubner R. Ratio scales of sensory and affective verbal pain descriptors. Pain 1978; 5:5–18.

Graham C, Bond SS, Gerkovich MM, Cook MR. Use of the McGill pain questionnaire in the assessment of cancer pain: replicability and consistency. Pain 1980; 8:377–387.

Greenfield S, Kaplan SH, Silliman RA, Sullivan L, Manning W, D'Agostino R, Singer DE, Nathan DM (1994) The uses of outcomes research for medical effectiveness, quality of care, and reimbursement in type II diabetes. Diabetes Care 1994; 17(Suppl 1):32–39.

Greenfield S, Nelson EC. Recent developments and future issues in the use of health status assessment measures in clinical settings. Med Care 1992:MS23–MS41.

Grond S, Zech D, Diefenbach C, Bischoff A. Prevalence and pattern of symptoms in patients with cancer pain: a prospective evaluation of 1635 cancer patients referred to a pain clinic. J Pain Symptom Manage 1994; 9:372–382.

Guo H, Fine PG, Mendoza TR, Cleeland CS. A preliminary study of the utility of the brief hospice inventory. J Pain Symptom Manage 2001; 22:637–648.

Hall JA, Roter DL, Katz NR. Meta-analysis of correlates of provider behavior in medical encounters. Med Care 1988; 26:657–675.

Hearn J, Higginson IJ. Outcome measures in palliative care for advanced cancer patients: a review. J Public Health Med 1997; 19:193–199.

Hearn J, Higginson IJ. Development and validation of a core outcome measure for palliative care: the palliative care outcome scale. Palliative Care Core Audit Project Advisory Group. Qual Health Care 1999; 8:219–227.

Herrmann C. International experiences with the Hospital Anxiety and Depression Scale–a review of validation data and clinical results. J Psychosom.Res 1997; 42:17–41.

Higginson IJ. Evidence based palliative care. There is some evidence-and there needs to be more. BMJ 1999; 319:462–463.

Higginson IJ, Carr AJ. Measuring Quality of Life: Using quality of life measures in the clinical setting. BMJ 2001; 322:1297–1300.

Higginson IJ, Finlay I, Goodwin DM, Cook AM, Hood K, Edwards AG.K, Douglas HR, Normand CE (2002) Do hospital-based palliative teams improve care for patients or families at the end of life. J Pain Symptom Manage 2002; 23:96–106.

Higginson I, McCarthy M. Measuring symptoms in terminal cancer: are pain and dyspnoea controlled. J R Soc Med 1989; 82(26):4–7.

Higginson IJ, McCarthy M. Validity of the support team assessment schedule: do staffs' ratings reflect those made by patients or their families. Palliat Med 1993; 7:219–228.

Higginson IJ, McCarthy M. A comparison of two measures of quality of life: their sensitivity and validity for patients with advanced cancer. Palliat Med 1994; 8:282–290.

Higginson IJ, Wade AM, McCarthy M. Effectiveness of two palliative support teams. Palliative Medicine 1992; 14:50–56.

Holzner B, Kemmler G, Sperner-Unterweger B, Kopp M, Dunser M, Margreiter R, Marschitz I, Nachbaur D, Fleischhacker WW, Greil R (2001) Quality of life measurement in oncology–a matter of the assessment instrument. Eur J Cancer 2001; 37:2349–2356.

Hotopf M, Chidgey, J, Addington-Hall J, Ly KL. Depression in advanced disease: a systematic review Part 1. Prevalence and case finding. Palliat Med 2002; 16:81–97.

Hunt SM, McEwen J. The development of a subjective health indicator. Sociol Health Illn 1980; 2:231–246.

Hunt SM, McKenna SP, McEwen J, Williams J, Papp E. The Nottingham Health Profile: subjective health status and medical consultations. Soc Sci Med.[A] 1981; 15:221–229.

Hwang SS, Chang VT, Kasimis BS. A comparison of three fatigue measures in veterans with cancer. Cancer Invest 2003; 21:363–373.

Ibbotson T, Maguire P, Selby P, Priestman T, Wallace L. Screening for anxiety and depression in cancer patients: the effects of disease and treatment. Eur J Cancer 1994; 30A:37–40.

Ingham JM, Brown MD, Lawrence WF, Mangan PA, Yabroff R, Taylor KL. The validity of the distress thermometer for detecting psychological distress in informal caregivers of patients with advanced cancer. Abstract American Society of Clinical Oncology, 2003.

Ita D, Keorney M, O'Slorain L. Psychiatric disorder in a palliative care unit. Palliat Med 2003; 17:212–218.

Jack B, Hillier V, Williams A, Oldham J. Hospital based palliative care teams improve the symptoms of cancer patients. Palliat Med 2003; 17:498–502.

Jacobsen PB, Donovan KA, Trask PC, Fleishman SB, Zabora J, Baker F, Holland JC (2005) Screening for psychological distress in ambulatory cancer patients. Cancer 103:1494–1502.

Jacobson SF. Evaluating instruments for use in clinical nursing research. In: Frank-Stromborg M, Olsen SJ (eds). Instruments for Clinical Health-Care Research, second edition, Jones and Bartless Publishers, Boston, 1997:3–19.

Jacox AK, Carr DB, Payne R, et al. Management of Cancer Pain. Clinical Practice Guideline No. 9. AHCPR Pub. No. 94-0592. Agency for Health Care Policy and Research, Public Health Service, U.S. Department of Health and Human Services, Rockville, MD, 1994.

Jadad AR. Pain relief in the information age: let's meet our childrens' expectations. Proceedings of the 10th World Congress on Pain. IASP Press, Seattle, pp 2003; 4:9–60.

Jensen MP, Karoly P, Braver S. The measurement of clinical pain intensity: a comparison of six methods. Pain 1986; 27:117–126.

Jensen MP, McFarland CA. Increasing the reliability and validity of pain intensity measurement in chronic pain patients. Pain 1993; 55:195–203.

Jensen MP, Smith DG, Ehde DM, Robinsin LR. Pain site and the effects of amputation pain: further clarification of the meaning of mild, moderate, and severe pain. Pain 2001; 91:317–322.

Jensen MP, Turner JA, Romano JM, Fisher LD. Comparative reliability and validity of chronic pain intensity measures. Pain 1999; 1999; 83:157–62.

Jones PW, Bogardus CR, Anderson DW. Significance of initial "performance status" in patients receiving halfbody radiation. Int J Radiat Oncol Biol Phys 1984; 10:1947–1950.

Kaasa S, de Conno F. Palliative care research. Eur J Cancer. 37, Suppl 2001; 8:S153–S159.

Kaasa T, Loomis J, Gillis K, Bruera E, Hanson J. The Edmonton Functional Assessment Tool: preliminary development and evaluation for use in palliative care. J Pain Symptom Manage 1997; 13:10–9.

Kaasa T, Wessel J. The Edmonton Functional Assessment Tool: further development and validation for use in palliative care. J Palliat Care 2001; 17:5–11.

Kaasa T, Wessel J, Darrah J, Bruera E. Inter-rater reliability of formally trained and self-trained raters using the Edmonton Functional Assessment Tool. Palliat Med 2000; 14:509–517.

Kahn KL, Malin JL, Adams J, Ganz PA. Developing a reliable, valid, and feasible plan for quality-of-care measurement for cancer: how should we measure. Med Care 2002; 40: III73–III85.

Kane, R.L,. Klein SJ, Bernstein L, Rothenberg R, Wales J. Hospice role in alleviating the emotional stress of terminal patients and their families. Med Care 1985; 23:189–197.

Kaplan SH, Greenfield S, Ware JE. Assessing the effects of physician-patient interactions on the outcomes of chronic disease. Med Care 1989; 7(suppl):S110–S127.

Karnofsky DA, Abelmann WH. C. L.F, Burchenal JH. The use of nitrogen mustards in the palliative treatment of cancer. Cancer 1948; 1:634–656.

King MT, Dobson AJ, Harnett PR. A comparison of two quality-of-life questionnaires for cancer clinical trials: the functional living index–cancer (FLIC) and the quality of life questionnaire core module (QLQ-C30). J Clin Epidemiol 1996; 49:21–29.

Klee M, Groenvold M, Machin D. Using data from studies of health-related quality of life to describe clinical issues. Quality of Life Research 1999; 8:733–742.

Kremer E, Atkinson JH, Ignelzi RJ. Measurement of pain: patient preference does not confound pain measurement. Pain 1981; 10:241–248.

Kristjanson LJ. Validity and reliability testing of the FAMCARE Scale: Measuring family satisfaction with advanced cancer care. Social Science Medicine 1993; 36:693–701.

Kuenstner S, Langelotz C, Budach V, Possinger K, Krause B, Sezer O. The comparability of quality of life scores: a multitrait multimethod analysis of the EORTC QLQ-C30, SF-36 and FLIC questionnaires. Eur J Cancer 2002; 38:339–348.

Kutner JS, Kassner CT, Nowels DE. Symptom burden at the end of life: hospice providers' perceptions. J Pain Symptom Manage 2001; 21:473–480.

Kyriaki M, Eleni T, Efi P, Ourania K, Vassilios S, Lambros V. The EORTC core quality of life questionnaire (QLQ-C30, version 3.0) in terminally ill cancer patients under palliative care: validity and reliability in a Hellenic sample. Int J Cancer 2001; 94:135–139.

Lichter I, Hunt E. The last 48 hours of life. J Palliat Care 1990; 6:7–15.

Lipman A, Jackson K, Tyler L. Evidence Based Symptom Control in Palliative Care: Systematic Reviews and Validated Clinical Practice Guidelines for 15 Common Problems in Patients with Life Limiting Disease. Pharmaceutical Products Press, The Hawarth Press, New York, 2000.

Lipscomb J, Snyder CF. The Outcomes of Cancer Outcomes Research: focusing on the National Cancer Institute's quality-of-care initiative. Med Care 2002; 40:III3–10.

Llobera J, Esteva M, Benito E, Terrasa J, Rifa J, Pons O, Maya A (2003) Quality of life for oncology patients during the terminal period. Validation of the HRCA-QL index. Support Care Cancer 2003; 11:294–303.

Lloyd-Williams M, Friedman T, Rudd N. An analysis of the validity of the Hospital Anxiety and Depression Scale as a screening tool in patients with advanced metastatic cancer. J Pain Symptom Manage 2001; 22:990–996.

Majani G, Tiengo M, Giardini A, Calori G, De Micheli P, Battaglia A. Relationship between MPQ and VAS in 962 patients. A rationale for their use. Minerva Anestesiol 2003; 69:67–73.

Marvel MK, Epstein RM, Flowers K, Beckman HB. Soliciting the patient's agenda: have we improved. JAMA 1999; 281:283–287.

Max MB. How to move pain and symptom control from the margin to the mainstream. J Pain 2003; 4:355–360.

Max MB, Lynch SA, Muir J, Shoaf SE, Smoller B, Dubner R. Effects of desipramine, amitriptyline,and fluoxetine on pain and diabetic neuropathy. N Engl J of Med 1992; 326:1250–1256.

Mazzocato C, Sweeney C, Bruera E. Clinical research in palliative care: patient populations, symptoms, interventions and endpoints. Palliative Medicine 2001; 15:163–168.

McArthur JC, Yiannoutsos C, Simpson DM, Adornato BT, Singer EJ, Hollanfer H, Marra C, Rubin M, Cohen BA, Tucker T, Navia BA, Schifitto G, Katzenstein D, Rask C, Zaborski L, Smith ME, Shriver S, Millar L, Clifford DB, Karalnik IJ (2000) A phase II trial of nerve growth factor for sensory neuropathy associated with HIV infection. Neurology 2000; 54:1080–1088.

McCorkle R, Benoliel JQ, Donaldson G, Georgiadou F, Moinpour C, Goodell B. A randomized clinical trial of home nursing care for lung cancer patients. Cancer 1989; 64:1375–1382.

McCorkle R, Cooley ME, Shea JA. A user's manual for the Symptom Distress Scale. University of Pennsylvania, Philadelphia, 1998.

McCorkle R, Cooley ME, Shea JA. A user's manual for the symptom distress scale [on-line]. Available: www.qlmed. org/SDS/index.html ..

McCorkle R, Jepson C, Malone D, Lusk E, Braitman L, Buhler-Wilkerson K, Daly J (1994) The impact of post hospital home care on patients with cancer. Res Nurs Health 1994; 17:243–251.

McCorkle R, Young K. Development of a symptom distress scale. Cancer Nurs 1978; 1:373–378.

McDowell I, Newell C. Measuring Health: A Guide to Rating Scales and Questionnaires. Oxford University Press, New York, 1996.

McGee HM, O'Boyle CA, Hickey A, O'Malley K, Joyce CR. Assessing the quality of life of the individual: the SEIQoL with a healthy and a gastroenterology unit population. Psychol Med 1991; 21:749–759.

McNair DM, Lorr M, Droppleman LF. Edits manual for the profile of mood states. Educational and Industrial Testing Service, San Diego, CA, 1971.

McQuay HJ, Moore A. An Evidence-based Resource for Pain Relief. Oxford University Press, Oxford, 1998.

McQuillan R, Finlay, I. Branch C, Roberts D, Spencer M. Improving analgesic prescribing in a general teaching hospital. Journal of Pain & Symptom Management 1996; 11:172–180.

Melzack R. The McGill Pain Questionnaire: major properties and scoring methods. Pain 1975; 1:277–299.

Melzack R. Re: Discriminative capacity of the McGill Pain Questionnaire. Pain 1985; 23:201–203.

Melzack R. The short-form McGill Pain Questionnaire. Pain 1987; 30:191–197.

Melzack R, Mount BM, Gordon JM. The Brompton mixture versus morphine solution given orally: effects on pain. Can Med Assoc J 1979; 120:435–438.

Melzack R, Ofiesh JG, Mount BM. The Brompton mixture: effects on pain in cancer patients. Can Med Assoc J 1976; 115:125–129.

Mendoza TR, Wang XS, Cleeland CS, Morrissey M, Johnson BA, Wendt JK, Huber SL (1999) The rapid assessment of fatigue severity in cancer patients: use of the Brief Fatigue Inventory. Cancer 1999; 85:1186–1196.

Miller MG, McCarthy N, O'Boyle CA, Kearney M. Continuous subcutaneous infusion of morphine vs. hydromorphone: a controlled trial. J Pain Symptom. Manage 1999; 18:9–16.

Mock V, Atkinson A, Barsevick A, Cella D, Cimprich B, Cleeland C, Donnelly J, Eisenberger MA, Escalante C, Hinds P, Jacobsen PB, Kaldo P, Knight SJ, Peterman A, Piper BF, Rugo H, Sabbatini P, Stahl C (2000) NCCN Practice Guidelines for Cancer-Related Fatigue. Oncology (Huntingt) 2000; 14:151–161.

Montazeri A, Gillis CR, McEwen J. Quality of life in patients with lung cancer: a review of literature from 1970 to 1995. Chest 1998; 113:467–481.

Montgomery C, Pocock M, Titley K, Lloyd K. Individual quality of life in patients with leukaemia and lymphoma. Psychooncology 2002; 11:239–243.

Mor V, Laliberte L, Morris JN, Wiemann M. The Karnofsky Performance Status Scale. An examination of its reliability and validity in a research setting. Cancer 1984; 53:2002–2007.

Morris JN, Suissa S, Sherwood S, Wright SM, Greer D. Last days: a study of the quality of life of terminally ill cancer patients. J Chronic Dis 1986; 39:47–62.

Morrow GR, Lindke J, Black P. Measurement of quality of life in patients: psychometric analyses of the Functional Living Index-Cancer (FLIC). Qual.Life Res 1992; 1:287–296.

Mulrow CD, Lohr KN. Proof and policy from medical research evidence. Journal of Health Politics, Policy & Law 2001; 26:249–266.

National Comprehensive Cancer Network. NCCN practice guidelines for the management of psychosocial distress. Oncology (Huntingt) 1999; 13:113–47.

Ng K, Von Gunten CF. Symptoms and attitudes of 100 consecutive patients admitted to an acute hospice/palliative care unit. J Pain Symptom Manage 1998; 16:307–316.

Nolan MT, Mock V. Measuring Patient Outcomes. Sage Publications, Thousand Oaks, CA, 2000.

Nunnally J. Psychometric theory. McGraw-Hill, New York, 1978.

O'Boyle CA, Waldron D. Quality of life issues in palliative medicine. J.Neurol. 244, Suppl 1997; 4:S18–S25.

O'Brien T, Welsh J, Dunn FG. ABC of palliative care. Non-malignant conditions. BMJ 1998; 316:286–289.

Oken MM, Creech RH, Tormey DC, Horton J, Davis TE, McFadden ET, Carbone PP (1982) Toxicity and response criteria of the Eastern Cooperative Oncology Group. Am J Clin Oncol 1982; 5:649–655.

Okuyama T, Wang XS, Akechi T, Mendoza T, Hosaka T, Cleeland CS, Uchitomi Y (2003) Validation study of the Japanese version of the Brief Fatigue Inventory. J Pain Symptom Manage 2003; 25:106–117.

Olt GJ. Managing pain and psychological issues in palliative care. Best Practice & Research Clinical Obstetrics & Gynaecology 2001; 15:235–251.

Osoba D. A taxonomy of the uses of health-related quality-of-life instruments in cancer care and the clinical meaningfulness of the results. Med Care 2002; 40: III31–III38.

Osse BH, Vernooij-Dassen MJ, de Vree BP, Schade E, Grol RP. Assessment of the need for palliative care as perceived by individual cancer patients and their families: a review of instruments for improving patient participation in palliative care. Cancer 2000; 88:900–911.

Passik SD, Lundberg JC, Rosenfeld B, Kirsh KL, Donaghy K, Theobald D, Lundberg E, Dugan W (2000) Factor analysis of the Zung Self-Rating Depression Scale in a large ambulatory oncology sample. Psychosomatics 2000; 41:121–127.

Patrick DL, Curtis R, Engelberg RA, Nielsen E, McCown BA. Measuring and improving the quality of dying and death. Ann Intern Med 2003; 139:410–415.

Patrick DL, Deyo RA. Generic and disease-specific measures in assessing health status and quality of life. Med Care 1989; 27:S217–S232.

Patrick DL, Engelberg RA, Curtis JR. Evaluating the quality of dying and death. J. Pain Symptom Manage 2001; 22:717–726.

Patton MQ. Qualitative research and evaluation methods. (3rd edition)., Sage Publications, Thousand Oaks, CA, 2002.

Peruselli C, Camporesi E, Colombo AM, Cucci M, Mazzoni G, Paci E. Quality-of-life assessment in a home care program for advanced cancer patients: a study using the Symptom Distress Scale. J Pain Symptom Manage 1993; 8:306–311.

Philip J, Smith WB, Craft P, Lickiss N. Concurrent validity of the modified Edmonton Symptom Assessment System with the Rotterdam Symptom Checklist and the Brief Pain Inventory. Support.Care Cancer 1998; 6:539–41.

Piper BF, Dibble SL, Dodd MJ, Weiss MC, Slaughter RE, Paul SM. The revised Piper Fatigue Scale: psychometric evaluation in women with breast cancer. Oncol Nurs Forum 1998; 25:677–684.

Piper BF, Dodd M, Ream E. Improving the clinical measurement of cancer treatment related fatigue. American Nurses Association, Washington D.C., pp 1999; 9:9.

Piper BF, Lindsey A, Dodd M. Fatigue mechanisms in cancer patients: developing a nursing theory. Oncology Nursing Forum 1987; 14:17–23.

Polit DF, Hungler BP. Nursing Research Principles and Methods. (Sixth Edition), Lippincott, Philadelphia, 1999.

Portenoy RK, Thaler HT, Kornblith AB, Lepore JM, Friedlander-Klar H, Kiyasu E, Sobel K, Coyle N, Kemeny N, Norton L, et al (1994) The Memorial Symptom Assessment Scale: an instrument for the evaluation of symptom prevalence, characteristics and distress. Eur J Cancer 1994; 30A:1326–1336.

Pransky G, Himmelstein J. Outcomes research, implications for Occupational Health. American Journal of Industrial Medicine 1996; 29:573–83.

Radbruch L, Sabatowski R, Elsner F, Everts J, Mendoza T, Cleeland C. Validation of the German version of the Brief Fatigue Inventory. J Pain Symptom Manage 2003; 25:449–458.

Radloff LS. A self-report depression scale for research in the general population. Applied Psychological Measurement 1977; 1:385–401.

Ragsdale D, Marrow JR. Quality of life as a function of HIV classification. Nursing Research 1990; 39:355–359.

Ransom S, Jacobsen PB, Booth-Jones M (2006) Validation of the Distress Thermometer with bone marrow transplant patients. Psycho-Oncology 15:604–612.

Rogers WH, Wittink HM, Ashburn MA, Cynn D, Carr DB. Using the "TOPS" an outcomes instrument for multidisciplinary outpatient pain treatment. Pain Medicine 2000; 1:55–67.

Rogers W, Wittink HM, Wagner A, Cynn D, Carr DB. Assessing individual outcomes during outpatient, multidisciplinary chronic pain treatment by means of an augmented SF-36. Pain Medicine 2000; 1:44–54.

Roth AJ, Kornblith AB, Batel-Copel L, Peabody E, Scher HI, Holland JC. Rapid screening for psychologic distress in men with prostate carcinoma: a pilot study. Cancer 1998; 82:1904–1908.

Rucker KS, Metzler HM, Kregel J. Standardization of chronic pain assessment: a multiperspective approach. Clinical Journal of Pain 1996; 12:94–110.

Rudy TE, Kerns RD, Turk DC. Chronic pain and depression: toward a cognitive-behavioral mediation model. Pain 1988; 35:129–140.

Sackett DL, Rosenberg WM, Gray JA, Richardson WS. Evidence based medicine: How to practice and Teach EBM. (2nd edition), Churchill-Livingstone Inc., NY, 1999.

Sanders C, Egger M, Donovan J, Tallon D, Frankel S. Reporting on quality of life in randomised controlled trials: bibliographic study. BMJ 1998; 317:1191–1194.

Sarna L. Correlates of symptom distress in women with lung cancer. Cancer Pract 1993; 1:21–28.

Schipper H, Clinch J, McMurray A, Levitt M. Measuring the quality of life of cancer patients: the Functional Living Index-Cancer: development and validation. J Clin Oncol 1984; 2:472–483.

Serlin RC, Mendoza TR, Nakamura Y, Edwards KR, Cleeland CS. When is cancer pain mild, moderate or severe? Grading pain severity by its interference with function. Pain 1995; 61:277–284.

Shacham S. A shortened version of the Profile of Mood States. J Pers Assess 1983; 47:305–306.

Shannon MM, Ryan MA, D'Agostino N, Brescia FJ. Assessment of pain in advanced cancer patients. J Pain Symptom Manage 1995; 10:274–278.

Shaver PR, Brennan KA. Measures of depression and loneliness. In: Robinson JP, Shaver PR, Wrightsman LS (eds). Measures of Personality and Social Psychological Attitudes Academic Press, Inc, San Diego, CA, 1991:221–215.

Singer PA, Martin DK, Kelner M. Quality end-of-life care: patients' perspectives. JAMA 1999; 281:163–168.

Skeel RT. Quality of life assessment in cancer clinical trials– it's time to catch up. J Natl Cancer Inst 1989; 81:472–473.

Spitzer WO, Dobson AJ, Hall J, Chesterman E, Levi J, Sheperd R, Battista RN, Catchlove BR (1981) Measuring the quality of life of cancer patients: a concise QL-index for use by physicians. J Chronic Dis 1981; 34:585–597.

Standing Medical Advisory Committee, Standing Nursing and Midwifery Advisory Committee. The principles and provision of palliative care. Standing Medical Advisory Committee and Standing Nurse and Midwifery Advisory Committee, London, 1992.

Steinhauser KE, Christakis NA, Clipp EC, McNeilly M, McIntyre L, Tulsky JA. Factors considered important at the end of life by patients, family, physicians, and other care providers. JAMA 2000; 284:2476–2482.

Sterkenburg CA, King B, Woodward CA. A reliability and validity study of the McMaster Quality of Life Scale (MQLS) for a palliative population. J Palliat Care 1996; 12:18–25.

Stewart AL, Teno J, Patrick DL, Lynn J. The concept of quality of life of dying persons in the context of health care. J Pain Symptom Manage 1999; 17:93–108.

Storey P. Symptom control in advanced cancer. Semin Oncol 1994; 21:748–753.

Stromgren AS, Groenvold M, Pedersen L, Olsen AK, Sjogren P. Symptomatology of cancer patients in palliative care: content validation of self-assessment questionnaires against medical records. Eur J Cancer 2002; 38:788–794.

Sutton LM, Porter LS, Keefe FJ. Cancer pain at the end of life: a biopsychosocial perspective. Pain 2002; 99:5–10.

Tanenbaum SJ. What physicians know. N Engl J Med 1993; 329:1268–1271.

Tarlov AR, Ware JE Jr., Nelson S, Greenfield EC, Perrin E, Zubkoff M. The Medical Outcomes Study. An application of methods for monitoring the results of medical care. JAMA 1989; 262:925–930.

Tashakkori A, Teddlie C. Mixed methodology combining qualitative and quantitative approaches. Sage Publications, Thousand Oaks, CA, 1998.

Tashakkori A, Teddlie C. Handbook of mixed methods in social & behavioral sciences. Sage Publications, Thousand Oaks, CA, 2003.

Tranmer JE, Heyland D, Dudgeon D, Groll D, Squires-Graham M, Coulson K. Measuring the symptom experience of seriously ill cancer and noncancer hospitalized patients near the end of life with the memorial symptom assessment scale. J Pain Symptom Manage 2003; 25:420–429.

Twycross R, Harcourt J, Bergl S. A survey of pain in patients with advanced cancer. J Pain Symptom Manage 1996; 12:273–282.

Varricchio CG. Measurement issues concerning linguistic translation. In: Frank-Stromborg M, Olsen SJ (eds). Instruments for Clinical Health-Care Research, (second edition), Jones and Bartlett Publishers, Boston, 1997:3–19.

Ventafridda V, Conno F, Ripamonti C, Gamba A, Tamburini M. Quality-of-life assessment during a palliative care programme. Ann Oncol 1990; 1:415–420.

Verger E, Salamero M, Conill C. Can Karnofsky performance status be transformed to the Eastern Cooperative Oncology Group scoring scale and vice versa. Eur J Cancer 1992; 28A:1328–3130.

Von Korff M, Jensen MP, Karoly P. Assessing global pain severity by self-report in clinical and health services research. Spine 2000; 25:3140–3151.

Wagner AK, Vickrey BG. The routine use of health-related quality of life measures in the care of patients with epilepsy: rationale and research agenda. Qual Life Res 1995; 4:169–177.

Wales J, Kane R, Robbins S, Bernstein L, Krasnow R. UCLA hospice evaluation study. Methodology and instrumentation. Med Care 1983; 21:734–744.

Wallen GR, Berger A. Mixed methods: In search of truth in palliative care medicine. J Palliat Med 2004; 7:403–404.

Walsh D, Donnelly S, Rybicki L. The symptoms of advanced cancer: relationship to age, gender, and performance status in 1,000 patients. Support Care Cancer 2000; 8:175–179.

Walsh D, Rybicki L, Nelson KA, Donnelly S. Symptoms and prognosis in advanced cancer. Support Care Cancer 2002; 10:385–388.

Wang XS, Hao X, Wang Y, Guo H, Jiang Y, Mendoza TR, Cleeland CS (2004) Validation study of the Chinese version of the Brief Fatigue Inventory. J Pain Symptom Manage 2004; 27:322–332.

Ware J Jr., Kosinski M, Keller SD. A 12-Item Short-Form Health Survey: construction of scales and preliminary tests of reliability and validity. Med Care 1996; 34:220–233.

Ware JE Jr.. Conceptualizing and measuring generic health outcomes. Cancer 1991; 67:774–779.

Ware JE Jr., Sherbourne CD. The MOS 36-item short-form health survey (SF-36). I. Conceptual framework and item selection. Med Care 1992; 30:473–483.

Wenk R, Diaz C, Echeverria M, et al. Argentina"s WHO Cancer Pain Relief Program: a patient care model. J Pain Symptom Manage 1991; 6:40–43.

Wester JP, de Valk HW, Nieuwenhuis HK, Brouwer CB, van ser Graaf Y, Meuwissen OJ, Hart HC, Sixma JJ, Banga JD (1996) Risk factors for bleeding during treatment of acute venous thromboembolism. Thromb Haemost 1996; 76:682–688.

Wiffen P. The Cochrane pain, Palliative and Supportive Care Group: life history of a Cochrane review. Palliative Medicine 2003; 17:719–720.

Witteveen PO, Jacobs HM, van Groenestijn MA, et al. Assessment of the quality of life of patients with advanced and end-stage cancer or serious infections with a symptom-based or an impact-based instrument. Support Care Cancer 1999; 7:64–70.

World Health Organization. Constitution of the WHO, Basic Documents. World Health Organization, Geneva, 1948.

World Health Organization. Cancer pain relief and palliative care. Technical Report Series 804. World Health Organization, Geneva, 1990.

World Health Organization. The International Classification of Functioning, Disability and Health (ICF). 2nd Edition, WHO, Marketing and Dissemination, Geneva, Switzerland, 2001.

Yates JW, Chalmer B, McKegney FP. Evaluation of patients with advanced cancer using the Karnofsky performance status. Cancer 1980; 45:2220–2224.

Yellen SB, Cella DF, Webster K, Blendowski C, Kaplan E. Measuring fatigue and other anemia-related symptoms with the Functional Assessment of Cancer Therapy (FACT) measurement system. J Pain Symptom Manage 1997; 13:63–74.

Zigmond AS, Snaith RP. The hospital anxiety and depression scale. Acta Psychiatr Scand 1983; 67:361–70.

Zubrod CG. Appraisal of methods for the study of chemotherapy of cancer in man: comparative therapeutic trial of nitrogen mustard and triethylene thiophosphoramide. J Chronic Dis 1960; 11:7–33.

Zwahlen A. Palliative care unit in a district hospital: analysis of two years experience multidisciplinary palliative care teams [French]. Rev.Med.Suisse Romande 1991; 111:761–769.

CHAPTER
24

Why pain control matters in a world full of killer diseases

Sir Michael Bond • Harald Breivik

PAIN: A SILENT DIMENSION OF THE GLOBAL TOP 10 DISEASES

In 2003, the World Health Organization (WHO) released its latest statistics on the leading causes of death and disease burden worldwide (WHO 2003). Although pain itself does not appear as a cause of either global mortality (Table 24.1) or disease burden (Table 24.2), pain researchers and clinicians know that pain can kill (European Federation of IASP Chapters).

Acute pain causes complications from immobility and often is the starting point for persistent pain. Cancer-related pain and chronic noncancer pain increase suffering and diminish all aspects of quality of life. Pain is likewise an important detractor from healthy life years in high-burden conditions such as HIV/AIDS (Breitbart et al. 1996), depression (Wörz 2003), violence such as from war and landmines (de Smet et al. 1998), and from stroke, and diabetes mellitus. Health policy makers have, at times, overlooked the importance of pain as a disease per se (Siddall and Cousins 2004). This chapter traces the joint efforts of the International Association for the Study of Pain (IASP) and WHO to remedy this oversight as these efforts enter a new and exciting phase.

PREVALENCE OF CHRONIC PAIN

In *developed countries* chronic pain afflicts about 20% of the adult population, particularly women and the elderly, but even children can suffer from recurrent or persistent pain. In only 1–2% of adults with chronic pain does the pain result from cancer. About 30–40% suffer pain from musculoskeletal and joint disorders. Neck and back pain accounts for another 30%. Headache and migraine account for less than 10% of cases of persistent pain (Blyth et al. 2001; Harstall and Ospina 2003; Breivik et al. 2006). A worldwide study indicates that pain in primary care is at least as prevalent in developing countries as in developed ones (Gureje et al. 1998).

PAIN AS A DISEASE

Acute pain after trauma or surgery signals actual or imminent tissue damage. Long-term pain from chronic disease such as degenerative arthritis remains a symptom that normally subsides after successful treatment, such as joint

Table 24.1 Leading causes of mortality among adults worldwide, 2002

Rank	Cause	Deaths (000)
Ages 15–59		
1	HIV/AIDS	2279
2	Ischemic heart disease	1332
3	Tuberculosis	1036
4	Road traffic injuries	814
5	Cerebrovascular disease	783
6	Self-inflicted injuries	672
7	Violence	473
8	Cirrhosis of the liver	382
9	Lower respiratory infections	352
10	Chronic obstructive pulmonary disease	343
Ages 60+		
1	Ischemic heart disease	5825
2	Cerebrovascular disease	4689
3	Chronic obstructive pulmonary disease	2399
4	Lower respiratory infections	1396
5	Trachea, bronchus, lung cancers	928
6	Diabetes mellitus	754
7	Hypertensive heart disease	735
8	Stomach cancer	605
9	Tuberculosis	495
10	Colon and rectum cancers	477

Source: Adapted from WHO (with permission) (WHO 2003).

chapters). Chronic pain as a disease in its own right should be diagnosed only when all signs of the original cause have disappeared or where curative treatment of the initial condition is not possible. Dysfunctional chronic pain has been termed "maldynia" in contrast to "eudynia," pain that appropriately warns of tissue injury (Lippe 2000).

CANCER PAIN IN THE DEVELOPED NATIONS

About 80% of the 6–7 million patients dying of cancer annually suffer from pain, and most had far from

Table 24.2 Leading causes of disease burden among adults worldwide, 2002

Rank	Cause	DALYs* (000)
Ages 15–59		
1	HIV/AIDS	68661
2	Unipolar depressive disorders	57843
3	Tuberculosis	28380
4	Road traffic injuries	27264
5	Ischemic heart disease	26155
6	Alcohol use disorders	19567
7	Hearing loss, adult onset	19486
8	Violence	18962
9	Cerebrovascular disease	18749
10	Self-inflicted injuries	18522
Ages 60+		
1	Ischemic heart disease	31481
2	Cerebrovascular disease	29595
3	Chronic obstructive pulmonary disease	14380
4	Alzheimer and other dementias	8569
5	Cataracts	7384
6	Lower respiratory infections	6597
7	Hearing loss, adult onset	6548
8	Trachea, bronchus, lung cancers	5952
9	Diabetes mellitus	5882
10	Vision disorders, age-related and other	4766

Source: Adapted from WHO (with permission) (WHO 2003).
*Estimates are expressed as disability-adjusted life years (DALYs). A condition that produces 50% disability in one person for 1 year carries a burden of 0.5 DALYs.

replacement. However, when pain persists long after its usefulness as an alarm signal has passed – after damaged tissue has healed – then it is no longer merely a symptom.

In that case, chronic pain is no longer directly related to evolving injury. Instead, it reflects pathophysiologic changes within the nociceptive system and psychosocial responses that perpetuate the chronic pain problem. These changes may transcend the specific disease condition that caused the acute pain (Table 24.3).

Therefore, persistent pain and the many physical and psychosocial changes and complications associated with it constitute a major health care problem: "Chronic pain is a specific health care problem, a disease in its own right" (European federation of IASP

Table 24.3 Signs and symptoms of chronic pain once it has evolved into a disease per se (EFIC; Siddall and Cousins 2004)

1. Immobility and consequent wasting of muscle, joints, etc.

2. Depression of the immune system and increased susceptibility to disease

3. Disturbed sleep

4. Poor appetite and nutrition

5. Dependence on medication

6. Overdependence on family and other caregivers

7. Overuse and inappropriate use of health care providers and systems

8. Poor performance on the job, or disability

9. Isolation from society and family

10. Anxiety and fear

11. Bitterness, frustration, depression, and suicide

optimal pain relief until representatives of the IASP joined with WHO to influence medical practice and improve the availability of analgesic drugs (Stewart and Kleinhues 2003). Pioneering members of IASP, John J. Bonica and Vittorio Ventafridda, met with Jan Stjernswärd from WHO and others in 1985 to develop the first guidelines on management of pain in patients with cancer (WHO 1986). WHO published the landmark booklet *Cancer Pain Relief* in 1986. This publication began a major worldwide movement – a revolution – with tremendous impact on the evaluation and treatment of cancer pain.

Because it is a simple, strong message, the WHO three-step analgesic ladder has had immense pedagogic value. It uses the simple, cheap, widely available, and effective non-opioid analgesics acetaminophen (paracetamol) or aspirin (acetylsalicylic acid) for mild or moderate pain, adds a weak opioid such as codeine for more severe pain, and adds morphine when pain is still more severe. Morphine consumption increased after publication of the booklet's first edition, but only in Australia and some Western countries.

The booklet's second, 1996, edition also addressed opioid availability (WHO 1996). This publication resulted in wider availability of morphine for cancer pain, progress emphasized in the WHO's national cancer control program recommendations of 1997 and 2002 (WHO 2002).

WHO's 2000 publication on achieving balance in regulation of opioids and improving their availability for pain relief was a further major step forward. It overcame legal barriers in some of the many parts of the world where legal restrictions and misconceived regulations of morphine availability, intended to reduce illegal abuse, remained obstacles to cancer pain relief. WHO-sponsored workshops were organized by David Joranson, Kathleen Foley, and others in Latin America, India, and eastern and southern Europe. They used the WHO publication as a "how-to" manual to promote access to and availability of morphine and similar drugs for cancer pain relief. The resulting progress otherwise would have been much slower (Rajagopal et al. 2001; Joranson 2004).

WHO's immense impact on health care policies and in changing the culture of pain relief is clear for cancer pain and symptom control. WHO and many IASP members have been directly and indirectly involved in this effort (WHO 1998). Still, in many parts of the world, even simple analgesics are not available for cancer pain, let alone morphine (Rajagopal et al. 2001; WHO 2002; Stewart and Kleinhues 2003; Joranson 2004). In developing countries, available resources for health care understandably focus on the prevention and treatment of "killer" diseases. Yet most such conditions are accompanied by unrelieved pain that increases suffering, functional disabilities, and loss of quality of life (WHO 2003). These conditions include HIV/AIDS, cancer, tuberculosis, malaria and other infectious diseases, and injuries caused by road traffic accidents, war, torture, and other forms of violence (WHO 2003).

BROADENING IASP'S MISSION: THE WHO LIAISON

The first IASP–WHO liaison officer, Kathleen Foley, was a major contributor to the WHO's efforts to improve management of cancer pain. Subsequent IASP–WHO liaisons Troels S. Jensen and Harald Breivik, together with Jean-Marie Besson and Sir Michael Bond acting as IASP presidents, have increased WHO's awareness of acute and chronic noncancer pain as equally serious health care problems. It is less well known that acute pain from all causes, including trauma, accidents, acts of war, surgery, childbirth, cancer, and HIV/AIDS, is poorly managed, even in the well developed part of the world. Unrelieved acute pain after surgery and trauma increases the risk of postoperative and posttraumatic cardiac, respiratory, and gastrointestinal complications. It also results in greater morbidity, higher costs, and even mortality. Even more important regarding health care costs and patients' quality of life is the high risk of unrelieved acute pain triggering chronic pain (Crombie et al. 1999; Perkins and Kehlet 2000).

Acute and chronic pain underlies much of the economic burden and loss of quality of life and functioning associated with the "killer" diseases, especially when nerve damage from surgery or trauma progresses to chronic neuropathic pain. These pain problems are frequently misunderstood and misdiagnosed, patients are stigmatized, and their pain condition is poorly managed (Carr 2001). Their chronic pain has become a disease in its own right (European Federation of IASP Chapters).

A BROAD POLICY FRAMEWORK ON ACUTE AND CHRONIC PAIN CONTROL

Representing IASP, we have recently been working with WHO to increase global awareness of poorly relieved acute pain as a major factor contributing to delayed recovery of health and function after surgery and trauma and to highlight the immense burden of chronic pain unrelated to cancer. In meetings with WHO department directors and program leaders in October 2001, and at yearly meetings at WHO headquarters with nongovernmental organizations (NGOs) related to neurologic disorders, pain as a major health care problem has been a focus of attention and discussion (Breivik 2002).

WHO considers acute and chronic pain control integrated into the management of different relevant conditions such as cancer and HIV/AIDS. Clearly, this development is of major importance. WHO's influence on governments worldwide and on national health care programs and policies will lay the groundwork for better management of acute and chronic pain and improved health-related quality of life in a number of major diseases and conditions that involve pain.

THE IASP AND EFIC GLOBAL DAY AGAINST PAIN COSPONSORED BY WHO

Our knowledge of the nature and management of pain has increased dramatically over the past 30 years. Facilities for the management of acute and chronic pain disorders have been improving, especially in developed countries. Even so, access to these facilities is patchy, and the quality of pain management varies.

In the developing countries, a lack of resources, poor medical education, opposition to the use of opioids, political intransigence, and other difficulties mean that there has been little or no consistent development of programs for the management of pain, with the exception of pain associated with cancer or at selected sites such as those served by NGOs including Douleurs Sans Frontières (www.douleurs-sans-frontieres.org).

IASP and the European Federation of IASP Chapters (EFIC) have been concerned for some time about improving facilities for pain education, research, and management in Europe and other developed countries.

In 2002, IASP announced its plans to address the problems faced by pain sufferers in developing countries. Most of those who would benefit from pain relief and palliative care live in developing countries, and the demand for such care will rise dramatically in the future. The need to involve those responsible for health care provision as well as the professions concerned with health care delivery led EFIC to establish a European Week against Pain in 2001 and for IASP to organize a pilot Global Day against Pain in 2003. The two organizations combined their efforts to host a Global Day against Pain on Monday, October 11, 2004, subtitled "Pain relief should be a human right."

The Global Day against Pain as well as the fourth European Week against Pain (October 11–16) was launched in Geneva with a European press conference in the morning, designed to reach as many European journalists as possible with networking worldwide, followed in the afternoon by a global press conference in the form of a live webcast. The timing of the conference allowed residents of five continents to watch the proceedings and participate in them through internet-based discussions.

The objectives of the Global Day against Pain were to:

- Increase awareness of acute and chronic pain and its treatment.
- Publicize major developments in pain research and treatment.
- Emphasize the human right for the treatment of pain, as reported in the companion issue of *Pain: Clinical Updates* (Brennan and Cousins 2004).
- Raise awareness of pain problems in developing countries, with the aim of improving their resources in this and other respects.

THE DEVELOPING WORLD AND IASP'S FUTURE STRATEGY

In 2002, the president of IASP, Sir Michael Bond, committed his term of office to increasing IASP's support to developing countries in recognition of the imbalance in educational and clinical resources between "the West" and those countries. IASP already offered visiting lectureships and consultancies, an "Adopt-a-Member" program, and grants for translation and publication of IASP publications in various languages. IASP also distributes all its publications free to libraries in currency restricted countries and provides grants to support travel to its World Congresses on Pain. To extend such support, IASP has formed a task force to assist an educational program in Kenya, and developed two other educational projects in 2004. IASP gave financial support to WHO's Five African Countries Project, which focused on HIV/AIDS, cancer pain relief, and palliative care (Sepulveda et al. 2002, 2003).

CONCLUSION

Although IASP's name focuses on the "study" of pain, since its inception many members have been energetically involved in pain education, in raising standards for pain care, and in improving access to such care. The IASP–WHO collaboration has met with success in the area of cancer pain control and is now seeking to broaden its scope to encompass other types of pain, particularly in less developed countries. The leadership of IASP is profoundly grateful to its hard-working members and national chapters, and invites their participation in all the activities described above.

For more information see also the following websites:

http://www.painreliefhumanright.com/ ("Relief of pain should be a human right" website)
http://www.iasp-pain.org/ (International Association for the Study of Pain® website)
http://www.efic.org/ (European Federation of IASP Chapters website).

THE INTERNATIONAL ASSOCIATION FOR THE STUDY OF PAIN

IASP was founded in 1973 as a nonprofit organization to foster and encourage research on pain mechanisms and pain syndromes, and to help improve the care of patients with acute and chronic pain. IASP brings together scientists, physicians, dentists, nurses, psychologists, physical therapists, and other health professionals who have an interest in pain research and treatment. Information about membership, books, meetings, etc., is available from the address below or on the IASP web page: www.iasp-pain.org. Free copies of back issues of the IASP's newsletter are available on the IASP web page.

REFERENCES

Blyth FM, March LM, Brnabic AJ, et al. Chronic pain in Australia: a prevalence study. Pain 2001; 89:127–134.
Breitbart W, Parr RB, Passik SD, et al. Pain in AIDS: a call for action. Pain: Clin Updates 1996; 4(1).
Breivik H. International Association for the Study of Pain: update on WHO–IASP. J Pain Sympt Manage 2002; 24:97–101.
Breivik H, Collett B, Ventafridda V, et al. Survey of chronic pain in Europe: prevalence, impact on daily life, and treatment. Eur J Pain 2006; 10:287–333.
Brennan F, Cousins MJ. Pain relief as a human right. Pain: Clin Updates 2004; 12(5).
Carr DB. The development of national guidelines for pain control: synopsis and commentary. Eur J Pain 2001; 5 (suppl A):91–98.
Crombie IK, Croft PR, Linton SJ, et al. Epidemiology of Pain. IASP Press, Seattle, WA, 1999.

de Smet J, Charlton J, Meynadier J. Pain and rehabilitation from landmine injury. Pain: Clin Updates 1998; 6(2).
Gureje O, Von Korff M, Simon GE, et al. Persistent pain and well-being: a World Health Organization Study in Primary Care. JAMA 1998; 280:147–151.
Harstall C, Ospina M. How prevalent is chronic pain? Pain: Clin Updates 2003; 11(2).
Joranson DE. Improving availability of opioid pain medications: testing the principle of balance in Latin America. J Palliat Med 2004; 7:105–114.
Lippe PM. The decade of pain control and research. Pain Med 2000; 1:286.
Perkins FM, Kehlet H. Chronic pain as an outcome of surgery. A review of predictive factors. Anesthesiology 2000; 93:1123–1133.
Rajagopal MR, Joranson DE, Gilson AM. Medical use, misuse, and diversion of opioids in India. Lancet 2001; 358:139–143.
Sepulveda C, Marlin A, Yoshida T, et al. Palliative care: the World Health Organization's global perspective. J Pain Sympt Manage 2002; 24:91–96.
Sepulveda C, Habiyambere V, Amandua J, et al. Quality care at the end of life in Africa. Br Med J 2003; 327:209–213.
Siddall PJ, Cousins MJ. Persistent pain as a disease entity: implications for clinical management. Anesth Analg 2004; 99:510–520.
Stewart BW, Kleinhues P. World Cancer Report. WHO and International Agency for Research on Cancer, IARC Press, Lyon, 2003:297–301.
World Health Organization. Cancer Pain Relief. WHO, Geneva, 1986.
World Health Organization. Cancer Pain Relief: With a Guide to Opioid Availability, 2nd edn. WHO, Geneva, 1996.
World Health Organization. Cancer Pain Relief and Palliative Care in Children. WHO, Geneva, 1998.
World Health Organization. Achieving Balance in National Opioids Control Policy: Guidelines for Assessment. WHO, 2000. Available at: http://www.who.int/medicines/library/qsm/who-edm-qsm-2000-4/who-edm-qsm-2000-4.shtml.
World Health Organization. National Cancer Control Programmes: Policies and Management Guidelines, 2nd edn. WHO, Geneva, 2002.
World Health Organization. The World Health Report: Shaping the Future. WHO, Geneva, 2003.
Wörz R. Pain in depression: depression in pain. Pain: Clin Updates 2003; 11(5).

FURTHER READING

European Federation of IASP Chapters. EFIC's declaration on pain as a major health problem, a disease in its own right, 2004. Available at: www.efic.org/about_pain.htm#efic_declaration.
International Association for the Study of Pain. Desirable characteristics for pain treatment facilities: report of the IASP Taskforce. In: Bond MR, Charlton JE, Woolf CJ (eds). Proceedings of the 6th World Congress on Pain. International Association for the Study of Pain, Seattle, WA, 1991:411–415. Available at: http://www.iasp-pain.org/desirabl.html.

GLOSSARY

Activity: execution of specific tasks or actions by an individual.

Agreement represents lack of measurement error. It expresses how close the values of two different measurements are in absolute terms. Examples of parameters which express agreement is kappa for nominal or ordinal scales, and the Bland and Altman approach is a typical method to calculate and visualize the measurement error for interval scales (Bland and Altman 1986; De Vet 1998).

Alternative modes of administration: these include self-report, interview-administered, trained observer rating, computer-assisted, interviewer administered, performance based measures (Lohr 2002).

Battery: a collection of measures.

Bias: any systematic error in an epidemiological study that results in an incorrect estimate of the association between exposure and risk of disease. **Recall bias:** cases remember exposure differently than controls.

Burden: the time, effort and other demands placed on those to whom the instrument is administered (respondent burden) or on those who administer the instrument (administrative burden) (Lohr and SAC 2002).

Capacity: refers to a person's physical ability to do a task. Questions with capacity wording ask whether the respondent could do a task.

Ceiling effect: occurs when a score distribution is skewed so that a large proportion of respondents score at the highest level on the measure. When ceiling effects occur, the measure cannot detect changes in a higher direction. The opposite is a floor effect; this occurs when a large proportion of the respondents score at the lowest level of the measure. When a respondent worsens the instrument cannot detect deterioration.

Clinimetrics: literally means the measurement of clinical phenomena. Clinimetrics is concerned with all health measurements with respect to diagnosis, prognosis and evaluation of treatment.

Coarse: a measure that has relatively few scale levels.

Concept: the phenomenon or attribute that the measure attempts to capture. For instance, the concept of health in HRQoL measures.

Conceptual and measurement model: the rationale for and description of the concept and the populations that a measure is intended to assess and the relationship between these concepts (Lohr and SAC 2002).

Computer-adaptive testing (CAT) is an extension of IRT and is a technologically advanced method of assessment in which the computer selects and presents test items to patients according to the estimated level of the patients' ability.

Cost-benefit analysis (CBA): measures the benefit of a treatment in monetary terms.

Cost-consequence analysis (CCA): the impact of the treatment of interest on resource use, costs and health outcomes for an individual or group of pain patients are estimated and reported separately.

Cost-effectiveness analysis (CEA): examines the cost and effectiveness of two or more treatment interventions.

Cost-minimization analysis (CMA): employed when the effectiveness of two or more interventions is assumed to be equivalent.

Cronbach's alpha: an estimate of internal consistency reliability based on the average inter-item correlation and number of items (Ware et al. 1993).

Cultural and language adaptations or translations: Involves two primary steps: (1) assessment of conceptual and linguistic equivalence and (2) evaluation of measurement properties (Lohr 2002).

Culturally sensitive: in the context of culturally sensitive measures, measures that consider the perspective of a cultural subgroup in framing a concept or writing an item. Thus, concepts and measures account for the experiences, beliefs, values, expectations, perceptions, and language of a cultural group (Lohr and Skillman 2000).

Dichotomous items: refers to items that have only 2 response categories (e.g., yes/no).

Dimension: a distinct component of a multidimensional construct that can be theoretically or empirically specified (for instance, physical, mental and social functioning are dimensions of HRQoL).

Disability-adjusted life-year (DALY): refers to the summary measure of population health status originally developed for use by the World Health Organization to quantify the global burden of diseases, injuries, and risk factors on human population, in the form of lost years of healthy life due to either disability or premature death. The calculation of DALYs is rooted in the disability weights (from zero for perfect health to 1 for death) assigned to each of the 107 categories of health states. An expert panel used the person trade-off technique to derive the specific disability weights. The

relative importance of healthy life at different ages is also reflected in the calculation of DALYs by the incorporation of separate age weights.

Disease or condition-specific tools: instruments that are used exclusively for the assessment the health status of populations with a specific disease or condition (e.g., back pain, post-herpetic neuralgia).

Domain: a domain identifies a particular focus of attention (e.g., physical functioning, mental or general health, patient satisfaction with care) and may comprise the response to a single item or responses to several related items. May consist of one scale (a collection of related items) or multiple scales that measure the same construct.

Domain or dimension specific instrument: a one domain or dimension instrument, e.g., the VAS scale for pain.

Effect size: the difference or change caused by an intervention and most commonly expressed as a proportion of the standard deviation associated with (1) sampling variability (usually the between-individual standard deviation at baseline) or (2) measurement error (the standard deviation of change during stable treatment or no intervention); the change in health-related quality of life caused by a treatment. Interpretation of effect sizes is often facilitated by the use of global ratings of change or importance of improvement, relating effects to treatments of known effectiveness, relating changes to clinical measures or large changes in clinical condition, or interpreting observed changes in terms of elements of those measures that are more meaningful to stakeholders (Lohr and Skillman 2000).

Effectiveness: how a treatment works under ordinary conditions by the average practitioner and delivery system for the typical patient.

Efficacy: how a treatment works in ideal circumstances, when delivered to selected patients by providers most skilled at providing it. Often demonstrated using randomized clinical trials with relatively restrictive selection criteria.

Efficiency: a measure of sensitivity to change: Efficiency (E) = d (mean change)/SDd (SD of the change measures) (Fischer et al. 1999).

Empirical validity: evidence of validity based on the analysis of data (Ware et al. 1993).

External validity: generalizability of results.

Floor effect: when a score distribution is skewed so that a large proportion of respondents score at the lowest level on the measure. When floor effects occur, the measure cannot detect changes in a lower direction.

Functional status: an individual's effective performance of or ability to perform those roles, tasks, or activities that are valued, e.g., going to work, playing sports, or maintaining the house. Most often, functional status is divided into physical, emotional, mental, and social domains, although much finer distinctions are possible. Deviations from usual performance or ability indicate dysfunction.

Generic HRQOL tools: instruments that estimate an individual's overall health status that can be used to compare HRQOL between groups of patients with different diseases.

Global rating of change: a single item assessing the respondent's perception of the extent to which some characteristic (eg, pain) has changed since some referent point (e.g., 2 weeks ago, when treatment began). Response scale can be a 5- or 7-point scale, e.g., improved a lot, improved a little, no change, worsened a little, worsened a lot. Alternatively, 15-point scales are used after screening for improved, stayed the same, and worsened, with follow-up questions on how much improved and how much worsened. Global ratings are used to help interpret findings from health-related quality-of-life results to define small, medium, and large changes (Lohr and Skillman 2002).

Guttman scale: a cumulative scale in which each item consists of progressively more severe or extreme items.

Health preferences: see "utility" and "utility measurement."

Health-related quality of life (HRQOL): personal health status. It usually refers to aspects of our lives that are dominated or significantly influenced by our mental or physical well-being (Ware et al. 1993). The value assigned to duration of life as modified by the impairments, functional states, perceptions, and social opportunities that are influenced by disease, injury, treatment, or policy. Some measures include only 1 or 2 components with or without incorporation of survival or preference weights (Lohr and Skillman 2000).

Health status: most often defined by the World Health Organization's definition: "A state of complete physical, mental, and social well-being, and not merely the absence of disease or infirmity" (World Health Organization 1948).

Impairments: limitations in functions of body systems or anatomical elements.

Instrument: a group of items used for the collection of desired data. An instrument may contain a single item or multiple items that may or may not be divided into domains (Gill and Feinstein 1994).

Index: an aggregation of two or more distinct health measures into an overall summary measure.

Internal consistency: the extent to which a set of items in a scale measure the same attribute; also called homogeneity.

Internal consistency reliability: see Cronbach's alpha.

Interval scale: a scale in which the distances between all levels along the scale have known numerical values (Ware et al. 1993).

Internal validity: evidence that findings are correct within the context of a single study and takes into account the rigor with which the study was conducted (e.g., the study's design, the care taken to conduct measurements, and decisions concerning what was and was not measured) and the extent to which the designers of a study have taken into account alternative explanations for any causal relationships they explore (Huitt 1999).

Interpretability: the degree to which one can assign easily understood meaning to an instrument's quantitative scores (Lohr and SAC 2002). The ability to know what a value on a scale or measure means (i.e., where it falls in the range and distribution of possible scores, what a high score indicates, and where the score falls along population or subgroup norms on that measure). Also includes the assignment of meaning to observed changes in functional status, health status, health-related quality of life, and quality-of-life measures to interpret the clinical significance of change.

Item: a single question or statement and its standardized set of responses.

Item bank: a large collection of questions that are organized, calibrated, and matched to a given construct or task (contrasted to "item pool").

Item homogeneity or consistency: a measure of reliability. Internal consistency reliability is a method for estimating reliability from the correlations among the items in a multi-item scale (usually expressed in terms of Cronbach's alpha).

Item pool: a loosely collated set of terms from which criteria are used to abstract a subset of items known as an item bank (see "item bank").

Item response theory (IRT): a field of inquiry in the methodology of measurement in which the characteristics of the items composing a test, assessment, or scale are the locus of the study, and the characteristics of the items and the underlying individual abilities or traits can be analytically parsed.

Life-event score: weights assigned to different life events indicating the perceived seriousness of the event either from the perspective of a community or an individual.

Likert scale: a type of survey question where respondents are asked to rate the level at which they agree or disagree with a given statement. Guyatt et al. (1987) compared a 7-point Likert scale and a visual analogue scale (VAS) and concluded that although the responsiveness of the scales was similar the Likert scale was easier to administer and interpret. Nagata et al. (1996) also found no difference between 4-, 5- and

7-point scales and the VAS scale. They concluded that the 5-point scale was the easiest to complete, had the least frequent item omission and was the most useful when measuring health status.

Limitation: a problem (or symptom) that interferes with performance.

Longitudinal construct validity: a method to evaluate responsiveness and facilitate interpretation in which the logical relations between changes in a health status measure and changes in a theoretically related external variable are correlated to provide an interpretation of score changes and the definition of a minimally important difference (Lohr and Skillman 2000).

Meaningful category intervals: the ordinal scaled intervals across the range of a continuous health outcome scale that correspond to recommended changes in action (e.g., delivery of care, therapeutic intervention, or reimbursement). Employs the "minimally important difference" (see below) to construct categories.

Minimal clinically important difference: alternative term for "minimally important difference." Some have dropped the use of the word "clinically" because it suggests the perspective of the clinician rather than the patient. (See "minimally important difference.")

Minimally important difference: a clinically meaningful change (Jaeschke et al. 1989). That difference in score on a health-related quality-of-life instrument that corresponds to the smallest change in status that stakeholders (persons, patients, significant others, or clinicians) consider important. Assessments of minimally important difference need not and do not always agree among different stakeholders in the health decision (Lohr and Skillman 2000).

Nominal scale: a scale in which the numeric values assigned to scale levels are arbitrary and have no numeric meaning. Categories are classifications rather than ordered values (e.g., 1 = male, 2 = female).

Norm: an empirical benchmark, based on the scores obtained for a defined sample (e.g., the general population mean), used in interpreting the score for an individual or group.

Normative data: data "pertaining to the normal, usual, accepted standard or values" (Last 1995).

Number needed to treat (NNT): the number of patients one needs to treat with a particular therapy for a specified period of time to prevent 1 adverse event, such as a death, stroke, or myocardial infarction.

Ordinal scale: a scale in which the numbers reflect levels ordered form "most to least" with respect to some attribute. The relative distance between each level differs throughout the scale and the number assigned to each level does not reflect an exact quantity. For example: the rating of health as excellent, good, fair or poor is an ordinal scale (Ware et al. 1993).

Outcome: "all possible results that may stem from exposure to a casual factor, or from a preventative or therapeutic intervention" (Last 1995).

Outcome research: the measurement of the (end) result of healthcare (not just medical care) interventions.

Participation: involvement in life situation with emphasis on the person's involvement in society.

Patient administered measures: respondents read and answer questions by themselves, without assistance.

Performance: refers to whether a person does a task. Questions with performance wording ask "do you?"

Pharmacoeconomics: discipline concerned with establishing the relative value of health care interventions to health care systems and society and provides evidence of the relative risks, benefits and costs of health care interventions.

Precision: extent to which an instrument is able to detect small differences.

Psychometrics: an approach to developing and analyzing measures that is based on the statistical relationships between the items and the scales.

Quality-adjusted life-year (QALY): a QALY is a composite endpoint that incorporates both quality and quantity improvements in life. The "quality" portion of the QALY represents society's or patients' preference for health states. Note that the terms "years of healthy life," "well years," "well life expectancy," and "health life-years" are synonyms for quality-adjusted life-years, although differences exist depending on the exact measurement and method (Lohr and Skillman 2000).

Quality of life: encompasses the entire range of human experience, states, perceptions, and spheres of thought concerning the life of an individual or a community. Both objective and subjective, quality of life can include cultural, physical, psychological, interpersonal, spiritual, financial, political, temporal, and philosophical dimensions. Quality of life implies a judgment of value placed on the experience of communities, groups such as families, or individuals (Lohr and Skillman 2000).

Questionnaire: a set of questions for obtaining statistically useful or personal information from individuals. It includes standardized questions and response choices. Synonyms are measure, test, tool, survey, or instrument (Ware et al. 1993).

Range: the full number of levels for a given variable or domain.

Rasch model: the simplest item response theory model, with 1 parameter in which items are assumed to vary only with respect to their difficulty.

Ratio scale: a scale with all the properties of an interval scale, but, in addition, has an absolute zero.

Rating scale: sometimes called category rating, the method of equal-appearing intervals, or Visual Analogue Scale, this is a numerical rating scale used to place preferences on health states from 0, indicating least desirable (usually assigned to death), to 1, indicating most desirable (usually assigned to health as perfect as you can imagine). These methods are used both in psychophysics and decision analytic sciences and are direct methods of preference assignment under conditions of certainty (Lohr and Skillman 2000).

Recall period: the interval of time the respondent is instructed to consider in rating a given item e.g., "today"/"in the past month."

Receiver operating curve (ROC curve): a measure of sensitivity. A graphical description of test performance plotted as the relation between the true-positive rate (y axis = sensitivity) against the false-positive rate (x axis = 1-specificity). A ROC curve visually demonstrates the tradeoff between sensitivity and specificity for a single test. It uses an external criterion, such as patient global ratings, as a gold standard to evaluate responsiveness. An instrument that classifies most patients correctly as improved versus not improved has a larger area under the ROC curve.

Reliability: the extent to which a measure is free of measurement or random error; the ratio of true score variance to observed score variance. Two basic forms of reliability are reproducibility and item homogeneity or consistency. Internal consistency reliability is a method for estimating reliability from the correlations among the items in a multi-item scale (usually expressed in terms of Cronbach's alpha).

Reproducibility: the stability of a score over time (test–retest) and inter-rater and intra-rater agreement at one point in time. In test–retest reproducibility two different concepts can be distinguished: agreement and reliability (De Vet 1998).

Respondent: person answering questions or completing a questionnaire.

Response item: item or question in a questionnaire.

Response scale: the response choices presented to a respondent with which to answer a particular question (1 = yes, 2 = a little, 3 = no).

Response shift: patients confronted with a life-threatening or chronic disease are faced with the necessity to make accommodations for their illness. An important mediator of this adaptation process is response shift, which involves changing internal standards, values, and the conceptualization of quality of life. Integrating response shift into quality-of-life research

would allow a better understanding of how quality of life is affected by changes in health status and would direct the development of reliable and valid measures for assessing changes in quality of life (Lohr and Skillman 2000).

Responsiveness: refers to the extent to which an evaluative instrument (one designed to measure within-person change over time) can detect differences in score that are clinically important or meaningful, even if those differences are small (see "minimally important difference"). It implies a noticeable change that is of value to the patient (Liang 2000). In a short period of time, 25 definitions and more than 31 different formulae have been developed to calculate responsiveness (Terwee et al. 2003).

Scale: a range of available responses to an item. A scale can be categorical (e.g., excellent, very good, good, fair, poor), numerical, or consist of a visual analogue scale.

Scale: an item or aggregation of one or more items to obtain information concerning a variable or domain. For instance; 10 of the 36 questions of the SF-36 relate to physical functioning, together they from the physical functioning scale.

Sensitivity to change: the ability of an instrument to measure change in a state regardless of whether it is relevant or meaningful to the decision maker (Liang 2000). Examples are: (1) standardized response mean (SRM): compares magnitude of change with the standard deviation of change; (2) effect size: compares magnitude of change with standard deviation at baseline; (3) standard error of measurement (SEM) is the standard error in an observed score that is estimated by multiplying the standard deviation of the instrument by the square root of 1 minus its reliability quotient; (4) smallest detectable difference (SDD) = $1.96 \times$ square root $(2) \times$ SEM.

Skewness: the extent of asymmetry in a frequency distribution.

Stability: the consistency of results of a questionnaire on repeated administration.

Treatment effectiveness evaluation: the evaluation of 1 or more health programs, clinical interventions, or regulatory practices to establish the magnitude of benefits, disseminate the results, and eliminate ineffective interventions.

Universality: a concept or measure that applies equally to all segments of a population, i.e., is equivalent and relevant across cultures.

Utility: a concept in economics, psychology, and decision analysis referring to the preference for, or desirability of, a particular outcome. In the context of health-related quality-of-life measurement, utility refers to the preference of the rater (usually a patient or a member of the general public) for a particular health outcome or health state (Lohr and Skillman 2000).

Utility measurement: by convention, utility is usually measured on a 0.0 to 1.0 scale in which 0.0 is the least desirable state, associated with being dead, and 1.0 is the most desirable state, associated with perfect health (see for instance the EuroQOL).

Validity: the degree to which the instrument measures what it purports to measure and does not reflect concepts that it is not supposed to measure.

1. **Content validity** concerns judgment whether all important aspects or dimensions of the construct to be measured are covered by the instrument. A clear definition of the construct to be measured is a prerequisite.
2. **Face validity** is the extent to which a measure "looks like" what it is intended to measure. Face validity implies an overall judgment of adequacy on the face of it, without necessarily paying close attention to the component parts. For example, to assess the intensity of the pain a visual analogue scale (VAS) on which the intensity of the pain is scored has a high face validity.
3. **Criterion validity** is the extent to which a measure corresponds to an accurate or previously validated measure of the same concept or to an external criterion established by the investigators.
4. **Construct validity** for many clinical phenomena no 'gold standard' exists. This is also the case for pain. In the absence of an acceptable "gold standard," construct validity is the next-best option. In that case, one measure of the construct "pain intensity" may be compared with another measure of pain intensity. To examine construct validity it is necessary to define hypotheses about how the scores on the instrument under study will correlate with the scores on other instruments. Confirmation of these hypotheses gives support to the validity of a measurement instrument. However, by absence of a "gold standard," we are never sure that the level of pain that is measured is the "true" level of pain.
   a. **Convergent validity** is a form of construct validity in which the strength of association between 2 measures of a similar construct is determined.
   b. **Discriminate validity** (a form of construct validity) is the lack of a relationship among measures which theoretically should not be related.
   c. **Predictive validity** is a form of construct validity in which the hypothesis being tested is whether the measure can forecast the likelihood of another event or state (eg, hospitalization). According to

Bowling (2000) this is a form of criterion validity.
   d. **Concurrent validity** similarly tests an association of measures that are both assessed at the same point in time (Lohr 2002). According to Bowling (2000) this is a form of criterion validity.

Well-being: subjective bodily and emotional states; how an individual feels; a state of mind distinct from functioning that pertains to behaviors and activities.

REFERENCES

Bland JM, Altman DG. Statistical methods for assessing agreement between two methods of clinical measurement. Lancet 1986; 1:307–310.

Bowling A. Research Methods in Health. Investigating Health and Health Services. Open University Press, Buckingham, UK, 2000.

de Vet HC, Terwee CB, Knol DL, Bouter LM. When to use agreement versus reliability measures. J Clin Epidemiol. 2006 Oct; 59(10):1033–1039.

Fischer D, Stewart AL, Bloch DA, et al. Capturing the patient's view of change as a clinical outcome measure. JAMA 1999; 282:1157–1162.

Gill TM, Feinstein AR. A critical appraisal of the quality of quality-of-life measurements. JAMA 1994; 272:619–626.

Guyatt GH., Townsend M, Berman LB, et al. A comparison of Likert and visual analogue scales for measuring change in function. J Chronic Dis 1987; 40:1129–1133.

Huitt W, Hummel J, Kaeck D, 1999 Internal and External Validity. General Issues. http://chiron.valdosta.edu/whuitt/col/intro/valdgn.html accessed 27-08-07

Jaeschke R, Singer J, Guyatt GH. Measurement of health status. Ascertaining the minimal clinically important difference. Control Clin Trials 1989; 10:407–415.

Last JM. A Dictionary of Epidemiology. Oxford University Press, Oxford, 1995.

Liang MH. Longitudinal construct validity: establishment of clinical meaning in patient evaluative instruments. Med Care 2000; 38(9 suppl):II84–II90.

Lohr K, SAC. Assessing health status and quality-of-life instruments: attributes and review criteria. Qual Life Res 2002; 11:193–205.

Lohr K, Skillman S. Glossary. Health outcomes methodology. Med Care 2000; 39(9).

Nagata C, Ido M, Shimizu H, et al. Choice of response scale for health measurement: comparison of 4, 5, and 7-point scales and visual analog scale. J Epidemiol 1996; 6:192–197.

Terwee CB, Dekker FW, Wiersinga WM, et al. On assessing responsiveness of health-related quality of life instruments: guidelines for instrument evaluation, Qual Life Res 2003; 12:349–362.

Ware J, Snow K, Kosinski M, et al. SF-36 Health Survey. Manual and Interpretation Guide. The Health Institute, New England Medical Center, Boston, MA, 1993.

World Health Organization. Constitution of the WHO, Basic Documents. WHO, Geneva, 1948.

Questionnaires included on accompanying CD-ROM

Important note: Please see individual questionnaires for source details to contact for reproduction

ARTHRITIS

Arthritis Impact Measurement Scales 2 (AIMS2)
Childhood Health Assessment Questionnaire – Disability and Discomfort sections (CHAQ)
Fibromyalgia Impact Questionnaire (FIQ)
Health Assessment Questionnaire (HAQ) – Disability Index and Pain Scale
Juvenile Arthritis Status Index (JASI) Examples of Items
Juvenile Arthritis Status Index (JASI) Examples of response options
Juvenile Arthritis Functional Assessment Scale Scoring Form
McMaster Toronto Arthritis Patient Disability Questionnaire (MACTAR)
Quality of Life-Rheumatoid Arthritis Scale (QOL-RA)
Western Ontario Arthritis of the Shoulder (WOOS) Index

CANCER

Brief Fatigue Inventory (BFI)
Brief Pain Inventory (BPI)
Descriptor Differential Scale (Gracely scale)
Eastern Cooperative Oncology Group (ECOG) Performance Status Functional Assessment of Cancer Therapy-Anemia (FACT-An) (Version 3)
Karnofsky Performance Scale
Memorial Symptom Assessment Scale – Short Form (MSAS-SF)
Memorial Symptom Assessment Scale Subscales – Scoring
Quality of Life Index
Rotterdam Symptom Checklist
Symptom Control and Palliative Care Symptom Assessment (Edmonton Scale)

GENERIC INSTRUMENTS

Barthel ADL Index
Center for Epidemiologic Studies Depression Scale (CES-D)
Descriptor Differential Scale
Disability Rating Index
Global Rating Scale of perceived change
Hospital Anxiety and Depression Scale

Karnofsky Performance Scale
McGill Pain Questionnaire
McGill Pain Questionnaire and Pain Diagram Short Form
Nottingham Health Profile
Radboud Skills Questionnaire (RASQ)
Rand-36 Health Survey: refer to www.rand.org/health/surveys_tools/mos/mos core_36item.html
Zubrod Functionality Scoring System
Zung Self-rating Depression Scale

GERIATRICS

Geriatric Depression Scale

HEADACHE

Headache Disability Index
Migraine Disability Assessment (MIDAS)
Migraine-specific Quality of Life Questionnaire (MSQ)

MUSCULOSKELETAL

Aberdeen Low Back Pain Questionnaire (ALBPQ)
Aberdeen Back Pain scale – Scoring
Copenhagen Neck Functional Disability Scale
Barthel ADL Index
Disability Rating Index (DRI)
Fear-avoidance Beliefs Questionnaire (FABQ)
Functional Rating Index (FRI)
Health Assessment Questionnaire – Disability Index (HAQ)
Low Back Pain Outcome Score (LBOS)
Low Back Pain Rating Scale
Neck Disability Index (NDI)
Neck Pain and Disability Visual Analogue Scale
Northwick Park Neck Pain Questionnaire
Oswestry Disability Index 2.0 (ODI)
Pain Disability Index (PDI)
Quebec Back Pain Disability Scale (QBPDS)
Roland-Morris Disability Questionnaire (RDQ)
Treatment Outcomes in Pain Survey (TOPS)
Waddell Disability Index

NEUROPATHIC PAIN

Leeds Assessment of Neuropathic Symptoms and Signs (LANSS) Pain Scale

McGill Pain Questionnaire
McGill Pain Questionnaire Short Form and Pain Diagram
Neuropathic Pain Questionnaire – Short Form (NPQ-SF)
Neuropathic Pain Symptom Inventory (NPSI)
Neuropathy Pain Scale (NPS)
Pain Quality Assessment Scale (PQAS)

PALLIATIVE CARE

Brief Hospice Inventory (BHI)
Center for Epidemiologic Studies Depression Scale (CES-D)
Descriptor Differential Scale (Gracely scale)
Eastern Cooperative Oncology Group (ECOG) Performance Status
Functional Assessment Tool
Hebrew Rehabilitation Center for Aged Quality of Life (HRCA-QL) Index
Hospital Anxiety and Depression Scale (HADS)
Karnofsky Performance Scale
Memorial Pain Assessment Card (MPAC)
Memorial Symptom Assessment Scale – short form (MSAS-SF)
Memorial Symptom Assessment Scale Subscales – scoring
Palliative Care Outcome Scale (POS) Staff Questionnaire
Zubrod Functionality Scoring System
Zung Self-rating Depression Scale

PEDIATRICS

Child Total Pain Quality Management
Childhood Health Assessment Questionnaire – Disability and Discomfort sections (CHAQ)
Children's Hospital Eastern Ontario Pain Scale (CHEOPS)
COMFORT Pain Scale
CRIES scale
Faces Pain Scale
FLACC Scale
Functional Disability Inventory
Juvenile Arthritis Status Index (JASI) Examples of Items

Juvenile Arthritis Status Index (JASI) Examples of response options
Juvenile Arthritis Functional Assessment Scale Scoring Form
Neonatal Facial Coding System (NFCS) for Pain Evaluation in Newborn Infants
Neonatal Infant Pain Scale (NIPS)
Non-Communicating Children's Pain Checklist Postoperative Version (NCCPC-PV)
N-PASS - Neonatal Pain, Agitation and Sedation Scale
Objective Pain Scale (OPS) for Postoperative Pain Assessment
Oucher Scale
Pain Coping Questionnaire
Pain Response Inventory for Children
Pediatric Pain Coping Inventory
Poker Chip Tool
Postoperative Pain Measure for Parents in Children 7–12 years of age

PSYCHOLOGICAL

Davidson Trauma Scale
Distress Thermometer
Fear-avoidance Beliefs Questionnaire (FABQ)
Fear Questionnaire
Impact of Event scale
Pain Catastrophizing Scale for Children
Pain Coping Questionnaire
Pain Response Inventory for Children
Pediatric Pain Coping Inventory
Post-traumatic Stress Disorder (PTSD) Checklist – Civilian Version
West Haven-Yale Multidimensional Pain Inventory (MPI) – Quality of Life Instruments
West Haven-Yale Multidimensional Pain Inventory (MPI) – Measure
West Haven-Yale Multidimensional Pain Inventory (MPI) – Subscales, Normative Data
Sample Items from the Pain Anxiety Symptoms Scale (PASS)

Index

Figures in **Bold**; Tables in *Italics*